770-7a

# Comprehensive
# Cancer Nursing Review

# Comprehensive
# Cancer Nursing Review

## FOURTH EDITION

EDITED BY

**Susan L. Groenwald, RN, MS**
Assistant Professor of Nursing, Complemental
Department of Medical Nursing
Rush University College of Nursing

Rush Presbyterian St. Luke's Medical Center
Chicago, Illinois

**Margaret Hansen Frogge, RN, MS**
Assistant Professor, Associate Faculty
Rush University College of Nursing

Rush Presbyterian St. Luke's Medical Center
Chicago, Illinois

Vice President, Strategic Development
and System Integration

Riverside Medical Center
Kankakee, Illinois

**Michelle Goodman, RN, MS, OCN®**
Assistant Professor of Nursing
Rush University College of Nursing
Oncology Clinical Nurse Specialist
Section of Medical Oncology
Rush Cancer Institute

Rush Presbyterian St. Luke's Medical Center
Chicago, Illinois

**Connie Henke Yarbro, RN, MS, FAAN**
Editor, *Seminars in Oncology Nursing*

Clinical Associate Professor
Division of Hematology/Oncology
Adjunct Clinical Assistant Professor
Sinclair School of Nursing

University of Missouri, Columbia
Columbia, Missouri

**JONES AND BARTLETT PUBLISHERS**
*Sudbury, Massachusetts*
BOSTON          LONDON          SINGAPORE

*Editorial, Sales, and Customer Service Offices:*
Jones and Bartlett Publishers, Inc.
40 Tall Pine Drive
Sudbury, MA 01776
978-443-5000
1-800-832-0034
info@jbpub.com
http://www.jbpub.com

Jones and Bartlett Publishers International
Barb House, Barb Mews
London W6 7PA
United Kingdom

*Design:* Wordbench
*Editorial Production Services:* Wordbench
*Composition:* Wordbench
*Cover Design:* Dick Hannus
*Printer and Binder:* Bawden Printing
*Cover Printer:* Bawden Printing

**Library of Congress Cataloging-in-Publication Data**

Comprehensive cancer nursing review / Susan Groenwald . . . [et al.]. —
    4th ed.
            p.    cm. — (The Jones and Bartlett series in oncology)
    Companion v. to: Cancer nursing. 4th ed. c1997.
    Includes index.
    ISBN 0-7637-0541-1
    1. Cancer—Nursing—Outlines, syllabi, etc.  2. Cancer—Nursing—
Examinations, questions, etc.   I. Groenwald, Susan L.   II. Cancer
nursing.   III. Series.
    [DNLM: 1. Neoplasms—nursing—examination questions.   WY 18.2
C737  1998]
RC266.C356 1997 Suppl.
610.73'698'076—dc21
DNLM/DLC
for Library of Congress                                         97-42396
                                                                     CIP

Printed in the United States of America.

99 98 97 96 95        10 9 8 7 6 5 4 3 2

# Contents

## Part VI    Issues in Cancer Survivorship

## Part VII    Delivery Systems for Cancer Care

## Part VIII    Professional Issues in Cancer Care

# Preface

This review guide accompanies *Cancer Nursing: Principles and Practice*, Fourth Edition, by Groenwald, Frogge, Goodman, and Yarbro. We are pleased to note that this review guide, while valuable as an instructor's aid or a student's review of the text book, has, over the last number of years, distinguished itself as a very popular guide for those nurses preparing for the Oncology Nursing Certification Examinations. In this edition, we have applied more of the education theory concepts that have been proven to work so well in preparation for nursing and other board exams.

## Cancer Updates

New features in this guide include, in Part I, a straightforward, easy-to-follow synthesis of diagnostic-related information into two related chapters: "Biology of Cancer" and "Carcinogenesis." At the same time, Part II, Prevention, Detection, and Diagnosis, has added a valuable chapter on "Dynamics of Cancer Prevention." In Part III, the treatment section, our discussion of bone marrow transplantation has been expanded into two chapters, one dedicated to allogeneic BMT (Chapter 18) and one on autologous bone marrow and bone cell transplantation (Chapter 19).

In Part IV, our coverage of symptom management has also been expanded with the addition of Chapter 26, "Paraneoplastic Syndromes." Specific cancer discussions in Part V have combined coverage of bladder and kidney cancers, while focusing on testicular germ cell and prostate cancers in two separate chapters. We have also offered extended coverage of gallbladder cancer. Part VII places new emphasis on issues in cancer survivorship, with the following new chapters: Chapter 48, "Psychosocial Responses to Cancer"; Chapter 49, "Physical, Economic, and Social Adaptation of the Cancer Survivor"; and Chapter 50, "Spiritual and Ethical End-of-Life Concerns."

Finally, in Part VIII, our discussion of cancer economics has been dramatically updated in Chapter 55, "Impact of Changing Health Care Economics on Cancer Nursing Practice." Chapter 61 reflects on the cultural diversity seen in cancer patients.

## Study Outlines

This guide takes advantage of key ways in which adults learn: specifically, through **summary integration** and **fact concentration**—skills that are reinforced in the **Study Outlines** through such tools as condensing materials to those facts and concepts that a cancer nurse will be expected to know in practice, in class, and on the Oncology Nursing Certification Examinations. These outlines also focus on the text's numerous figures, tables, boxes, and other summary materials. Such graphics have been demonstrated, in education research, to be especially valuable to *adult* learners; in fact, more valuable than educators had originally known. Although this summary integration and fact concentration is valuable—even essential—in exam preparation (when using this guide independent of the text), students and instructors find these tools just as valuable for reinforcing materials stressed in the classroom and course literature.

## Practice Questions

A second tool used in this edition of the review guide is seen in the use of the more demanding and useful **Application/Analysis** type questions, while keeping a significant quantity of the traditional **Knowledge/Comprehension**-based questions. These questions, sometimes grouped together as continuing case studies, demand more of the adult thinker than memorization and basic comprehension. Instead, **Application** questions require integration and synthesis of concepts, engage the user in analysis, and apply concepts to real-life situations. Application questions are, of course, frequently seen on board exams.

## Answer Explanations

The answer explanations, so popular in our last edition, serve three important functions: (1) Naturally, they provide the letter of the correct answer to each Practice Question; (2) they also explain and reinforce information covered in the Study Outline and text; and (3) they cite the page or pages in the text where a more detailed discussion of the answer can be found. These explanations should help clarify points the reader may have overlooked or misunderstood in the text, especially many important distinctions between closely related terms or concepts. Of course, for those who are using the guide without the text, questions and answers are designed so that they may be used without reference to the outlines or text.

If you have any comments about the guide or any suggestions for improving its value to cancer nurses, please write to the publisher at the following address:

Jones and Bartlett Publishers
40 Tall Pine Drive
Sudbury, MA 01776

# Contributors to
# Cancer Nursing:
# Principles and Practice,
## 4th edition

**Barbara A. Barhamand, RN, MSN, AOCN**
Oncology Clinical Nurse Specialist/Practice Manager
Hematology-Oncology Consultants Ltd.
Naperville, IL

**Andrea M. Barsevick, RN, DNSc**
Director of Nursing Research
Fox Chase Cancer Center
Philadelphia, PA

**Karen Belford, RN, MS, OCN®, CCRN**
Clinical Instructor, Department of Nursing Education
Memorial Sloan-Kettering Cancer Center
New York, NY

**Connie Yuska Bildstein, RN, MS, CORLN**
Vice President of Operations
Northwestern Memorial Home Health
    Care/Services, Inc.
Chicago, IL

**Carol Blendowski, RN, BS, OCN®**
Oncology Clinical Nurse
Rush Cancer Institute
Rush Presbyterian St. Luke's Medical Center
Chicago, IL

**Karen Smith Blesch, RN, PhD**
Documentation Specialist
Hoffman-LaRoche
Nutley, NJ

**Debra L. Brock, RNC, MSN, CS, AOCN, ANP**
Nurse Practitioner
Nashville Family Medicine
Nashville, IN

**Patricia Corcoran Buchsel, RN, MSN**
Senior Research Associate
University of Washington
Transplantation Consultant
Issaquah, WA

**Dawn Camp-Sorrell, RN, MSN, AOCN, FNP**
Oncology Nurse Practitioner
University of Alabama at Birmingham Hospital
Birmingham, AL

**Brenda Cartmel, PhD**
CPS/CARET: Yale University
Occupational Health Center
Groton, CT

**David Cella, PhD**
Associate Professor of Psychology and Social Sciences
Director, Psychosocial Oncology
Rush Presbyterian St. Luke's Medical Center
Chicago, IL

**Dianne D. Chapman, RN, MS, OCN®**
Coordinator, Comprehensive Breast Center
Genetic Counselor
Rush Inherited Susceptibility for Cancer (RISC)
    Program
Rush Cancer Institute
Rush Presbyterian St. Luke's Medical Center
Chicago, IL

**Rebecca F. Cohen, RN, EdD, MPA, CPHQ**
Associate Professor
Rockford College, Department of Nursing
Rockford, IL

**JoAnn Coleman, RN, MS, CRNP, OCN®**
Case Manager for Pancreas and Biliary Surgery
Department of Surgical Nursing
Johns Hopkins Hospital
Baltimore, MD

**Mary Cunningham, RN, MS**
Clinical Nurse Specialist
Department of Neuro-Oncology
Pain and Symptom Management Section
M.D. Anderson Cancer Center
Houston, TX

**Diane Scott Dorsett, RN, PhD, FAAN**
Director
Comprehensive Cancer Support Services
San Francisco, CA

**Jan M. Ellerhorst-Ryan, RN, MSN, CS**
Oncology/HIV Clinical Nurse Specialist
Vitas Health Care Corporation
Cincinnati, OH

**Jayne I. Fernsler, RN, DSN, AOCN**
Associate Professor
College of Nursing
University of Delaware
Newark, DE

**Ann T. Foltz, RN, DNS**
Breast and Cervical Cancer Program Director
Louisiana Office of Public Health
New Orleans, LA

**Susan M. Fox, RN, MS, OCN®**
Oncology Research Nurse
Indiana University Cancer Pavilion
Indianapolis, IN

**Marilyn Frank-Stromborg, EdD, JD, NP, FAAN**
Professor and Acting Chair
School of Nursing
Northern Illinois University
Dekalb, IL

**Margaret Hansen Frogge, RN, MS**
Assistant Professor, Associate Faculty
Rush University College of Nursing
Rush Presbyterian St. Luke's Medical Center
Chicago, IL
Vice President
Strategic Development and System Integration
Riverside Medical Center
Kankakee, IL

**Annette Galassi, RN, MA, CANP, AOCN**
Adult Nurse Practitioner
Instructor in Medicine
Lombardi Cancer Center
Georgetown University Medical Center
Washington, DC

**Barbara Holmes Gobel, RN, MS**
Oncology Clinical Nurse Specialist
Gottlieb Memorial Hospital
Melrose Park, IL
Instructor, Complemental
Rush University College of Nursing
Chicago, IL

**Michelle Goodman, RN, MS, OCN®**
Assistant Professor of Nursing
Rush University College of Nursing
Oncology Clinical Nurse Specialist
Section of Medical Oncology
Rush Cancer Institute
Rush Presbyterian St. Luke's Medical Center
Chicago, IL

**Susan L. Groenwald, RN, MS**
Assistant Professor of Nursing, Complemental
Rush University College of Nursing
Rush Presbyterian St. Luke's Medical Center
Chicago, IL

**Carol Guarnieri, RN, MSN, AOCN**
Oncology Clinical Nurse Specialist
Samitivej Srinakarin Hospital
Bangkok, Thailand

**Irene Stewart Haapoja, RN, MS, OCN®**
Oncology Clinical Nurse Specialist
Rush Cancer Institute
Rush Presbyterian St. Luke's Medical Center
Chicago, IL

**Mel Haberman, RN, PhD, FAAN**
Director of Research
Oncology Nursing Society
Pittsburgh, PA
Assistant Staff Scientist
Fred Hutchinson Cancer Research Center
Seattle, WA

**Lynne Hagan, RN, BSN, CETN**
Enterostomal Therapy
USC Kenneth Norris, Jr. Cancer Hospital
Los Angeles, CA

**Gloria A. Hagopian, RN, EdD**
Associate Professor of Nursing
Department of Adult Health Nursing
University of North Carolina, Charlotte
Charlotte, NC

**Pamela J. Haylock, RN, MA, ET**
Cancer Care Consultant
Kerrville, TX

**Jeanne Held-Warmkessel, RN, MSN, CS, AOCN**
Instructor of Roxborough Memorial Hospital
School of Nursing
Philadelphia, PA

**Laura J. Hilderley, RN, MS**
Clinical Nurse Specialist, Radiation Oncology
Radiation Oncology Services of Rhode Island
Warwick, RI

**Linda Hoebler, RN, MSN**
Oncology Clinical Nurse Specialist
Allegheny General Hospital
Pittsburgh, PA

**Rebecca J. Ingle, RN, MSN, FNP, AOCN**
Oncology Clinical Specialist
The Dan Rudy Cancer Center
Saint Thomas Hospital
Adjunct Instructor of Nursing
Vanderbilt University School of Nursing
Nashville, TN

**Joanne K. Itano, RN, PhD, OCN®**
The University of Hawaii at Manoa
School of Nursing
Honolulu, HI

**Barbara Hansen Kalinowski, RN, MSN, OCN®**
Clinical Research Nurse
Joint Center for Radiation Therapy
Boston, MA

**Marsha A. Ketcham, RN, OCN®**
Senior Research Nurse
Arizona Cancer Center
Tucson, AZ

**Paula Klemm, RN, DNSc OCN®**
Assistant Chair
University of Delaware, College of Nursing
Newark, DE
Clinical Nurse
Department of GYN/OB
Johns Hopkins Hospital
Baltimore, MD

**Linda U. Krebs, RN, PhD, AOCN**
Nursing Oncology Program Leader and Senior
  Instructor
University of Colorado Cancer Center
University of Colorado School of Nursing
Denver, CO

**Luana Lamkin, RN, MPH, OCN®**
Senior Vice President
Rose Medical Center
Denver, CO

**Jennifer Lang-Kummer, RN, MN, CS, FNP**
Oncology Case Management Services
Pitt County Memorial Hospital
Adjunct Assistant Professor of Nursing
East Carolina University
Greenville, NC

**Paul J. LeMarbre, MD**
Medical Oncology/Hematology
Waukesha Memorial Hospital
Waukesha, WI

**Julena Lind, RN, MN, MA, PhD(c)**
Assistant Professor of Clinical Nursing
University of Southern California
Los Angeles, CA

**Lois J. Loescher, RN, MS**
Senior Research Specialist
Cancer Prevention and Control
Arizona Cancer Center
Tucson, AZ

**Jeanne Martinez, RN, MPH**
Clinical Nurse Manager
Northwestern Hospice Program
Chicago, IL

**Mary B. Maxwell, RN, C, PhD**
Clinical Specialist/Nurse Practitioner in Oncology
Veterans' Affairs Medical Center
Adjunct Assistant Professor of Nursing
Oregon Health Sciences University
Portland, OR

**Katherine McDermott, RN, MPA, OCN®**
Clinical Nurse Specialist
Division of Nursing
Memorial Sloan-Kettering Cancer Center
New York, NY

**Mary Ellen McFadden, RN, MLA, OCN®**
Clinical Support Specialist
Amgen
Baltimore, MD

**Deborah B. McGuire, RN, PhD, FAAN**
Edith Folsom Honeycutt Chair in Oncology Nursing
Associate Professor
Nell Hodgson Woodruff School of Nursing
Emory University
Altanta, GA

**Joan C. McNally, RN, MSN, OCN®, CRNH**
Director, Health Care Services
Karmanos Cancer Institute Home Care and Hospice
  Programs
Detroit, MI

**Mary Ann Miller, RN, PhD**
Associate Professor, College of Nursing
University of Delaware
Newark, DE

**Ida Marie (Ki) Moore, RN, DNSc**
Assistant Professor
College of Nursing
University of Arizona
Tucson, AZ

**Theresa A. Moran, RN, MS**
AIDS/Oncology Clinical Nurse Specialist
University of California, San Francisco/
    San Francisco General Hospital
Assistant Clinical Professor
Department of Physiological Nursing
University of California
San Francisco, CA

**Judie Much, MSN, CRNP, AOCN**
Oncology Clinical Nurse Specialist
Psychosocial Support Nurse
Fox Chase Cancer Center
Philadelphia, PA

**Lillian M. Nail, RN, PhD, FAAN**
Associate Professor
Associate Dean for Research
University of Utah College of Nursing
Salt Lake City, UT

**Cathleen A. O'Conner-Vaccari, RN, MSN, OCN®**
Manager/Clinical Nurse Specialist
Memorial Sloan-Kettering Cancer Center
New York, NY

**Sharon Saldin O'Mary, RN, MN, OCN®**
Director of Hospice Services
Nations Health Care Hospice
San Diego, CA

**Diane M. Otte, RN, MS, ET, OCN®**
Alegent Health
Administrative Director, Cancer Center
Immanuel Medical Center
Omaha, NE

**Lawrence F. Padberg, PhD**
Vice President for Planning and Enrollment
    Management
Marymount University
Arlington, VA

**Rose Mary Padberg, RN, MA, OCN®**
Nurse Consultant
Division of Cancer Prevention and Control
National Cancer Institute
National Institutes of Health
Bethesda, MD

**Patricia A. Piasecki, RN, MS**
Clinical Coordinator, Orthopedic Oncology
Rush Presbyterian St. Luke's Medical Center
Chicago, IL

**Sandra Purl, RN, MS, AOCN**
Oncology Clinical Nurse Specialist
Lutheran General Hospital
Park Ridge, IL

**Mary Reid, RN, MSPH**
Research Specialist
Department of Family and Community Medicine
University of Arizona
Tucson, AZ

**Mary Beth Riley, RN, MS**
Oncology Clinical Specialist
Rush Cancer Institute
Rush Presbyterian St. Luke's Medical Center
Chicago, IL

**Kimberly Rohan, RN, MS, OCN®**
Patient Services Coordinator
Edward Hospital
Naperville, IL

**Kathleen S. Ruccione, RN, MPH**
Division of Hematology/Oncology
Children's Hospital of Los Angeles
Los Angeles, CA

**Valinda Rutledge, RN, MSN, MBA**
Administrator
Brandon Regional Medical Center
Brandon, FL

**Vivian R. Sheidler, RN, MS**
Clinical Nurse Specialist—Neuro-Oncology
Johns Hopkins Oncology Center
Baltimore, MD

**Carol A. Sheridan, RN, MSN, AOCN**
Clinical Support Specialist
Amgen
New York, NY

**Joy Stair, RN, MS**
Director, Oncology Services
McAuley Cancer Care Center
St. Joseph Mercy Hospital
Ann Arbor, MI

**Carole Sweeney, RN, MSN, OCN®**
Fox Chase Cancer Center
Philadelphia, PA

**Karen N. Taoka, RN, MN, AOCN**
Clinical Nurse Specialist
The Queens Medical Center
Honolulu, HI

**Elizabeth Johnston Taylor, RN, PhD**
Assistant Professor
University of Southern California
Department of Nursing
Los Angeles, CA

**David C. Thomasma, PhD**
The Fr. Michael I. English S.J. Professor of Medical
  Ethics
Director, Medical Humanities Program
Loyola University of Chicago Medical Center
Maywood, IL

**Peter V. Tortorice, Pharm D, BCPS**
Oncology Clinical Pharmacist
Illinois Masonic Cancer Center
Chicago, IL

**Steven Wagner, RN, BSN**
Nurse Clinician
Northwestern Hospice Program
Chicago, IL

**Janet Ruth Walczak, RN, MSN**
Clinical Nurse Specialist
The Johns Hopkins Oncology Center
Clinical Associate
The Johns Hopkins University, School of Nursing
Baltimore, MD

**Vera S. Wheeler, RN, MN, OCN®**
Consultant
Cancer Nursing and Biotherapy
Vancouver, WA

**Rita Wickham, RN, PhD(c), AOCN**
Assistant Professor, College of Nursing
Rush University
Rush Presbyterian St. Luke's Medical Center
Chicago, IL

**Debra Wujcik, RN, MSN, AOCN**
Clinical Director
Affiliate Network Office
Vanderbilt Cancer Center Clinical Trials Office
Adjunct Instructor
Vanderbilt University School of Nursing
Nashville, TN

**Connie Henke Yarbro, RN, MS, FAAN**
Editor, *Seminars in Oncology Nursing*
Clinical Associate Professor
Division of Hematology/Oncology
Adjunct Clinical Assistant Professor
Sinclair School of Nursing
University of Missouri—Columbia
Columbia, MO

**John W. Yarbro, MD, PhD**
Professor Emeritus, School of Medicine
University of Missouri—Columbia
Columbia, MO
Editor, *Seminars in Oncology*

# Chapter 1     Milestones in Our Understanding of Cancer

## INTRODUCTION

- Multicellular life forms depend on the meticulous balance and regulation of reproduction, growth, development, tissue repair, response to injury, and regeneration. Cancer results from an imbalance of these mechanisms.

## THE AGE OF REASON

- During the Age of Reason, Bernardino Ramazzini noted the high incidence of breast cancer in nuns and hypothesized this was in some way related to their celibate lifestyle; the age of cancer epidemiology had begun.
  - John Hill of London was the first to recognize the dangers of tobacco.
  - The description of scrotal cancer in chimney sweeps by Percival Pott of St. Bartholomew's Hospital in London is the most frequently cited example of cancer epidemiology and has influenced our view of cancer epidemiology and etiology.

## NINETEENTH CENTURY DEVELOPMENT

- The nineteenth century saw the birth of scientific oncology as science shifted from anatomy to pathology.
  - Virchow established the microscopic basis for the characterization of cancer.
  - Halsted and Handley's doctrine that cancer is contained within anatomical compartments and can be cured by radical resection en bloc became the basis of the "cancer operation" for almost a century.
  - Paget concluded that cancer cells spread by way of the bloodstream and that cancer cells from a primary tumor are able to grow in only certain other organs.
  - Beatson illustrated the potential for systemic treatment of cancer in his tests of oophorectomy and breast cancer.
  - Huggins reported dramatic regression of metastatic prostate cancer following castration.
  - Roentgen devised the use of x-rays for diagnosis; within three years radiation was used in the treatment of cancer.
    - Delivering radiation over a protracted period of time by use of daily fractions was found to greatly improve therapeutic response.

## TWENTIETH CENTURY ANSWERS

- Peyton Rous' experiments led to the discovery of the Rous virus as the source of the first well-characterized oncogene.
- Yamagiwa and Ichikawa launched the field of chemical carcinogenesis with a firm scientific foundation and a research technique.

### Cancer Progression Explored

- For the second half of the nineteenth century, cancer surgery was synonymous with the Halsted radical resection of a cancer and its draining lymph node groups. Progress was held back by a failure t understand multistage carcinogenesis and to grasp the relationship of clonal selection during progression to metastasis.

- Peyton Rous defined the difference between *initiation* and *promotion*.
- Berenblum and Shubik formed the prototype for the way carcinogenesis was conceptualized. This led to the concept of *initiation* by one agent followed by *promotion* by another and finally *progression* of the tumor to a more malignant form.
  - The initiator was viewed as able to cause cancer but only after a prolonged time.
  - The promoter alone was viewed as not always able to cause cancer but able to potentiate the effects of the initiator.
  - The term *progression* was said by Rous to designate "the process by which tumors go from bad to worse."
- Foulds codified and expanded the concept of multistage carcinogenesis.

## Development in Chemotherapy

- Exactly 100 years after the beginning of the "century of the surgeon" (which began in 1846), the first anticancer activity of a chemical was reported.
- German scientist Paul Ehrlich is called the "father of chemotherapy."
  - Nitrogen mustard was developed by the chemical warfare research division of the U.S. Army. It proved to have remarkable activity against lymphomas.
  - Two years later Sidney Farber of Boston reported the efficacy of aminopterin. Subsequently, Hitchings and Elion developed the antimetabolite 6-mercaptopurine, and Charles Heidelberger developed 5-fluorouracil. The era of chemotherapy had begun.
    - The first cure of metastatic cancer was obtained in 1956 by the use of methotrexate in choriocarcinoma.

## Mutagens and Carcinogenesis

- It was not until 1944 that DNA was demonstrated to be the chemical mediator of heredity.
  - A key discovery was made by Ames, who developed a classic assay system to measure carcinogens based on the fact that most carcinogens are mutagens (i.e., they damage DNA).
- Two surgeons, Fisher and Veronesi, led the way to the overthrow of the classic "cancer operation" by their demonstration that survival in breast cancer and melanoma is independent of the extent of surgical resection. This led to the reevaluation of our notion of the anatomic containment of cancer and to an understanding that it is our *biology,* not our anatomy, that restricts cancer spread.
  - Scientists learned that cancer cells spread throughout the body from the time the first capillaries are attracted into the growing tumor, but are unable to establish metastatic deposits because the cells have not yet evolved the capacity to proliferate outside the site of the primary tumor.
  - Time is indeed a factor; however, the time is required not to overcome some anatomic containment but to allow evolution of the cells of the primary tumor into subclones capable of metastatic growth.

## Identification of Oncogenes and Retroviruses

- Researchers in chemical carcinogenesis were identifying mutagens, but the target genes of the mutagens were unknown. Virologists were identifying cancer-causing viruses, but their mechanism of carcinogenesis was obscure.
- Increasing numbers of oncogenic viruses were discovered in animal systems. They were originally called *type C viruses* and later *retroviruses*; the latter term applied because they were RNA viruses that were converted to DNA by the enzyme reverse transcriptase.
  - Retroviruses add their genes to the cell and in this way influence the cell's behavior.

- Huebner and Todaro focused attention on the word *oncogene* in 1969 when they proposed that RNA viruses somehow placed viral genes in the human genome that were then genetically transmitted.
  - The basic experiments in retroviral carcinogenesis demonstrated that the intact virus and isolated genes were able to induce malignant transformation. This allowed the identification of oncogenes. A host of retroviruses that caused cancers were identified.
  - Genes are usually designated by a three-letter code in lowercase italics, sometimes preceded by a *v-* for a viral gene or a *c-* for a cellular gene.
  - Two discoveries led to a better understanding of how oncogenes relate to growth factors and provided strong support for the hypothesis that the oncogenes found in retroviruses were the same as the growth factor and growth factor receptor genes found in normal cells.
    - It is now known that experimental retroviruses obtain their oncogenes by capture of normal genes from the host cell.
    - Retroviral oncogene research did allow the identification of many human oncogenes that code for normal growth-promoting substances; this improved our understanding of the way in which oncogenes promote normal and neoplastic growth.
    - We now know that it is the human growth control genes, first identified as oncogenes in retroviruses, that are the long-sought-after targets of the mutating chemicals and radiation that contribute certain critical lesions leading to human cancer. But mutated oncogenes alone are not sufficient to cause human malignancies.
  - Unlike the retroviruses, the oncogenes of DNA viruses are not recently captured cellular genes, and thus they do not have such a close structural relationship to human genes. Their products do, however, react with the products of human genes.
  - The mechanisms of carcinogenesis by the DNA viruses are more complex than is the case for the retroviruses.
  - Work with the oncogenes of the DNA viruses led to discovery of several viruses causing human cancer and to a better understanding of normal cellular control mechanisms.

## Antioncogenes

- Oncogenes code for proteins that induce malignant growth by "turning on" cell division. There are proteins with an opposite function, to "turn off" cell growth. These suppressor proteins were discovered because the oncogenic DNA viruses had oncogenes whose products bound to and inactivated them; thus, they were called *antioncogenes*. Because they suppressed malignant growth, they were also called *cancer-suppressor genes*.
- It is likely that for each "up-regulating" function coded by an oncogene there is a balancing "down-regulating" function coded by a cancer-suppressor gene.
  - The scientific basis for our understanding of this mechanism was laid in 1971 when Alfred Knudson argued, on the basis of a statistical model, that one of the two mutations required for the development of familial retinoblastoma was inherited and the second occurred in the retinal cells of the affected eye.
    - The gene has been identified on chromosome 13 and named the *retinoblastoma gene (RB)*.
      - The function of the gene is to prevent malignant growth.
- Transcription factors are proteins that bind specifically to DNA and initiate expression of a set of genes controlled by the binding site.
- As human cancers were being studied for mutations of the oncogenes and cancer-suppressor genes, it became clear that the number of such mutations was too large to be explained by the simple action of carcinogens on human cells.
- One of the most important of the cancer-suppressor genes is the gene that codes for a protein designated *p53*. The *p53* gene is the most frequently mutated gene in human cancer.

- The protein product of *p53* may detect the presence of damaged DNA and arrest the cell cycle in $G_1$ until the damage is repaired or, if not repaired, induces cell suicide (apoptosis).
- DNA viruses produce proteins that inactivate the *p53* protein.

# PRACTICE QUESTIONS

1.  Oncogenes found in retroviruses:
    a.  are obtained by the capture of normal genes from the host cell and are the targets of the mutating chemicals and radiation that contribute critical lesions.
    b.  create more complex mechanisms of carcinogenesis than those created by DNA viruses.
    c.  are enough on their own to cause human malignancies.
    d.  do not have a close structural relationship to human genes.

2.  A patient asks, "What are cancer-suppressor genes?" As part of your answer, you explain that cancer-suppressor genes code for proteins that _____ growth-promoting factors.
    a.  enhance
    b.  fuel
    c.  inactivate
    d.  duplicate

3.  Transcription factors:
    a.  initiate expression of a set of genes controlled by the binding site.
    b.  bind specifically to the *myc* oncogene.
    c.  are referred to as retinoblastoma genes (RBs).
    d.  bind specifically to RNA.

4.  The *p53* gene:
    a.  is a potent oncogene.
    b.  is the most frequently mutated gene in human cancer.
    c.  is the "guardian of the oncogene."
    d.  is protected from DNA viruses.

# ANSWER EXPLANATIONS

1.  **The answer is a.** Experimental retroviruses obtain their oncogenes by capture of normal genes from the host cell. Many human retroviral oncogenes code for normal growth-promoting substances and are the targets of mutating chemicals and radiation that contribute critical lesions leading to human cancer. But mutated oncogenes alone are not sufficient to cause human malignancies. It is the oncogenes of DNA viruses that do not have a close structural relationship to human genes. (p. 11)

2.  **The answer is c.** Suppressor proteins "turn off" cell growth. Since the genes coding for these proteins have an opposite function to that of oncogenes, they are called antioncogenes; because they suppress malignant growth, they are also called cancer-suppressor genes. (p. 12)

3.  **The answer is a.** Transcription factors are proteins that bind specifically to DNA and initiate the expression of a set of genes controlled by the binding site. The *myc* oncogene produces a transcription factor that stimulates cell division; it is not a binding site but a producer of transcription factor. (p. 12)

4.  **The answer is b.** The *p53* gene is one of the most important of the cancer-suppressor genes. Not only is it the most frequently mutated, but when it is not mutated, another abnormal gene blocks the *p53* protein. The protein product of *p53* is the "guardian of the genome." DNA viruses produce proteins that inactivate the *p53* protein. (pp. 12–13)

# Chapter 2        Biology of Cancer

## RESEARCH MODELS

### Limitations of Study of Human Tissues

- A major technical difficulty in studying cancer cells is that researchers cannot be sure of the actual normal cell counterpart for a cancer cell in a given tissue.

### Transformed Cell Models

- Cell lines can be developed from a single cell to provide a certain level of uniformity.
  - Cell lines may or may not become continuous; they do so when they develop the ability to propagate indefinitely in tissue culture. Many normal cell lines will cease growing and die after a span of time. This phenomenon is believed to be related to a "programmed" or defined number of cell divisions that a normal cell will make before it stops proliferating (*senescence*).
- Occasionally a cell line will continue to grow indefinitely; this pattern of prolonged growth is more likely to occur if the cells are exposed to carcinogenic agents, and the cells are thus considered to be *transformed*. They often resemble neoplastic cells and can be studied experimentally; more practically, they represent a self-renewing population that saves researchers time and effort.

## DIFFERENCES IN THE FEATURES OF NORMAL AND CANCER CELLS

- The primary difference between cancer cells and normal cells relates to abnormal growth regulation—cancer cells will grow even at the expense of outstripping their blood supply and destroying the host.
- Rapidity of growth is not a discriminating factor.
- Tumor doubling times are variable, but an average of two months is generally accepted.
- In cancer, masses continue to expand beyond normal boundaries, with continued cell division overbalancing any cell loss. ✓

### Immortality of Cancer Cells

- A potential counting mechanism to limit the number of doublings involves *telomeres,* which are DNA segments at the ends of chromosomes. Telomeres protect the chromosomal ends from damage, and the telomere length shortens a little bit with each chromosomal replication (during the phase of DNA synthesis).
- Many cancers contain an enzyme, *telomerase,* which replaces the segments trimmed away during cell division, enabling the cell to replicate indefinitely.

### Loss of Contact Inhibition

- Normal cells typically will grow in a continuous single layer on a plastic surface, stopping at the boundaries of the chamber; at that point the population stabilizes and cell loss approximates cell growth. Transformed cells will grow in multiple layers or clusters, reaching higher densities in culture.
- One salient reason to explain why normal cells do not form multilayers is the requirement for optimal utilization of nutrients; access to nutrients may well be compromised when normal cells crowd each other. The term *density-dependent growth* has replaced the term *contact inhibition*.

• Cancer cells form irregular masses. There typically appears to be no contact inhibition.

## Diminished Growth Factor Requirements of Cancer Cells

• On occasion, an abnormal growth factor receptor on the surface of a transformed cell can activate the signal pathway spontaneously without exposure to a growth factor. Alternatively, transformed cell lines may grow in media without serum, suggesting that they can synthesize and secrete their own growth factors.

## Ability to Divide Without Anchorage

• Transformed cells can exist in a suspension or gel; this unique property is most closely associated with the ability to form tumors.

## Loss of Restriction Point in the Cell Cycle

• Cellular proliferation occurs as the result of mitosis and the duplication of DNA within the cell. These two events make up what is known as the cell cycle.
    • The cycle is made up of four stages: the $G_1$, S phase, $G_2$, and the M phase (or mitosis).
    • Cells can begin the growth sequence anew, or they may divert themselves into a resting or quiescent state called $G_0$. Most of the cells in the adult body are in $G_0$.
    • A critical step in the cell cycle occurs late in $G_1$, when the cell has to decide whether it will go through with the entire sequence or delay and rest—a sort of "point of no return." This threshold is called the *restriction point*.
    • Normal cells will often leave $G_1$ and enter $G_0$ at the restriction point if there is a shortage of nutrients or growth factors. Many cancer cells lack this degree of control, particularly if they have too little of the pRb protein.

## DIFFERENCES IN THE APPEARANCE OF NORMAL AND CANCER CELLS

• Transformed cells have variable sizes and shapes (*pleomorphism*). The nuclei of cancer cells stain darker (*hyperchromatism*); they are disproportionately larger; cancer cells frequently exhibit a variety of abnormal mitotic figures.

## DIFFERENCES IN DIFFERENTIATION OF NORMAL AND CANCER CELLS

• Transforming growth factor-beta (TGF-β) may stimulate differentiation in some cells and inhibit it in others, while in human tumor cell populations it may inhibit tumor growth and promote more differentiation in the remaining cells.
• Cancer cells tend to be less differentiated than cells from surrounding normal tissue. Some cancer cells are so poorly differentiated (or anaplastic) that the tissue origin cannot be ascertained.
• Normal cells may undergo a gradual transition to malignancy, passing through the stages of *metaplasia, dysplasia, carcinoma in situ*, and finally invasive cancer.

## DIFFERENCES IN THE CELL SURFACES OF NORMAL AND CANCER CELLS

• The fluid nature of the membrane and the existence of mobile proteins within the membrane and on the surface was described as the *fluid mosaic model*.
• The cell surface and membrane are particularly important in cancer biology because they are involved in anchorage dependence, cell adhesion, and invasiveness, and literally hundreds of biochemical interactions.

## Glycoprotein Alterations

- In cell transformation changes are related to a lower protein content. The glycoproteins that remain are altered, mostly by becoming simpler.

### Fibronectin

- Fibronectin is a large glycoprotein found on normal cell surfaces.
- Cancer cells and transformed cells have low levels of fibronectin, causing them to attach poorly to the surface of the culture vessel; they do continue to grow, however.
- The lack of fibronectin in cancer cells is an important factor in the process of metastasis.

### Proteases

- Transformed cells secrete a variety of protein-degrading enzymes. Proteases are involved in metastasis by providing avenues through extracellular matrices and not by contributing to the transformation process itself.
- Proteolytic enzymes that have been implicated in matrix destruction include collagenases, plasminogen activators, stromelysin, cathepsin D, and procoagulants.

## Glycolipid Alterations

- Glycosphingolipid interacts with receptor proteins on the surface of normal cells to inhibit their responsiveness to growth factors. Transformed cells have less and/or altered glycosphingolipids on their cell surfaces, thus increasing their responsiveness to growth factors.

## Cell-Surface Antigens

- The great majority of human tumor antigens are *tumor-associated antigens* that have relative rather than absolute specificity.
- Tumor-associated antigens are of two basic types: *tumor-associated transplantation antigens* (TATAs) appear on the surface of cells transformed by carcinogens; *oncofetal antigens* (*embryonic antigens*) are normally found exclusively on embryonic cells that are reexpressed on certain tumors.
- Tumor-associated antigens are used clinically as markers for detection of tumors, assessment of patient prognosis, and evaluation of treatment measures.

## Altered Permeability and Membrane Transport

- Transformed cells transport materials across the cell membrane at higher rates than do normal cells.

## BIOCHEMICAL DIFFERENCES BETWEEN NORMAL AND CANCER CELLS
## Cyclic AMP and Cyclic GMP

- Cyclic adenosine monophosphate (cAMP) levels are generally high in resting normal cells and low in dividing cells, including cancer cells. In addition, cAMP reduces the rate of division of certain normal and transformed cells in culture.
- A related substance, cyclic guanosine monophosphate (cGMP), also restricts growth.

## Nutrients

- Cancer cells in culture have been shown to take up nutrients at greatly increased rates. This increased transport may be associated with alteration of transport sites of cancer cells.

## Growth Factors

- Transformed cells often will proliferate with growth factor levels that are too low for normal cell proliferation, as the normal cells will enter a resting state.

### Epidermal growth factor (EGF)

- High levels of EGF receptors are noted on many epithelial carcinomas, and mutant EGF receptors have been found on high-grade glioblastomas.

### Transforming growth factor-alpha (TGF-α)

- TGF-α is quite similar to EGF and binds avidly to the same receptor. TGF-α is angiogenic, stimulating endothelial cell proliferation.

### Transforming growth factor-beta (TGF-β)

- TGF-β inhibits the growth of many normal and transformed cells, and the development of a tumor may represent an escape from TGF-β influence. Differentiation of certain cell types may occur due to TGF-β, and it can also activate macrophages as well as increasing adhesion of cells to matrix proteins.

### Platelet-derived growth factor (PDGF)

- PDGF is produced by some tumor cells that lack a receptor for it. Combined with another growth factor such as EGF or insulin-like growth factor 1, PDGF can stimulate cell division in cultures; it cannot accomplish this effect alone. PDGF appears to play a role in the development and support of brain tumors.

### Basic fibroblast growth factor (bFGF)

- bFGF has strong angiogenic properties and can bind heparin (thus giving rise to the title *heparin-binding growth factor*). This molecule acts also through a cell-surface receptor with tyrosine kinase activity.

### Insulin-like growth factors (IGF-I and IGF-II)

- IGF-I is also known as *somatomedin C* and mediates the effect of human growth hormone.

### C-ERBB 2 (or HER2/NEU) receptor

- Although technically not a growth factor, this receptor is very similar to the EGF receptor and is amplified in many adenocarcinomas; presence may be a poor prognostic indicator.

## GENETIC DIFFERENCES BETWEEN NORMAL AND CANCER CELLS

- When a regulatory gene becomes altered and has the capacity to contribute to the development of a malignant clone, it is called an *oncogene*. The normal precursor gene (before it is altered) is called a *proto-oncogene*. A proto-oncogene is actually a normal gene.
- Multiple mutations are generally necessary for a cell to achieve a malignant character.
- Cells progressively become more unstable with each genetic change, and the rate of further genetic alterations may actually increase.
- Each human cell has the capacity to program itself for cell death in the event of serious damage or loss of regulation; this action is called *apoptosis*.
- *DNA repair genes* encode proteins that are able to rapidly fix damaged DNA. These so-called *mismatch repair genes* recognize areas in DNA where nucleotide base pairs are mistakenly aligned.

- Mutations may involve the *p53* protein (a relatively common development in human cancers).
- Two new growth-suppressor genes, *BRCA1* and *BRCA2*, have been identified; mutations in these two genes are inherited randomly and can be diagnosed with blood testing.

## THE CLINICAL PROBLEM OF METASTASIS

- Most cancer deaths are related to the uncontrolled progression of metastasis.

## FACTORS CONTRIBUTING TO METASTATIC POTENTIAL

- The metastatic process is selective, favoring the survival of certain tumor cell subpopulations already existing in a heterogeneous group of cells constituting a primary tumor.
- The property of abnormal proliferation in transformed cells does not guarantee invasion and metastasis. Tumorigenicity and metastasis have both overlapping and separate features.

### Tumor Cell Factors
#### Oncogenes

- Progression of tumors from benign to malignant is associated with structural alterations in genes and with changes in gene expression.
- Invasion and metastasis have at least somewhat different genetic controls than those for proliferation alone.

#### Heterogeneity

- Tumor cells are heterogeneous within the same tumor, among cancers of different histological origins, and among tumors of the same histological origin but in different individuals.

#### Production of angiogenic factors

- Once a tumor has been initiated, any subsequent increase in cell population must be preceded by an increase in new capillaries that converge on the tumor. The stimulus for and development of these new capillaries are initiated and supported by a group of peptide proteins called *angiogenic factors*. These polypeptides include FGF, angiogenin, TGF, and tumor necrosis factor.

#### Motility

- Motility factors produced by tumor cells and neighboring tissue cells stimulate tumor cells to move toward new destinations.

#### Specific cell-surface receptors

- Cells express specific surface receptors that recognize a vast array of proteins in their extracellular environment, including matrix proteins.

### Host Factors
#### Deficient immune response

- Cytotoxic T cells are capable of interacting with tumor-associated antigens on tumor cells. Natural killers are large, granular lymphocytes that can naturally lyse a broad range of tumor cell targets. Macrophages are the tissue-based counterpart to the blood monocyte; they have a natural antitumor activity that is enhanced when they are "activated" by various substances.
- Interleukin-2 can heighten the antitumor actions of cytotoxic T cells and NK cells, while gamma-interferon is a classic activator of macrophages.

- How tumors escape immune destruction is still somewhat mysterious, but a number of potential mechanisms are known, such as the presence of variants, antigenic modulation, immunosuppressive substances such as TGF-β, chemotherapy and radiation treatments, and dense, fibrous tissue stroma.
- In advanced stages of cancer, a general immunosuppression is not uncommon. Reactivity to common antigens by skin testing may be lost; common patterns of immunologic deficiency have been associated with tumor stage and grade.

### Intact hemostatic mechanism

- Normal platelet function is required for optimal tumor cell metastasis.

## THE METASTATIC SEQUENCE

- From the initial cell division of a malignant clone will arise a pair of cells that will reside in a specific site.
- In the majority of human malignancies the growth of a tumor restricted to its primary site is not fatal; the process of tumor spread to distant body locations is a more dangerous threat.
- Although the metastatic sequence is a continuum of integrated events, an understanding of the most important facets is facilitated by dividing the process into specific steps:
  1. tumor growth and neovascularization
  2. tumor cell invasion of the basement membrane and other extracellular matrices
  3. detachment and embolism of tumor cell aggregates
  4. arrest in distant organ capillary beds
  5. extravasation
  6. proliferation within the organ parenchyma

## Tumor Growth and Neovascularization

- An organizing population of tumor cells requires the development of new blood vessels.
  - Endothelial cells in the native vessels are stimulated to break through the endothelial basement membrane and to form new channels across parenchymal stroma, finally reaching the tumor and forming a network within it.
  - The process of tumor angiogenesis relies on the presence of various biological substances, both stimulatory and inhibitory; VEGF, which promotes growth and chemotaxis of endothelial cells in vitro, is overexpressed in many tumors. Most important, VEGF may be the final pathway through which other angiogenic agents exert their influence.
  - Inhibitory angiogenic compounds are as important as the stimulatory agents and include TGF-β$_1$, alpha interferon, and angiostatin.
  - The new and immature tumor vessels are disorganized, with prominent gaps in their walls. These gaps allow tumor cells in the vicinity to gain entrance and potentially travel away from the primary site.

## Invasion of Surrounding Tissue

- To survive, cancer cells must be able to spread beyond the boundaries of the tissue barriers that initially surround them.
  - As an early tumor develops, it is initially surrounded by the tissue of its native organ. The substance of the tissue is composed of interstitial stroma and basement membrane.
  - Cell-surface molecules, involved in anchorage to basement membrane are called *integrins*; cancer cells develop mechanisms to survive away from their normal position along a basement membrane.

- As an invasive tumor develops, the integrity of the basement membrane is compromised.
- Cancer cells will often have enhanced receptors for laminin, which allows them to begin an interaction that will eventually disintegrate the barrier.
- As the process of basement membrane deterioration progresses, an immune response may develop as tumor cells release chemoattractants for monocytes and lymphocytes.
- The resulting inflammatory milieu will often result in a dense, fibrous reaction around the tumor called *desmoplasia*, a development that causes tumors to become firmer.
- Tissue inhibitors of metalloproteinases (TIMPs) and plasminogen activator inhibitors (PAIs) represent the two most important families of inhibitors.
- The stimulus for the locomotion of cells as they push through tissue on their way to achieving an avenue for distant spread appears to reside in various chemoattractants in tissue, including complement-derived materials, collagen peptides, and other connective tissue components.
  - This abnormal motility is based on a substance secreted by tumor cells termed *autocrine motility factor* (AMF).
  - Dividing endothelial cells can release proteins such as interleukin-6 into the microenvironment to stimulate proliferation and motility while local growth factors such as GM-CSF and IGFs can direct tumor cell migration.
  - The fluctuations of growth factors, cytokines, and proteolytic enzymes will determine whether a tumor cell can break away and successfully traverse the distance to enter the lumen of a blood vessel or lymphatic duct.

## Detachment and Embolism of Tumor Cell Aggregates

- A common pathway of tumor dissemination involves the lymphatic system; invading cells may stagnate in the first lymph node they reach or may pass through to other nodes or into small blood vessels.
- A relative protective effect occurs if tumor cells form aggregates either with each other or with platelets, as it is less likely that immune cells will be able to penetrate the conglomerate.

## Arrest in Distant Organ Capillary Beds

- Unless circulating tumor cells are able to stop safely in capillary beds, they may circulate indefinitely until they die. In order to maximize the ability to arrest in a blood vessel, malignant cells may secrete substances that cause platelets to aggregate around them; in turn, platelets elaborate growth factors that favor continued survival.
- In addition to selective target tissue adhesion, specific chemotactic factors or growth factors may lure circulating malignant cells to a particular site.

## Extravasation

- Approximately 1 in 10,000 circulating tumor cells will successfully arrest and penetrate the vessel wall to establish a niche in another organ. Negotiating a passage through the vessel wall is called *extravasation*.

## Proliferation Within the Organ Parenchyma

- Once a malignancy has demonstrated the capacity to successfully complete the process of metastasis, overcoming all the natural obstacles in place, there would appear to be no significant reason that further metastases could not develop naturally.

## GENETIC CONTROL OF THE METASTATIC CONTINUUM

- Current evidence suggests that invasion and metastasis require activation of a set of effector genes over and above those required for unrestrained growth alone. A metastasis suppressor gene, *NM23*, may be a most important factor in determining metastatic potential. To date, however, the exact nature of the gene's actions requires further elucidation.

## ANTIMETASTASIS THERAPY

- Failure of one step in the metastatic process may be enough to provide a survival advantage or to maximize the current effects of conventional systemic treatment.

### Prevention of Tumor Invasion

- An inhibitor of proteinase activity would be a likely candidate to interrupt the metastatic cascade.

### Antiadhesive Therapy

- Certain synthetic peptides with a sequence of Arg-Gly-Asp are capable of blocking tumor cell adhesion reactions and decreasing metastases in experimental animals.

### Monoclonal Antibodies

- Monoclonal antibodies are pure preparations of a specific antibody directed against a particular cell or cell structure.

### Modulation of Tumor Vascularization

- One of the most promising areas for future trails involves the area of angiogenesis inhibition. It is very likely that a successful blockade of tumor blood vessel formation would significantly affect the frequency of metastases and the success of conventional treatment. There are currently a number of promising agents: Razoxane; TNP-470, the first antiangiogenic drug; thalidomide; CAI; and captopril.

### Anticoagulation Therapy

- There has been a long history of efforts to modify the hemostatic mechanism in order to change the course of cancer, using both anticoagulants and antiplatelet agents.
- Antiplatelet agents can prevent platelet activation and secretion as well as inhibiting experimentally induced metastases.

### Genetic Manipulation

- Should certain genes such as *NM23* be found to have a significant impact on the metastatic character of cancer cells, it will be possible in the near future to place normal copies of missing *NM23* genes or replace abnormal *NM23* genes in tumor cells.

## CONCLUSION

- We still need to know how to predict the metastatic potential of a tumor at the time of diagnosis.

## PRACTICE QUESTIONS

1. Problems arise when experimental transformed cell models are applied to human cancer because:
   a. transformed cells do not have features identical to those of cancer cells.
   b. transformed cell lines are characterized by uncontrolled growth and immortality.
   c. human cancers evolve because of exposure to chemical, viral, or radiation carcinogens.
   d. there are too many human cancers to develop transformed cell lines.

2. The phenomenon of normal cell division ceasing upon achievement of a monolayer across a petri dish or vessel is called:
   a. density-dependent growth.
   b. senescence.
   c. cell-cell growth.
   d. prototype development.

3. The "decision" of the cell whether to enter $G_0$ (the resting state) or to continue in $G_1$ occurs at a point in $G_1$ called the:
   a. anchorage-dependent growth phase.
   b. restriction point.
   c. contact inhibition point.
   d. differentiation point.

4. What is the name given to transformed cells that have variable sizes and shapes because of unpolymerized proteins?
   a. transforming growth factors
   b. hyperchromaticism
   c. pleomorphism
   d. unequal segregation

5. Which of the following statements about cell differentiation is true?
   a. Cancer cells are more differentiated than normal cells.
   b. Cancer cells are less differentiated than normal cells.
   c. Cancer cells are completely undifferentiated.
   d. Cancer cells are at the same level of differentiation as the tissues from which they derive.

6. Fibronectin is a glycoprotein found on the surface of normal cells and in low levels on cancer cells. Which of the following is one of its numerous functions in normal cells?
   a. It provides constant sources of nutrients.
   b. It inhibits cell responsiveness to growth factors.
   c. It promotes cell-to-cell adhesion.
   d. It degrades attachment proteins.

7. A tumor-associated antigen that is normally found only on embryonic cells is:
   a. human chorionic gonadotropin.
   b. oncofetal antigen.
   c. testosterone.
   d. estrogen.

8. In order for metastasis to occur, a sequence of events takes place. The initial mechanism in the metastatic sequence is:
   a. imbalance in motility and proteolysis and loss of control over growth.
   b. abnormal proliferation and access to the circulatory system.
   c. the completion of differentiation.
   d. loss of angiogenesis and provision of motility factors.

9. Invasion and metastasis:
   a. have the same genetic controls as those for motility.
   b. are initiated by the destruction of angiogenic factors.
   c. have different genetic controls than those for proliferation alone.
   d. have different genetic controls.

10. What percentage of individuals have metastatic disease at the time of their initial diagnosis?
    a. 10%
    b. 30%–40%
    c. 60%
    d. 80%

11. An organizing population of tumor cells requires the creation of capillaries and development of a circulatory system through the process of:
    a. proliferation.
    b. diversification.
    c. angiogenesis.
    d. intravasation.

12. In order to enter underlying interstitial stroma and gain access to lymphatics and the bloodstream, tumor cells must first:
    a. stimulate endothelial cells to break through epithelial basement membranes.
    b. choose an organ to which to metastasize.
    c. differentiate.
    d. enter the progression phase of metastasis.

13. The stimulus for the locomotion of cells as they spread through tissue is *not* found in:
    a. chemoattractants in the tissue.
    b. complement-derived materials.
    c. integrins in the cell surfaces.
    d. collagen peptides.

14. An immune response to tumor cells' release of chemoattractants often results in a dense, fibrous, sometimes palpable reaction around the tumor called:
    a. pus.
    b. desmoplasia.
    c. TIMP.
    d. cytokine profusion.

15. _____ can direct tumor cell migration.
    a. Cytokines
    b. Local growth factors like GM-CSF and IGFs
    c. Proteolytic enzymes
    d. Interleukin-6

16. The process by which a tumor cell negotiates a passage through the vessel wall is called:
    a. invasion.
    b. vascularization.
    c. extravasation.
    d. circulation.

17. A metastasis suppressor gene, _____, may be a most important factor in determining metastatic potential.
    a. RGD
    b. Arg-Gly-Asp
    c. *NM23*
    d. CAI

## ANSWER EXPLANATIONS

1. **The answer is a.** For the cancer cell prototype, normal cells derived from normal tissue are established in culture under controlled conditions. These cells can be transformed into cells that behave like malignant cells when they are exposed to chemical, viral, or radiation carcinogens. Not all transformed cell lines exhibit all the characteristics generally found in transformed cells. Two factors–uncontrolled growth and immortality–are observed in all cancer cells. While transformed cells provide the best model for studying the differences between normal and malignant cells, the model is not a perfect duplication of what actually occurs in a human being. (pp. 18–19)

2. **The answer is a.** Density-dependent growth refers to a monolayer of cell growth in a vessel or culture that ceases growing upon achievement of the monolayer. Recent experiments have shown that when cells crowd each other, their access to nutrients necessary for cell division is inhibited. This phenomenon may explain why normal cells stop dividing when a contained area is filled with a monolayer of cells. (p. 20)

3. **The answer is b.** The cell's decision whether to enter $G_0$ or to continue in $G_1$ occurs at a point in $G_1$ called the restriction point. Once the cell passes this point, it must continue through all phases of the cell cycle and return to $G_1$. (p. 20)

4. **The answer is c.** Normal cells have a well-organized and extensive cytoskeleton made up of bundles of microfilaments and microtubules. These bundles consist of polymerized subunits of proteins that provide the structure and shape of the cell. Transformed cells contain the subunits of proteins, but the proteins are not polymerized, which causes transformed cells to have variable sizes and shapes, a condition known as pleomorphism. (p. 21)

5. **The answer is b.** As the human organism develops, cells become different and specialized for various structural and functional purposes. This process is called differentiation. Cancer cells may arise at any point during differentiation. Cancer cells tend to be less differentiated than cells from surrounding normal tissue, and some cancer cells are so poorly differentiated (anaplastic) that the tissue of origin cannot be identified. (p. 22)

6. **The answer is c.** Fibronectin is a large glycoprotein found on normal cell surfaces. Together with various proteoglycans, collagen, and elastin, fibronectin forms the matrix in which cells are embedded and that anchors cells in place within tissues. (p. 23)

7. **The answer is b.** Alpha-fetoprotein (AFP) is an oncofetal antigen normally found on embryonic cells that are reexpressed on certain tumors. AFP can be found in liver cancers and in some testicular, pancreatic, and gastrointestinal tract tumors. (p. 24)

8. **The answer is a.** The property of abnormal proliferation in transformed cells does not guarantee invasion and metastasis. Tumorigenesis and metastasis have both overlapping and separate features. For invasion and metastasis to occur, imbalances in motility and proteolysis leading to tissue barrier breakdown are required, in addition to loss of growth control. Tumor cells must also avoid the dynamic assaults of the immune system to succeed in establishing distant colonies. Finally, *angiogenesis* (new blood vessel formation) is necessary. (p. 27)

9. **The answer is c.** Progression of tumors from benign to malignant is associated with structural alterations in genes and with changes in gene expression. There exists a question as to whether the genes controlling abnormal cell proliferation are the same as the genes involved in conferring an ability to metastasize. Current evidence supports the concept that separate mechanisms underlie these two characteristics of transformed cells. Thus it appears that invasion and metastasis have at least somewhat different genetic controls than those for proliferation alone. (p. 27)

10. **The answer is c.** Although many tumors are now treated successfully by surgery alone or in combination with chemotherapy, radiotherapy, or immunotherapy, metastasis is the most frequent cause of cancer treatment failure. It is estimated that up to 60% of individuals with solid tumors have metastatic disease at the time of their initial diagnosis, even though many of the metastases are microscopic lesions that remain undetected until later in the individual's disease course. (p. 28)

11. **The answer is c.** The formation of new blood vessels (or angiogenesis) is an integral part of embryology; similarly, an organizing population of tumor cells requires the development of new blood vessels. While not sufficient alone to guarantee a viable metastatic result, angiogenesis is a natural beginning. Malignant cells (and normal cells of the surrounding tissue, such as fibroblasts and macrophages) are able to elaborate substances that encourage nearby native blood vessels to form new branches extending toward the enlarging tumor mass. (p. 29)

12. **The answer is a.** Malignant cells (and normal cells of the surrounding tissue, such as fibroblasts and macrophages) are able to elaborate substances that encourage nearby native blood vessels to form new branches extending toward the enlarging tumor mass. Endothelial cells in the native vessels are stimulated to break through the endothelial basement membrane and to form new channels across parenchymal stroma, finally reaching the tumor and forming a network within it. (p. 29)

13. **The answer is c.** Cell-surface molecules, involved in anchorage to basement membrane are called *integrins*; unless cultured cells can attach to a surface via these molecules, they will not be able to reproduce and eventually will undergo apoptosis. In order for normal cells to survive and flourish, they must have the right matrix code and the correct integrin. Cancer cells overcome this frailty by developing mechanisms to survive away from their normal position along a basement membrane. The stimulus for the locomotion of cells as they push through tissue on their way to achieving an avenue for distant spread appears to reside in various chemoattractants in tissue, including complement-derived materials, collagen peptides, and other connective tissue components. (p. 30)

14. **The answer is b.** As the process of basement membrane deterioration progresses, an immune response may develop as tumor cells release chemoattractants for monocytes and lymphocytes. The resulting inflammatory milieu will often result in a dense, fibrous reaction around the tumor called *desmoplasia*, a development that causes tumors to become firmer and more easily appreciated on physical examination. (p. 30)

15. **The answer is b.** Local growth factors such as CM-CSF and IGFs can direct tumor cell migration. The fluctuations of growth factors, cytokines, and proteolytic enzymes will determine whether a tumor cell can break away and successfully traverse the distance to enter the lumen of a blood vessel or lymphatic duct. (p. 31)

16. **The answer is c.** Historically, it has been estimated from experimental systems that approximately 1 in 10,000 circulating tumor cells will successfully arrest and penetrate the vessel wall to establish a niche in another organ. Negotiating a passage through the vessel wall is called *extravasation*. (p. 31)

17. **The answer is c.** Current evidence suggests that invasion and metastasis require activation of a set of effector genes over and above those required for unrestrained growth alone. A metastasis suppressor gene, *NM23*, may be a most important factor in determining metastatic potential. (p. 32)

# Chapter 3    Carcinogenesis

## INTRODUCTION

- Cancer is the process by which some of the cells of the organism attempt to destroy the organism itself.
- *Oncogenes* are growth-promoting genes, and *cancer-suppressor genes* are growth-inhibitory genes. Carcinogenesis is the process by which these genes are damaged to the extent that clones of cells lose the normal control mechanisms of growth and proliferate out of control.
- Cancer develops and evolves by the process of *clonal selection.* Mutation in the genome of a cell may confer a survival advantage on that cell. If a second mutation also confers a survival advantage, this new clone grows even more vigorously.
- Damage to the genome may result from exposure to chemicals, radiation, asbestos, or certain viruses. The path of action, though, will be through oncogenes and cancer-suppressor genes.
  - Oncogenes must be mutated or relocated so as to be activated, and cancer-suppressor genes must be mutated or lost so as to be inactivated.
  - Oncogenes usually act as dominant genes; that is, only one gene of each pair needs to be mutated to have an effect; cancer-suppressor genes usually act as recessive genes, that is, both genes of a pair must be mutated or lost to abolish their cancer-suppressor effect.
- Cancer may be thought of as a defect in the control of the cell cycle.
- Cancer may also be thought of as being related to a defect in programmed cell death (apoptosis), which is a mechanism by which defective cells are disposed of.
  - The cancer cell reproduces in an uncontrolled manner, does not undergo normal programmed cell death, and seems to lack the normal "biological clocks" called *telomeres*, which are not completely copied when the chromosome is duplicated during cell division. With age the telomeres grow progressively shorter until the chromosome can no longer replicate.
    - Cancer cells also develop the enzyme telomerase, which contributes to their immortality.

## STAGES OF CARCINOGENESIS

- In humans carcinogenesis is much more complex than in well-studied animal laboratory models. The distinction among the three stages of initiation, promotion, and progression is blurred, and there are many more steps.
- Carcinogenesis is ordinarily classified as chemical, viral, physical, or familial, even though it is likely that human carcinogenesis involves a combination of factors. Carcinogenesis can also be classified as occupational, dietary, environmental, lifestyle, and so forth.

## CHEMICAL CARCINOGENESIS

- Classic work by the Millers led in 1951 to the understanding that covalent binding within the cell was essential for carcinogenic activity; the active metabolite of the carcinogen was later identified to be an electrophilic reactant that bound to DNA. Carcinogens are converted by a series of metabolic steps into free radicals, that is, compounds with a single unpaired electron. Free radicals are electrophilic, that is, highly reactive with macromolecules that are rich in electrons, such as DNA. Compounds called *antioxidants* inhibit carcinogenesis because they react with free radicals before the free radicals damage DNA.

- Because different organisms have different metabolic systems, potential carcinogens are metabolized in one way in some organisms and in other ways in other organisms, with the result that some chemicals are carcinogenic for one species but not for another.
- Ames developed a classic assay system to measure carcinogens. The assay employs bacteria and is based on the fact that most carcinogens are mutagens, that is, they damage DNA.
- The metabolism of a carcinogen leads to the final active chemical, called the *proximate carcinogen*, that reacts with the DNA.
- The specific targets of carcinogens are the oncogenes and cancer-suppressor genes, the "on" and "off" switches for cell growth.
- There still remain few chemicals (other than tobacco) for which there is strong evidence of causation of the common cancers in man.
- Only 4% of all cancer deaths in the United States are due to occupational causes. Cancer chemotherapeutic agents are carcinogenic, and cured cancer patients are at risk for leukemia and some other tumors.

## FAMILIAL CARCINOGENESIS

- A variety of sources estimate that up to 15% of all human cancers may have a hereditary component.
- Genes have now been isolated for several of the classic family cancer syndromes.
- Familial carcinogenesis is based in large part on a group of genes that, when mutated, cause cancer by their absence, that is, they seem to *prevent* cancer when they are functioning normally. These protective genes are the *cancer-suppressor genes*.
- The loss of the normal copy of a gene by the process of mitotic recombination is referred to as *loss of heterogeneity* or *reduction to homozygosity* because the cell becomes homozygous for the abnormal gene, thus losing its ability to prevent malignant growth.

## PHYSICAL CARCINOGENESIS

- Physical carcinogens are agents that damage the same oncogenes and cancer-suppressor genes that are attacked by chemicals, but they exert their action by physical rather than chemical means.
- There are two forms of radiation that induce cancer: ultraviolet radiation and ionizing radiation.

### Ultraviolet Radiation

- Ultraviolet radiation (UVR) from the sun leads to malignant transformation. The basal cell and squamous cell carcinomas of the exposed areas of the skin are the result.
- Melanoma is also linked to ultraviolet exposure, though not as tightly as basal and squamous cancers. The most active carcinogenic wavelength of UVR is 280–320 nm, which is referred to as ultraviolet B (UVB).
- Appropriate preventive techniques include avoidance of direct sunlight and the use of sunblocks that block out UVB radiation.

### Ionizing Radiation

- Ionizing radiation leads to permanent mutations in DNA. When these mutations involve oncogenes or cancer-suppressor genes, transformation of a cell to malignant growth may occur.
- Minimizing exposure to man-made radiation hazards and stopping smoking provide the greatest potential for prevention of radiation-induced cancer of the lung, since radon exposure acts synergistically with tobacco smoke.
- The large unavoidable radiation doses from our natural environment dwarf the small medical exposure.
- Of particular public concern is exposure from mammography.

### Asbestos

- Asbestos, the major carcinogenic fiber, is believed to be related to about 2000 cases of mesothelioma annually in the United States. Actually, asbestos causes more bronchogenic cancers than mesotheliomas, perhaps 6000, because of its synergism with tobacco smoke. Lung cancer is rare in asbestos workers who do not smoke.
- Data do not support an association between gastrointestinal cancer and asbestos.
- Only certain forms of asbestos increase the risk of mesothelioma.

## VIRAL CARCINOGENESIS

- The epidemiological evidence for the viral etiology of cancer is strongest for a relationship between hepatitis B virus (HBV) and hepatocellular carcinoma and between human T-cell leukemia virus type 1 (HTLV-1) and T-cell lymphoma.
- The mechanism of carcinogenesis may be insertion of the virus into the host genome in such a way as to activate host proto-oncogenes; or, as is the case with HPV, there may be HTLV-coded proteins that interfere with the cell cycle.
- HBV is endemic in Asia and Africa, where large numbers of people are chronic carriers. Epidemiological studies have established HBV to be etiologic in hepatocellular carcinoma (HCC).
- HCC may be induced by a mechanism that does not involve HBV, such as the natural carcinogen aflatoxin.
- EBV, a double-stranded DNA virus of the herpes family, causes infectious mononucleosis in the United States and Burkitt's lymphoma in Africa.
- HPVs are double-stranded circular DNA viruses that infect squamous epithelium.
- HPV is etiologic in genital warts.

## BACTERIAL CARCINOGENESIS

- A relationship between *H pylori* and MALT lymphoma has now been noted; the early proliferation is reversible by eradication of the bacteria with antibiotics, whereas the later tumor is not and requires conventional anticancer therapy.

## COLON CANCER AS A MODEL OF HUMAN CARCINOGENESIS

- In nonfamilial colorectal cancer the sequence of events required for carcinogenesis and progression has been worked out more completely than for any other neoplasm.
- In colorectal cancer, two familial syndromes have been matched with their genes.

## PRACTICE QUESTIONS

1. In clonal selection:
   a. mutation in the genome of a cell may confer a survival advantage on that cell.
   b. a cell becomes weaker with each mutation.
   c. oncogenes are destroyed.
   d. telomeres develop, which are completely duplicated during cell division.

2. A patient asks you to describe the "types of things that cause cancer." Because of her interest in "types" of causes, you might begin by explaining that carcinogenesis is *ordinarily* classified as:
   a. biological, viral, physical, or chemical.
   b. occupational, viral, dietary, or familial.
   c. chemical, viral, physical, or familial.
   d. viral, chemical, familial, occupational, or lifestyle.

3. Antioxidants:
   a. are converted by a series of metabolic steps into free radicals.
   b. react with free radicals before the free radicals damage DNA.
   c. are electrophilic.
   d. are highly reactive with macromolecules that are rich in electrons, such as DNA.

4. Mr. Henderson's cancer is said to have been induced by familial carcinogenesis. From this you can assume that in his case certain genes:
   a. caused cancer by functioning to excess.
   b. caused cancer by their absence.
   c. acted as growth promoters.
   d. lost their ability to prevent malignant growth by their loss of homozygosity.

5. Mr. Buck's cancer is reportedly related to his years of exposure to asbestos when he was working in construction. Mr. Buck is 67, worked in construction for 50 years, drinks beer occasionally, and smoked "off and on over the years." From this you can infer that Mr. Buck *most likely* has:
   a. mesothelioma.
   b. bronchogenic cancer.
   c. gastrointestinal cancer.
   d. lung cancer.

6. Ms. Harris has hepatocellular carcinoma, which is apparently viral. The most likely assumption, then, is that she was exposed somehow to:
   a. HTLV-1.
   b. ATL.
   c. HCC.
   d. HBV.

7. Ms. Linhorst is diagnosed with an early proliferation of MALT lymphoma, apparently due to her exposure to *H pylori*. The most likely course of treatment for Ms. Linhorst is:
   a. a course of antibiotics.
   b. a course of radiation and antiviral agents.
   c. antiviral agents alone.
   d. conventional anticancer therapy.

## ANSWER EXPLANATIONS

1.  **The answer is a.** In clonal selection, mutation in the genome of a cell may confer a survival advantage on that cell. The cell grows stronger, not weaker, with each mutation. The cancer cell is immortal because it seems to lack the "biological clocks" like *telomeres*, which are not completely duplicated during cell division, and thus grow progressively shorter until the chromosome can no longer replicate. In cancer, the final common path of action is through oncogenes, the growth-promoting genes: oncogenes must be mutated or relocated so as to be activated. (p. 40)

2.  **The answer is c.** Carcinogenesis is ordinarily classified as chemical, viral, physical, or familial, even though it is likely that human carcinogenesis involves a combination of factors. Carcinogenesis can also be classified as occupational, dietary, environmental, lifestyle, and so forth. (p. 41)

3.  **The answer is b.** Carcinogens are converted by a series of metabolic steps into free radicals—that is, compounds with a single unpaired electron. Free radicals are electrophilic; this means they are highly reactive with macromolecules that are rich in electrons, such as DNA. Compounds called antioxidants inhibit carcinogenesis because they react with free radicals before the free radicals damage DNA. (p. 41)

4.  **The answer is b.** Familial carcinogenesis is based in large part on a group of genes that, when mutated, cause cancer by their absence; that is, they seem to prevent cancer when they are functioning normally. These protective genes are the cancer-suppressor genes. The loss of the normal copy of a gene by the process of mitotic recombination is referred to as *loss of heterogeneity* or *reduction to homozygosity* because the cell becomes homozygous for the abnormal gene, thus losing its ability to prevent malignant growth. (p. 42)

5.  **The answer is b.** Asbestos, the major carcinogenic fiber, is believed to be related to about 2000 cases of mesothelioma annually in the United States. However, asbestos causes more bronchogenic cancers than mesotheliomas, perhaps 6000, because of its synergism with tobacco smoke. Lung cancer is rare in asbestos workers who do not smoke. Data do not support an association between gastrointestinal cancer and asbestos. (p. 43)

6.  **The answer is d.** The epidemiological evidence for the viral etiology of cancer is strongest for a relationship between hepatitis B virus (HBV) and hepatocellular carcinoma and between human T-cell leukemia virus type 1 (HTLV-1) and T-cell lymphoma. (p. 44)

7.  **The answer is a.** The early proliferation of MALT lymphoma is reversible by eradication of the bacteria with antibiotics, whereas the later tumor is not and requires conventional anticancer therapy. (p. 45)

# Chapter 4  Cancer Control and Epidemiology

## INTRODUCTION

- Cancer epidemiology examines the frequency of cancer in populations, the role of certain risk factors that contribute to cancer rates, and the interrelationships or associations that exist between the host, the environment, and other conditions that may contribute to the development or inhibition of cancer.

## BASIC CONSIDERATIONS IN EPIDEMIOLOGICAL RESEARCH

### Study Designs

#### Experimental studies

- An experimental study design attempts to control the variability of all factors except for the exposure of interest. These studies are conducted when a research hypothesis is being developed.

#### Ecological studies

- In this design, trends are examined in disease distribution among humans across ecological or geographic areas.

#### Cross-sectional studies

- In this study design a onetime view of a population is taken, and the rates of existing (prevalent) cases of the disease, the degree of exposure, and other demographic characteristics of interest are measured. While cross-sectional studies cannot establish a causal relationship, they do provide the prevalence rates for the disease in that population.

#### Case-control studies

- The information gained from case-control studies does not establish a causal relationship between the disease and the exposure, but it does explore the concurrent association between the two.
- *Control subjects* are defined as people who do not have the disease at present but who, if the disease did develop, would have the same opportunity to be diagnosed as the case subjects.
- In *matching,* certain demographic characteristics of the cases are matched to those of the controls.
- The advantage of matching and analyzing the data in pairs of subjects is that fewer subjects are required in each group to see a relationship between the exposure and the disease. The major disadvantage of matching is that any variable used in matching cannot be studied in relation to the disease.
- A commonly used alternative to matching is the recruitment of more than one control subject per case subject. This technique affords an increase in statistical power without limiting the variables that can be investigated.

### Cohort studies

- The cohort, or group of subjects, included in this type of study design represents individuals who do not have the disease of interest. Once the cohort is selected, the exposures of interest are assessed and the subjects monitored for a designated *period of time* to record development of the disease.
- Cohort studies can be retrospective, prospective, or ambidirectional.
    - *Retrospective* studies use a previously defined cohort, identify individuals who developed the disease, and assess the level of exposure.
    - In *prospective* studies a current population of disease-free individuals is selected and the exposure(s) measured. This study population is then followed into the future and evaluated for development of the disease.
    - The *ambidirectional* cohort study starts with a previously established cohort and continues subject follow-up into the future. This design carries the same advantages and disadvantages as the retrospective and prospective designs combined.

### Clinical trials and intervention studies

- The clinical trial or intervention study tests the effect of an intervention on the rates of disease development. Two groups of subjects are created within the study population: a treatment group and a control group.
- The design is called *double-blind* when the assignment of the treatment group is kept from the subject and the immediate clinical personnel.

## Defining the Population

- The *source population* for the study is the larger group or population from which the study subjects are recruited.

### Eligibility criteria

- These are designed to create a population of subjects with a sufficient prevalence of the disease to test the hypothesis efficiently, and for whom the intervention is safe.

### Defining the disease and the exposure

- An *exposure* is a contact that a subject has had with the variable of interest that may influence the development of or improvement in disease status.
- The characteristics of the exposure that are most important to clarify are the *dose* of the exposure, the *duration* or length of time of the exposure, and *characteristics* that are specific to the exposure.
- *Dose* refers to a standardized, measured amount of exposure issued.

## Statistical Plan

- A major goal of epidemiological research is to make inferences to the larger population based on information obtained from the study population.

## Potential Sources of Bias and Confounding

- The potential sources of bias are examined to determine if the differences seen between the two groups can be explained by influences other than the research hypothesis.

## Data Sources

- Data sources relating to cancer and risk factors for cancer are listed in Table 4-4 on text page 57.

## ENVIRONMENTAL FACTORS ASSOCIATED WITH CANCER CAUSATION
### How Do We Decide What Causes Cancer?

- The criteria to be considered are the following: magnitude of association, consistency of findings, biological credibility, temporal association between the risk factor and the disease.

### Tobacco

- Tobacco use is still the most important known cause of cancer in the United States. Tobacco causes about 30% of cancer deaths, and cigarette smoking causes 90% of lung cancers.
  - A clear linear relationship exists between the number of cigarettes smoked and the risk of lung and oropharyngeal cancers.
- There is a gradual decrease in the ex-smoker's risk of dying from lung cancer; eventually the risk is almost equivalent to that of a nonsmoker.
  - The rate of decline of the risk after cessation of smoking is determined by the cumulative smoking exposure prior to cessation, the age when smoking began, and the degree of inhalation.

### Diet

- Case-control and cohort studies of diet and cancer present several methodological problems:
  - Accurate assessment of dietary intake is very difficult.
  - Individual nutrients are often highly correlated because they are strongly related to calorie intake.
  - Frequently, the range of nutrient intake within the study population is narrow.
  - Recall bias may be present if dietary assessment is being conducted after the presentation of the disease.

#### Colon cancer and fat intake

- Studies have shown a strong association between per capita meat consumption or dietary fat and incidence of colorectal cancer. However, a causal association cannot be assumed.

#### Colon cancer and fiber intake

- High fiber intake is protective for colon cancer in studies where the source of fiber has been examined: fiber from vegetables appears protective against colon cancer, whereas the data for cereal fiber are less supportive of a protective effect.

#### Colon cancer and calcium intake

- To reduce the risk of colon cancer, calcium intake for females should be 1500 mg and for males, 1800 mg.

#### Breast cancer and fat intake

- Ecological studies that use data from many countries show a strong positive relationship between per capita fat intake and breast cancer mortality rates. However, case-control and cohort studies give conflicting results.
- Current dietary recommendations are for women to reduce fat intake to less than 30% of calories.

#### Cancer, micronutrients, and intake of fruits and vegetables

- One of the most consistent dietary findings with regard to cancer is a protective effect of fruits and vegetables.

- Relatively high levels of the carotenoid beta-carotene, vitamin A, vitamin E, and selenium have been found to be associated with lower cancer risk.
- National Research Council recommendations include eating at least five servings of fruit and vegetables a day, reducing fat intake to 30% or less of calories, maintaining protein intake at moderate levels, and balancing food intake and physical activity to maintain appropriate body weight.

## Alcohol

- Alcohol has been causally linked to cancers of the oral cavity, pharynx, larynx, esophagus, and liver, and may be linked to cancers of the breast and rectum. It is estimated that 3% of cancer deaths are attributable to alcohol.
- Rectal cancer appears to be associated specifically with beer consumption.

## Physical activity

- Increased physical activity consistently has been found to be protective for colon cancer and pre-cancerous colon polyps. Mounting evidence suggests that increased physical activity is protective for breast cancer.

## Occupational exposures

- It is estimated that 4%–9% of cancer deaths can be attributed to exposure to occupational carcinogens. The lung is the most commonly affected site.

## Pollution

- Pollution accounts for less than 1%–5% of cancer deaths in the United States.
- Epidemiological studies of pollution present a difficult methodological problem.
- Associations between air and water pollution and site-specific cancer risk are unproved.
- Chlorofluorocarbons (CFCs) may indirectly increase cancer risk.

## Reproductive factors and sexual behavior

- In cervical cancer, having multiple sexual partners has been identified as a risk factor.
- In general, the reproductive risk factors associated with breast, endometrial, and ovarian cancers are unavoidable. Furthermore, there are no other proven risk factors for these cancers that can be avoided. Thus, early detection of these cancers is very important.

## Viruses and other biological agents

- Worldwide, 15% of cancer incidence is due to viruses. Table 4-7 on text page 62 lists several putative human cancer viruses and their associated cancers.

## Radiation

### Ionizing radiation

- For most of the earth's population, over 80% of exposure to ionizing radiation is from natural sources, such as the food chain, air, water, minerals on or near the earth's crust, and cosmic rays.
- Man-made sources are x-rays, fallout from nuclear explosions, and emissions and waste from nuclear power stations.
- Determining the effect of low-dose exposure—the level at which most exposures occur—is difficult.

- Occupational exposure to ionizing radiation is highest among underground uranium miners, commercial nuclear power plant workers, fuel fabricators, physicians, flight crews and attendants, industrial radiographers, and well loggers.

### Ultraviolet radiation

- Ultraviolet radiation (UVR) is the major cause of nonmelanoma skin cancer, with cumulative exposure and number of lifetime sunburns being predictive of risk.

### Nonionizing radiation

- Nonionizing electromagnetic fields (EMF) are generated from a variety of electrical power, radar, and microwave sources and have only recently been suspected of increasing cancer risk.

## Drugs

- Antineoplastic drugs damage cellular DNA. A late effect of this damage can be the development of a second malignancy. Second tumors most frequently involve hematopoietic and lymphatic systems, but solid tumors also can occur.

## Exogenous hormones

- Diethylstilbestrol has been associated with vaginal and cervical cancers in the daughters of treated women. This is the only known carcinogen to act transplacentally.
- In contrast, use of combined oral contraceptives has been associated with a decreased risk of endometrial and ovarian cancer.
- An increased risk of liver cancer in young women also has been associated with oral contraceptive use. Oral contraceptive use has been associated with an increased risk of breast cancer in women diagnosed at young ages.
- Estrogen replacement therapy (ERT) in postmenopausal women has been shown to increase the risk of endometrial cancer. A small increase in breast cancer risk has been associated with long-term ERT.

## HOST CHARACTERISTICS INFLUENCING CANCER SUSCEPTIBILITY

### Age

- Although cancer can occur at any age, it is very much a disease of the elderly, with those over age 65 being ten times more likely than those under 65 to develop cancer.
- Leukemia is the leading cause of death for children under 15 years of age but is no longer among the five leading causes of cancer death after the age of 35.

### Sex

- The incidence of cancers that are not sex-specific is generally lower in females. In part this is due to the differences in lifestyles between the sexes.

### Genetic Predisposition

- Two genes have recently been discovered that are associated with susceptibility to breast cancer, *BRCA1* and *BRCA2*.
  - The *BRCA1* gene is associated with increased susceptibility to both breast and ovarian cancer, whereas *BRCA2* is associated only with an increase in breast cancer.
- Familial polyposis of the colon is an example of an autosomal dominant syndrome.
- Cancer aggregates in some families.

- Some gene defects may increase a person's risk for cancer because they have an impact on carcinogen metabolism.

## Ethnicity and Race

- Ethnicity and race are both prone to misclassification.
- Ethnicity and race are often highly correlated with SES.
- There are four main racial/ethnic groups in the United States: African-Americans (blacks), Hispanic Americans, Asian/Pacific Islanders, and Native Americans.

## Socioeconomic Factors

- Socioeconomic status is usually assessed by data on income, education, or percent below the poverty level, and has been found to be associated with some cancers, independent of race.

## OTHER APPLICATIONS OF EPIDEMIOLOGY IN ONCOLOGY
### Survival

- Survival analysis is the calculation of the probability that an individual with a specific disease will be alive at a particular time point after diagnosis.
  - For most cancers the survival rate is greatly affected by the stage of cancer at diagnosis.
  - Survival analysis is also used to assess the effectiveness of new treatment modalities.

## CANCER CONTROL

- *Cancer control* has been defined as "the reduction of cancer incidence, morbidity, and mortality through an orderly sequence, from research to systematic application of the research results."
- In the Healthy People 2000 Study, high-priority research needs for cancer control science in the United States were identified.

## Screening

- Screening refers to the detection of disease by use of tests, examinations, or other procedures prior to the development of symptoms.

## Barriers to Participation in Screening Programs

- General barriers to participation in screening programs include cost, availability, discrimination, time, and patient characteristics such as culture and knowledge.

### Behavioral change

- Groups with differing characteristics may require differing interventions to achieve behavioral change.

### Government policy

- National, state, and local government legislation may indirectly or directly affect cancer control.
- Cancer control efforts are affected by the monies specifically appropriated to cancer control in the National Institutes of Health budget by the government.

## THE APPLICATION OF EPIDEMIOLOGY TO NURSING PRACTICE

- Within their roles in cancer prevention and control, nurses apply epidemiological data and research principles to three main phases of their work: The *development phase*, the *planning phases of research and prevention programs*, and the *evaluation phase*.

# PRACTICE QUESTIONS

**Questions 1–6 pertain to the cases of two specific research teams.**

1. Eric is a member of a research team that conducts an epidemiologic study. They determine that in a given year approximately 1 of every 12,000 American men suffers from prostate cancer. This figure represents a(n):
   a. incidence rate.
   b. mortality rate.
   c. prevalence rate.
   d. survival rate.

2. Eric's team switches to a cross-sectional study design. They are no doubt using this to assess:
   a. demographic data.
   b. the rates of disease and exposure in a population.
   c. causal relationships between exposures and diseases.
   d. trends in disease distribution.

3. Jana's research attempts to measure the strength of the association between a suspected carcinogen and a certain type of cancer. She will use the _____ ratio.
   a. prospective risk
   b. attributable risk
   c. retrospective risk
   d. relative risk

4. A year later Jana's team has identified the relative risk and the frequency of a suspect etiologic factor in an entire defined population. A case-control study is conducted. What is the study *most* likely to be seeking to establish?
   a. causation
   b. attributable risk
   c. a survival risk
   d. prevalence

5. Jana's next project is an epidemiologic study of workers in asbestos mines who are free of any cancer. Subjects are to be followed over a 10-year period, and the incidence rates of certain types of cancers are to be determined. This design is an example of a:
   a. prospective study.
   b. retrospective study.
   c. historical prospective study.
   d. historical retrospective study.

6. Eric's project is a retrospective study. Compared with Jana's, Eric's study has the advantage of being:
   a. less subject to bias from individuals' knowledge of the disease.
   b. less subject to bias from incomplete or faulty medical records.
   c. less time-consuming, less expensive, and quicker.
   d. more generalizable to the population from which it is drawn.

**Questions 7–8 apply to a specific cohort study.**

7. Jeffrey is screening subjects for a cohort study. He is looking for:
   a. a cross section of the general population.
   b. individuals who have the disease of interest.
   c. individuals who do not have the disease of interest.
   d. family members of individuals who have the disease of interest.

8. Given the information you have so far, you know that a primary goal in Jeffrey's study will be to:
   a. evaluate the effect of time on the emergence of some outcome.
   b. relate clusters to a common etiologic agent or to genetic or cultural factors.
   c. reconstruct descriptive data from available historical documents.
   d. trace changes in cancer incidence that occur through migration.

**Questions 9–12 apply to the case of Mr. Jantzen, a smoker.**

9. Mr. Jantzen says he just cannot believe that the number of cigarettes he smokes "makes any difference. Either you're a smoker or you're not," he says. You explain that the risk of developing _____ is directly correlated with the number of cigarettes smoked.
   a. bladder cancer
   b. pancreatic cancer
   c. oropharyngeal cancer
   d. kidney cancer

10. Mr. Jantzen quits smoking. He asks, "How much will my risk be affected?" You explain that the rate of decline in his risk of developing lung cancer is determined by the cumulative smoking exposure prior to cessation, the age when smoking began, and the:
    a. degree of inhalation.
    b. amount of passive smoke previously exposed to.
    c. brand of cigarettes smoked.
    d. amount of time that has passed since quitting.

11. As long as he is making lifestyle changes, Mr. Jantzen's wife wants him to eat more fiber because his brother had colon cancer. Which of the following sources of fiber has been shown to provide the *most* protection against colon cancer?
    a. cereals
    b. vegetables
    c. fruits
    d. bread

12. Mr. Jantzen says, "I heard that beer causes cancer in some people. Is that true?" You answer that:
    a. Yes, a variety of beers and whiskeys have been linked to oropharyngeal cancer.
    b. Yes, beer and vodka have definitely been linked to liver cancer.
    c. Yes, beer is associated with esophageal cancer.
    d. Yes, beer is specifically associated with rectal cancer.

13. Increased physical activity has been consistently found to be protective against:
    a. head and neck cancer.
    b. esophageal cancer.
    c. colon cancer.
    d. bone cancer.

14. Sources of ionizing radiation include:
   a. air.
   b. light bulbs.
   c. flowering plants.
   d. microwaves.

15. Which of the following variables appears to be the *best* descriptive determinant of cancer risk?
   a. gender
   b. age
   c. ethnicity or race
   d. genetic predisposition

16. Which of the following host characteristics does *not* influence susceptibility to cancer?
   a. age
   b. ethnicity
   c. sex
   d. hair color

17. Which of the following is the *best* example of the role of genetic predisposition in the development of cancer?
   a. The mortality rates for Japanese Americans with stomach cancer are significantly higher than those for the white American population.
   b. As more women smoke, more women are developing lung cancer.
   c. A study of Johns Hopkins medical students found that 55 students who later developed cancer perceived themselves as less close to their parents than did their healthy counterparts.
   d. Familial aggregates of cancer have been found to occur.

18. Effective cancer control is influenced *most* by which of the following?
   a. government policy
   b. routine chest X rays
   c. hygiene
   d. a low-fat diet

## ANSWER EXPLANATIONS

1. **The answer is c.** The prevalence rate is the total number of cases–new and existing–in a given population during a specific time period, in this case 1 year. It is a function of both incidence and duration. In other words, the higher the survival rate (duration) for a type of cancer, the higher its prevalence rate will be. (p. 52)

2. **The answer is b.** The cross-sectional study is another design that allows an investigator to assess the rates of disease and exposure in a population. A one-time view of a population is taken, and the rates of existing (prevalent) cases of the disease, the degree of exposure, and other demographic characteristics of interest are measured. Although they cannot establish a causal relationship between the exposure and the disease, cross-sectional studies do provide descriptive statistics for the population. (p. 53)

3. **The answer is d.** Relative risk is expressed as a ratio comparing the rate of the disease among exposed individuals with the rate of the disease among unexposed individuals. A high relative risk suggests a strong correlation between the exposure and the disease. Unlike attributable risk, however, relative risk is not intended to measure the probability that an exposed person will develop the outcome. (p. 52)

4.  **The answer is b.** Attributable risk is the difference in the incidence or death rates between the group exposed to some factor and unexposed groups. It is used to evaluate the magnitude of change in an outcome (e.g., respiratory cancer) with the removal of the suspect antecedent factor (e.g., smoking). Provided that the relative risk and the frequency of the suspect factor in the entire defined population are known, attributable risk can be estimated from a case-control study. Otherwise, it must be calculated directly from a prospective study. (p. 52)

5.  **The answer is a.** In this prospective study, subjects (miners) are being selected with varying degrees of exposure to the suspected factor (asbestos). They have not experienced the outcome thought to be associated with the factor (lung cancer or some other cancer). They are then being followed over time to see whether the outcome (e.g., a type of cancer) occurs. (p. 55)

6.  **The answer is c.** A well-done retrospective study is statistically less time-consuming, more economical, and quicker than a prospective study, but it is subject to bias from several sources, including the effect of subjects' knowledge of the disease on their recollection of factors associated with the condition, incomplete medical records, and the determination of the risk associated with exposure to some factor. It is also harder to generalize the conclusions of a retrospective study to the population from which it is drawn. (p. 55)

7.  **The answer is c.** The cohort, or group of subjects, that is included in this type of study design represents individuals who do not have the disease of interest. An initial cross-sectional study or assessment of a population can identify and eliminate all active cases of the disease. Once the cohort is selected, the exposures of interest are assessed, and the subjects are monitored for a designated period of time to record development of the disease. (p. 54)

8.  **The answer is a.** In cohort studies, several cohorts are compared at the same time to evaluate the effect of time on the emergence of some outcome, often mortality. This method is used to determine whether common exposure to a suspected etiologic factor resulted in an increased incidence of disease and to measure how prevention or treatment has altered the course of the disease over time. (p. 55)

9.  **The answer is c.** Active tobacco use has been linked to many cancer types (lung, oropharyngeal, bladder, pancreatic, cervical, and kidney), and a clear linear relationship exists between the number of cigarettes smoked and the risk of lung and oropharyngeal cancers. (p. 57)

10. **The answer is a.** There is a gradual decrease in the former smoker's risk of dying from lung cancer; eventually the risk is almost equivalent to that of a nonsmoker. The rate of decline of risk after cessation of smoking is determined by the cumulative smoking exposure prior to cessation, the age when smoking began, and the degree of inhalation. (p. 57)

11. **The answer is b.** A majority of studies of differing epidemiologic designs support the hypothesis that high fiber intake is protective against colon cancer, although not all studies are supportive. In studies where the source of fiber has been examined, fiber from vegetables appears protective against colon cancer, whereas the data for cereal fibers are less supportive of a protective effect. (p. 59)

12. **The answer is d.** Alcohol has been causally linked to cancers of the oral cavity, pharynx, larynx, esophagus, and liver, and it may be linked to cancers of the breast and rectum. It is estimated that 3% of cancer deaths are attributable to alcohol. For most cancer sites, alcohol appears to act synergistically with smoking. Although cancers at most sites do not appear to be associated with any particular type of alcohol, rectal cancer appears to be associated specifically with beer consumption. (p. 60)

13. **The answer is c.** Increased physical activity consistently has been found to be protective against colon cancer and precancerous colon polyps. Increased physical activity also may be protective against breast cancer. Increased physical activity is known to be protective against heart disease, and a general increase in physical activity throughout the population would be beneficial. (p. 60)

14. **The answer is a.** For most of the earth's population, over 80% of exposure to ionizing radiation is from natural sources, such as the food chain, air, water, minerals on or near the earth's crust, and cosmic rays. Human-made sources include x-rays, fallout from nuclear explosions, and emissions and waste from nuclear power stations. (p. 62)

15. **The answer is b.** The vulnerability of the host to different cancers changes throughout each phase of the life cycle, with an overall sharp and steady increase in cancer incidence occurring from childhood to old age as a result of intrinsic psychological states and exposure to different social, cultural, and environmental conditions. (p. 64)

16. **The answer is d.** Cancer is very much a disease of the elderly, with those over age 65 being ten times more likely than those under 65 to develop cancer. The incidence of cancers that are not sex-specific is generally lower in females, in part because of the differences in lifestyle between the sexes. Ethnicity and race can be important issues to assess in epidemiologic research, and they are often highly correlated with socioeconomic status. (pp. 64–66)

17. **The answer is d.** Data from a number of sources, including familial patterns, have been studied in an attempt to elicit features of genetic predisposition to cancer. (p. 66)

18. **The answer is a.** The national, state, and local governments have an impact on cancer control through legislation. Cancer control efforts are affected by the monies specifically appropriated to cancer control in the National Institutes of Health budget. The government can influence advancement in this area by setting national goals for cancer control, such as those in the Healthy People 2000 document. (p. 70)

# Chapter 5   Factors Affecting Health Behavior

## INTRODUCTION

- Promotion of health care has become a national initiative.

## NATIONAL INITIATIVES

- Major initiatives to influence health behavior:
  - National Cancer Institute (NCI) objectives for 1985–2000
  - American Cancer Society (ACS) priorities
  - U.S. Department of Health and Human Services objectives

## DEFINITIONS
### Health Behavior

- *Health behaviors* are "those personal attributes, such as beliefs, expectations, motives, values, perceptions, and other cognitive elements; personality characteristics, including affective and emotional states and traits; and overt behavior patterns, actions and habits that relate to health maintenance, to health restoration and to health improvement."
- *Health protective behavior* is "any behavior performed by a person, regardless of his or her perceived or actual health status, in order to protect, promote or maintain his or her health, whether or not such behavior is objectively effective toward that end."
- *Health promotion activities* are those directed toward increasing the level of well-being that already exists.

### Illness Behavior

- *Illness behavior* is "any activity, undertaken by a person who feels ill, to define the state of his health and to discover a suitable remedy."

### Sick Role Behavior

- *Sick role behavior* is the activity taken by individuals who believe themselves (or whom others believe) to be ill in order to get well.

## MODELS AND THEORIES OF HEALTH BEHAVIOR
### Social Learning Theory

- Bandura's social cognitive theory provides a framework for analyzing health behavior in terms of a continuous, mutual interaction among cognitive, behavioral, and environmental determinants (reciprocal determinism).

### Sources of influence

- Three interdependent sources that influence behavior are antecedent determinants, cognitive determinants of behavior, and consequent outcomes.
    - Antecedent determinants stem from objects or events that precede behavior change.
    - Cognitive factors partly determine which external events will be observed, how they will be perceived, and how information they convey will be organized for future use.
    - Most behavior is maintained by anticipated rather than by immediate consequences.

### Efficacy and outcome expectations

- An *outcome expectation* is defined as a personal belief that a given behavior will lead to certain outcomes.
- An *efficacy expectation* is the conviction that one can successfully execute a specific behavior required to produce a specific outcome.
- The types of outcomes that people anticipate are strongly influenced by efficacy expectations, the most important prerequisite for behavior change.
- The most dependable and powerful source of efficacy expectations is personal experience.
- Other sources include the actions of others, verbal persuasion, and one's own physiological state or emotional arousal in threatening situations.

### Application of beliefs about self-efficacy to cancer care

- Generally, a strong belief in one's ability to carry out a required activity is a powerful influence in the decision to engage in healthy behavior.

## Health Belief Model

- The Health Belief Model (HBM) was originally developed in the 1950s by Rosenstock and Hochbaum to explain preventive health behavior using psychosocial variables and psychological theories of decision making.
- The HBM is based on the assumption that an individual's subjective perception of the environment determines behavior. See Table 5-1, text page 81, for variables of the HBM.
    - *Perceived barriers* are the most powerful single predictor of behavior, although *perceived susceptibility* and *benefits* are strong also. *Perceived severity* is the weakest predictor, but appears to be strongly related to sick role behaviors.
    - Adding self-efficacy to the HBM increases its explanatory power.

### Application of the Health Belief Model to health behavior

- The HBM is one of the most widely used and influential approaches to explaining health-related behavior. It is based on premise that health is a valued goal for all.

### Application of the Health Belief Model to cancer care

- The HBM has been used to identify individuals who engage in behaviors to prevent and detect cancer.
- Health motivation and/or perceived barriers are strong predictors of people's intentions and behaviors related to cancer prevention and screening activities.

## Theory of Reasoned Action

- The Theory of Reasoned Action is a value-expectancy theory to predict a person's intention to perform a behavior in a specific situation.
- Two factors contribute to the strength of the intention to perform a specific behavior: attitude toward the behavior, and the influence of the social environment or general subjective norms on the behavior.
  - Attitude is determined by an individual's belief that a specific outcome will occur if he or she performs the behavior and by an evaluation of the outcome (cost/benefit analysis).
  - The influence of norms stems from a person's belief about what significant others believe that he/she should do, weighted by the individual's motivation to comply with their wishes (social pressure to perform).

### Application of the Theory of Reasoned Action to cancer care

- The Theory of Reasoned Action has been used in research on BSE, mammography screening, women's beliefs, attitudes, and behaviors regarding Pap tests, seeking care for symptoms of breast cancer, and adolescents' intention to chew tobacco.

## Theory of Planned Behavior

- The Theory of Planned Behavior extends the Theory of Reasoned Action to include a dimension of perceived control.
- Perceived control reflects past experience as well as perceived ease or difficulty in achieving a behavioral goal.

### Application of the Theory of Planned Behavior to cancer care

- The Theory of Planned Behavior has been used to support research in the area of colorectal cancer, BSE frequency, and adherence to a program of BSE or TSE in young adults.

## Social Support

- The relationships individuals have with others in daily living form their social or personal network.
- Affect, affirmation, and aid are three components of supportive transactions.

### Relevance of social support to health behavior

- Social support, particularly that provided by the patient's family, has a positive influence on compliance with medical advice.

### Application of social support to cancer care

- Social support is influential in women's participation in screening for breast cancer and in cessation of smoking behavior.

## Locus of Control/Health Locus of Control

### Locus of control

- Internal locus of control = Degree to which individuals perceive events in their lives as consequences of their own actions, and thereby controllable.
- External locus of control = Degree to which individuals perceive events in their lives as unrelated to their own behavior, and therefore beyond personal control.
  - External locus of control is represented by two constructs, that of chance (health determined by fate) and *powerful others* (health determined by externals such as health professionals).

- Health locus of control = A generalized expectation about whether health is controllable by one's own behavior or by forces external to oneself.

### Application of health locus of control to cancer care

- The influence of beliefs about health locus of control has been examined in relation to BSE behavior, seeking medical care for breast symptoms, and adjustment to cancer.
- BSE was practiced more frequently by women with an internal locus of control.

## Attribution Theory

- Attribution Theory involves the explanations that individuals use to make sense of their world.
- Attributions can be used to predict behavior, feelings, and expectancies, and can serve to maintain self-esteem and reduce anxiety.
- There are four dimensions of causal attributions: locus of cause, controllability, stability, and globality. (See Table 5-2, text page 85.)

### Application of Attribution Theory to cancer care

- The influence of beliefs about attribution has been examined in relation to adjustment or response to cancer.

## Transtheoretical Model of Change

- The Transtheoretical Model of Change is based on the assumption that a continuum of readiness to change applies to behavior. There are five stages in this process:
  - Precontemplation (not considering change and resistant to outside pressures to change)
  - Contemplation (starting to think about changing behavior within the next six months; more open to feedback and information; ambivalent about costs/benefits—can remain in this stage for years)
  - Preparation (taking some steps toward action and planning to change within the next month)
  - Action (initiating the new behavior and maintaining it for a minimal time)
  - Maintenance (sustaining the change for more than six months)
- The model also includes ten basic processes of change, overt and covert cognitive and behavior strategies that individuals use to move through the five stages of change and elements of decision making.

### Application of the Transtheoretical Model of Change to cancer care

- The Transtheoretical Model of Change has been applied extensively to smoking.

## Combined Theoretical Approaches to Health Behavior

- In an attempt to enhance the explanatory power of the models described previously, many researchers have combined models or selected variables from the models.

## RELATED FACTORS

### Sociodemographics

#### Knowledge and educational level

- Being knowledgeable about a specific cancer or cancer detection or screening measure has been found to relate positively to health behaviors.
- On the other hand, being knowledgeable and/or having a high level of education is not associated consistently with positive health behaviors.

### Socioeconomic status

- Educational level is sometimes used as an indicator of socioeconomic status (SES).
- People of low SES have been found to be less likely than people of high SES to report symptoms and participate in screening.

### Age

- Age is an important influence on health behavior.
- Age modifies the influence of health beliefs, and confidence in one's ability to carry out a task is influential regardless of age.

### Race

- Differences in cancer incidence, mortality, and survival rates among people of different races have stimulated researchers to examine the health behaviors of these groups.
  - The influence of race, exclusive of SES and educational level, is not evaluated easily.

## Family Factors

- Families in the childbearing years may be more likely than older families to hear health-related messages directly from providers.
- Family ethnicity can be a powerful influence on health behavior.

## Social Factors

- Social support, social roles, and social stigma all influence health behavior of individuals with regard to cancer prevention, detection, and treatment.
- Cultural factors have been found to influence people's decisions both to participate in screening and to delay seeking help for symptoms of cancer.

## Institutional Factors

- Health care delivery systems and health care providers influence people's health behavior.

## IMPLICATIONS FOR NURSING PRACTICE

- Nurses can apply some of the empirically validated concepts and propositions of health behavior by incorporating them into the nursing process.

## PRACTICE QUESTIONS

1. After her father's death from colon cancer, Ellen takes the initiative in preventing colon cancer for herself by eating less fat and more produce and by taking up running. She is engaged in:
   a.  illness behavior.
   b.  sick role behavior.
   c.  health protective behavior.
   d.  information seeking behavior.

2. Henry's persistent cough begins to concern him so he sees his physician to determine what's causing it. Henry is engaged in application of:
   a.  social learning theory.
   b.  illness behavior.
   c.  cancer control behavior.
   d.  environmental influence.

3. The *majority* of health behavior is maintained by:
   a.  immediate consequences.
   b.  delayed consequences.
   c.  anticipated consequences.
   d.  outcome consequences.

**Questions 4–6 look at the case of Karen, who hopes to quit smoking.**

4. Karen knows that cessation of smoking will decrease her cancer risks, but she doubts that she can do it. This demonstrates that the *most* important prerequisite for behavior change that involves an individual's beliefs is:
   a.  reactions of others.
   b.  verbal persuasion.
   c.  outcome expectation.
   d.  efficacy expectation.

5. In trying to help, Karen reach her goal, you keep in mind the fact that the *most* powerful source of efficacy expectations is:
   a.  personal experience.
   b.  what others have experienced.
   c.  verbal persuasion.
   d.  physiologic state.

6. Karen recognizes that she needs some sort of support system while she quits smoking. She lists possible supports in her life. These include "my sister and my mom, my doctor, my friends in the book club, and my two close friends at work." Which will probably be her best support?
   a.  Her work friends.
   b.  Her book club.
   c.  Her mother and sister.
   d.  Her physician.

7. The Health Belief Model attempts to explain health behavior and is guided by:
   a. the assumption that an individual's subjective perception of the environment determines behavior.
   b. the assumption that people expect treatment and care.
   c. the assumption that people change their behaviors in response to familial pressures and familial patterns of disease.
   d. the assumption that people will perform a specific behavior in response to intense education and peer pressure.

8. Predictors of behaviors are determined by three variables. These variables are:
   a. belief in self, perceived susceptibility, and support systems.
   b. support systems, perceived barriers, and perceived benefits.
   c. perceived barriers, perceived benefits, and belief in self.
   d. perceived barriers, perceived susceptibility, and perceived benefits.

9. Marion performs BSEs on a regular basis; Ginny does not. Marion is more likely to have a(n):
   a. external locus of control.
   b. low perceived susceptibility.
   c. high perceived benefits.
   d. internal locus of control.

10. Jeff demonstrates an increased effort and an enhanced participation, even exerting some enthusiasm for his own role in recovery therapy. Applying attribution therapy, one might predict that Jeff is demonstrating the _____ dimension of causal attributions.
    a. controllability
    b. locus of cause
    c. stability
    d. globality

11. Factors that influence health behaviors include knowledge and education level, socioeconomic status, race, and:
    a. residential location.
    b. marital status.
    c. age.
    d. employment status.

## ANSWER EXPLANATIONS

1. **The answer is c.** Health protective behavior consists of actions taken by people in order to protect, promote, or maintain their health. (p. 78)

2. **The answer is b.** Illness behavior is any activity that a person who feels ill undertakes to define the state of her or his health and to discover a suitable remedy. (p. 78)

3. **The answer is c.** Anticipated consequences, rather than immediate consequences, determine most health behaviors. (p. 80)

4. **The answer is d.** Efficacy expectations are the most important prerequisite for behavior change since stronger efficacy expectations produce more active and sustained efforts in the face of adverse conditions. (p. 80)

5.  **The answer is a.** Personal experience is the most powerful and dependable source of efficacy expectations, followed by seeing what others have experienced and accomplished in similar circumstances. (p. 80)

6.  **The answer is c.** Family relationships and support have a positive influence on compliance with medical advice. (p. 84)

7.  **The answer is a.** The Health Belief Model attempts to explain health behavior and is guided by the assumption that an individual's subjective perception of the environment determines behavior. (p. 81)

8.  **The answer is d.** Perceived barriers, perceived susceptibility, and perceived benefits are strong predictors of behavior; perceived barriers are the most powerful single predictor. Perceived severity is the weakest predictor but appears to be strongly related to sick role behaviors. (p. 81)

9.  **The answer is d.** In studies of breast self-examination behavior, women who practiced breast self-examination more frequently were those who perceived an internal locus of control. This locus of control is often seen in combination with beliefs in high susceptibility and benefits. (p. 85)

10. **The answer is a.** Believing in and controlling one's level of effort (controllability) usually results in increased effort or enhanced performance. (p. 85)

11. **The answer is c.** Age has an influence on health behaviors. (pp. 86–88)

# Chapter 6    Dynamics of Cancer Prevention

## DEFINITIONS OF CANCER PREVENTION

- The definition of cancer prevention is evolving.
- Generally, cancer prevention is achieved when modulation or modification of self-care behaviors or exogenous factors results in reduced cancer risk.
- Thus, *primary prevention* is the avoidance of exposure to carcinogens.
- *Secondary prevention* is the prevention of promotion by mechanisms that might inhibit the activation of cancer.
- *Tertiary prevention* consists of arresting, removing, or reversing a premalignant lesion to prevent recurrence or progression to cancer.

## MODERN APPROACHES TO CANCER PREVENTION

- There are three main approaches to achieve primary, secondary, and tertiary prevention: (1) education and knowledge, (2) regulation, and (3) host modification.

### Education and Knowledge

- Education focuses on changing lifestyle behaviors to reduce cancer incidence.
- *Cancer Control Objectives for the Nation: 1985–2000* target four areas of prevention: smoking, diet, sun exposure, counseling. (See Table 6-1, text page 96.)
- Education must persuade people to adopt preventive behaviors. Persuasion depends on the following factors:
  - recipients of the information need to receive it from a source that is credible and is similar and attractive to the recipient
  - the quality, quantity, and timing of messages are critical
  - channels for communicating messages must maximize exposure or coverage of at-risk populations, speed of transmission, cost, and message function; and
  - the characteristics of the receiver (e.g., age, culture, ethnicity, developmental level, gender) must be considered.

### Regulation

- Regulation occurs in the form of legislation (e.g., prohibiting sale of alcohol and tobacco to minors).

### Host Modification

- Host modification is the alteration of the body's internal environment to prevent initiation or progression of cancer by immunization and chemoprevention.

#### Immunization

- Table 6-2, text page 96, lists viral mechanisms involved in cancer development.
- The discovery of cancer-causing viruses in humans shows some promise for cancer prevention in

that similar viruses in animals have been eliminated by vaccines made from the attenuated (inactivated) viruses.

- Clinical trials of cancer vaccines are in various phases of testing.

## Chemoprevention

- Chemoprevention is the use of defined, noncytotoxic nutrients and/or pharmacological agents to inhibit or reverse the process of carcinogenesis.
- Chemopreventive agents enhance the inactivation of carcinogens, modify the expression of oncogenes, or interfere with cell proliferation.

### Chemoprevention and carcinogenesis

- Proto-oncogenes, which code for proteins involved in normal cell growth and differentiation, most likely are involved in initiation and promotion of cancer. The theoretical disruption of carcinogenesis at several points provides the rationale for use of chemopreventive agents.
- Agents that inhibit carcinogenesis generally are classified by the point in the process at which they are effective.

### Biological end points of chemoprevention

- Assessing efficacy of chemoprevention uses *biomarkers*, *genetic markers*, *proliferation markers*, *differentiation markers*, *immunologic markers*, and *micronutrient markers*.
- Table 6-3, text page 99, lists some biomarkers of end points.

## CHALLENGES OF CONDUCTING CANCER PREVENTION TRIALS

## Comparisons of Prevention and Treatment Trials

- Cancer prevention trials commonly involve more collaboration with biology, epidemiology, and behavioral sciences than do treatment trials.
- The specific goals of cancer chemoprevention trials are safety and efficacy.
- Clinical cancer chemoprevention trials have specific phases.
  - Phase I trials develop pharmacokinetic safety and toxicity profiles
  - Phase II trials demonstrate efficacy and develop biomarkers of efficacy.
  - Phase III trials demonstrate modulation of surrogate end points of cancer or demonstrate cancer incidence reduction.

## Design

- Cancer prevention trials usually are randomized, single- or double-blinded studies, generally of a high-risk population.
- Chemoprevention trials usually combine the chemopreventive agent or placebo with corresponding behavioral interventions.

## Recruitment

- Finding people at high risk for a certain cancer is much more difficult than finding people at ordinary risk.
- Criteria for trial eligibility or ineligibility may pose some barriers to recruitment.
- In most chemoprevention trials, participants are randomly assigned to either an intervention (treatment) arm using a chemopreventive agent or a placebo arm. Thus, potential participants need to be well-informed about the short- and long-term toxicities of the chemopreventive agents under study.

### Enrollment

#### Toxicity monitoring

- Early identification of toxicity is critical and entails carefully following the trial protocol and seeing that participants undergo proper testing to evaluate toxicity.

#### Adherence

- Study personnel also monitor and promote short- and long-term adherence to the assigned regimen.
- Some trials build a run-in period into the design to assess likely adherence. If their adherence is unacceptable during the run-in period, the potential participants are not enrolled in the trial.
- Enrolled participants who are assigned to the intervention group and fail to adhere to the regimen are called dropouts, whereas participants in the control group who adopt the intervention are called *drop-ins*.

## CHEMOPREVENTION RESEARCH

- In 1982 the NCI established the Chemoprevention Research Program, which is divided into two broad categories: chemoprevention, and diet and nutrition.

### Chemoprevention Trials

- See Table 6-5, text pages 102 and 103, for a summary of trials.

#### Breast Cancer Prevention Trial

- This randomized, double-blind trial is testing the ability of tamoxifen to prevent breast cancer in healthy women at high risk.

#### Prostate Cancer Prevention Trial

- Initiated in 1993, the PCPT is a double-blind, randomized, intergroup trial testing the ability of finasteride to prevent prostate cancer in healthy men aged 55 and older.

### Diet and Nutrition Research

- The NCI is sponsoring several studies targeting diet and nutrition in cancer prevention.

## CANCER PREVENTION CONTROVERSIES AND DILEMMAS

### Incomplete Knowledge

- Interventions aimed at reducing risks often are implemented before the relationship among the factors is known.
- Lack of evidence from randomized, controlled trials for an intervention's efficacy should not prevent us from recommending the intervention if other evidence is compelling.

### Overselling Prevention

- Prevention campaigns should be evaluated for their ability to determine the potential and practical consequences of prevention strategies, including social, legal, and ethical factors.

### Attribution of Responsibility

- Participants in prevention and screening campaigns need to be reminded that observance of guidelines does not guarantee a cancer-free existence, particularly when guidelines are based on incomplete knowledge.

## CANCER PREVENTION AND CHANGES IN HEALTH CARE

- For cancer prevention to be successful, the health care community and policy makers need first to change the existing treatment-oriented model to one that is prevention-oriented.
- Historically in the United States, cancer prevention services have not been reimbursed by payers at all levels.
- The growth of managed care and capitation and the increasing use of primary health care providers as gatekeepers are driving the coverage of preventive services.

## IMPLICATIONS FOR NURSING

- Nurses must strive to keep pace with the science of cancer prevention.
- To understand and participate in these advances in cancer prevention, nursing education, clinical practice, and research will need to have a stronger foundation in genetics, carcinogenesis, bioethics, behavioral change strategies, health policy, and environmental health.
- Given the opportunity, nurses can be instrumental in developing cancer prevention standards of care along with developing, supporting, and steering health policies related to cancer prevention.

## PRACTICE QUESTIONS

**Questions 1–3 follow the research work of Jan, a member of a research team focusing on smoking cessation.**

1. A Baltimore study group focuses on smoking cessation among a specific target population. This group's research is focusing on _____ prevention.
   a. primary
   b. secondary
   c. tertiary
   d. integrated

2. Jan, a member of the Baltimore research team discussed in question 1, wants to correlate the group's findings with related objectives from the DCPC's *Cancer Control Objectives for the Nation: 1985–2000*. Which is not a target area of prevention addressed by the DCPC?
   a. Smoking
   b. Exercise
   c. Counseling
   d. Sun exposure

3. One aspect of Jan's research includes the study of precancerous lesions, which can serve as:
   a. proliferation markers.
   b. differentiation markers.
   c. tissue markers.
   d. biologic markers.

4. One encouraging aspect of research into tumor-associated viruses is the discovery of:
   a. their direct tumor causation.
   b. their promise for prevention through development of vaccines from animal forms of the viruses.
   c. their promise for prevention through inactivation.
   d. similar viruses in animals that have been eliminated by vaccines made from attenuated viruses.

5. Which of the following is *not* true of carcinogenesis and chemoprevention?
   a. Chemoprevention is the most promising form of host modification, using nutrients or pharmacological agents to inhibit or reverse carcinogenesis.
   b. Proto-oncogenes are most likely involved in initiation and promotion of cancer.
   c. Chemoprevention has the potential for both secondary and tertiary prevention, but by definition, it cannot be useful in primary prevention.
   d. Agents that inhibit carcinogenesis generally are classified by the point in the process at which they are effective.

6. Trent is involved in analysis of differentiation markers, which include:
   a. Ki 67 antigen.
   b. ornithine decarboxylase.
   c. DNA adducts.
   d. cytokeratins.

7. Rachel is involved in a study that demonstrates cancer incidence reduction. This study is most likely a:
   a. cancer treatment trial.
   b. Phase I trial.
   c. Phase II trial.
   d. Phase III trial.

8.  The Breast Cancer Prevention Trial (BCPT), which will be completed in the year 2002, tests the ability of _____ to prevent breast cancer in healthy women at high risk for the disease.
    a.  sulindac
    b.  retinoic acid
    c.  tamoxifen
    d.  beta-carotene

9.  The Prostate Cancer Prevention Trial tests the ability of _____ to prevent prostate cancer in healthy men.
    a.  finasteride
    b.  DFMO
    c.  beta-carotene
    d.  retonoic acid

10.  The growth of managed care and capitation have contributed to:
    a.  a dramatic drop in coverage of prevention-oriented services.
    b.  driving the coverage of preventive services.
    c.  reducing funding for immunologic studies.
    d.  fewer eldercare provisions.

# ANSWER EXPLANATIONS

1.  **The answer is b.** Primary prevention is the avoidance of exposure to carcinogens; secondary prevention is the prevention of promotion by smoking cessation, changes in diet, and administration of chemopreventive agents presumed to act on promotion. Tertiary prevention consists of arresting, removing, or reversing a premalignant lesion to prevent recurrence or progression to cancer. (p. 95)

2.  **The answer is b.** The four areas of prevention targeted by the DCPC's Cancer Control Objectives for the Nation: 1985–2000 include smoking, diet, sun exposure, and counseling. (pp. 95–96)

3.  **The answer is a.** As proliferation markers, precancerous lesions can show regression to a lower degree of precancer, progression to a higher degree, and the status of surrounding unaffected tissue and its relation to the precancer (field cancerization effect). (pp. 98 and 99)

4.  **The answer is d.** Tumor-associated viruses probably are necessary but not sufficient for tumor causation. The discovery of cancer-causing viruses in humans shows some promise for cancer prevention in that similar viruses in animals have been eliminated by vaccines made from the attenuated (inactivated) viruses. (p. 97)

5.  **The answer is c.** Chemoprevention is the most promising form of host modification, using nutrients or pharmacological agents to inhibit or reverse carcinogenesis. Proto-oncogenes are most likely involved in initiation and promotion of cancer. The theoretical disruption of carcinogenesis at several points provides the rationale for use of chemopreventive agents. Agents that inhibit carcinogenesis generally are classified by the point in the process at which they are effective. Chemoprevention has the potential for primary, secondary and tertiary prevention. (p. 98)

6.  **The answer is d.** Differentiation markers include growth factors and epithelial markers such as cytokeratins, involucrin, and certain blood-related antigens of epithelial cells. (p. 99)

7. **The answer is d.** Phase III cancer prevention trials demonstrate modulation of surrogate end points of cancer or demonstrate cancer incidence reduction. Phase I trials develop pharmacokinetic safety and toxicity profiles on potential chemopreventive agents. Phase II trials demonstrate efficacy and develop biomarkers of efficacy. Cancer treatment trials do not deal with prevention or incidence reduction. (p. 99)

8. **The answer is c.** The BCPT is testing tamoxifen as a chemopreventive agent in a randomized, double-bind trial. (p. 101)

9. **The answer is a.** Initiated in 1993, the PCPT is a double-blind, randomized, intergroup trial testing the ability of finasteride to prevent prostate cancer in healthy men aged 55 and older. (p. 103)

10. **The answer is b.** Historically in the United States, cancer prevention services have not been reimbursed by payers at all levels. The growth of managed care and capitation and the increasing use of primary health care providers as gatekeepers are driving the coverage of preventive services. Quality-control efforts by health plans carefully monitor whether patients received necessary preventive services. However, funding for preventive services remains inadequate, even in prepaid health systems. (p. 105)

# Chapter 7    Cancer Risk and Assessment

## INTRODUCTION

- Risk models are successful in differentiating high-, medium-, and low-risk individuals and in estimating relative risk, but are much less successful in estimating absolute risk in individuals or across populations.
- Health risk assessment (HRA) has a number of very desirable qualities for clinicians and health educators: preventive orientation, systematic approach, ability to emphasize modifiable factors, and a scientific knowledge base. However, a major concern is the value of quantitative estimates of absolute risk.

## DEFINITIONS OF RISK

- *Risk* is the potential realization of unwanted consequences of an event. Both a probability of occurrence of an event and the magnitude of its consequences are involved.
- Decisions made about whether to bear the risks or to minimize them by reducing their source or taking protective actions are often referred to as *risk evaluation*.
- *Relative risk* is a ratio that compares the rate of the disease among exposed persons with the rate of the disease among unexposed persons.
- The *attributable risk* is the difference in the disease rates between the group exposed to the factor and unexposed groups.

## CANCER RISK FACTORS

- Cancer prevention strategies can be divided into two major areas: (1) identification of the contributors to the cause(s) of cancer, and (2) the action taken in response to this knowledge.
- Cancer risk factors are categorized as those that are under a person's control and those outside a person's control. Risk factors have also been divided according to whether they are unique to an individual or shared by a group of persons.
- The two biggest challenges for the cancer research establishment are (1) the implementation of interventions to prevent cancers from known or proven causes, and (2) the verification of highly suspected causes of major types of cancer.
- See text page 110, column 1 for the categories of risk factors responsible for 70% to 90% of cancers.

## CANCER RISK FACTORS IN MINORITY POPULATIONS
### Racial/Multifactorial Aspects

- There are differences in cancer incidence and mortality rates among ethnic and cultural groups. See Table 7-1, text page 111 for list of high-incidence cancers for specific ethnic groups.

### Socioeconomic/Educational Factors

- Poor Americans, regardless of race, are at a disproportionate risk of dying of cancer.
- Several factors contribute to the increased mortality and morbidity from cancer among the poor. These factors include the following:
  - inadequate education
  - lack of employment

- substandard housing
- lack of access to medical care
- chronic malnutrition
- fatalistic attitudes about cancer
- obstacles in obtaining and using health insurance
- personal sacrifices needed to obtain and pay for health care
- insensitive cancer education and outreach efforts

## Ethnic/Cultural Factors

- Cancer screening and prevention methods must be ethnically and culturally based.

## Gender Differences

- Six cancers account for almost 70% of cases in women and more than 60% of deaths, namely, breast, lung, colorectal, cervix uteri, corpus uteri, and ovarian cancers.

## RISK FACTORS FOR SPECIFIC CANCERS

- It appears that the actual risk from a single factor depends on (1) the number and intensity of other coexisting factors in a given individual, and (2) the intensity of the factor itself.
- Risk factors for specific cancers are summarized in Table 7-2, text pages 113–115.

## Bladder Cancer

- The strongest risk factors for bladder cancer involve occupational exposures and lifestyle practices. In some cohorts of chemical workers exposed to aromatic amines, more than 80% have died of bladder cancer.
- Cigarette smoking is the most important known risk factor for bladder cancer.
- As many as 60% of bladder cancers result from smoking.
- There is conflicting information concerning the role of coffee drinking and the use of artificial sweeteners and the risk of bladder cancer.

## Breast Cancer

- The primary risk factors for breast cancer are increasing age, family history of breast cancer, history of benign breast disease, late age at first live birth, nulliparity, early age at menarche, late age at menopause, higher socioeconomic status, being Jewish, estrogen replacement therapy, exposure of the female breast to ionizing radiation in infancy, mammographic parenchymal patterns that are dense, having complex fibroadenomas, and being single.
- All women 35 or older should be treated as being at-risk for breast cancer.
- A strong family history of breast cancer is generally defined as having four or more genetically related women affected with the disease; about 40% of their cancers are caused by an inherited mutation in the gene *BRCA1* and another 40% by *BRCA2*.

## Cervical Cancer

- Race, personal factors, and venereal disease are the major risk factors associated with cervical cancer. Personal risk factors include early age at first coitus, multiple marriages or sexual partners, and use of nonbarrier contraceptives.
- A smoker's risk of developing cervical cancer is four times greater than that of nonsmokers.

## Colorectal Cancer

- High rates of colorectal cancer are found in highly developed countries, and low rates are found in Asia, Africa, and most countries of Latin America.
- The risk factors for colorectal cancer include obesity, high fat intake, diet low in fiber and fruits and vegetables containing vitamins A and C, a sedentary lifestyle, age, familial and hereditary factors, adenomatous polyps, and ulcerative colitis.

## Liver Cancer

- The risk factors for hepatocellular carcinoma (HCC) include hepatitis B virus, cirrhosis, hepatitis C virus, being a man between the third and fifth decades of life, and the chemical vinyl chloride. "Chronic hepatitis B virus infection is probably the leading cause of HCC throughout the world, accounting for 75%–90% of the world's cases."

## Lung Cancer

- The major risk factors for lung cancer are cigarette smoking, occupation, air pollution, environmental tobacco smoke, and radon exposure. Cigarette smoking in the United States contributes to the majority of lung cancers. Studies have also found an elevated risk of lung cancer as well as heart disease among individuals who have never smoked but are living with a spouse who smokes cigarettes.
- Radon exposure may be responsible for about 10,000 lung cancer deaths per year, while smoking accounts for 85% of the lung cancer deaths annually.
- High-risk occupations are those in which persons work with asbestos, polycyclic hydrocarbons, chromium, mustard gas, chloromethyl ethers, radon, nickel, and inorganic arsenic.

## Oral Cancer

- Tobacco is a major risk factor for oral cancer. The habitual smoking of cigarettes, cigars, and pipes and the use of chewing tobacco or snuff have long been associated with oral cancer.
- Other significant risk factors for oral cancer are excessive alcohol intake, nutritional deficiencies, and poor dentition.
- Occupations related to long-term exposure to the sun have been associated with cancer of the lip.

## Ovarian Cancer

- Ovarian cancer tends to be more common among white upper-income groups in highly industrialized countries.
- The risk of ovarian cancer is associated with delayed age at first pregnancy, a smaller number of pregnancies, or the absence of childbearing.
- Oral contraceptive use might protect against ovarian cancer.

## Endometrial (Uterine Corpus) Cancer

- Estrogen, history of menstrual irregularities and infertility, obesity, high socioeconomic status, hypertension, and diabetes mellitus have been correlated with the development of endometrial cancer.
- Long-term use of conjugated estrogens as hormone replacement therapy (HRT) may reduce the risk of coronary heart disease and fractures but greatly increase the risk of endometrial cancer.
- The use of oral contraceptives (containing both estrogen and progesterone in each pill) for at least one year has a protective effect against endometrial cancer.

## Prostate Cancer

- Age and race are significant risk factors for prostate cancer. Black Americans have the highest prostate cancer incidence rate in the United States, and Japanese American men have the lowest incidence rate.
- Prostate cancer affects the elderly more than the young to a greater extent than any other cancer. 80% of cases are found in men over 65.
- A high-fat diet may increase the risk of clinically significant prostate cancer.

## Skin Cancer

- The chief risk factor for the development of basal cell and squamous cell carcinomas of the skin is exposure to ultraviolet radiation (UVR).
- Melanoma is also related to UVR, but there are several other influential risk factors: familial predisposition, hormonal factors, dysplastic nevus syndrome, and nearness to the equator.
- Overall, those at greatest risk of skin cancer are fair-skinned white persons, particularly those with reddish or blond hair and blue or light eyes, those with a tendency to freckle or burn easily, and individuals who have spent considerable time in the sun.

## Testicular Cancer

- A significant risk factor for testicular cancer involves race and age. This cancer occurs about 4.5 times more frequently in whites than in blacks and in men between the ages of 20 and 40 years and again in late adulthood over age 60.
- Another significant risk factor is undescended testicles, especially in men who have a testicle that descended after the age of 6 or a testicle that never descended (cryptorchidism).

## Vaginal Cancer

- A risk factor for vaginal cancer is the use of diethylstilbestrol (DES) by the mother during pregnancy.

## CANCER RISK ASSESSMENT

- The purposes of a cancer risk assessment include:
  - providing an individual with information about his or her health-related behavior that may increase cancer risk;
  - serving as an effective aid for educating patients about the relationship between risk factors and the likelihood of cancer; and
  - stimulating a person to participate in activities aimed at changing lifestyle and improving health.
- Before information is provided about an individual's specific risks, however, it is important that there be an understanding of the risk to an average person in the population. One of the problems that exists in assessment of cancer risks is that some persons are unwilling to seriously consider what their risks might be.
- According to the American Cancer Society, *risk assessment* is a two-step process: The first step, *hazard identification*, evaluates the chemical or physical nature of hazards and their oncogenicity. The second step, exposure measurement, determines the levels of hazards in the environment and the extent to which people are actually exposed.
- A comprehensive risk analysis should include (1) the identification of risks and the estimation of the likelihood and magnitude of risk occurring, and (2) an evaluation that measures *risk acceptance* and *risk management*.
- Risk assessment not only is a part of cancer prevention but also must be included in detection procedures.
- See Table 7-4, text pages 121–126 for a list of health risk assessment instruments.

### Evaluation

- The history is helpful in identifying signs and symptoms.
- In addition, the history helps to identify factors, such as a family history of genetic susceptibility, that may increase an individual's risk of specific cancers.
- For individuals identified as having a high risk of cancer, advice should be given about avoiding additional exposure to carcinogens, and rigorous intervention may be indicated.

## EDUCATION

- The aims of public education are to inform and educate about treatable forms of cancer; and to persuade people to undertake preventive action, to undergo early detection tests, or to seek medical advice quickly.
- Topics that should be covered in educational programs include tobacco, alcohol, occupations and cancer, environmental pollutants, sexual activity, radiation, infective and genetic factors, and diet.
- See Table 7-5, text page 128, for the recommended schedule of prevention and detection procedures for the general population, as suggested by the American Cancer Society.

## CONCLUSION

- More than 80% of the causes of cancer are avoidable.
- Increased knowledge about cancer risk factors and how they affect the body are necessary.

## PRACTICE QUESTIONS

1. In general, health risk assessment models are *most* effective in estimating what type of risk?
   a. relative risk
   b. quantitative risk
   c. empirical risk
   d. absolute risk

2. Dorothy, a colleague, is teaching a class of student nurses about cancer risk assessment. She defines risk as "the probability of occurrence of an event." What other component of risk is she leaving out?
   a. consequences if the event does not occur.
   b. magnitude of the event itself.
   c. protective reactions to the event.
   d. magnitude of the consequences of the event.

3. Four patients arrive at a clinic for cancer risk assessment. The most significant risk factor for each patient is listed below. Based on this information you determine that one risk factor is both specific to the individual and yet outside of the individual's control. This patient's risk factor is:
   a. cigarette smoking.
   b. exposure to asbestos.
   c. air pollution.
   d. familial polyposis.

4. Mr. Frank's cancer has been associated with occupational exposure to a carcinogen. Of these choices, which type of cancer is he most likely to have, based on this small clue?
   a. bladder cancer.
   b. colorectal cancer.
   c. testicular cancer.
   d. cervical cancer.

5. The leading cause of liver cancer throughout the world is:
   a. chronic hepatitis B virus.
   b. chronic hepatitis C virus.
   c. chronic cirrhosis.
   d. chronic hepatitis A virus.

6. Ms. Ellis tells you that her adult daughter is pressuring her to give up sun tanning. "I've had a good tan for over twenty years," she says. "I like it. Is my daughter being a little hysterical?" You explain that long-term exposure to the sun has been associated with skin cancer and also with:
   a. colorectal cancer.
   b. breast cancer.
   c. cancer of the lip.
   d. uterine cancer.

7. Primary risk factors for breast cancer include:
   a. being in the 30- to 45-year age group.
   b. late age at first live birth.
   c. two or more heterosexual relationship.
   d. lower socioeconomic status.

8. Risk factors for colorectal cancer include:
   a. obesity.
   b. high level of exercise.
   c. African-American heritage.
   d. infection with hepatitis B virus.

9. Erika is concerned about the number of years she used birth control pills. Although these are associated with some degree of cancer risk, you are able to tell her that the long-term use of oral contraceptives containing both estrogen and progesterone in each pill has been found to offer protection against:
   a. vaginal cancer.
   b. colorectal cancer.
   c. breast cancer.
   d. endometrial cancer.

10. Ms. Ellis asks, "What is the purpose of a cancer risk assessment?" Your answer will be influenced by the fact that each of the following is one of the primary purposes of cancer risk assessment *except*:
   a. identifying the distribution and determinants of diseases and health problems in human populations.
   b. providing individuals with information about their health-related behaviors that may increase cancer risk.
   c. educating patients about the relationship between risk factors and the likelihood of cancer.
   d. stimulating individuals to participate in activities aimed at changing lifestyle and improving health.

11. If Ms. Ellis is identified as having a high risk of cancer, one of the outcomes of the evaluation stage of her cancer risk assessment may be rigorous intervention involving a surgical procedure that reduces the risk of a cancer developing. Another outcome may be:
   a. generating a health history that provides subjective data on her health.
   b. screening her more frequently and in greater detail than in low-risk patients.
   c. asking her to undergo a thorough physical examination that provides objective data on her health.
   d. educating her about the relationship between risk factors and quality of life.

## ANSWER EXPLANATIONS

1. **The answer is a.** Risk models have been successful in distinguishing low-, medium-, and high-risk persons and in estimating relative risk but are much less successful in estimating absolute risk in individuals or across populations. Despite the value of a health risk assessment (HRA) in "prospective health assessment," a major concern with HRA is the value of quantitative estimates of absolute risk. The text suggests that more qualitative measures may have more valuable purposes in risk assessment. (p. 109)

2. **The answer is d.** Risk is the potential realization of unwanted consequences of an event, and it involves both a probability of occurrence of an event (e.g., what are the chances of getting cancer) and the magnitude of its consequences (e.g., how life-threatening is it likely to be). (p. 109)

3. **The answer is d.** Choice **a** is individual but under the person's control; choice **b** is typically a group risk factor shared by persons from the same occupation; choice **c** is typically a group risk factor shared by persons from the same geographic residence. Only choice **d**, an inherited condition, is

both specific to the individual and, at the same time, outside the person's control. (p. 110)

4.   **The answer is a.** One of the strongest risk factors for bladder cancer involves occupational exposure to 2-naphthylamine, benzidine, and aniline dyes. Workers exposed to aromatic amines have a fourfold greater risk of bladder cancer. (p. 113)

5.   **The answer is a.** Chronic hepatitis B virus infection is the leading cause of hepatocellular carcinoma throughout the world. (p. 114)

6.   **The answer is c.** Long-term exposure to the sun has been associated with cancer of the lip, an oral cancer. (p. 114)

7.   **The answer is b.** The primary risk factors for breast cancer are increasing age, family history of breast cancer, history of benign breast disease, late age at first live birth, nulliparity, early age at menarche, late age at menopause, higher socioeconomic status, being Jewish, estrogen replacement therapy, exposure of the female breast to ionizing radiation in infancy, mammographic parenchymal patterns that are dense, having complex fibroadenomas, and being single. (p. 115)

8.   **The answer is a.** Obesity, sedentary lifestyle, high fat intake, low fiber intake, and a dearth of fruits and vegetables containing vitamins A and C have been identified as risk factors for colorectal cancer (Table 7-2, p. 114)

9.   **The answer is d.** The long-term use of combination oral contraceptives has been found to offer some protection against both ovarian and endometrial cancer. Long-term use of conjugated estrogens, on the other hand, is an iatrogenic risk factor for endometrial cancer. (p. 118)

10.   **The answer is a.** Choice **a** is the definition of epidemiology, a study related to but distinct from cancer risk assessment. Categorizing risk factors is an important preliminary step in risk assessment. From this data base of risk factors an individual's cancer risk profile can be developed and specific interventions for risk reduction can be planned. Choices **b** through **d**, however, are the primary objectives of cancer risk assessment. (p. 120)

11.   **The answer is b.** The patient will also be given advice about avoiding additional exposure to carcinogens, even when surgical intervention or more frequent screening are not called for. Note that choices **c** and **d** are the initial stages of the evaluation process. It is on the basis of data generated by the health history and physical examination that recommendations are made. (p. 127)

# Chapter 8    Assessment and Interventions for Cancer Detection

## INTRODUCTION

- Cancer was among the first chronic diseases recognized as potentially "controllable" and amenable to public health strategies.

### Can We Prevent Cancer?

- It is apparent that the best treatment of cancer is its prevention.
- Screening holds the greatest promise for a major impact on reducing mortality and is an important prevention strategy. Screening is defined as looking for disease in asymptomatic populations while early detection is looking for disease in asymptomatic and symptomatic patients (case finding).
- In order for early detection to be useful, there must be a test or procedure that will detect cancers earlier, and there must be evidence that earlier treatment will result in an improved outcome.
- Of screening measures, the greatest benefit includes improved prognoses for some patients whose disease is detected by screening.
- Several disadvantages to screening exist. Earlier detection can create a longer period of morbidity for patients whose prognosis is unaltered.
- Several obstacles exist that may prevent screening from making a major contribution to cancer control: (1) an unfavorable natural history of some cancers, (2) poor organization of screening programs, and (3) poor compliance of those at risk.

## DETECTION OF MAJOR CANCER SITES

- Physical assessment techniques enable the nurse to assume an active role in the early detection of cancer.

### Lung Cancer

- Of all the known risk factors the most important environmental carcinogen related to the increased incidence of lung cancer is cigarette smoking.
- Cigarette smoking is the largest single preventable cause of premature death and disability and the major single cause of cancer mortality.

#### History assessment

- Smoking habits, including marijuana use
- Occupational history, including shipyard work and exposure to asbestos. Certain occupations require special scrutiny because of possible exposure of workers to suspected carcinogens (e.g., clothing and textiles).
- The general respiratory environment of both the workplace and home, including exposure to a smoke environment
- See Figure 8-1, text page 137, for a systematic approach to the occupational and environmental health history.
- See text pages 137–139 for questions that should be included in the history.

- The first symptoms are usually not alarming and can easily be overlooked or attributed to other causes.
  - The most common symptom is a cough that is productive and often associated with hemoptysis and chest pain. A nonproductive cough may indicate a cancer that is centrally located or that involves the main carina only.
  - Later symptoms include a combination of coughing, wheezing, pleuritic pain, hoarseness, local nerve disorders, edema of head, neck, or arms, dysphagia, and persistent pneumonitis.

## Physical examination

- See Figure 8-5, text page 141, for a synopsis of physical findings commonly seen with tumors of different anatomic sites in the lungs.
- The only early physical finding is wheezing localized to a single lobe of the lung in an elderly person with a long history of smoking.
- Later findings may include finger clubbing (Figure 8-2, text page 139), barrel chest (associated with emphysema), abnormal breathing, bulges of the thorax, breathlessness, and superior vena cava obstruction.
- Palpation of the thorax includes testing for vocal fremitus, respiratory excursion, and compression, and compression and determining the position and moveability of the trachea. Symptoms to look for include:
  - A deviated or fixed trachea
  - Decreased or absent vocal fremitus
- Percussion and auscultation may provide final clues to assessment of the individual who is at high risk for lung cancer. Physical signs to look for include:
  - Dullness, indicating pleural effusion (text page 140, Figure 8-4)
  - Decreased or absent breath sounds
  - Unilateral wheezing and the bagpipe sign
  - Presence of whispered pectoriloquy, bronchophony, and egophony

## Screening tests for asymptomatic individuals

- No screening programs or tests for lung cancer have been shown to reduce mortality significantly.

## Screening tests for asymptomatic individuals

- Studies show no evidence of a significant reduction in mortality from these programs.

## Smoking cessation

- Educational level is the major demographic predictor of both smoking and cessation of smoking.

### The role of the nurse

- Monitor most aggressively those who smoke, who have had a history of heavy smoking, or who were employed in high-risk occupations. These individuals should undergo a complete respiratory assessment.
- Assist smokers in their efforts to stop smoking. See Table 8-1, text page 142, for a list of specific steps the nurse should follow.
- Remind smokers that smoking cessation results in improved sensory, respiratory, and cardiovascular status. The effects of smoking are partially reversible.
- Remain nonjudgmental in dealing with those who refuse or are unable to stop smoking. Nicotine is addictive, and the smoker may need repeated attempts before he or she is successful.
- Disseminate information on the disease potential of smoking whenever possible.
- Serve as a positive role model by not smoking.

- Take advantage of opportunities to advise smokers to quit both in health care settings and in the community.
- Work with physicians and others on a team approach to delivering individualized advice on multiple occasions and using multiple smoking cessation interventions.
- See Tables 8-1 and 8-2 (text pages 142 and 143) for guidelines to be used by physicians and nonphysicians to improve smoking cessation rates in patients.
- Multiple smoking cessation interventions include the following:
    1. direct, face-to-face advice
    2. self-help materials
    3. referral to community smoking cessation programs
    4. drug therapy when appropriate (nicotine gum, nicotine patch)
    5. scheduled reinforcement
- Antismoking policies appear to have a dramatic effect on the nation's smoking habits by increasing the social pressure against it and by restricting the time available for it.

## Gastrointestinal Cancer

- Colorectal cancer incidence and mortality in the United States are second only to those for lung cancer.

### History assessment

- Several conditions and health practices cause symptoms that mimic gastrointestinal cancer.
- The signs and symptoms of cancers of the colon and rectum often are related to the portion of intestine involved.
- Signs to look for are rectal bleeding, anorexia, constipation, weight loss.

### Physical examination

Inspection

- Findings that may suggest cancer of the gastrointestinal system include the following:
    - Nodular umbilicus
    - Masses that distort the abdominal profile and indicate organomegaly
    - Subcutaneous nodules visible with tangential lighting
    - Distention
    - Venous distention (edema of the eyelids, a bluish face and lips, prominent neck veins, and pitting edema of the arms and large veins over the upper portions of the chest and shoulders)
    - Visible peristaltic waves
    - Bulging of the flanks may signal intraabdominal fluid

Auscultation

- Bowel sounds heard with the stethoscope bell range from absent to frequent. Significant types of bowel sounds include the following:
    - High-pitched, long, intense peristaltic rushes
    - High-pitched "tingling" sounds
    - Extremely weak or infrequent sounds
    - Absent bowel sounds
- Succussion splash is produced by a combination of air and fluid in the gut.
- Some abdominal circulatory sounds also signal cancer.
- Auscultation of the abdomen may indicate a bowel obstruction, a hepatoma, or pancreatic carcinoma.

## Palpation and percussion

- The following findings on palpation and percussion merit further attention, and may signal colorectal cancer:
  - Hepatomegaly (enlarged liver)
  - Splenomegaly (enlarged spleen)
  - Enlargement of the colon
  - Fluid
- The presence of intraperitoneal fluid is suspected when there is abdominal distention with bulging flanks and possibly an everted umbilicus.

## Rectal examination

- Half the cancers that occur in the rectum and colon are within reach of the examining finger.
- On palpation the examiner may feel a rectal shelf. The shelf indicates a carcinoma that has metastasized to the pelvic floor.
- Several physical findings in other parts of the body, which are not revealed in the abdominal examination, are typical in abdominal carcinoma.
  - For instance, enlargement of a single node called Virchow's node, is frequently behind the clavicular head of the left supraclavicular group. The Valsalva maneuver causes the node to rise.
  - Another physical finding associated with abdominal carcinoma is *acanthosis nigricans*, a skin lesion. It is a velvety, brownish skin eruption that strongly suggests an intestinal malignancy when it occurs in patients older than 40 years of age.
  - Jaundice and accompanying steady pain may indicate hepatic or pancreatic lesions.
- Findings that most strongly suggest cancer of the colorectal area are (1) a mass palpated in the rectum, (2) a palpable mass in the abdomen, and (3) evidence of blood in the feces.

## Screening tests for asymptomatic individuals

- The two most important screening tests for asymptomatic individuals are examination of the feces for occult blood and the digital rectal examination.
- The American Cancer Society, the National Cancer Institute, and the American College of Surgeons recommend that asymptomatic individuals have a sigmoidoscopic (preferably flexible) examination every three to five years in conjunction with an annual fecal occult blood test beginning at age 50.
- The American Cancer Society further advocates an annual digital rectal examination starting at age 40.
- The role of fecal occult blood tests in the early detection of colorectal cancer is still being evaluated.
- The carcinoembryonic antigen (CEA) assay is not conclusive in the diagnosing of colorectal cancer.
- See Figure 8-8, text page 148, for a diagnostic guide for asymptomatic patients.

## Additional nursing interventions

- As educators, nurses can play an important role in colorectal cancer detection by (1) informing the general public, as well as high risk groups, and (2) encouraging the participation of the general public and high-risk groups in early detection of the disease through the use of a stool guaiac slide test, digital rectal examination, and, after 50 years of age, proctosigmoidoscopic examination.
- The nurse should promote the following dietary recommendations of the American Cancer Society and the National Cancer Institute to lower overall cancer risk including colorectal cancer:

- Avoid obesity.
- Decrease total fat intake to 30% of total calories.
- Consume more high-fiber foods, such as whole grain cereals, fruits, and vegetables.
- Include foods rich in vitamins A and C in the daily diet.
- Be moderate in the consumption of alcoholic beverages.
- Be moderate in the consumption of salt-cured, smoked, and nitrite-cured foods.
- Include cruciferous vegetables in the diet.

## Prostate Cancer

- Prostate cancer is currently the second most common cancer in American men.
- Prostate cancer increases in incidence with age more rapidly than any other cancer.

### History assessment

- Most symptoms are related to late complications of stage III or IV prostate cancer.
- The most frequent initial symptoms of prostate cancer are frequency of urination, difficult or painful urination, pain, complete urinary retention, and hematuria.
- See text page 150, column 1, for a list of assessment questions.

### Physical examination

- An early diagnosis of prostate cancer can be done only by rectal palpation of the prostate.
- The normal prostate on palpation is usually rounded, about 4 cm in diameter, and firm.
- Cancer of the prostate typically appears as a stony-hard nodule, whereas benign prostatic hypertrophy usually results in a diffuse enlargement of the prostate without masses.
- It is common to find in older men a diffusely enlarged prostate gland without masses (benign prostatic hypertrophy).

### Screening tests for asymptomatic individuals

- The American Cancer Society and the American Urological Association recommend that men older than 50 years be tested annually using digital rectal examination and PSA.
- PSA is a tumor marker that the Food and Drug Administration in 1994 approved for use with digital rectal examination for early detection of prostate cancer.
- All men older than 40 years of age, especially African-American men, should be informed of the importance of and rationale for yearly or biannual rectal examinations. Men with strong family histories of prostate cancer should be urged to request and expect rectal examinations and a PSA blood test at their annual physical.

## Breast Cancer

- Breast cancer is the most common cancer in women in the western world. It is the leading cause of cancer deaths in American women aged 40 to 55 and the second cause of cancer deaths in women older than 55 years of age.
- The most common presenting complaint of women with breast cancer is a painless lump or mass in the breast. About 90% of all palpable breast tumors are discovered by women themselves.

### History assessment

- See text page 153 for a list of questions to ask.

## Physical examination

- Breasts should be examined from several positions. See Figure 8-11, text page 153.

### Inspection

- The physical examination begins with inspection of the breast with the woman sitting relaxed with arms at sides, then sitting with arms at sides pressed against body, hands on waist pressed against body, and then sitting with arms overhead.
  - Visible signs of cancer of the breast include the following:
  - Dimpling of the breast
  - Unilateral flattening of the nipple
  - Abnormal contours or flattening
  - Peau d'orange
  - Increased venous prominence
  - Scaling or eczematoid lesions
- The initial inspection must include all positions, including having the woman lean forward to observe abnormal contours; omitting a position may cause the nurse to miss important pathological findings.

### Palpation

- Palpation for thickening is done very lightly and slowly toward the nipple. First palpate the normal breast.
- Cancer occurs as a hard, poorly circumscribed nodule, fixed to the skin or underlying tissue.
- A malignant tumor that may be attached to the deep fascia will limit the mobility of the breast on the chest wall.
- The breasts need to be thoroughly palpated while the woman is supine with her arms above her head.
- Any mass that is felt should be charted.
- The nipple should be gently compressed in all directions for the presence of discharge.
- Because carcinoma of the breast may metastasize to regional lymph nodes, a careful palpation of the axillae and the supraclavicular regions is necessary.
- The physiological changes that normally occur with aging may simulate cancer of the breast.
- In conclusion, the physical signs that most strongly suggest cancer of the breast are dimpling, peau d'orange, abnormal contours of the breast, flattening of the nipple, palpable hard, poorly circumscribed nodules that are fixed to the skin or underlying tissue, and palpable hard, fixed nodes in the axillae or supraclavicular region.

## Screening tests for asymptomatic individuals

- Three methods used in screening for breast cancer are physical examination of the breast by the health professional, teaching the woman BSE, and mammography.
- The American Cancer Society's revised recommendations for screening for breast cancer are as follows:
  - All women from age 20 years should perform BSE monthly.
  - Women 20–40 years of age should have a breast physical examination every three years, and women older than 40 years should have a breast physical examination every year.
  - Screening mammography should begin by age 40; women 40–49 years of age should have a mammogram every one to two years; and women older than 50 years of age should have a mammogram every year.

Breast self-examination

- The importance of BSE is based on the fact that approximately 95% of breast cancers are self-discovered either accidentally or through planned examination.
- Because approximately 10% of cancers termed interim cancers will become apparent within a year of an examination with negative results, reliance has been placed on BSE to find these lesions.
- Self-instruction includes teaching a woman to do BSE by using her own hand on her breast under the direct guidance of a professional.

## Testicular Cancer

- Although testicular cancer is relatively rare, it is the most common solid tumor in young men between 20 and 34 years of age.

### History assessment

- The most common presenting complaint is a painless enlargement of the testis. Nodules are typically small, hard, and usually painless.
- See text page 157 for a list of questions to ask.

### Physical examination

- Cancer of the testes may be manifested by asymmetry of the scrotum. Another clue is scrotal skin that appears stretched and thin over the tumor.
- Diffuse induration of the testis in the absence of discrete nodularity may be the initial abnormality.
- The most common sites for tumors are on the testicular anterior and lateral surfaces.
- Transillumination is helpful in distinguishing cystic from solid masses.
- Hydroceles may develop as a result of a tumor.

### Education: testicular self-examination (TSE)

- Nurses who work in the military in occupational health settings, in physicians' offices, and in educational settings are in ideal clinical settings for teaching TSE.
- A nursing assessment of any male younger than 40 years of age should include a health history to elicit any subjective symptoms and established risk factors.
- See Table 8-5, text page 160, for what should be taught regarding TSE.

## Skin Cancer

- Cancers of the skin are the most common cancers in humans.
- Malignant melanoma accounts for about 74% of all deaths that result from cutaneous cancers. The mortality rate from malignant melanoma is increasing faster than that of any other cancer except lung cancer.
- The majority of individuals with malignant melanoma are relatively young: the median age at diagnosis is 45 years.

### History assessment

- When obtaining a health history, the nurse must inquire whether any changes in moles have occurred.
- See text pages 160–161 for a list of questions to ask.

## Physical examination

- Areas that have been chronically exposed to sunlight are common sites for basal cell and squamous cell carcinomas.
- Melanomas are found on head, neck, and trunk, which may or may not be exposed to sun, and on the legs in women.
- If a skin lesion is detected, the nurse has three responsibilities: accurate documentation, referral of the patient to a physician for diagnosis, and follow-up for recurrent disease.
- There are three types of skin cancer: basal cell carcinoma, squamous cell carcinoma, and melanoma. See Tables 8-6 and 8-7, text page 162, for further information about these conditions.
- The nurse should be aware of the following precancerous skin lesions: leukoplakia, senile and actinic keratoses, and dysplastic nevi.

## Education

- Of all the known risk factors, ultraviolet radiation from the sun is the leading cause of skin cancer. The most carcinogenic of the ultraviolet wavelengths can be blocked by sunscreening agents. Sunscreens are rated according to sun protection factor (SPF), on a scale currently ranging from 2 to 35.
- Routine self-examination of the skin is the best defense against skin cancer, especially malignant melanoma. It is recommended that individuals older than 30 years of age who have fair skin and are subject to heavy sun exposures be taught skin self-assessment. See Figure 8-17, text page 164, on how to do a skin self-examination.
- Melanoma is more likely to develop in individuals and families with a history of dysplastic nevus syndrome (DNS) than it is in most people.

## Oral Cancer

- Approximately 95% of all oral malignancies begin in the surface mucosa.

## History assessment

- See text page 163 for a list of questions to ask.

## Physical examination

- The majority of oral cancers cause no symptoms in their early stages. Most individuals notice a white or bright red spot, "sore," or a swelling in their mouth.
- Physical examination of the mouth includes inspection, digital palpation, and olfaction of the oral cavity.
- Limitation of normal movement could indicate that a tumor is interfering with muscle action.
- Palpation of a hard lesion should be referred for biopsy to establish the diagnosis. Most tongue cancers appear on the lateral surfaces.
- Squamous cell carcinomas frequently are found on the floor of the mouth.
- Inspection of the mouth may reveal snuff keratosis, nicotine stomatitis, leukoplakias, or erythroplakia.
- Solar keratoses occur on sun-exposed surfaces and are flat, reddish-to-tan plaques that are usually scaly.
- An odor of sourness may indicate obstruction and fermentation, whereas fetid and foul odors may signal necrotic neoplasms indicative of advanced disease.
- Palpate the parotid, submandibular, and submental areas and the cervical lymph nodes.

## Screening

- Because alcoholics who smoke constitute the largest risk group for oral cancers, screening programs should be geared to this population.
- Instruct individuals 40 years of age and older that it is necessary to have a complete oral and dental examination on a periodic basis.

## Gynecologic Cancer

- The risk of endometrial cancer is age-related; the disease usually occurs in women 50–60 years old.
- Ovarian cancer accounts for about 26% of all gynecologic cancer and about 52% of all genital cancer deaths. The greatest number of cases of ovarian cancer are found in the age group of 55- to 74-year-old women.

### History assessment

- See text page 166 for a list of questions to ask.

### Physical examination

- Ovarian cancer usually has no early manifestations.
- The majority of patients with endometrial cancer have unexplained bleeding. A malodorous watery discharge may be noticed as an early sign.
- The symptoms of cervical cancer typically are abnormal vaginal discharge, irregular bleeding, elongation of menstrual period, or bleeding.

#### Abdomen

- A mass in the upper portion of the abdomen may suggest the presence of omental cake.

#### Vulva

- Infection with human papillomavirus (HPV) may produce the typically raised exophytic tumors (warts) that can be seen with simple inspection of the vulva.

#### Vagina

- The vagina should be inspected and palpated for cancer—masses, vaginal bands, texture changes, ulcers, erosions, leukoplakia, pink blush, induration, telangiectasis, and erythematosus.
- The nurse may elect to do a Schiller's test on any suspicious area of the vagina or cervix.

#### Cervix

- The cervix is freely movable, firm, and smooth, and if it has been invaded by cancer, it becomes hard and immobile. Malignancy produces a rough, granular surface and is likened to both the feel and appearance of a cauliflower.
- An annual suction curettage is recommended for menopausal women and women who have taken estrogen without progestational modification for a prolonged period after menopause.

#### Uterus and adnexa

- Uterine tenderness, immobility, or enlargement merits further investigation. An enlarged boggy uterus is an indication of advanced disease.

### Ovaries

- Palpation of the ovaries in prepubertal girls or postmenopausal women also merits investigation because (1) normal ovaries and tubes are usually not palpable, (2) ovaries in these two groups of women are smaller than the usual ovarian size of 4 cm, and (3) three to five years after menopause the ovaries usually have atrophied and are no longer palpable.

### Rectovaginal palpation

- Thickening of the peritoneal rectovaginal pouch, or Douglas' cul-de-sac, occurs from spread of cervical carcinoma.

## Screening of asymptomatic individuals

### Cervical smears

- Because of the Pap test, the death rate from invasive cervical cancer has decreased by at least 70% over the last 40 years.
- The ACS recommends that all women who are, or who have been, sexually active or who have reached 18 years of age have an annual Pap smear and pelvic examination.
- Several factors contribute to false-negative results from Pap smears and other errors: patient error, physician error, and laboratory error.

## Additional nursing interventions

- Nurses should discuss the myths about menopause with women who are in their late 30s and early 40s.
- Nurses must conduct educational programs in community settings that dispel these myths that surround menopause and aging and provide factual information on the early signs and symptoms of the common gynecologic cancers in older women.
- Nurses need to be aware that older women are at high risk for endometrial, vulvar, vaginal, and ovarian cancer.
- Young women who have had venereal disease must be alert to the necessity of having regular Pap smears.

# PRACTICE QUESTIONS

1. The best treatment of cancer is:
   a. prevention.
   b. early detection.
   c. radiation and excision.
   d. new developments in chemotherapy.

2. Mr. Allen has been exposed to asbestos in the workplace for most of his adult life (he is now 75); Mr. Eliot, 64, has smoked since he was 17; Ms. Frank, 43, calls herself "a dedicated suntanner." Which patient is probably at greatest risk for cancer mortality?
   a. Mr. Allen
   b. Mr. Eliot
   c. Ms. Frank
   d. the two men

**Questions 3–6 follow the case of Mr. Eliot, a patient who presents with an undifferentiated neoplasm in the proximal right bronchus.**

3. Mr. Eliot (from question 2) has an undifferentiated neoplasm arising in the proximal right bronchus. Which symptom most typically reflects this?
   a. barrel chest
   b. bulges on the thorax
   c. breathlessness
   d. superior vena cava obstruction

4. In examining Mr. Eliot, you hear a dullness on percussion. What might this indicate?
   a. tumor in the main bronchus
   b. bagpipe sign
   c. bronchophony
   d. pleural effusion

5. On continuing your examination of Mr. Eliot, you discover that he is exhibiting the only early physical finding that is usually suggestive of lung cancer. Which of the following signs must Mr. Eliot be exhibiting?
   a. whispered pectoriloquy
   b. egophony
   c. wheezing localized to a single lobe
   d. bagpipe sign

6. Mr. Eliot's son, Ted, who has also smoked for a number of years, is inspired by his father's situation to quit smoking. In encouraging him, you tell Ted that if he succeeds, he may find that his _____ status will improve.
   a. sensory
   b. respiratory
   c. cardiovascular
   d. all of the above

**Questions 7–10 follow the case of Ms. Harris, who is being assessed for a possible gatrointestinal cancer.**

7. Ms. Harris is being assessed for a possible gastrointestinal cancer (according to the patient's own suspicions). Which of the following factors could cause signs that might mimic signs of GI cancer?
   a. ADHD in adolescence
   b. depression (anorexia, weight loss)
   c. use of the tumor marker PSA
   d. all of the above

8. On inspection, you note that Ms. Harris exhibits edema and a bluish tint to the face, and that her neck veins seem too prominent. What might be causing these symptoms?
   a. blockage of the inferior vena cava
   b. nodular umbilicus
   c. distention
   d. intraabdominal fluid

9. On auscultation of Ms. Harris's abdomen, you hear very loud splashes. What might be causing this?
   a. partial obstruction
   b. bowel immobility
   c. air and fluid in the gut
   d. all of the above

10. During Ms. Harris' rectal examination, you detect a stony hard mass in the cul-de-sac. What does this indicate?
    a. Ms. Harris has small amounts of intraabdominal fluid forming a "puddle sign" on the pelvic floor.
    b. Ms. Harris has pancreatic or hepatic lesions pressing on the pelvic floor.
    c. Ms. Harris has a carcinoma that has metastasized to the pelvic floor.
    d. Ms. Harris has metastasis at Virchow's node.

**Questions 11 and 12 concern Mr. Vincennes, who is being screened for colon cancer.**

11. Mr. Vincinnes is 40 and is being screened for possible colon cancer. He is asymptomatic. What tests are most important for this patient?
    a. Shifting dullness and fluid wave tests are used first on asymptomatic patients.
    b. Fecal occult blood test and digital rectal exam are the two most important tests for asymptomatic patients.
    c. Hemoccult test and urinalysis are the two standard tests for screening asymptomatic individuals.
    d. None of these answers is completely correct.

12. Mr. Vincinnes does not have cancer. Before he goes home, however, you gather materials to discuss ways that he can lower his overall cancer risk (including the colorectal cancer for which he was screened). Which of the following should *not* be part of your teaching plan for Mr. Vincinnes?
    a. "Avoid obesity; decrease your total fat intake to less than a third of your total calories."
    b. "Eating at least one helping of salt-cured or smoked fish or seaweed per day keeps your metabolism in balance and helps purify your system, thus reducing cancer risk."
    c. "Be moderate in your consumption of beer and alcohol."
    d. "Include more high-fiber foods and cruciferous vegetables in your daily diet."

13. Mr. Benson presents with some pain and frequency of urination. During a rectal palpation, the examiner detects a diffuse enlargement of the prostate. There seems to be no mass, however. With no other information, one might infer that Mr. Benson is most likely to have:
    a. nephritis.
    b. cancer of the prostate.
    c. cancer of the bladder.
    d. benign prostatic hypertrophy.

14. A student nurse you have befriended is about to perform her first breast exam on a patient. You know she is ready when she tells you:
    a. "I should palpate the normal breast first."
    b. "It is important to press firmly but gently to detect subtle differences beneath the cutaneous layers."
    c. "After the patient is supine, I will start at the armpit and palpate in increasingly small circles, slowly moving in toward the center and finishing at the nipple area."
    d. "To avoid false-positive diagnoses, it is important to avoid charting every single mass that is felt; charting only masses confirmed to be either cancerous or precancerous ensures accuracy."

15. Alexis, 27, brings her mother Margie, 48, in for a breast exam. During the course of the interview, you discover that neither is familiar with the rationale behind regular BSEs or mammography. As part of your patient education plan, you intend to tell them that:
    a. Alexis should have a breast exam every year but should perform BSE monthly; her mother should do both every six months.
    b. Alexis should begin getting mammograms annually. Her mother should get one every two years.
    c. Margie is the only one who should be getting BSEs at this time; Alexis will, too, at 30 years of age.
    d. Alexis should have a breast exam every three years; Margie, every year.

16. The most common sites for testicular tumors are:
    a. the anterior and lateral surfaces.
    b. the medial and lateral surfaces.
    c. the posterior and medial surfaces.
    d. the anterior and medial surfaces.

**Questions 17–19 concern Ms. Allison, who presents with a skin lesion.**

17. Ms. Allison notices a "funny discoloration" on her arm and comes in for an examination. She tells you that her brother died several years ago from a common skin cancer. He was only 42. Ms. Allison's brother most likely had:
    a. squamous cell carcinoma.
    b. basal cell carcinoma.
    c. melanoma.
    d. leukoplakia.

18. Ms. Allison turns out to have a skin lesion that appears to be possibly cancerous. The action least likely to be part of your response is:
    a. documenting the size, location, and description of the lesion.
    b. teaching Ms. Allison appropriate routine self-examination of the skin.
    c. referring Ms. Allison to a physician for diagnosis.
    d. following Ms. Allison up for recurrent disease.

19. Mr. Finkle reports a "rash of some kind" in his mouth. He reports that he likes spicy foods, but says that his wife predicts the rash has been caused by his habit of smoking a pipe. The type of irritation you might be most likely to discover on inspecting Mr. Finkle's mouth is:
    a. snuff keratosis.
    b. nicotine stomatitis.
    c. leukoplakias.
    d. erythroplakia.

20. Which of the following women should have an annual Pap smear and pelvic examination?
    a. Lisa, 15, who is sexually active
    b. Marilyn, 55, a widow who has not been sexually active
    c. Glynnis, 17, who is not yet sexually active
    d. Both Lisa and Marilyn

## ANSWER EXPLANATIONS

1. **The answer is a.** The best treatment of cancer is its prevention. About 90% of the 800,000 skin cancers that were expected to be diagnosed in 1996 could have been prevented by protection from the sun. All cancers caused by cigarette smoking and heavy use of alcohol could be prevented completely. (p. 135)

2. **The answer is b.** Mr. Eliot is at greatest risk. Cigarette smoking is the largest single preventable cause of premature death and disability and the major single cause of cancer mortality. Individuals like Mr. Allen who are exposed to high levels of asbestos and other respiratory carcinogens in the workplace also have an increased risk, but it is not the single major cause of cancer mortality. Cancers of the skin—most often caused by excessive sun exposure—are the most common cancers in humans, but they too are not the major single cause of cancer mortality. (pp. 136 and 160)

3. **The answer is d.** Superior vena cava obstruction is a common complication of lung cancer; approximately 80% of these cases are caused by undifferentiated neoplasms arising in proximal right bronchi. Barrel chest is associated with pulmonary emphysema or normal aging. Bulges on the thorax is often a manifestation of a neoplasm on the ribs. Breathlessness is a more generalized indication of obstruction of the lungs. (p. 138)

4. **The answer is d.** Dullness on percussion indicates either pleural effusion or a consolidated lung. Lung cancer is the most common cause of hemorrhagic pleural effusion in middle-aged and elderly male smokers. Mr. Eliot has smoked since he was 17. (p. 140)

5. **The answer is c.** The only early physical finding that most strongly suggests lung cancer is wheezing localized in a single lobe of the lung in an elderly person with a long history of smoking. (p. 140)

6. **The answer is d.** Smoking cessation results not only in improved respiratory status, but improved sensory and cardiovascular status as well. Those who have given up smoking for five years demonstrate a lung cancer mortality rate approximately 40% that of a current smoker. After 15 years without smoking, the mortality rate of ex-smokers was only slightly greater than that of nonsmokers. The point is, of course, that it is never too late to benefit from smoking cessation. (p. 141)

7. **The answer is b.** Conditions that might affect the patient's gastrointestinal system include advanced age (not adolescence), depression, nutritional disturbances (again, in the elderly), and drug intake. (p. 143)

8.  **The answer is a.** Venous distention is caused by blockage of the inferior vena cava, which can occur from spread of cancer. In this condition there is edema of the eyelids, a bluish face and lips, prominent neck veins, and pitting edema of the arms and large veins over the upper portions of the chest and shoulders. (pp. 144–45)

9.  **The answer is c.** Succussion splash in the small intestines is produced by a combination of air and fluid in the gut when the examiner shakes the stomach or vigorously moves the abdomen. The sound resembles very loud splashes. (p. 145)

10. **The answer is c.** On palpation during a rectal exam, the examiner may feel a rectal shelf. In women it is felt as a stony hard mass in the cul-de-sac. The shelf indicates a carcinoma that has metastasized to the pelvic floor and therefore is a sign of advanced malignancy. (p. 146)

11. **The answer is b.** The two most important screening tests for asymptomatic individuals are examination of the feces for occult blood and the digital rectal examination. At age 40, the American Cancer Society advocates an annual digital rectal exam. Beginning at age 50, the ACS, the National Cancer Institute, and the American College of Surgeons recommend that asymptomatic individuals have a sigmoidoscopic exam every 3 to 5 years in conjunction with an annual fecal occult blood test. (pp. 146–47)

12. **The answer is b.** Patients should be counseled to reduce their risk of colorectal cancer by avoiding obesity, decreasing total fat intake to less than a third, by being moderate in consumption of alcohol, and by including more high-fiber foods and cruciferous vegetables. One should be moderate in the consumption of salt-cured, smoked, and nitrite-cured foods. (p. 149)

13. **The answer is d.** The normal prostate on palpation is usually a rounded structure about 4 cm in diameter that feels firm. Cancer of the prostate typically appears as a stony-hard nodule, whereas benign hypertrophy usually results in a diffuse enlargement of the prostate without masses. (p. 150)

14. **The answer is a.** The examiner should palpate the normal breast first. It is important to press very lightly (not firmly) and gently to detect subtle differences. When the patient is supine, the examiner will start at the areolar area and palpate in increasingly wider concentric circles. Finally, it is important to chart every mass that is felt. (pp. 154–55)

15. **The answer is d.** All women from age 20 should perform BSE monthly. Women in Alexis' age category (20–40 years of age) should have a breast physical exam every three years, and women older than 40 years should have a breast physical examination every year. (pp. 154–55)

16. **The answer is a.** The most common sites for tumors of the testes are on the anterior and lateral surfaces. Initially, cancer of the testes may be manifested by asymmetry of the scrotum or scrotal skin that appears stretched and thin over the tumor. Diffuse induration of the testis in the absence of discrete nodularity also may be the initial abnormality. (p. 158)

17. **The answer is c.** There are three types of skin cancer: basal cell carcinoma, squamous cell carcinoma, and melanoma. However, melanoma is the most common. Leukoplakia is one of the precancerous skin lesions, along with senile and actinic keratoses and dysplastic nevi. (pp. 160–61)

18. **The answer is b.** If a skin lesion is detected, the nurse has three responsibilities: accurate documentation of size, location, and description of the lesion; referral of the patient to a physician for diagnosis, and follow-up for recurrent disease. (p. 161)

19. **The answer is b.** Nicotine stomatitis is a diffuse white condition that contains numerous red dots. This lesion usually covers the entire hard palate and is almost always associated with pipe smoking. It has minimal or no malignant potential. Complete resolution should occur with cessation of smoking. (p. 165)

20. **The answer is d.** The American Cancer Society recommends that all women who are, or who have been, sexually active or who have reached 18 years of age have an annual Pap smear and pelvic examination. (p. 168)

# Chapter 9    Diagnostic Evaluation, Classification, and Staging

## DIAGNOSTIC EVALUATION

### Factors That Affect the Diagnostic Approach

- The major goals of the diagnostic evaluation for a suspected cancer are to determine the tissue type of the malignancy, the primary site of the malignancy, the extent of disease within the body, and the potential for tumor recurrence.
- The worst prognosis can be expected in those people who delay seeking medical evaluation at the onset of their symptoms, in those cancers for which technological methods are unavailable to make an early diagnosis, and in people for whom the primary lesion cannot be found.
- The proper test is one that yields information on the suspicious site of malignancy and complements rather than merely confirms known information.
- Third-party payers, prospective payment systems, and managed care networks play an important role as gatekeepers in the diagnostic evaluation.

### Nursing Implications in Diagnostic Evaluation

- Seven warning signals of cancer include the following: change in bowel or bladder habits; unusual bleeding or discharge; a sore that does not heal; obvious change in wart or mole; thickening or lump in breast or elsewhere; nagging cough or hoarseness; and indigestion or difficulty in swallowing. (See Table 9-1 on text page 177.)
- Oncology nurses play a key role in providing information and support to reduce the stress of going through a diagnostic evaluation for a suspected malignancy.
- Nurses also must be cognizant of any potential for complications during or after a procedure.
- Including the family members in all aspects of the diagnostic evaluation is helpful to the individual and family and to the health care team.

### Laboratory Techniques

- The accuracy of a particular laboratory study or imaging technique often is reported in terms of sensitivity or specificity. *Sensitivity* establishes the percentage of people with cancer who will have positive (abnormal) test results, known as *true-positive* results. Test results of people with cancer that are negative (normal) are *false-negative* findings.
- Specificity establishes the percentage of people without cancer who will have negative (normal) test results, known as *true-negative* results. People who are free of disease and show positive (abnormal) results are considered to have false-positive results. The *predictive value* of a test establishes the probability that a test result correctly predicts the actual disease status.
- Ideally, a tumor marker is produced exclusively by the tumor cell and not in other conditions (highly specific), is present and detectable in early, occult disease (highly sensitive), is detectable in levels directly reflecting tumor mass (proportional), predicts disease response and recurrence (predictive), and is cost effective and commercially available (feasible).
- The only marker that approaches this ideal is human chorionic gonadotrophin in gestational trophoblastic tumors. Table 9-2, text page 181, identifies several tumor markers and their clinical significance.

- Techniques to produce monoclonal antibodies that detect specific tumor antigens have been important to the diagnosis, classification, localization, and treatment of several solid tumors, T- and B-cell lymphomas, and leukemia.
- Radioimmunoassay determines the amount of tumor antigen in a serum sample.
- Flow cytometry rapidly measures and identifies DNA characteristics and cell surface markers that correlate with patient prognosis.

## Tumor Imaging

### Radiographic techniques

- Radiographic studies, or x-ray films, allow visualization of internal structures of the body. See Table 9-3, text page 182, for preferred imaging procedures for various sites.
- Mammographic examination incorporates a tissue compression device or cone that improves the quality of the image and reduces the amount of primary and scatter radiation.
- Diagnostic mammography is indicated when symptoms or clinical findings exist that suggest an abnormality.
- Tomography provides a radiographic image of a selected layer or plane of the body that would otherwise be obscured by shadows of other structures.
- Computerized axial tomography (CT or CAT) also provides sectional views of structures in the body.
- Angiography, venography, cholangiography, and urography, in addition to computerized tomography, all rely on the intravascular administration of iodinated contrast agents for optimal visualization of body structure and function.
- An oily iodinated contrast material is employed in lymphangiography (LAG). The lymphatic vessels in each foot (or hand) are injected to allow visualization of the lymphatic vessels and nodes. This is indicated in the diagnosis and staging of Hodgkin's and non-Hodgkin's lymphomas and in some pelvic cancers.
- Intrathecal contrast agents are used in myelography and in computerized tomography.
- Barium sulfate is a nonabsorbable, radiopaque agent used to enhance the contrast between the lumen of the gastrointestinal tract and adjacent soft tissues. Studies that use barium include esophagraphy, upper gastrointestinal (UGI) series, small-bowel series, barium enema, and hypotonic duodenography.

### Nuclear medicine techniques

- Nuclear medicine imaging involves the intravenous injection or the ingestion of radioisotope compounds followed by camera imaging of those organs or tissues that have concentrated the radioisotopes. Nuclear medicine studies often will detect sites of abnormal metabolism or early malignancy several months before changes are seen on a radiograph.
- Positron emission tomography (PET) provides information based on the biochemical and metabolic activity of tissue.
- Nuclear imaging with radio-labeled monoclonal antibodies visualizes microscopic sites of metastasis or suspected malignancy.

### Ultrasonography

- Ultrasonography (US) uses sound waves to distinguish a cyst from a solid mass. A limitation of the examination is its inability to visualize through bone or air. Ultrasonography is most applicable in detecting tumors within the breast, pelvis, the retroperitoneum, and the peritoneum.

### Magnetic resonance imaging

- Magnetic resonance imaging creates sectional images of the body, but does not expose the patient to ionizing radiation.
- Magnetic resonance imaging is most applicable in the detection, localization, and staging of malignant disease in the central nervous system, spine, head and neck, and musculoskeletal system.

## Invasive Diagnostic Techniques

### Endoscopy

- Endoscopy is a method of directly visualizing the interior of a hollow viscus by the insertion of an endoscope into a body cavity or opening.
- Visual inspection, tissue biopsy, cytological aspiration, staging the extent of disease, and the excision of pathological processes are possible through the endoscope.
- Endoscopic retrograde cholangiopancreatography combines the diagnostic procedures of endoscopy and contrast-enhanced radiography to evaluate biliary tract obstruction and pancreatic masses.
- The endoscopic ultrasound (EUS) may prove superior to other imaging modalities for assessing direct depth of tumor invasion and local lymph node status.
- EUS is indicated to distinguish benign from malignant lesions, to stage neoplasms, to establish operability and surgical approach, and to determine response or recurrence.

### Biopsy

- The importance of obtaining histological or cytological proof of malignancy cannot be overstated.
- The cytological examination of aspirated fluid, secretion, scrapings, or washings of body cavities may reveal malignant cells that have exfoliated from a primary or metastatic tumor.
- The fine-needle aspiration biopsy is available in the ambulatory setting. It provides not only cytological information but also microhistologic information if adequate tissue fragments are obtained.
- Stereotactic localization is another diagnostic tool to establish the coordinates of a lesion and accurately position a needle for the tissue biopsy.
- The following are commonly recognized techniques for obtaining a biopsy: needle biopsy, incisional biopsy, excisional biopsy, punch biopsy, and bone marrow aspiration.

## CLASSIFICATION AND NOMENCLATURE

### Basic Terminology

- A *tumor* is a swelling or mass of tissue that may be benign or malignant. *Cancer*, synonymous with *malignant neoplasm*, is an uncontrolled "new growth" capable of metastasis and invasion. The term *primary tumor* is used to describe the original histological site of tumorigenesis. A *secondary*, or *metastatic tumor* resembles the primary tumor histologically. A *second primary lesion* refers to an additional, histologically separate malignant neoplasm in the same patient.

### Benign and Malignant Tumor Characteristics

- The *benign* tumor is relatively slow-growing. Growth occurs as the tumor expands locally within a capsule of fibrous tissue. Benign tumors do not invade adjacent tissues, destroy normal tissue, or metastasize elsewhere in the body.
- The *malignant* tumor is characterized by its generally high mitotic rate, rapid growth, invasion of local tissues, and the ability to metastasize.

## Tumor Classification System

- An early occurrence in the life of the embryo is the development of three primary germ layers: the ectoderm, the mesoderm, and the endoderm. The cells within these layers divide, specialize, and give rise to all cells, tissues, and organs within the body. Virtually every cell type in the body is capable of transforming into a malignant cell.
- In the histogenetic classification system benign tumors usually end in the suffix *-oma*. Most malignant tumors end in either the suffix *-sarcoma* or the suffix *-carcinoma*. (See Table 9-6, text page 193.)
- *Sarcoma* specifies a malignant tumor of the connective tissues.
- *Carcinoma* specifies a malignant tumor arising from epithelial tissues.
- Carcinomas are further delineated by the prefixes *adeno-*, for tumors that arise from glandular epithelial tissue, and *squamous*, for tumors that originate from squamous epithelial tissues.
- The suffix that refers to malignant tumors that resemble the primitive blastula phase in embryonic development is *-blastoma*.
- Teratoma and its malignant counterpart, teratocarcinoma, arise from tissue of all three germ layers and have no relationship to the site of origin.
- Lymphoma, melanoma, and hepatoma are malignant tumors with the *-oma* suffix.

## Tumors of Unknown Origin

- The patient with a tumor of unknown origin presents with metastatic disease and generally poor prognosis.
- Most frequently the histological classification will be adenocarcinoma, but the site of origin may never be determined.
- Most tumors of unkown origin arise from the lung, breast, or pancreas.

## STAGING AND GRADING CLASSIFICATIONS

### Staging the Extent of the Disease

- The staging process is a method of classifying a malignancy by the extent of its spread within the body. Staging is based on the premise that cancers of similar histological features and site of origin will extend and metastasize in a predictable manner. There are multiple objectives of solid-tumor staging, but the most important is to provide the necessary information for individual treatment planning.
- The TNM committee of the International Union Against Cancer (UICC) and the American Joint Committee on Cancer (AJCC) have agreed on the TNM staging system. The TNM staging system classifies solid tumors by the anatomic extent of disease.
- Three categories are quantified, with gradations representing progressive tumor size or involvement.
  - The extent of the primary tumor (T) is evaluated on the basis of depth of invasion, surface spread, and tumor size.
  - The absence or presence and extent of regional lymph node (N) metastasis are considered, with attention to the size and location of the nodes.
  - The absence or presence of distant metastasis (M) is assessed.
- The TNM system is further classified by whether the assessment is obtained clinically (cTNM), after pathological review (pTNM), at the time of retreatment (rTNM), or at autopsy (aTNM). Table 9-7, text page 194, presents the nomenclature of the TNM system.
- The cTNM is based on a clinical exam.
- The pTNM is determined after surgery when the true extent of the disease is known and treatment decisions can be made.
- Persons with leukemia, lymphoma, or myeloma have different methods of staging based on cellular characteristics.

- Numerical values are assigned to the T, N, and M categories; they are clustered into one of four stages (I through IV), or stage O for carcinoma in situ. Stage IV consistently includes distant metastases (M1) and predicts the worst prognosis.

## Patient Performance Classification

- The most prevalent performance scales are the Karnofsky Performance Status scale, the Eastern Cooperative Oncology Group (ECOG) scale, and the World Health Organization (WHO) scale. In an attempt to standardize this classification, the American Joint Committee on Cancer (AJCC) developed a simplified performance scale. Each seeks to objectively define a person's ability to perform activities of daily living.

## Grading

- For selected tumors the grade is considered more significant than anatomic staging in terms of prognostic value and treatment.
- The AJCC recommends the following grading classification.
  - GX    grade cannot be assessed
  - G1    well differentiated
  - G2    moderately well differentiated
  - G3    poorly differentiated
  - G4    undifferentiated

## PRACTICE QUESTIONS

1. You are preparing for an initial meeting with Mr. Jennings, who is about to undergo diagnostic screening for a suspected abdominal cancer. In describing this process, you intend to tell him that major goals of the diagnostic evaluation may be to establish, among other things, the:
   a. tissue type of the malignancy.
   b. primary type of the malignancy.
   c. extent of disease within the body.
   d. all of the above.

2. Four patients have recently been assessed for possible cancers. Which patient's symptom seems least likely to be a warning signal of cancer?
   a. Mr. Jennings reports that he "goes to the bathroom more" and says that the color and consistency of the stools have changed.
   b. Ms. Harris has a painful lump in her breast; it is tender on palpation, especially a week before her menstrual cycle.
   c. Twelve-year-old Jill has developed a new mole on her shoulder that is large with an unusual shape or pattern to it. Her mother thinks it's getting larger.
   d. Mr. Traynor has a sore on his forehead that "just won't clear up."

3. Mr. Smith has an ultrasound of a mass in his abdomen, and it accurately determines that he does not have cancer; therefore, Mr. Smith's test results are:
   a. true-positive.
   b. true-negative.
   c. false-positive.
   d. false-negative.

4. Mr. Hall is receiving chemotherapy for metastic colon cancer. Since he started treatment, his cancer has gotten much smaller and his tumor marker has greatly declined. The tumor marker is capable of demonstrating response to treatment. This particular quality of the tumor marker makes it:
   a. highly specific.
   b. highly sensitive.
   c. proportional.
   d. predictive.

5. Mr. Phillips has cancer of the liver. The preferred procedure for imaging the abdomen is usual
   a. ultrasonography.
   b. CT scan.
   c. thermography.
   d. x-ray.

6. Intravascular iodinated contrast agents are needed in:
   a. cholangiography.
   b. venography.
   c. CT scan.
   d. all of the above.

**Questions 7–8 concern Mrs. Plyman, who is to have an ultrasonographic examination.**

7. Mrs. Plyman is about to undergo ultrasonography to evaluate a possible pelvic tumor. She asks you for information on the procedure. Which of the following statements will *not* be part of your education plan?
   a. Ultrasonography can be used to discriminate masses.
   b. The procedure is most applicable in detecting tumors within the pelvis, retroperitoneum, and peritoneum.
   c. It is an excellent means of visualizing through bone or air, especially in comparison with radiography or CT scans.
   d. Ultrasonography is non-invasive, directing reflecting echoes of high-frequency sound waves into specific tissues.

8. Mrs. Plyman says, "I don't like the idea of ultrasonography. Why can't I be examined using MRI?" Your best explanation is that:
   a. MRI is most helpful in detecting and staging cancer in the central nervous system, spine, head and neck, and musculoskeletal system.
   b. MRI is more dangerous than ultrasonography because it uses radio-labeled monoclonal antibodies to visualize microscopic sites of metastasis.
   c. MRI exposes patients to ionizing radiation and therefore is not safer than ultrasonography—although both are easily used within safe limits.
   d. there is no way to enhance MRI imaging, as there is with ultrasonography.

9. Which of the following is/are *not* true?
   a. Endoscopic ultrasound is used to assess direct depth of tumor invasion.
   b. Endoscopy is used primarily to visualize body cavities rather than to obtain biopsies.
   c. Fine-needle aspiration biopsy not only provides cytological information, but it can be used to obtain microhistologic information.
   d. It is acceptable to use an anesthetic in stereotactic localization.

10. Mr. Jones has colon cancer and is found to have an additional, histologically separate malignant neoplasm in his thyroid. This is referred to as a:
    a. malignant neoplasm, primary.
    b. metastasis.
    c. second primary lesion.
    d. secondary, metastatic tumor.

**Questions 11–14 refer to three patients whose cancers are being classified and staged.**

11. Ms. Hilliard has a lipoma; Mr. Mayle has cancer of the connective tissues; and Mr. Fleischman has cancer of the epithelial tissues. Which of the following is true?
    a. Ms. Hilliard and Mr. Mayle each have a type of teratocarcinoma.
    b. Ms. Hilliard has a benign tumor; Mr. Fleischman a sarcoma.
    c. Mr. Mayle has a sarcoma, while Mr. Fleischman has a carcinoma.
    d. Mr. Fleischman and Ms. Hilliard both have a teratocarcinoma.

12. In the TNM staging system:
    a. cTNM indicates that assessment has been obtained clinically.
    b. cTNM indicates whether carcinogenesis has occurred.
    c. rTNM indicates that remission of the cancer is occurring.
    d. aTNM indicates that the cancer has been detected on first assessment (a).

13.  Mr. Mayle's clinical exam reveals evidence of an extensive primary tumor with fixation to a deeper structure, bone invasion, and lymph nodes of a similar nature. The lesion is operable but not resectable, and gross disease is left behind. There is some chance of survival. How would you classify Mr. Mayle's cancer?
     a.  Stage IV, T4, N3, M+
     b.  Stage I, T1, NO, MO
     c.  Stage II, T2, N1, MO
     d.  Stage III, T4, N2, MO

14.  Mr. Fleischman's cancer is given an AJCC classification of G2. This means his cancer is:
     a.  undifferentiated.
     b.  well differentiated.
     c.  poorly differentiated.
     d.  moderately well differentiated.

# ANSWER EXPLANATIONS

1.  **The answer is d.** The major goals of the diagnostic evaluation for a suspected cancer are to determine the tissue type of the malignancy, the primary site of the malignancy, the extent of disease within the body, and in addition, the tumor's potential to recur in the future. (p. 176)

2.  **The answer is b.** Breast lumps commonly seen in cancer tend to be painless; this is not to say that it is impossible for Ms. Harris to have cancer, but that her sign is less definitive than the others'. The seven classic warning signals of cancer include the following: changes in bowel or bladder habits; unusual bleeding or discharge; a sore that does not heal; obvious changes in warts or moles; painless thickening or lump in the breast or elsewhere; nagging cough or hoarseness; and indigestion or difficulty swallowing. (p. 177)

3.  **The answer is b.** When an individual who is cancer free has negative (normal) test results, these are called true-negative results. Test results of people with cancer that are negative (normal) are false-negative results. People who are free of disease and show positive (abnormal) results are considered to have false-positive results. (p. 179)

4.  **The answer is c.** Ideally, a tumor maker is produced exclusively by the tumor cell and not in other conditions (highly specific), is present and detectable in early, occult disease (highly sensitive), is detectable in levels directly reflecting tumor mass (proportional), predicts disease response and recurrence (predictive), and is cost effective and commercially available (feasible). (p. 179)

5.  **The answer is b.** In the case of liver cancer, CT has been preferred for imaging, but MRI with contrast may be equivalent. Ultrasound is preferred for differentiating biliary obstruction from hepatic parenchymal disease. (p. 182)

6.  **The answer is d.** Angiography, venography, cholangiography, and urography, in addition to computerized tomography, all rely on the intravascular administration of iodinated contrast agents for optimal visualization of body structure and function. (p. 186)

7.  **The answer is c.** Ultrasonography (US) can be used to discriminate masses. A *limitation* of the exam is its *inability* to visualize through bone or air. US is most applicable in detecting tumors within the pelvis, the retroperitoneum, and the peritoneum of patients with cancer. (p. 188)

8.  **The answer is a.** MRI is most applicable in the detection, localization, and staging of malignant disease in the CNS, spine, head and neck, and musculoskeletal system. This imaging method creates sectional images of the body but does not expose the patient to ionizing radiation. It is nuclear imaging, and not MRI, that uses radio-labeled monoclonal antibodies to visualize microscopic sites

of metastasis or suspected malignancy. MRI can be enhanced with IV contrast agents. (p. 188)

9. **The answer is b.** Visual inspection, tissue biopsy, cytological aspiration, disease staging, and excision of pathological processes are all possible through the endoscope. EUS may prove superior to other imaging modalities for assessing direct depth of tumor invasion. Fine-needle aspiration biopsy not only provides cytological information, but it can be used to obtain microhistologic information. It is acceptable to use an anesthetic in stereotactic localization. (pp. 189–90)

10. **The answer is c.** A second or subsequent histologically separate malignant neoplasm in the same patient is referred to as a second primary lesion. The original histological site of tumorigenesis is the primary tumor; a secondary, or metastatic, tumor resembles the primary tumor histologically. (p. 191)

11. **The answer is c.** Mr. Mayle has a malignant tumor of the connective tissues, which is a sarcoma, while Mr. Fleischman has a malignant tumor arising from epithelial tissues, or, in other words, a carcinoma. Ms. Hilliard's lipoma is a benign tumor of fat tissue. (p. 192)

12. **The answer is a.** In the TNM system, the extent of the primary tumor (T) is evaluated on the basis of depth of invasion, surface spread, and tumor size. The absence or presence and extent of regional lymph node (N) metastasis are considered and the presence of distant metastasis (M) is assessed. The system is further classified by whether the assessment is obtained clinically (cTNM or TNM), after pathological review (pTNM), at the time of retreatment (rTNM), or on autopsy (aTNM). (p. 194)

13. **The answer is d.** A stage grouping of Stage III, T4, N2, M0 is consistent with a clinical exam that reveals evidence of an extensive primary tumor with fixation to a deeper structure, bone invasion, and lymph nodes of a similar nature. Typically, in such a stage, the lesion may be operable but not resectable, and gross disease is left behind. (p. 195)

14. **The answer is d.** A G2 rating means the tumor is moderately well differentiated. The AJCC recommends the following grading classification:

GX = grade cannot be assessed

G1 = well differentiated

G2 = moderately well differentiated

G3 = poorly differentiated

G4 = undifferentiated  (p. 197)

# Chapter 10    Quality of Life as an Outcome of Cancer Treatment

## INTRODUCTION

- The term *quality of life* (QL or QOL) or *health-related quality of life* (HQL) has emerged to organize and galvanize a collection of outcome evaluation activities in cancer treatment research over the past two decades.
- *Quality* of survival is as important as *quantity* of survival.
- HQL evaluation differs from classic toxicity ratings in two important ways: (1) it incorporates more aspects of function and (2) it focuses on the patient's perspective.

## EVALUATING METHODS OF ASSESSMENT

### Construct Definition as a Frame for Measurement

- Definitions of HQL may differ across study groups and still be measured reliably and validly within the parameters of a definition.
- There may well be a distinction between social *well-being* (perceived social support, satisfaction with relationships, etc.) and social *functioning* (ability to see friends, leisure activity).

## APPROACHES TO MEASURING HEALTH-RELATED QUALITY OF LIFE

- Over time, two approaches to measuring HQL have evolved: psychometric and utility.

### Psychometric Approach

- The *psychometric approach* includes generic health profile measurement and specific instruments to measure impact of a specific disease, treatment, or condition.
  - The psychometric approach places heavy emphasis on an individual's response and response variability across individuals. It measures subjective or perceived well being.
  - Psychometric measures may or may not include a summary or total score. When available, only rarely have these summary scores been connected to patients' values for their current health status.

### Utility Approach

- The *utility approach* is explicitly concerned with treatment decision making, usually at a policy level. Treatments typically are evaluated as to their benefit compared in some way to their cost.
- The *cost-utility approach* extends the cost-effectiveness approach conceptually by evaluating the HQL benefit produced by the clinical effects of a treatment, thereby including the patient's (presumed) perspective.
- In the *standard gamble* approach, people are asked to choose between their current state of health and a "gamble" in which they have various probabilities for death or perfect health.
- The *time trade-off* method involves asking people how much time they would be willing to give up in order to live out their remaining life expectancies in perfect health.
- All utility approaches share in common the use of 0–1 scale in which 0 = death and 1 = perfect health.
- The psychometric approach provides the detailed perspective of the patient, but it does not tell us how important a given problem or set of problems is to a group of patients.

- The utility approach informs us about the relative value of various health states; however, because of its emphasis on a single summary score, it fails to reflect the specific problems that might emerge.

## EVALUATING PSYCHOMETRIC MEASURES
## Reliability

- *Repeatability* refers to the extent to which a measure, applied two different times or in two different ways produces the same score.
- Consistency refers to the homogeneity of the items of a scale.

### Reliability is a matter of degree

- Reliability is not a fixed property of a measure but rather a property of a measure used with certain people under certain conditions. Reliability cannot be assumed to be generalizable.

### Reliability depends on the number of items

- As the number of items goes up, so too does the reliability coefficient.

### Reliability is increased by heterogeneous samples

- Heterogeneous samples produce a greater spread of scores.

## Validity

- *Validity* refers to a scale's ability to measure what is purports to measure.
- Validity generally has been subdivided into three types: content, criterion, and construct.
- *Content validity* is further divided into face validity (the degree to which the scale superficially appears to measure the construct in question, and *true content validity* (the degree to which the items accurately represent the range of attributes covered by the construct).
  - Content validity does not include statistical evidence to support inferences.
  - Content coverage should cut across at least three broad domains in order to be considered valid from the perspective of item content.
- *Criterion validity* is also subdivided into two types, *concurrent validity* and *predictive validity*.
  - Criterion data that are collected simultaneously with the scale data provide evidence of concurrent validity.
  - Data that are collected some time after the scale data provide evidence for predictive validity.
- Construct validity extends criterion-related validity into a broader arena in which the scale in question is tested against a theoretical model and adjusted according to results that can, in turn, help refine theory.
- The ability of an instrument to differentiate groups of patients expected to differ in HQL is also an important validation of its sensitivity.

### Validity is not absolute

- Validity data are cumulative, requiring ongoing updates and refinements. Validity is relative, in that a given measure might be valid in one setting and not in another.
  - An HQL measure should assess well-being in addition to impairment.
  - Statistical significance is not always clinically meaningful.

## Acceptability of Measures

- Intrusiveness or inappropriateness of items can damage the integrity of an HQL measure that might otherwise be quite sound.

• While reliability and validity are certainly important, they are not static standards.

## QUALITY-OF-LIFE MEASURES FOR USE IN ONCOLOGY

### Psychometric Measures

#### Quality-of-Life Index (QLI)

• The QLI was developed originally as a 10-point physician rating of five areas of functioning (activity, daily living, health, support, outlook). Since then, many have used this observer rating scale as a patient-rated scale, with reasonable success.

• The QLI has demonstrated the ability to distinguish cancer patients with terminal disease from either patients with recent disease or ones who were engaged in active treatment.

#### European Organization for Research and Treatment of Cancer Quality-of-Life Questionnaire—Core (EORTC-QLQ)

• This measure is a 36-item instrument consisting of both dichotomous responses (yes/no) and responses that utilize a 4-point rating scale ranging from "not at all" to "very much."

• The 36-item QLQ has been replaced with a 30-item version that reduces the number of physical- and emotional-functioning items and replaces the single concentration and memory item with two separate items.

#### Functional Living Index—Cancer (FLIC)

• This is a 22-item scale on which patients indicate the impact of cancer on "day-to-day living issues that represent the global construct of functional quality of life," using a 7-point Likert-type rating.

#### Functional Assessment of Cancer Therapy (FACT) scales

• This instrument is a 29–49 item compilation of a generic core (29 items) and over 20 specific sub-scales, which reflect symptoms or problems associated with different diseases, treatments, or other concerns.

• The FACT-G (general core) is able to distinguish metastatic from nonmetastatic disease. It also distinguishes between stage I, II, III, and IV disease, and between inpatients and outpatients from different centers.

• A unique feature of the FACT scales is that they provide supplemental valuative ratings that allow patients to provide domain-specific utility weights.

#### Ferrans and Powers Quality of Life Index (QLI)

• The QLI is a 68-item index of overall quality of life, which provides a summary score of four health domains: health and physical functioning; social and economic; psychological/spiritual; and family. A unique feature of the instrument is its two-part response format, which allows people to rate satisfaction with 34 areas and then has them rate their perceived importance of those same areas.

#### Cancer Rehabilitation Evaluation System—Short Form (CARES—SF)

• This is a 59-item self-administered rehabilitation and HQL instrument composed of a list of statements reflecting problems encountered by cancer patients.

#### Linear Analogue Self-Assessment (LASA) scales

• LASA scales use a 100-mm line with descriptors at each extreme. Respondents are required to mark their current state somewhere along that line, which is then measured as a score in centimeters or millimeters from the 0 point.

- Items include ten on symptoms and side effects, five on physical functioning, five on mood, and five on social relationships.
- Linear analogue scales are appealing because they are easy to administer and are usually presumed to have robust sensitivity due to interval scaling and a wide range of scores. They have also been criticized on the grounds that their sensitivity may be illusory and that it is difficult to know the minimal clinically significant difference.

### Medical Outcomes Study—Short-Form Health Status Survey (MOS SF-36)

- The Medical Outcomes Study—Short-Form Health Status Survey (MOS SF-36) is a self-administered 36-item measure of eight health concepts: physical functioning, limitations in role functioning due to physical health problems, social functioning, bodily pain, general mental health, limitations in role functioning due to emotional problems, vitality, and general health perceptions.

## Utility Measures

### Quality of Well-Being (QWB) Scale

- The QWB is a utility-based measure of HQL. Kaplan and Anderson focus on the qualitative dimension of functioning rather than exclusively on the psychological and social attributes of health outcomes, and use the term *health-related QL* to refer to the impact of health conditions on function. The Quality of Well-Being (QWB) scale is a 25-item list of symptom/problem complexes (CPX) covering the domains of mobility, physical activity, and social activity, each representing related but distinct aspects of daily functioning.

### Quality-Adjusted Time Without Symptoms and Toxicity (Q-TWiST)

- The only utility approach developed specifically for assessing cancer patients, the Quality-Adjusted Time Without Symptoms and Toxicity (Q-TWiST) approach, attempts to evaluate the effectiveness of treatments relative to one another by partitioning posttreatment time into distinct health states.

## OTHER APPLICATIONS OF HQL DATA

- There are other important applications of HQL data. These include rehabilitation planning, predicting survival and treatment response, and predicting treatment preferences.
- Survival prediction is a feature common to virtually every HQL assessment tool that has tested this component of prediction validity.

## PRACTICE QUESTIONS

1. You have been asked to conduct a seminar stressing the values and limitations of an approach that uses quality of life as an outcome of cancer treatment. As part of your opening discussion, you intend to stress that the psychometric approach:
   a. tells us how important a given problem or set of problems is to a group of patients.
   b. places heavy emphasis on an individual's response and response variability.
   c. is explicitly concerned with treatment decision making, usually at a policy level.
   d. extends the cost-effectiveness approach by evaluating the HQL benefit, thereby including the patient's perspective.

2. The reliability of a measure can be said to depend on:
   a. the homogeneity or consistency of the items on the scale.
   b. the extent to which it produces the same score when applied to two different times or in two different ways.
   c. test-retest or alternate form and interrater repeatability.
   d. all of the above.

3. Content validity:
   a. need not depend on the degree to which the scale superficially appears to measure the contruct.
   b. includes the degree to which the items represent the range of significant attributes.
   c. includes statistical evidence to support inferences.
   d. must include the physical and psychological domains, but not the social (which is covered under construct validity).

4. The QLI:
   a. was originally a patient-rated scale of five areas of functioning (activity, daily living, health, support, and outlook).
   b. cannot be expected to distinguish cancer patients with terminal illness from those with recent disease or active treatment, as was once popularly assumed.
   c. is probably the best example of a "cancer-specific" scale that in reality measures generic health concepts.
   d. all of the above.

5. Evelyn uses the FLIC scale to assess a group of patients to determine the impact of cancer on daily issues. The degree to which this scale superficially appears to measure the construct in question is referred to as:
   a. face validity.
   b. true content validity.
   c. construct validity.
   d. criterion validity.

6. Evelyn discovers that validity data:
   a. are cumulative.
   b. require ongoing updates and refinements.
   c. are relative.
   d. all of the above.

## ANSWER EXPLANATIONS

1.  **The answer is b.** The psychometric approach places heavy emphasis on an individual's response and response variability. While it provides the detailed perspective of the patient, it does not tell us how important a given problem or set of problems is to a group of patients. It is HQL evaluation in general that differs from classic toxicity ratings by incorporating more aspects of function (of which mood, affect, and social well-being are parts) than those typically attributed to treatment. The utility approach is explicitly concerned with treatment decision making, usually at a policy level, and the cost-utility approach extends the cost-effectiveness approach by evaluating the HQL benefit, thereby including the patient's perspective. (p. 205–206)

2.  **The answer is d.** Two synonyms for reliability are repeatability and consistency. Repeatability refers to the extent to which a measure, applied two different times (test-retest) or in two different ways (alternate form and interrater), produces the same score. Consistency refers to the homogeneity of the items of a scale. Reliability is not a fixed property of measure and it cannot be assumed to be generalizable. (p. 206)

3.  **The answer is b.** Content validity includes both face validity (the degree to which the scale superficially appears to measure the construct in question), and true content validity (the degree to which the items accurately represent the range of attributes covered by the construct). Content validity does not include statistical evidence to support inferences made from tests, but it should cut across at least three broad domains (e.g., the physical, psychological, and social) to be considered valid from the perspective of item content. (p. 207)

4.  **The answer is c.** The QLI is probably the best example of a "cancer-specific" scale that in reality measures generic health concepts. It was originally a physician-rated scale of five areas of functioning (activity, daily living, health, support, and outlook). It has been shown to distinguish cancer patients with terminal illness from those with recent disease or active treatment, as was once popularly assumed. (p. 208)

5.  **The answer is a.** The degree to which a scale superficially appears to measure the construct in question is referred to as face validity. The degree to which the items accurately represent the range of attributes covered by the construct is called true content validity. Criterion validity includes both concurrent and predictive validity: data collected simultaneously with the scale data provide evidence of concurrent validity. Data collected after the scale data provide evidence for predictive validity. Construct validity extends criterion validity to test the scale in question against a theoretical model and adjusts it according to results to help refine theory. (p. 207)

6.  **The answer is d.** Validity data are cumulative, requiring ongoing updates and refinements. Validity is relative, in that a given measure might be valid in one setting and not in another. (p. 208)

# Chapter 11    Principles of Treatment Planning

## INTRODUCTION

- Therapeutic decisions in oncology are based on the location, cell type, and extent of the malignancy, with established modes of therapy directed toward the particular disease presentation.
- The aim of treatment is to cure or to palliate, causing minimal structural or functional impairment of the individual.
- The sequence in treatment planning consists of gathering information, planning, executing the plan, and evaluating.
- The recipient of cancer treatment is a unique human being; every aspect of the design and evaluation of therapeutic activities must take the individual's unique needs into consideration.

## HISTORICAL PERSPECTIVES ON CANCER TREATMENT

- Survival rates for cancer during the first 50 years of this century improved dramatically as methods for detecting and surgically removing primary tumors improved and morbidity from treatment decreased. However, by the 1950s cancer survival plateaued as cancers believed to be localized were shown to have micrometastases at diagnosis.
- Traditionally, surgeons managed the treatment of most cancer patients. Over the past 80 years a number of developments have marked a new approach to cancer therapy.
  - Treatment involving a combination of surgery, radiotherapy, and chemotherapy began to emerge.
  - Medical oncology became a specialty.
  - Oncology nursing became more sophisticated and carried greater responsibility for all aspects of patient management.
  - Consultation by oncology specialists became freely available.
  - Patients could often be treated in the community.
  - Care became increasingly palliative and research-oriented.
  - Special oncology units and cancer rehabilitation programs in local hospitals and hospice development in local communities became common.
- Control has joined cure and palliation as a part of cancer treatment. Control refers to keeping cancer within bounds for increasingly longer periods through a combination of therapies.

## FACTORS INVOLVED IN TREATMENT PLANNING

### The Patient Presents

- Any unexplained pain or energy loss, any irregularity in a body system, and any lumps or bumps should be investigated.

### A Diagnostic Workup Is Begun

- A detailed history, physical exam, and hematological, biochemical, and radiological studies must be performed.

### A Biopsy Is Done

- Histological proof of malignancy is the cornerstone of diagnosis and treatment.

- A biopsy is also a useful guide to prognosis.
- Treating without a tissue diagnosis could lead to disaster if the lesion were later found to be benign.

## The Biopsy Establishes the Diagnosis

- The pathologist's report is crucial in oncology because it conveys the significance of a given neoplasm.
- The two major agencies involved in the standardization of the language of malignant disease are the International Union Against Cancer (UICC) and the American Joint Committee on Cancer (AJCC).

## Classifying the Tumor

- Cancers are classified, or staged, via two main approaches: *pathological*, based on information about the tumor, and *clinical*, based on information about the host (patient).
- See Table 11-1, text page 219.

### Pathological classification

- The current and best pathological classification system includes critical information, anticipated biological behavior, histogenesis (tissue of origin), and grade.
- In terms of *biological behavior*, tumors can be divided into benign or malignant groups.
  - A benign tumor is well circumscribed or encapsulated: it is made up of cells similar to those of its parent tissue.
  - A malignant tumor invades the organs from which it originated and eventually surrounding tissues or distant sites; it is made up of cells that vary greatly in size and shape.
- The suffix *oma* implies, simply, tumor.
- Malignant tumors arising in epithelial tissues are known as *carcinoma*. *Sarcoma* refers to malignant tumors involving mesenchymal tissues.
- *Histopathological type* is a qualitative assessment whereby a neoplasm is categorized in terms of the tissue or cell type from which it has originated.
- A lesion with the same cell type but at a site other than the original site would indicate a *metastatic* tumor.
- A different cell type originating from another lesion anywhere in the body would indicate a second primary cancer.
- *Histopathological grade* is a quantitative assessment of the extent to which the tumor resembles the tissue of origin.
- Grade is expressed in both numerical and descriptive terms: well differentiated (grade I), moderately differentiated (grade II), poorly differentiated (grade III), or undifferentiated (grade IV).
- Cytogenetic analysis plays an important part, particularly in hematological neoplasms.

### Clinical classification

- Further testing is needed to assess the clinical extent of the disease. This process is called *staging*.
- By following the TNM system, the extent of disease is evaluated separately with respect to the primary tumor site (T), the regional lymph nodes (N), and the presence or absence of metastasis (M). The basic TNM model is expanded by using subcategories to describe how far the disease has progressed and the extent of metastasis, if any.
- *Stage groupings* involve combining the various classification elements of defined T, N, and M.
- There are two main staging periods: (1) before treatment starts and (2) retreatment.
  - *Pretreatment staging* is based on tests and evidence gathered before the first treatment is begun.
    - There are two aspects to pretreatment staging of a previously undiagnosed cancer: *clinical-diagnostic* staging, for patients who have had a biopsy and *postsurgical resection-pathological* staging, which includes a complete evaluation of the surgical specimen by a pathologist.

- *Retreatment staging* occurs if the patient has a recurrence following a disease-free interval and needs further treatment. Restaging, or reevaluation, may be done after a prescribed course of treatment to document remission.
- *Autopsy staging* may occur to assess the extent of disease at death.

## DETERMINING THE TREATMENT PLAN

- A series of crucial decisions are made regarding prognosis, anticipated response, and individual condition.
- The most effective, most definitive treatment aimed at cure for a given cancer is called *primary therapy.*

### Should Treatment Be Aimed at Cure?

- Generally, oncologists tend to think of tumors with 5-year survival probabilities in the range of 1%–5% as having no or minimal chance for cure.
- The risks involved with any method must also be related to the person's age and condition.
- A correct decision on whether to treat for cure is one of the most important decisions that the oncologist must make.
- The patient's feelings and values are crucial to the decision.

### Which Modality Should Be Used?

- After the decision to treat for cure, the next decision involves choosing the optimal modality or combination thereof. *Multimodality therapy* is the treatment strategy most often utilized.
- Basic principles for treatment selection that have evolved include the following:
  - When tumors are large, locally aggressive, and contiguous to adjacent structures, radiotherapy might be given prior to surgery.
  - Both *radiation* and *chemotherapy* may be given after surgery.
    - Radiation will usually be indicated if the tumor is found to be invading nearby tissues that cannot be surgically resected. Chemotherapy would be used to eliminate micrometastasis.
    - Radiation and chemotherapy have been combined in an attempt to produce a more powerful antitumor effect than either treatment can produce alone. Chemotherapy is sometimes used prior to radiotherapy to shrink a lesion, since radiation has a more effective tumoricidal action against smaller lesions.
  - The new biological therapies are being blended with standard radiotherapy and chemotherapy.
- The best approach for treatment planning and evaluation is for an interdisciplinary group to share in the decision-making process.
- Nurses may be involved in any number of ways: as staff nurses, enterostomal therapists, clinical specialists, nurse practitioners, case managers, or discharge planners, to name a few.
- See Table 11-3, text page 223, and Table 11-4, text page 224.

### The Benefit of Clinical Trials

- Clinicians turn to clinical trials for guidance in making therapeutic decisions. These constitute the only sure foundation for therapeutic progress.
- A randomized clinical trial is defined as a carefully and ethically designed experiment with the aim of answering a precisely framed question.
- The publication of results of clinical trials allows clinicians from around the world to build on treatment successes. Replication of the experiment at other institutions ensures that treatment outcomes are not serendipitous.
- However, no clinical trial can absolutely guarantee the best treatment for an individual.

## Selecting a Treatment Plan

- If a patient cannot be entered into an existing trial, which is the optimal choice, then other choices are as follows:
  - Conventional or standard regimens are those that have been studied extensively, used for a long time, and are widely accepted for common cancers.
  - If there is no conventional treatment program suitable for the case, the physician usually tries to find a study in the literature that documents a successful treatment program for the situation.
  - If all else fails, the physician will develop an individualized treatment plan.
- See Table 11-5, text page 225.

## ASSESSING RESPONSE TO TREATMENT

- Responses to treatment may be classified as *objective* or *subjective*. See Table 11-6, text page 226.
- Objective responses include:
  - *Complete response*: Complete disappearance of signs and symptoms of cancer, lasting at least 1 month.
  - *Partial response*: A 50% or more reduction in the sum of the products of the greater and lesser diameters of all measured lesions, lasting at least 1 month, without the development of any new lesions during therapy.
  - *Progression*: A 25% or more increase in the sum of the products of the greater and lesser diameters of all measured lesions, or the emergence of new lesions.
  - *Stable disease*: Not any of above.
- When treatment is completed, reevaluation, often called *restaging*, focuses particular attention on the disease parameters that were positive at diagnosis to signal a search for any remaining evidence that treatment should continue.
- Restaging does not imply that if a remission is obtained the patient reverts to a lesser disease stage. The stage ascribed at the time of diagnosis is the one referenced throughout the illness.

## Survival Statistics

- The only precise definition of cure is "no evidence of tumor at biopsy." However, most clinicians accept freedom from clinical evidence of recurrent metastatic disease during the person's lifetime as a reasonably reliable estimate.
- In oncology, "cure" is a statistical term that applies to groups of cancer patients rather than to an individual.
- The observation over time of individuals with cancer and the calculation of their probability of surviving over several time periods is called *survival analysis*.

## Patient Follow-up

- An integral part of a hospital's cancer program is a tumor registry or cancer data center where systematic follow-up of individuals with cancer facilitates evaluation of therapy.

## WHEN A CURE IS NOT ACHIEVED

- Should the disease recur, there may be a long period during which treatment is aimed at control. Cancer can thus be viewed as a chronic disease, similar to diabetes or heart disease, where cure is impossible and control is the objective.
- When relapse occurs, survival can be prolonged with proper treatment.
- *Palliative measures* may sometimes be used to minimize cost, discomfort, and compression of vital organs.

## FUTURE PROSPECTS

- The current era of cancer treatment features rather crude interventions based on our understanding of the disease: that cancer is usually systemic at presentation and that it involves a complex spectrum of host-tumor interrelations.
- Future strategies for cancer treatment may feature gene therapy, antineoplastic agents and delivery systems that exploit the differences between normal and malignant cells, the use of new and improved biologicals, and biological response modifiers.

# PRACTICE QUESTIONS

1. Mr. Axtel is about to begin combination chemotherapy. In the course of planning patient education, you intend to tell him that this therapy:
   a. eliminates the need for pulse dosing.
   b. involves concomitant use of drugs and radiotherapy.
   c. involves high doses of multiple drugs being given intermittently.
   d. a and b.

2. Mr. Vance has just had surgery and will need both radiation and chemotherapy. Why would these both be given after surgery?
   a. Sometimes it is difficult for the surgeon to assess before surgery whether invasion and excision is the best choice.
   b. Most likely, the tumor was found to be invading nearby tissues that could not be surgically resected, and micrometastasis is a potential problem.
   c. Radiotherapy before surgery is only appropriate as a first-line means of defense; the surgery was a second-line treatment that was unsuccessful, so a more aggressive third line—combination therapy—is now being employed.
   d. b and c

3. A benign tumor:
   a. is well circumscribed or encapsulated and appears orderly.
   b. is not made up of cells similar to those of its parent tissue.
   c. invades the organs from which it originated and is made up of cells that vary greatly in size and shape.
   d. a and b

4. Malignant tumors arising in glandular epithelial tissues are known as:
   a. sarcomas.
   b. osteosarcomas.
   c. transitional cell carcinomas.
   d. adenocarcinomas.

5. Histopathological type refers to:
   a. a qualitative assignment given to a lesion at a site other than the orginal site that is of the *same* cell type as the original; this is used to determine metastatic tumors.
   b. a quantitative assessment of the extent to which the tumor resembles the tissue of origin.
   c. a qualitative assessment whereby a neoplasm is categorized in terms of the tissue or cell type from which it has originated.
   d. a qualitative assignment that indicates that a lesion at a site other than the original site is of a *different* cell type than the original tumor; this is used to indicate a second primary cancer.

6. Stage groupings involve:
   a. combining the various classification elements of tumor site, regional lymph node involvement, and the presence or absence of metastasis.
   b. two main staging periods: pretreatment and posttreatment.
   c. two main staging periods: clinical diagnostic staging and pretreatment staging.
   d. a and b.

**Questions 7–9 concern Ms. Trent, who is newly diagnosed with cancer.**

7. Ms. Trent's cancer is being evaluated using the pathological classification system. You must keep in mind that this system:
   a. is effective only for malignant tumors, not for benign tumors.
   b. assesses the clinical extent of the disease.
   c. is based on information about the tumor, using a combination of anticipated biological behavior, histogenesis, and grade.
   d. is based on an accurate assessment of the host's susceptibility, receptiveness to agents, and possible resistance to chemotherapy.

8. Ms. Trent's physician is in the process of selecting her treatment plan. His order of preference for protocol, from most desirable to least desirable choice, is probably:
   a. conventional or standard treatment, a unique individualized treatment plan, a clinical trial, or (last choice) protocol from an abstract or journal article.
   b. clinical trial, conventional treatment, unique individualized treatment program, professional conference abstract, or (last choice) a journal article.
   c. unique individualized treatment plan, clinical trial, standard approach, or (last choice) journal article or abstract.
   d. clinical trial, conventional treatment plan, protocol from a journal article or abstract, and (last choice) a unique individualized treatment plan.

9. After a course of treatment, Ms. Trent's treatment response is evaluated. This reevaluation or restaging:
   a. makes possible the redesignation of a more appropriate stage to be referenced throughout the remaining course of the illness, replacing the stage ascribed at the time of diagnosis.
   b. focuses attention on the disease parameters that were positive at diagnosis.
   c. determines whether the patient is eligible to participate in a clinical trial.
   d. a and b.

10. In oncology, the tendency is to use the term "cure" to refer to:
   a. groups of cancer patients.
   b. an individual who has a normal recovery with the return to health.
   c. an individual who no longer exhibits symptoms, gains lost weight, and resumes normal activity.
   d. all of the above, but in differing circumstances.

11. Palliative treatment:
   a. is never used on asymptomatic individuals to minimize cost, risk and inconvenience to the patient.
   b. is used when impending development of a catastrophic problem can be predicted.
   c. is used only when the disease is incurable.
   d. a and c.

## ANSWER EXPLANATIONS

1. **The answer is c.** In combination chemotherapy, multiple drugs are given concurrently in pulse dosing (high doses are given intermittently). (p. 217)
2. **The answer is b.** Radiation is usually indicated if the tumor is found to be invading nearby tissues that cannot be surgically resected. Chemotherapy is used to eliminate micrometastasis. (p. 223)

3.  **The answer is a.** A benign tumor is well circumscribed or encapsulated: microscopically, it appears orderly and is made up of cells similar to those of its parent tissue. A malignant tumor invades the organs from which it originated and eventually the surrounding tissues; it is made up of cells that vary greatly in size and shape. (p. 219)

4.  **The answer is d.** Malignant tumors arising in glandular epithelial tissues are known as adenocarcinomas. (p. 219)

5.  **The answer is c.** Histopathological type is a qualitative assessment whereby a neoplasm is categorized in terms of the tissue or cell type from which it has originated. Histopathological *grade* is a quantitative assessment of the extent to which the tumor resembles the tissue of origin. A lesion with the same cell type but at a site other than the original site would indicate a metastatic tumor; and a different cell type originating from another lesion anywhere in the body would indicate a second primary cancer. (pp. 219–220)

6.  **The answer is a.** Stage groupings involve combining the various classification elements of tumor site, regional lymph node involvement, and the presence or absence of metastasis. It involves two main staging periods: pretreatment and retreatment. There are two aspects to pretreatment staging of a previously undiagnosed cancer: clinical diagnostic staging, for patients who have had a biopsy, and *postsurgical resection-pathological* staging, which includes a complete evaluation of the surgical specimen by a pathologist. (p. 221)

7.  **The answer is c.** The pathological classification system is based on information about the tumor, using a combination of anticipated biolocial behavior, histogenesis, and grade. By contrast, clinical classification is based on an accurate assessment of the host. A qualitative assessment whereby a neoplasm is categorized in terms of the tissue or cell type from which it has originated is not called staging; it is the histopathological type and is only one aspect of pathological classification. (pp. 218–19)

8.  **The answer is d.** The optimal treatment plan from the physician's point of view would have the patient entered into an existing clinical trial, if one fits the patient's stage of disease and the patient is eligible and willing. If this is not an option, conventional or standard regimens that have been studied for a long time are widely accepted for common cancers. If no conventional program is appropriate, the physician usually tries to find a study in the literature that documents a successful treatment program. Abstracts (synopses of oral presentations) are less detailed and thus less helpful. If all else fails, the physician will develop a protocol specific to the situation. (pp. 225–226)

9.  **The answer is b.** Restaging focuses particular attention on the disease parameters that were positive at diagnosis to signal a search for any remaining evidence that treatment should continue. Restaging does not imply that if a remission is obtained the patient reverts to a lesser disease stage. The stage ascribed at the time of diagnosis is the one referenced throughout the illness. (p. 226)

10. **The answer is a.** In oncology, "cure" is a statistical term that applies to groups of cancer patients rather than to individuals. An individual's normal recovery—with the return to health, weight gain, and the resumption of normal activity—is not conclusive evidence that a cure has been achieved. The nature of cancer is such that even after a long time interval of apparent health, the disease may reappear and the person may die. If at autopsy there is no evidence of tumor, a cancer can be said to have been cured, but this is of little practical value. (p. 226)

11. **The answer is b.** Palliative measures may sometimes be needed for people who are asymptomatic in whom the impending development of a catastrophic probem can be predicted, such as obstruction of the superior vena cava or a major bronchus, or a collapsing vertebral body. However, palliative treatment of most patients who are asymptomatic and incurable is usually deferred until the appearance of specific problems. (p. 227)

# Chapter 12    Surgical Therapy

## FACTORS INFLUENCING SURGICAL ONCOLOGY
### Ambulatory Surgery

- Over 50% of the surgical procedures performed in the United States today occur within the ambulatory setting.
- Individuals with cancer who have an ambulatory procedure for treatment or diagnosis usually need additional support and education.

### Technological Advances

- Lasers, laparoscopes, endoscopes, conscious sedation, and new anesthetic agents are among the leading approaches in ambulatory surgical care.

### Economic Forces

- Economic forces and managed care have precipitated development of aggressive measures to reduce lengthy and costly hospital stays.
- In many settings, nurses act as case managers to assist the patient and family in the complex negotiations necessary in the continuum of cancer care.

## FACTORS INFLUENCING TREATMENT DECISIONS
### Tumor Cell Kinetics

- Tumor cell characteristics such as growth rate, differentiation, metastatic potential, and metastatic pattern affect the treatment decision.

#### Growth rate

- The rate of growth of a tumor is expressed in terms of volume-doubling time.
- Tumors that are slow growing and that consist of cells with prolonged cell cycles lend themselves best to surgical treatment.

#### Invasiveness

- A surgical procedure intended to be curative involves resection of the entire tumor mass and normal tissue surrounding the tumor to ensure a margin of safety for removal of all cancer cells.

#### Metastatic potential

- Subclinical metastasis or occult disease is responsible for most recurrences when surgery has been the only treatment used. It is thought that micrometastases are present in 60% of individuals by the time a tumor is large enough to be detected clinically.

## Tumor Location

- Superficial and encapsulated tumors are more easily resected than those that are embedded in inaccessible or delicate tissues or those that have invaded tissues in multiple directions.

## Physical Status

- Evaluation of respiratory, cardiovascular, nutritional, immunologic, renal, and central nervous system (CNS) status is important.
- The health care team assesses the patient's rehabilitation potential.

## Quality of Life

- The goal of therapy for the patient with cancer varies according to the stage of disease.

# PREVENTING CANCER USING SURGICAL PROCEDURES

- Certain conditions, diseases, and genetic or congenital traits are known to be associated with a higher risk of developing cancer. In some instances, surgical removal of nonvital benign tissue responsible for predisposing the individual can lower incidence and possibly prevent occurrence of cancer.

# DIAGNOSING CANCER USING SURGICAL TECHNIQUES

- Surgical diagnostic techniques such as endoscopy, needle aspiration, incisional biopsy, excisional biopsy, and core needle biopsy are commonly used to procure cells or tissue specimens for histopathologic examination.
- Only positive biopsy findings are definitive.
- A negative biopsy finding can mean no cancer, but it can also mean that the biopsy specimen was not representative of the tumor.
- The placement and orientation of the biopsy incision should facilitate any further surgical resections deemed necessary.
- Minimum disruption or disturbance to the bulk of the tumor, while achieving an adequate specimen, requires careful consideration prior to biopsy.
- Important principles of biopsy include minimizing dissection and maintaining adequate hemostasis.

## Needle Biopsy: Fine Needle and Core Needle

- Needle biopsies are usually performed in an outpatient setting. Local or topical anesthesia is commonly used. Some needles have carriers that reduce the possibility of contaminating the needle tract with tumor cells from the specimen as the needle is withdrawn.
- Fine-needle aspiration or biopsy is the procedure of choice when there is a high index of suspicion for malignancy and the lesion is both accessible and solid.
- Core biopsies, which include percutaneous biopsies, are usually indicated when there is a need to confirm malignancy, yet there is clinical and diagnostic evidence that the disease will be treated with nonsurgical approaches.
- If surgery is likely, the biopsy approach selected is often the fine needle rather than the core biopsy.
- Regional biopsy involves obtaining several samples of tissue from different locations within a tumor or within a diseased organ.

## Surgical Biopsy: Excisional, Incisional, Endoscopic

- *Excisional biopsy* is performed on small, discrete, accessible tumors to remove the entire suspected mass with little or no margin of surrounding normal tissue.

- *Incisional biopsy* is generally selected for the diagnosis of a large tumor that will require major surgery for complete removal.
- *Endoscopy* is used to obtain biopsy specimens for diagnosis of tumors in accessible lumens.

## STAGING CANCER USING SURGICAL PROCEDURES

- Exploratory surgical procedures can be done to diagnose most intracavitary tumors or to define the extent of tumor growth, size, nodal involvement, implants, or multiorgan involvement.
- If distant metastases are present, radical surgery is usually not indicated, and the focus of treatment quickly shifts from local control to systemic treatment or palliation.

## SURGERY FOR TREATMENT OF CANCER

- Preoperative considerations include a thorough patient and family history and physical examination.

### Surgery Aimed at Cure

#### Resection—local and radical

- Local resection is used for small lesions if the entire tumor and an adequate margin of tumor-free tissue can be encompassed in the excision.
- Radical surgical resections are performed when the tumor is surgically accessible and there is hope that the tumor can be resected en bloc along with the necessary local or regional tissues and lymphatics.
- Striking a balance between length of life and quality of life is a major challenge in surgical oncology.
- Indications for extensive radical surgery include primary tumors that grow slowly, have wide local infiltration, and are large. The emotional and adaptive challenges to the patient receiving this type of surgery must be carefully assessed and evaluated before electing to proceed.
- During the preoperative period, it is important that the individual understand the anticipated outcomes of surgical therapy, as well as how surgery fits in the overall plan of therapy.

#### Surgery and adjuvant therapies

- Combination or adjuvant therapies are used to improve the rates of cure and disease-free survival.
- Surgery may be combined with radiotherapy for local and regional tumor control.
- Chemotherapy is given to provide systemic control of micrometastases and distant metastases.
- In some situations cytoreductive surgery is used to debulk or reduce the tumor mass to a size that enables combination therapy to be most effective.

#### Excision of metastatic lesions

- Surgery also may be used to resect a metastatic lesion if the primary tumor is believed to be eradicated, if the metastatic site is solitary, and if the patient can undergo surgery without significant morbidity.

### Surgery Aimed at Palliation

- The goal of palliative surgery is to relieve suffering and minimize the symptoms of the disease.
- Several surgical techniques are used for palliation of cancer: fulgeration, electrocoagulation, lasers, photodynamic therapy, shunts, and bone stabilization procedures.
- Palliative surgery is particularly useful in relieving suffering caused by an obstructive process.

## Surgery for Rehabilitation

- The development of various implants, microvascular surgery, allografts, and autogenous reconstructive techniques has enlarged the scope of reconstructive surgery.
- Rehabilitative teaching and counseling generally are begun before primary surgical therapy is initiated. Some people fear that their desire for rehabilitative surgical procedures will be interpreted as valuing their physical appearance or function as more important than the length of their life. Nurses can assist the patient to see that rehabilitation is desirable and sometimes necessary.

## SPECIAL CONSIDERATIONS FOR NURSING CARE

### Surgical Setting and Length of Stay

- Because the period of contact with health care professionals during surgical care is of such short duration, it is most important for patients and their families to know whom to contact and how to do so when they need help or further information.

### General Surgical Care and Oncological Emergencies

- The surgical patient may experience a complex set of reactions and responses to therapy that may be precipitated by the concomitant therapies or the complications of the underlying disease process itself.

### Autologous Blood Donation

- Nonanemic patients can donate up to 6 units of blood prior to surgery. Blood usually can be donated from 42 days to 72 hours prior to surgery.

### Anxiety and Pain Control

- Anxiety and pain control should be addressed prior to the actual operation to allow patients to verbalize fears, and to be made aware of advances in methods of pain relief.
- Health care professionals should make it a priority to encourage and teach methods of reducing anxiety and providing pain relief.
- In the preoperative period, nurses should be acutely aware of problems that can occur as a result of the cancer disease process itself, as well as anticipating possible postoperative complications.

### Nutritional Support

- Protein-calorie malnutrition is a common occurrence among cancer patients, especially those with advanced disease.
- The individual with cancer undergoing surgery may be experiencing the advanced symptoms of cachexia: a syndrome of weight loss, anorexia, and wasting of lean body mass.
- The nutritional plan is based on the metabolic needs of the patient, which can vary from hypermetabolic to hypometabolic.
- The route of administration of nutritional support should be considered in the following sequence:
  1. Enteral nutrition is the preferred route when the gastrointestinal (GI) tract is functioning.
  2. Total parenteral nutrition (TPN) for brief periods may be indicated in a severely malnourished patient who cannot be fed.
  3. Total parenteral nutrition for prolonged periods or home TPN is only indicated in situations where enteral feeding is not feasible because of advanced disease or severe toxicities.

### Hemostasis

- Elevated clotting factors and shortened partial thromboplastin and prothrombin times have been noted to occur in individuals with cancer.

- An individual with cancer is more likely to develop postoperative thrombophlebitis.
- The importance of early postoperative ambulation cannot be overemphasized. These individuals are at high risk for deep-vein thrombosis.

## Combined Modality Therapy

- Chemotherapy, radiation therapy, and biotherapy are being given for certain tumors in varied sequences, including preoperative, intraoperative, and postoperative treatment.
- Preoperative chemotherapy or radiotherapy, alone or in combination, is used with particular tumors.
- Wound healing may become a more significant problem with combined modality therapy.
- Surgical procedures sometimes become necessary during active radiation or chemotherapy treatment cycles.
- Preoperative assessment of the patient who is actively receiving combination therapy is specifically focused on those body systems and organs that are being affected by the current therapy.
- Intraoperative radiotherapy or intraoperative chemotherapy involves the delivery of a single, high dose directly to the surgically exposed tumor or tumor bed.
- Intraoperative treatments are administered for locally advanced abdominal and pelvic malignancies.
- Once the integrity of the tissue is damaged by radiation, additional trauma is not tolerated well. Postoperative wound dehiscence, infection, tissue necrosis, and bone necrosis are potential complications of surgery performed on previously irradiated tissue.
- Radiation itself will interfere with healing if it is administered in the early postoperative period.
- Critical phases of wound healing last for about 25 days following incision. During the proliferative phase of wound healing, which can last from 3 to 25 days following surgery, granulation tissue is formed and provides the characteristic strength of a wound.
- Most chemotherapy agents act by interfering with protein synthesis.
- Wound healing could be disrupted by the administration of most chemotherapeutic agents in the early phases of wound healing.

## CONCLUSION

- Adjuvant therapy can lengthen survival and disease-free intervals and improve the quality of life. The potential side effects of combination modality therapies present new challenges to health care practitioners.

# PRACTICE QUESTIONS

1. You have recently become part of a new, interdisciplinary oncological team. You are aware that situations lending themselves best to surgical treatment include such factors as:
   a. slow-growing tumors that consist of cells with prolonged cell cycles.
   b. an ability to achieve resection of the entire tumor mass as well as a margin of safety of normal, healthy tissue surrounding the tumor.
   c. embedded tumors.
   d. a and b.

2. The following patients have been recently diagnosed: Mr. Alexander has a superficial skin cancer; Ms. Jeffries has a musculoskeletal encapsulated tumor; Mrs. Myers' tumor is embedded deep within the abdomen and pelvis; Mr. Mitchell's tumor has invaded tissues and organs in multiple directions. Which of the following are true?
   a. Mr. Mitchell's and Ms. Jeffries' cancers need immediate resection.
   b. Mrs. Myers' tumor should be treated with radiation, and Mr. Alexander's should be treated only with a topical antineoplastic agent; neither will benefit from surgery at this point.
   c. Mr. Alexander and Ms. Jeffries will most likely benefit from surgical resection.
   d. None of the above offer the best treatment options.

**Questions 3–5 concern Mr. Kramer, who is about to undergo diagnostic biopsy.**

3. Mr. Kramer is about to have a diagnostic biopsy. He asks you how reliable this procedure is. You tell him that:
   a. only positive biopsy findings are definitive.
   b. a negative biopsy means no cancer.
   c. a positive biopsy can indicate that the specimen was not representative of the tumor.
   d. all of the above.

4. Mr. Kramer's physician tells you that there is a high degree of suspicion that Mr. Kramer has a malignancy and that she also believes surgery is likely. His lesion is both accessible and solid. Which biopsy procedure is Mr. Kramer most likely to receive?
   a. Large-needle biopsy
   b. Excisional biopsy
   c. Core biopsy
   d. Fine-needle biopsy

5. On further investigation, distant metastases are present in Mr. Kramer. Knowing nothing else, what would you predict will be the focus of treatment for Mr. Kramer?
   a. Radical surgery
   b. Local control
   c. Combined modality therapy
   d. Palliation only

6. Ms. Stein has a small lesion on her lip that is accessible. It is cancerous and must be eradicated. Which is most likely to be the treatment of choice?
   a. Simple radiation
   b. Local resection
   c. Radical resection
   d. Combined radiation and chemotherapy only

7.  Which of the following is *not* an example of palliative surgery?
    a.   Joshua's leg, which has a sarcoma, is amputated because it is nonfunctioning and painful.
    b.   Mary Ellen receives breast reconstruction following mastectomy.
    c.   Mike undergoes removal of an ulcerative lesion that is a likely source of infection.
    d.   Shante has undergone resection of her primary tumor to prevent obstruction.

8.  After surgery, a patient develops aspiration pneumonia. Which of the following symptoms may have caused this?
    a.   Difficulty in swallowing
    b.   Mechanical obstruction from cancer
    c.   Excessive sedation
    d.   All of the above

**Questions 9–12 concern Mr. Svensen, who has had complete eradication of a primary tumor.**

9.  Mr. Svensen has had treatment for a primary tumor, which was completely eradicated. Now, however, the surgeon discovers a metastatic lesion. The metastatic site seems to be solitary, and Mr. Svensen seems very healthy otherwise. Given these limited clues, what method of treatment would you predict will be used for Mr. Svensen's metastatic lesion?
    a.   Chemotherapy to provide systemic control of metastasis
    b.   Cytoreductive surgery to reduce the mass so combination therapy will be effective
    c.   Radiation and chemo combination therapy
    d.   Surgical resection

10. Mr. Svensen expresses an interest in autologous blood donation. You give him the following parameters needed to qualify. These include the following:
    a.   He must be nonanemic.
    b.   He can donate no more than 6 units of blood before surgery.
    c.   The blood can be donated from 42 days to 72 hours prior to surgery.
    d.   All of the above.

11. Review all information you have been given about Mr. Svensen so far. Based on this, which route of administration of nutritional support do you predict would be *most likely* to be appropriate for Mr. Svensen immediately following surgery?
    a.   Enteral nutrition
    b.   TPN for 7–10 days
    c.   Home TPN
    d.   None of the above

12. In the days *immediately* following Mr. Svensen's surgery:
    a.   one should not be surprised to see a temporary suppression of wound healing; healing will become more proliferative after 21 days.
    b.   chemotherapy agents can be used to best advantage.
    c.   granulation tissue is usually formed in the first 3 to 25 days following surgery, providing the characteristic strength of the wound.
    d.   b and c.

# ANSWER EXPLANATIONS

1.  **The answer is d.** Situations lending themselves best to surgical treatment include such factors as slow-growing tumors that consist of cells with prolonged cell cycles. A surgical procedure intended to be curative must involve resection of the entire tumor mass as well as a margin of safety of normal, healthy tissue surrounding the tumor. Superficial and encapsulated tumors are more easily resected than those that are embedded in inaccessible or delicate tissues. (p. 231)

2.  **The answer is c.** Superficial and encapsulated tumors are more easily resected than those that are embedded in inaccessible or delicate tissues or those that have invaded tissues and organs in multiple directions. (p. 231)

3.  **The answer is a.** Only positive biopsy findings are definitive. A negative biopsy finding can mean no cancer, but it can also mean that the specimen was not representative. (p. 232)

4.  **The answer is d.** Fine-needle aspiration or biopsy is the procedure of choice when there is a high index of suspicion for malignancy and the lesion is both accessible and solid. If surgery is likely, the approach selected is often, again, fine needle rather than the core biopsy. Core biopsies are usually indicated to confirm malignancy when there is clinical and diagnostic evidence that the disease will be treated with nonsurgical approaches. Excisional biopsy is performed on small, discrete, accessible tumors to remove the entire suspected mass with little or no margin of surrounding normal tissue. (p. 233)

5.  **The answer is c.** If distant metastases are present, radical surgery alone is usually not indicated, and the focus of treatment quickly shifts from local control to combined modality treatment. (p. 235)

6.  **The answer is b.** Local resection is used for small lesions if the entire tumor and an adequate margin of tumor-free tissue can be encompassed in the excision. Tumors of the ear, skin, or lip are typical lesions where local excision can be used as definitive therapy for cure. Radical surgical resections are performed when the tumor is surgically accessible, and there is hope that the tumor can be resected en bloc along with the necessary local or regional tissues and lymphatics. (p. 236)

7.  **The answer is b.** Breast reconstruction, while not curative, is considered a reconstructive rather than palliative procedure. The goal of palliative surgery is to relieve suffering and minimize the symptoms of the disease—for example, amputation of a nonfunctional, painful limb with sarcoma, or procedures like fulgeration, electrocoagulation, photodynamic therapy, and bond stabilization procedures. (p. 237)

8.  **The answer is d.** Aspiration pneumonia in the surgical oncology patient may be caused by difficulty in swallowing, mechanical obstruction from the cancer, or excessive sedation. (p. 239)

9.  **The answer is d.** Surgery may be used to resect a metastatic lesion if the primary tumor is believed to be eradicated, if the metastatic site is solitary, and if the patient can undergo surgery without significant morbidity. (p. 237)

10. **The answer is d.** Nonanemic patients can donate up to 6 units of blood prior to surgery. Blood usually can be donated from 42 days to 72 hours prior to surgery. (p. 241)

11. **The answer is a.** Because Mr. Svenson seems to be very healthy otherwise, enteral nutrition is the preferred route, assuming that his GI tract is functioning. Total parenteral nutrition (TPN) for brief periods (7–10 days) may be indicated in a severely malnourished patient who cannot be fed via the enteral route. Home TPN or prolonged TPN is only indicated in situations in which enteral feeding is not feasible because of advanced disease or severe toxicities. (p. 242)

12.  **The answer is c.** During the proliferative phase of wound healing, which lasts from 3 to 25 days following surgery, granulation tissue is formed and provides the characteristic strength of a wound. Most chemotherapy agents act by interfering with protein synthesis. Thus, wound healing could be disrupted by the administration of most chemotherapeutic agents in the early phases of wound healing. (p. 243)

# Chapter 13     Radiotherapy

## THE CURRENT APPLICATION OF RADIOTHERAPY IN THE MANAGEMENT OF THE PATIENT DIAGNOSED WITH CANCER

- Radiotherapy often is combined with surgery or chemotherapy and immunotherapy, as well as being the sole treatment for cancer in some instances.
- The goal or intent of radiotherapy may be curative, for control of the cancer, or for palliation.
- "Anticipatory" palliation is useful in treating potentially symptomatic lesions before they become a problem.

## APPLIED RADIATION PHYSICS

- The use of ionizing radiation in the treatment of cancer is based on the ability of radiation to interact with the atoms and molecules of the tumor cells to produce specific harmful biological effects. Ionization affects either the molecules of the cell or the cell environment.
- As unstable atoms break down into a more stable state, alpha, beta, or gamma rays may be emitted.
- Radium, radon, and uranium are examples of unstable atoms that produce ionizing radiation.
- Stable atoms also may be made to produce ionizing radiation through excitation, ionization, and nuclear disintegration.
- Radiation produced by these processes can be classified into two groups: *electromagnetic radiation* and *particulate radiation.*
- The electromagnetic spectrum can be further divided into five levels of decreasing wavelength:
    1. radio waves
    2. infrared radiation
    3. visible light
    4. ultraviolet radiation
    5. ionizing radiation
- Ionizing radiation has the shortest wavelength and the greatest energy of the electromagnetic spectrum and is therefore the form of energy used in radiotherapy.
- The terms *x-ray* and *gamma ray* both describe ionizing electromagnetic radiation and differ only in their means of production.
- X-rays are produced by specially designed equipment, and gamma rays are emitted by radioactive materials such as $^{60}$Co.
- Because they have no mass, x- and gamma rays can penetrate much deeper into tissue before releasing their energy.
- Particulate radiation, on the other hand, is composed of alpha and beta particles, as well as electrons and neutrons, which have mass.
- Alpha particles penetrate only a short distance into tissue before collision and energy release take place; beta particles, which are smaller than alpha particles, will penetrate deeper, but do not reach as deeply into tissues as do x- and gamma rays.
- X-rays are produced when a stream of fast-moving electrons, accelerated by the application of high voltage, strikes the target, and the electrons give up their energy.
- In addition to x-rays, some treatment machines (betatron, linear accelerator) are equipped to produce particle irradiation in the form of electrons.

- The time required for half the radioactive atoms present at any time to decay is known as the *half-life* of that radioactive element or isotope.
- Radioisotopes are referred to as artificial isotopes to distinguish them from naturally occurring radioisotopes.

## EQUIPMENT, BEAMS, AND MATERIALS USED IN RADIOTHERAPY

- Equipment can be classified according to use: external radiation, or *teletherapy* (radiation from a source at a distance from the body), and internal application, or *brachytherapy* (radiation from a source placed within the body or a body cavity).
- *Contact therapy* using $^{90}$Sr isotopes for conjunctival lesions and *surface (mould) therapy* for superficial skin lesions are additional applications of brachytherapy.

### Teletherapy (External Radiation)
#### Conventional or orthovoltage equipment

- Conventional or orthovoltage equipment produces x-rays of varying energies, depending on the voltage used.
- In selecting the proper beam for treatment of a particular lesion, the percentage depth of the beam must be known, as well as the depth of the lesion within the body.
- Disadvantages to orthovoltage beams, in addition to the poor depth of penetration, are the severe skin reactions and bone necrosis.

#### Megavoltage equipment

- The primary advantages of megavoltage therapy are (1) deeper beam penetration, (2) more homogeneous absorption of radiation, and (3) greater skin sparing.
- Linear accelerators are widely used in most hospital-based radiotherapy departments as well as in the private practice setting. Linear accelerators have distinct treatment advantages, including the speed with which treatments can be given.
- Linear accelerators accelerate electrons along a radio frequency electromagnetic wave, achieving energies equivalent to those that could be obtained only in a conventional x-ray tube at excessively high voltage.
- Some linear accelerators are also equipped to allow use of the electron beam (particulate radiation) itself. Electron beam therapy is useful for relatively superficial lesions. It may be used to provide a booster dose to a limited site following treatment with megavoltage therapy. Its limited penetration is a distinct advantage over x- or gamma radiation in that almost all the electron energy is expended at a particular tissue depth, thus sparing whatever structures lie beyond the tumor site.

#### High LET and charged particle radiation therapy

- There are two basic forms of radiation used in radiotherapy: low LET (linear energy transfer) radiation, such as x-rays, gamma rays, and electrons; and high LET radiation, such as neutron beams, heavy ions, and negative pi-mesons (pions).
- Basically, the difference between low and high LET radiation is in the rate of energy deposition in the tissue molecule. Low LET radiation could conceivably pass through a molecule without damaging it.
- In contrast, the number of ionizing events with high LET radiation is much greater and damage is invariably produced.
- High LET radiation has several advantages over low LET radiation:
  1. greater relative biological effectiveness (RBE)
  2. reduced relative radioresistance of hypoxic cells in tumors (low oxygen enhancement ratio [OER])
  3. less intertreatment recovery of tumor cells in fractionated dosage

### Neutron beam therapy

- Fast neutrons are produced by a cyclotron. Technological problems and the low dose rate (5–6 cGy/min) are among the disadvantages.

### Heavy charged particle therapy

- Heavy ions, such as protons, helium, and nitrogen, are mainly useful for small tumors. As the tumor size increases, treatment volume and OER will also increase.

### Negative pi-meson therapy

- Negative pi-mesons (pions) are small, negatively charged particles found in the nuclei of atoms that "cement" protons and neutrons together.
- The advantage of pion therapy, like other forms of high LET radiation, is that the beam can be shaped to fit the tumor precisely.
- Because of the cost and complexity of building and operating pion facilities, pion radiation will not likely be pursued in the future.

## Brachytherapy (Internal Radiation)

- *Brachytherapy*, the use of sealed sources of radioactive material placed within or near a tumor, is the treatment of choice for a variety of lesions. Brachytherapy frequently is combined with teletherapy and also may be used preoperatively and postoperatively.
- Radioactive isotopes for brachytherapy application are contained in a variety of forms, such as wires, ribbons or tubes, needles, grains or seeds, and capsules.
- The source is selected by the radiotherapist according to the site to be treated, the size of the lesion, and whether the implant is to be temporary or permanent.
- Intracavitary radiotherapy most often is employed in the treatment of gynecologic lesions.
- The afterloading method is most desirable because it prevents unnecessary radiation exposure for personnel.
- Use of high-dose-rate (HDR) sources for brachytherapy has distinct advantages over low-dose-rate (LDR) sources in that HDR produces the same radiobiological effect in a shorter period of time.
- HDR brachytherapy can be used for intralumenal, interstitial, intracavitary, and surface lesions.
- Major advantages of the remote afterloading HDR technique include reduced exposure of personnel, flexible techniques, shorter treatment time, and outpatient options.

## SIMULATION AND TREATMENT PLANNING

- One of the first steps in planning is localizing the tumor and defining the volume to be treated. Often it is necessary to employ a simulator to determine treatment volume accurately.
- A simulator contains a diagnostic x-ray unit for visualizing the proposed treatment site. Fluoroscopic examination also may be done. From radiographs taken on the simulator, the physician can determine the field of treatment.
- Treatment portals can be identified by several small tattoos placed at the corners of the field.
- For individuals receiving head and neck irradiation, tattoos may be substituted for inked lines. Injection molding equipment also can be employed to form head holders.
- Field markings can be placed on these masks rather than on the skin, avoiding conspicuous facial marks.
- Some simulators also are capable of transverse axial tomography, a radiographic technique for showing a three-dimensional view of the tumor and surrounding structures.

- Computerized tomography (CT scan) and magnetic resonance imaging (MRI) can provide the radiation oncologist with even finer detail for treatment planning.
- Some simulators are also equipped with an ultrasound device that produces an image of internal structures.
- Various restraining or positioning devices may be designed at the time of simulation to aid in immobilizing the patient.
- An important part of simulation and treatment planning is shaping the field and determining what structures are to be blocked and protected from radiation.
- Blocks to protect vital body organs and tissues are secured to a plastic tray that is then placed on the head of the treatment machine between the beam and the patient.
- *Portal films* (sometimes called *beam films*) are radiographs taken through the treatment machine to confirm the treatment field and the placement of blocks in the desired position.
- Working together, the physicist and radiation oncologist design the field arrangement, determine the dose calculations, monitor tumor response, and ensure accuracy of technical aspects.

## RADIOBIOLOGY

### Cellular Response to Radiation

- Radiation effect at the cellular level may be either direct or indirect, according to the target theory.
- A *direct hit* occurs when any of the key molecules within the cell, such as DNA or RNA, are damaged.
- An *indirect hit* occurs when ionization takes place in the medium (mostly water) surrounding the molecular structures within the cell.
- Radiation absorbed by the water molecules results in the formation of free radicals that trigger a variety of chemical reactions, producing compounds toxic to the cell.
- A direct hit accounts for the most effective and lethal injury produced by ionizing radiation. However, the probability of indirect damage through ionization of intracellular water is much greater.

### Cell cycle and radiosensitivity

- The maximum effect from radiation should occur just before and during actual cell division.
- Because the effect of radiation is known to be greatest during mitosis, undifferentiated cell populations generally are most sensitive to radiation. In contrast, well-differentiated cells are relatively radioresistant.
- Changes in mitotic activity due to radiation can be classified as either *delayed onset* or *complete inhibition*.
- *Delayed onset* of mitosis indicates that although damage occurred, repair was accomplished and division occurred.
- *Complete inhibition* of mitosis renders the cell incapable of division.

### Cell death

- There are three types of cell death: mitotic death, interphase death, and instant death.
  - *Mitotic death* occurs after one or more divisions and usually with much smaller radiation doses.
  - *Interphase death* occurs many hours after irradiation and before the cell begins the mitotic process.
  - *Instant death* occurs following extremely high doses of radiation.

## Contributory biological factors

### Oxygen effect

- Well-oxygenated tumors show a much greater response to radiation—that is, they are more radiosensitive than poorly oxygenated tumors.
- The clinical significance of the oxygen effect is that oxygen modifies the dose of radiation needed to produce a given degree of biological damage.

### Linear energy transfer

- Linear energy transfer (LET) describes the rate at which energy is lost from different types of radiation while traveling through matter.
- Low-LET radiations (x- and gamma rays) have a random pathway that results in few direct hits within the cell nucleus.
- Radiation of higher LET (alpha particles, neutrons, and negative pi-mesons) has a greater probability of interacting with matter and producing more direct hits within the cell.

### Relative biological effectiveness

- The term *relative biological effectiveness (RBE)* is used to compare a dose of test radiation with a dose of standard radiation that produces the same biological response.

### Dose rate

- Dose rate refers to the rate at which a given dose is delivered.

### Radiosensitivity

- Ionizing radiation is most effective on cells that are undifferentiated and undergoing active mitosis.

### Fractionation

- Fractionation, or the dividing of a total dose of radiation into a number of equal fractions, is based on four important factors: repair, redistribution, repopulation, and reoxygenation.

#### *Repair*

- The goal of fractionation is to deliver a dose sufficient to prevent tumor cells from being repaired while allowing normal cells to recover before the next dose is given.

#### *Redistribution*

- Redistribution of cell age (within the cell cycle) as a result of daily radiation is advantageous because more tumor cells are made radiosensitive.

#### *Repopulation*

- Fractionation of dose allows repopulation in normal tissues. Those tumor cells that do succeed in dividing while undergoing a fractionated course of radiotherapy usually are incapable of surviving.

#### *Reoxygenation*

- Radiosensitivity is closely related to oxygen tension in the tumor cell; hypoxic or anoxic cells generally are radioresistant, whereas oxygenated cells are radiosensitive. Fractionating the dose allows time between treatments for the tumor to reoxygenate.

- Tissue and organ response to radiation is based on the sensitivity of cellular components. Tissues and organs are composed of more than one cell category, each cell category having different degrees of radiosensitivity.
- If parenchymal tissue is relatively radioresistant, radiation response in that organ is due to the indirect effects on the stromal components (especially the vasculature) that support the parenchyma.
- Table 13-2, text page 260, lists various organs according to their degree of radiosensitivity as measured by parenchymal hypoplasia.

## CHEMICAL AND THERMAL MODIFIERS OF RADIATION

### Radiosensitizers and Radioprotectors

- Certain compounds increase the radiosensitivity of tumor cells or protect normal cells from radiation effect.
- Combined modality therapy with both radiation and certain cytotoxic agents takes advantage of enhanced tumor cell kill.
- *Enhancement* or *potentiation* describes any radiation effect that is greater in the presence of the chemical than in its absence.
- If the effect is less than that caused by the most active agent in the combination, then this is known as *interference*.
- *Antagonism* is the term used to describe an outcome less than that of the least effective agent in a given combination.
- In clinical radiotherapy, enhancement by noncytotoxic sensitizers is called *radiosensitization*. Antagonism by protective compounds is called *radioprotection*.
- *Radiosensitizers* are compounds that apparently promote fixation of the free radicals produced by radiation damage at the molecular level.
- Clinical trials thus far have failed to establish the overall efficacy of radiosensitizers as adjuncts to radiation therapy in the clinical setting.
- *Radioprotectors* are compounds that can protect oxygenated (nontumor) cells while having a limited effect on hypoxic (tumor) cells.
- The sulfhydryl groups contained in the nonprotein fraction of most cells aid in the reduction process following radiation damage.
- The compound that appears to be most useful at present is designated WR-2721.

### Combined Modality Therapy

- To increase or improve the therapeutic index, various combinations of chemotherapy and radiation have been studied.
- Ideally, a chemotherapeutic agent (or combination of agents) will shrink a tumor when given *prior* to local radiation (neoadjuvant chemotherapy); enhance or increase radiation cell kill when given *during* radiation (concomitant therapy); or control micrometastases and subclinical disease *after* a course of radiation (adjuvant therapy).
- Radiation and chemotherapy sometimes are given on a planned, alternating schedule using the so-called *sandwich technique*.
- Combined-modality therapy has the potential for enhanced side effects as well as enhanced tumor effect.

## Hyperthermia

- Heat is cytotoxic to cancer cells but is also destructive to healthy tissue if applied in excess of tolerable ranges. Controlled hyperthermia combined with radiation achieves tumor cell kill without excess toxicity.
- Tumor cells are *least* radiosensitive during S phase. Hyperthermia is most effective during S phase; therefore, the combined effect of radiation and hyperthermia on a tumor produces greater cell kill than either does alone.
- Similarly, hypoxic cells, which are generally radioresistant, have been found to be quite thermosensitive. Heat is also known to inhibit the repair of radiation damage, thus increasing the therapeutic ratio.
- Hyperthermia is achieved in various ways, including immersion of the local area in a heated bath, ultrasound, microwaves, interstitial implants, and perfusion techniques.
- Side effects of combined hyperthermia and radiation include local skin reaction, pain, fever, gastrointestinal effects, and cardiac arrhythmias.

## TISSUE AND ORGAN RESPONSE TO RADIATION

- The acute effects are seen within the first six months following treatment, and late effects are seen after six months.
- In general, acute effects are due to cell damage in which mitotic activity is altered. If early effects are not reversible, late or permanent tissue changes can be attributed to the organism's attempt to heal or repair the damage.
- The unit of radiation dose is called a *gray* (Gy). One Gy equals 100 *rad*. One cGy equals 1 rad (an acronym for *r*adiation *a*bsorbed *d*ose).
- Treatment volume, *dose rate* (number of cGy in a given unit of time), and *dose-time* factor (total number of cGy in a total number of days), as well as beam quality, may alter the tissue reaction.
- Side effects from radiation are specific, and therefore preparation, teaching, and care must be planned specifically for each individual. Radiation response is seen mostly in tissues and organs within or adjacent to the treatment field; i.e., they are site-specific.

## Integumentary System

- Continual reproductive activity accounts for the high radiosensitivity of skin. It is also irradiated whenever any other site within the body is treated.
  - Erythema may be the only manifestation, or the skin reaction may progress to dry and then moist desquamation.
  - Fibrosis and atrophy may occur after high doses, as may ulceration, necrosis, and skin cancer.
- Skin in certain areas (such as the groin, gluteal fold, axilla, and under the breasts) usually exhibits a greater and often earlier reaction to radiation due to the natural warmth and moistness in these areas and to friction caused by apposition of skin surfaces.
- Hair follicles and glands (sweat and sebaceous) are also radiosensitive. The radiosensitivity of the hair follicle is due to the relatively high rate of growth (mitotic activity) taking place.
- When the scalp is irradiated, the resulting inhibition of growth of new hair coupled with the accelerated hair loss due to damage to the follicle produces a net loss of hair, or *alopecia*. Epilation occurs in doses as low as a single dose of 500 cGy but is usually temporary. Regrowth may not begin for several months following the end of treatment, and the new hair may have a different quality or color.
- Higher doses (4500 cGy or greater) may produce permanent alopecia or delay regrowth for a year or more.
- Sebaceous and sweat glands usually will experience a decrease in activity during treatment and may cease functioning altogether at high doses (over 6000–7000 cGy).

## Hematopoietic System

- When large areas of red bone marrow (in the adult) are irradiated, the number of circulating mature cells decreases because production is suppressed.
- The patient receiving radiotherapy may have depressed blood counts if sufficient radiation was given to active red bone marrow, especially if prior or concomitant chemotherapy has been given.
- The usual pattern seen in individuals whose marrow has been affected is a decrease first in lymphocytes, then in neutrophils, and then in platelets and red blood cells.

## Gastrointestinal System

- A large proportion of the cells of the GI system are undifferentiated and highly mitotic and are thus extremely radiosensitive.
- The effect of radiation on glandular tissue can be summarized as follows:
  1. Initial swelling and edema of the epithelial lining of the ducts results in partial obstruction.
  2. Secretion is inhibited.
  3. Atrophy and fibrosis occur as healing takes place, with permanent reduction in secretion.
- Oral mucous membrane may develop a confluent mucositis. Salivary function is altered as damage to the serous and mucous acini occurs. Higher doses of radiation lead to atrophy of the salivary glands. Such changes in saliva production and acidity often are permanent.
- Alterations in the sense of taste occur early in treatment but are rarely permanent.
- The esophagus and stomach also develop dose-dependent reactions. Inflammation of the mucosa occurs with moderate to high doses and produces dysphagia, anorexia, and sometimes nausea and vomiting. Late changes may include atrophy, ulcerations, and fibrosis.
- The most sensitive area of the entire gastrointestinal tract is thought to be the small intestine.
- Radiation reaction in the small intestine is characterized by shortening of the villa and loss of absorptive surface.
- In individuals receiving 5000–6000 cGy to the abdomen or pelvis, shortening of the villi and denuding of the intestinal mucosa prevent adequate absorption of the end products of digestion. Late changes following high doses of radiation include fibrosis, ulcerations, necrosis, and hemorrhage.
- Intestinal obstruction is more likely to happen postoperatively.
- The effect of radiation on the colon and rectum is similar to that seen in the small intestine, with the addition of tenesmus.

## Liver

- The liver is moderately radiosensitive.
- The greatest damage produced by radiation to the liver is due to vascular injury.
- Radiation hepatitis is a possible consequence of doses over 2500 cGy.

## Respiratory System

- Hoarseness due to laryngeal mucous membrane congestion sometimes occurs.
- Radiation pneumonitis is usually a transient response to moderate doses.
- Late changes are manifested by fibrosis in the lung tissue itself plus some thickening of the pleura.

## Reproductive System

- The cervix and uterine body are quite radioresistant; however, vaginal mucous membrane responds with mucositis and inflammation.
- Following brachytherapy, vaginal stenosis due to permanent fibrotic changes is a potential problem. Radiation to the ovaries produces either temporary or permanent sterility.

- Permanent sterilization will occur at doses of 600–1200 cGy, and older women are sterilized at lower doses than younger women.
- Hormonal changes and early menopause may occur.
- Perhaps most significant in terms of late or long-term consequences of radiation to the gonads in both the male and female is the potential for genetic damage.
- Radiation to the male testes damages and prevents maturation of the immature spermatogonia. Sterility can be permanent even after a dose of 500–600 cGy.

## Urinary System

- Radiation-induced cystitis and urethritis are early and transient effects on the urinary tract that usually respond well to symptomatic treatment.
- Of major significance is damage to the kidneys in the form of nephritis. Early changes brought about by high doses of radiation lead to permanent fibrosis and atrophy. Renal failure and death can result. Protection of the kidneys is essential.

## Cardiovascular System

- Blood vessels may become occluded when excessive cell production takes place during repair and regeneration.
- Thrombosis may be induced by the thickening that occurs during regenerative activity. Late changes can be seen in the form of telangiectasia, petechiae, and sclerosis.
- At doses above 4000 cGy, pericarditis may occur in addition to the damage to the vasculature of the heart muscle.

## Nervous System

- The brain and spinal cord are considered to be relatively radioresistant.
- Doses between 3000 and 6000 cGy have produced transient symptoms in the CNS, resulting in a response called Lhermitte's syndrome, characterized by paresthesia in the form of shocklike sensations that radiate down the back and extremities when the neck is bent forward.
- Myelopathy usually is transient, but at higher doses may lead to paralysis or paresis.
- Damage that does occur following radiation probably relates to vascular insufficiency.

## Skeletal System

- Mature bone and cartilage are radioresistant.
- Late avascular necrosis can occur after high dose, causing pain and possible pathological fracture. This is a relatively rare complication.
- Of much greater clinical significance is the effect of radiation on growing bone and cartilage. Children are susceptible to deformity as a result of radiation to the vertebrae.

## Systemic Effects of Radiation

- The patient receiving radiotherapy may experience certain subjective systemic effects, including nausea, anorexia, and malaise.
- The release of toxic waste products into the bloodstream may cause nausea and anorexia, whereas the increased metabolic rate required to dispose of the waste products might be partially responsible for the frequent complaint of fatigue.

### Total-body and hemibody radiation

- Total body and hemibody irradiation are relatively infrequent therapeutic applications of radiation. The effect on the patient varies with the dose, dose rate, and dose-time factor.
- Total body irradiation for "conditioning" prior to bone marrow transplantation has three purposes: (1) myeloablation to create space for donor marrow, (2) immunosuppression to prevent graft rejection, and (3) clearing of residual malignant cells.
- Fractionation of the dose appears to be more beneficial and less likely to produce tissue tolerance and late effects.
- Acute effects of TBI include graft-versus-host disease, nausea, vomiting, diarrhea, mucositis, erythema, and alopecia.
- Chronic or late effects occurring up to three months after TBI include cataracts, growth disturbances, endocrine dysfunction, and nephrotoxicity. The single most significant chronic effect is interstitial pneumonitis, which carries a 70% mortality rate.
- *Hemibody radiation* refers to treatment of the upper, middle, or lower body in a single large fraction of approximately 500–800 cGy. This approach is used primarily for the patient with widespread bone metastases to achieve rapid palliation of pain.
- Lower hemibody radiation is better tolerated, although some patients experience brief periods of post-treatment nausea and occasional abdominal cramping or diarrhea. Bone marrow suppression is likely to occur.

### Altered fractionation schedules

- Standard treatment with radiation therapy calls for single daily fractions, given five days per week in daily doses in the range of 180–300 cGy.
- *Hyperfractionation* (HFX) involves an increased number of fractions delivered over the same total treatment time as in standard fractionation.
- *Accelerated fractionation* (AFX), on the other hand, uses three fractions per day to achieve the same total dose as HFX while shortening overall treatment time.
- In the *dynamic fractionation* approach, doses are escalated over the length of the treatment course.

### Chronic low-dose exposure

- Chronic low-dose radiation exposure occurs to all individuals, due to background radiation from naturally occurring radioactive substances and cosmic rays.

### Total-body radiation syndrome

- *Total-body radiation syndrome* refers to the effects of the acute exposure of the organism to doses of radiation received in a matter of minutes rather than hours or days.

### Radiation-induced malignancies in humans

- The carcinogenic effects of radiation, often called "late effects," can result from both chronic low-dose exposure and acute exposure to the whole body.
- The usually prescribed therapeutic doses (in the range of 2500–6500 cGy) are believed to be less carcinogenic than lower doses given over a much longer time period.
- The most common malignancies associated with radiation exposure are skin carcinoma and leukemia.
- Radiation carcinogenesis includes a latent period of from 1–30 years, radiation dose, concomitant factors in the radiated organism's environment, and the actual fate of the cell as it responds to radiation injury.

## NURSING CARE OF THE PATIENT RECEIVING RADIOTHERAPY

- Symptomatic relief of side effects, nutritional support, and social and financial assistance are all nursing concerns. Coordination of complex treatment schedules and protocols also may be part of the nurse's role.
- Expected side effects usually occur after 10–14 days, depending on dose, volume, and site. Individuals undergoing treatment frequently count the days and keep track of the number of treatments received.
- There are a number of reasons for adding to, subtracting from, or changing the plan, and if the patient understands this from the beginning, changes will not be interpreted as signs of recurrence or disease progression.

## SPECIFIC NURSING CARE MEASURES FOR PATIENTS RECEIVING RADIOTHERAPY

- During a course of radiotherapy, certain treatment-related side effects can be expected to develop, most of which are site specific as well as dependent on volume, dose fractionation, total dose, and individual differences.
- Many symptoms do not develop until approximately 10–14 days into treatment, and some do not subside until two or more weeks after treatments have ended.

### Fatigue

- Fatigue or malaise is common among individuals with cancer, and may be even more pronounced during and after a course of radiation treatment.
- Pain management is especially important, because chronic and uncontrolled pain is one of the most wearisome challenges faced by some patients.
- Extra rest and a reduction in the normal activity level may be necessary during treatment.

### Anorexia

- Anorexia, like fatigue, is probably related to the presence in the patient's system of the waste products of tissue destruction. Other possible causes include anemia, inactivity, medications, alterations in the individual's ability to ingest and digest foods, and psychological factors.
- The symptom must be treated utilizing all the techniques known to encourage adequate nutritional intake.

### Mucositis

- The reaction induced by radiation within the mucous membranes of the body is called mucositis, a patchy, white membrane that becomes confluent and may bleed if disturbed.
- It is important to enlist the patient's cooperation in avoiding irritants such as alcohol, tobacco, spicy or acidic foods, very hot or very cold foods and drinks, and commercial mouthwash products.
- One ounce of diphenhydramine hydrochloride (Benadryl) elixir diluted in one quart of water provides an ideal agent for mouth care in individuals with mucositis.
- Mouth care should be done as often as every three or four hours and is especially important before mealtime.
- Care should be taken not to dislodge the plaquelike formations of mucositis, because dislodgement will cause bleeding and denude the mucosal surface.
- Agents that coat and soothe the oral mucosa, such as Maalox, are sometimes used. Lidocaine hydrochloride 2% viscous solution may provide some relief from discomfort.
- Occasionally, a break from treatment will have to be given when reactions are excessive.

## Xerostomia

- The dry mouth resulting from radiation to the salivary glands or portions of them is known as xerostomia. Alterations in taste frequently accompany xerostomia. During the course of radiation, little can be done to relieve this annoying symptom. Frequent sips of water seem to be the best method of providing moisture. Frequent mouth care, especially before meals, will provide some relief.
- When a course of therapy has ended and any intraoral reaction has subsided, some individuals will benefit from the use of a saliva substitute to provide moisture and lubrication for two- to four-hour periods.

## Radiation Caries

- Radiation caries can be greatly reduced or avoided by proper care before, during, and after a course of treatment. Absence or decrease in saliva and the altered pH produced by treatment promote decay. Before the start of therapy, a thorough dental examination and prophylaxis should be carried out. If teeth are in good repair, a vigorous preventive program is begun to protect them from the late effects of radiation. This can include daily diphenhydramine hydrochloride mouth sprays followed by a 5-minute application of fluoride gel. Brushing the teeth with a soft-bristled brush several times daily is also important.

## Esophagitis and Dysphagia

- Esophagitis is a transient effect in which the esophageal mucous membrane becomes somewhat edematous, and mucositis can develop.
- The patient will first notice dysphagia, which may then progress to a definite esophagitis, which makes swallowing painful and can be responsible for a decrease in intake of foods and fluids.
- A mixture of Mylanta, lidocaine, and diphenhydramine provides temporary relief from radiation esophagitis.
- The patient receiving treatment should be encouraged to substitute high-calorie, high-protein, high-carbohydrate liquids and soft, bland foods for their regular meals.
- Blenderized foods from the patient's regular diet are less expensive than commercial products, and the patient with esophagitis should be encouraged to try this method.

## Nausea and Vomiting

- Of the potential side effects from radiotherapy, nausea or vomiting are probably the most distressing to the patient being treated. However, nausea and vomiting are not common.
- Generally, the patient receiving radiotherapy can be expected to experience some degree of nausea when treatment is directed to any of the following sites: whole abdomen or portions of it, large pelvic fields, hypochondrium, epigastrium, or para-aortic areas.
- When nausea does occur, it usually can be controlled by antiemetics administered on a regular schedule and by adjusting the eating pattern so that treatment is given when the stomach is relatively empty.
- Delaying intake of a full meal until three or four hours after treatment is helpful because nausea, if it occurs, will usually appear from one to three hours after treatment.

## Diarrhea

- Diarrhea is not an expected side effect in most individuals receiving radiotherapy. However, it does occur if areas of the abdomen and pelvis are treated after about 2000 cGy have been given.
- Some individuals experience only an increase in their usual number of bowel movements, whereas others develop loose, watery stools and intestinal cramping.
- For most individuals with radiation-induced diarrhea, a low-residue diet and prescription of loperamide hydrochloride usually are sufficient.

## Tenesmus, Cystitis, and Urethritis

- Although infrequent, tenesmus, cystitis, and urethritis do occur. Treatment consists of urinary antiseptics and antispasmodics for symptomatic relief. High fluid intake is encouraged.
- Tenesmus of the anal or urinary sphincter produces a persistent sensation of the need to evacuate the bowel or bladder. Relief sometimes can be obtained from gastrointestinal and urinary antispasmodics and anticholinergic preparations.
- Cystitis and urethritis resulting from radiation to the bladder area is distressing to the patient.
- Treatment consists of urinary antiseptics and antispasmodics for symptomatic relief. High fluid intake is encouraged.
- Sitz baths, which are commonly prescribed for tenesmus, cystitis, and urethritis, are contraindicated if the perineal area is being irradiated. The added moisture will only enhance any potential or actual skin reaction.

## Alopecia

- If patients are being prepared for radiotherapy that does not include the scalp, they should be reassured that hair loss will not occur as a result of treatment.
- During treatment of the whole brain, alopecia will occur and follows a typical pattern. At about 2500–3000 cGy, the patient will notice excessive amounts of hair in the brush or comb and a gradual thinning of the hair. Then quite suddenly most of the hair comes out, and the patient awakens to find the remainder of his or her hair on the pillow.
- Care of the hair and scalp while receiving radiation to the scalp includes very gentle brushing or combing and infrequent shampooing.
- Individuals should avoid any procedures on the hair that involve the use of harsh chemicals, because such substances may run down onto treated skin.
- As in the case of irradiated skin in general, the scalp should be treated with care and caution for several months to a year or more after healing has taken place.

## Skin Reactions

- The response of normal skin to radiation treatments varies from mild erythema to moist desquamation that leaves a raw surface similar to a second-degree burn.
- Individuals treated with electron beams will exhibit considerable skin reaction when the electron beam is intended for lesions located on the skin or a few centimeters below the surface.
- In some areas of the body, such as the groin, perineum, buttocks, inframammary folds, and axillae, skin has a relatively poor tolerance to radiation.
- Because moisture enhances skin reactions, the patient should be advised to keep the skin in the treated area as dry as possible.
- Treated skin should be bathed gently with tepid water and mild soap. The area should be rinsed thoroughly and gently patted (not rubbed) dry.
- Lines or markings placed on the skin at simulation should not be removed until the radiation therapist advises the patient to do so.
- General guidelines include:
  - Keep the skin dry.
  - Avoid using powders, lotions, creams, alcohol, and deodorants.
  - Wear loose-fitting garments.
  - Do not apply tape to the treatment site when dressings are applied.
  - Shave with an electric razor only. Do not use preshaves or aftershaves.
  - Protect the skin from exposure to direct sunlight, chlorinated swimming pools, and temperature extremes (e.g., hot water bottle, heating pad).

- When planning for skin care for the patient receiving radiotherapy, it should be remembered that individuals often are treated by parallel opposing portals and only one of these portals may be marked to indicate the field.
- During treatment and for a month or more afterward, treated skin should not be exposed to direct sunlight.
- When a course of radiotherapy has ended and after any reaction has subsided and healed, a cautious approach to sun exposure may be resumed, using a number 15 sunblock.

## Bone Marrow Suppression

- When large volumes of active bone marrow are irradiated (especially the pelvis or spine in the adult), the effect on the marrow can be quite significant.
- Weekly blood counts should be done on all individuals receiving radiotherapy and two to three times per week for individuals receiving concomitant chemotherapy or those who have had extensive chemotherapy before radiation.
- Individuals receiving total-body irradiation or splenic irradiation for chronic lymphocytic leukemia will require daily blood counts.
- Transfusions of whole blood, platelets, or other blood components may be necessary for the patient who has dangerously low blood counts. Treatment may have to be adjusted or interrupted. Nursing care should include observation of the patient for signs and symptoms of bleeding, anemia, and infection.

## Radiation Side Effects: Special Considerations

### Transient myelitis

- When lymph nodes in the cervical region are radiated, some individuals will experience paresthesia when flexing the neck. This is known as Lhermitte's syndrome and occurs after a latent period of two to three weeks after final treatment of the site.
- The temporary nature of this effect should be stressed and the patient reassured that this is a known side effect that sometimes occurs.

### Parotitis

- Parotitis is a painful swelling and inflammation of the parotid glands that sometimes occurs in individuals receiving radiation to the maxillomandibular area.
- The symptoms subside almost as quickly as they arise, and no specific treatment is necessary.

### Visual and olfactory disturbances

- During radiation to the pituitary area, some individuals occasionally experience visual or olfactory disturbances that can be distressing.

### Radiation recall

- *Radiation recall* can occur in a previously irradiated site that exhibited mucositis or erythema. Radiation recall occurs in response to the systemic administration of certain chemotherapeutic agents several months to a year or more after radiation was received.
- Treatment is symptomatic, and the drug dosage may be modified.

## NURSING CARE OF THE PATIENT WITH A RADIOACTIVE SOURCE

- In addition to being implanted in tissues or inserted into body cavities, some radioactive isotopes may be administered orally, intravenously, or by instillation, and specific safety precautions are required.

- Adsorbed or metabolized isotopes used most commonly include $^{131}$I, $^{32}$P, and $^{198}$Au, all of which are administered as colloids or solutions, which present a possibility of contamination of equipment, dressings, and linens.
- Sealed sources such as $^{137}$Cs and $^{226}$Ra for implantation through a mechanical device are not metabolized and therefore are not excreted in body fluids.
- Three primary factors in radiation protection should be foremost in the minds of all personnel involved in care of the patient: time, distance, and shielding.

## Time

- The amount of exposure to radiation that personnel receive is directly proportional to the time spent within a specific distance from the source.
- A team of providers with a clearly defined plan for care is a common approach used to minimize a nurse's exposure.

## Distance

- As radiation is emitted from a point source, the amount of radiation reaching a given area decreases according to the law of inverse square. Nurses can use distance creatively when noncontact care is being given.

## Shielding

- When a sheet of absorbing material is placed between a radiation source and a detector, the amount of radiation that reaches the detector decreases.
- Because shielding from gamma radiation requires lead or concrete of specific thicknesses, it is usually impractical to expect that much physical care can be given from behind such a shield.
- Shielding is not always possible or practical; time and distance are the two factors that nurses must incorporate into the care plan.

## Patient Education and Support

- Individuals who are isolated for radiation precautions often feel "unclean" or "contaminated."
- Planning and providing emotional support are major components of nursing care.
- Preparation for implants should include:
  1. Description of the procedure
  2. Possible change in appearance
  3. Anticipated pain or discomfort and measures available for relief
  4. Potential short-term and long-term side effects and complications
  5. Restrictions on activity while the radioactive sources are in place
  6. Visiting restrictions
  7. Radiation precautions observed by hospital personnel
- The patient also should be helped to prepare for such procedures by planning for suitable activities such as reading, handwork, television, and so on.

## ADVANCES IN RADIOTHERAPY

- *Radiolabeled antibody therapy* involves attaching a radioactive isotope to the tumor-specific antibody to deliver therapeutic radiation directly to the target tumor.
- *Intraoperative radiotherapy* (IOR) has the advantage of increasing tumor dose in relation to normal tissue dose.
- After surgically exposing the target volume, a single, large fraction of radiation is delivered directly to the tumor site.

- *Conformal radiation therapy* is an outgrowth of computer technology and the continued search to more precisely target the tumor site while sparing surrounding healthy tissue. By tightly conforming the zone of high-dose volume to the target volume, dose outside the target volume would be greatly reduced. Conformal therapy utilizes either a multifield technique or the newer multileaf collimator.
- *Stereotactic radioneurosurgery* uses multiple convergent beams via a coordinate system.
- The most common high-energy radiation technique employs a linear accelerator with a specially adapted collimator.
- The Gamma Knife is the second most common high-energy source for stereotactic radiosurgery.
- The third technique for delivering stereotactic radiation utilizes charged particle beams produced by cyclotrons or synchrotrons.

## Practice Questions

1. An important advantage of megavoltage equipment over conventional or orthovoltage equipment used in radiotherapy is that it:
   a. is more effective in treating surface lesions.
   b. reduces absorption of radiation by bone.
   c. delivers radioisotopes to the site of the tumor.
   d. limits release of dangerous heavy ions and negative pi-mesons.

2. An advantage that high LET (linear energy transfer) radiation has over low LET radiation is that:
   a. equipment used to produce high LET radiation is generally less costly.
   b. high LET radiation produces fewer ionizing events in molecules.
   c. it produces greater relative biological effectiveness (RBE).
   d. high LET radiation increases the radioresistance of hypoxic cells in tumors.

3. For which of the following would surface (mould) therapy using radioisotopes most likely be used?
   a. a skin carcinoma on the ear
   b. a brain tumor
   c. a metastatic abdominal tumor
   d. Hodgkin's disease

4. Simulators are used in treatment planning for radiotherapy in order to localize a tumor and to:
   a. define the volume to be treated with radiotherapy.
   b. remove a section of a tumor for a laboratory evaluation.
   c. reduce the size of a tumor prior to surgical resection.
   d. prepare a histopathologic profile of a tumor.

5. Radiation effects take place primarily at the level of:
   a. cells.
   b. tissues.
   c. organs.
   d. the whole body.

6. Which of the following cells is most likely to be most radiosensitive?
   a. a well-differentiated, nondividing, and well-oxygenated cell
   b. an undifferentiated, dividing, and poorly oxygenated cell
   c. a well-differentiated, nondividing, and poorly oxygenated cell
   d. an undifferentiated, dividing, and well-oxygenated cell

7. One of the primary goals of dose fractionation is to:
   a. redistribute cell age within the cell cycle, making normal cells less radiosensitive.
   b. allow tumor cells to repopulate, making them more vulnerable to the late consequences that occur if new growth was inhibited.
   c. deliver a dose sufficient to prevent tumor cells from being repaired while allowing normal cells to recover before the next dose is given.
   d. provide time between treatments for normal cells to reoxygenate, thus making them less radiosensitive.

8. The late effects of radiation that are often seen 6 months or more after radiotherapy are the result of:
   a. cell damage in which mitotic activity is temporarily altered in some way.
   b. acute damage that occurs to tissues and organs outside the treatment field.
   c. the organism's attempt to repair the damage inflicted by ionizing radiation.
   d. acute, site-specific reactions to treatment.

9. A patient being treated in an abdominal field is concerned about hair loss that she expects to experience following radiotherapy. You can best reassure her by telling her that
   a. hair follicles are relatively radioresistant due to their low rate of growth and mitotic activity.
   b. radiation response is seen mostly in tissues and organs that are within the treatment field.
   c. alopecia is permanent only when radiation is administered in low doses over an extended period of time.
   d. alopecia is more closely associated with brachytherapy than with teletherapy.

10. In tissues such as the liver or heart that are relatively radioresistant, damage from high doses of radiation is most likely to occur from damage to:
    a. parenchyma.
    b. vascular tissue.
    c. mucous membranes.
    d. rapidly dividing cells.

11. Subjective systemic reactions to radiation, including fatigue, anorexia, and nausea, are most often caused by:
    a. acute exposure of the organism to doses of radiation in a matter of minutes rather than hours or days.
    b. chronic exposure of the whole body to low doses of radiation.
    c. acute, site-specific reactions that occur at the cellular and molecular levels.
    d. the release of toxic wastes into the bloodstream resulting from tumor destruction.

12. A patient who has been treated with radiation to the mouth and oropharynx has developed mucositis. Effective management of this side effect would incorporate all of the following *except*:
    a. encouraging the patient to avoid alcohol and cigarettes.
    b. administering a Benadryl solution as a mouthwash or spray.
    c. removing the plaquelike tissue that forms with mucositis.
    d. administering Maalox to coat and soothe mucosa.

13. Management of tenesmus, cystitis, and urethritis that may result when radiation is given to the pelvic area involves several nursing options, including all of the following *except*:
    a. administering gastrointestinal and urinary antispasmodics.
    b. administering antibiotics if there is evidence of infection.
    c. encouraging high fluid intake by the patient.
    d. providing sitz baths if the perineal area is being irradiated.

14. Side effects of radiation to the skin are least likely to include:
    a. mild erythema and moist desquamation.
    b. fibrosclerotic changes that make skin smooth, taut, and shiny.
    c. permanent tanning.
    d. complete or patchy alopecia.

15. The possibility of contamination of equipment, dressings, and linens is greatest when radioactive isotopes are delivered:
    a.  as implants.
    b.  as colloids or solutions.
    c.  as moulds.
    d.  as ovoids separated by a spacer.

16. Compounds that assist in maximizing the tumor cell kill achieved with radiation, while minimizing injury to normal tissues, are called:
    a.  radioantagonists.
    b.  radiosensitizers.
    c.  oxygen enhancement ratios.
    d.  linear energy transfer.

17. Nurses are often involved with managing the side effects that result from radiotherapy. To minimize the degree of the symptoms experienced, the nurse should schedule to see most patients:
    a.  immediately after the first fractionated dose.
    b.  upon completion of the scheduled 5-week course.
    c.  at the end of the first week.
    d.  10–14 days after treatment has begun.

## ANSWER EXPLANATIONS

1.  **The answer is b.** Megavoltage equipment operates at 2 to 40 million electron volts (MeV) compared to orthovoltage equipment's 40 to 400 thousand electron volts (Kv). It has the advantages of deeper beam penetration, more homogeneous absorption of radiation (minimizing bone absorption), and greater skin sparing. Megavoltage equipment includes cobalt and cesium units, the linear accelerator, the betatron, and such experimental units as those producing neutron beams, heavy ions, and negative pi-mesons. (p. 251)

2.  **The answer is c.** High LET radiation has several advantages over low LET radiation: (1) greater relative biological effectiveness (RBE); (2) reduced relative radioresistance of hypoxic cells in tumors (low oxygen enhancement ratio [OER]); (3) less intertreatment recovery of tumor cells in fractionated dosage (p. 253)

3.  **The answer is a.** Mould (or surface) therapy is a type of brachytherapy involving close contact of radioactive seeds, often of radon, encased in a plastic mould. The mould is placed in close contact with the lesion. This method is most useful for surface lesions in irregularly contoured areas such as the face. (p. 250)

4.  **The answer is a.** Simulator machinery may involve the use of diagnostic X rays, fluoroscopic examination, transverse axial tomography, CT scans, and ultrasound, with the goal in mind of localizing a tumor and defining the volume to be treated with radiotherapy. Other aspects of treatment planning include the tattooing of the treatment area, installing various restraining and positioning devices to immobilize the person, shaping the field, and determining what structures are to be blocked and protected from radiation. (p. 255)

5.  **The answer is a.** The biologic effects of radiation on humans are the result of a sequence of events that follows the absorption of energy from ionizing radiation and the organism's attempt to compensate for this assault. Radiation effect takes place at the cellular level, with consequences in tissues, organs, and the entire body. (p. 257)

6. **The answer is d.** Ionizing radiation is most effective on cells that are undifferentiated and undergoing active mitosis (dividing). In addition, well-oxygenated cells show a much greater response to radiation than poorly oxygenated (hypoxic) cells. Other factors that affect cellular response to radiation include the type, strength, and biologic effectiveness of the irradiation used, and the frequency at which a dose is administered (fractionation). (p. 258)

7. **The answer is c.** All of the other choices are opposites of the actual goals of fractionation. Fractionation redistributes cell age within the cell cycle, making tumor cells more radiosensitive. It allows normal cells to repopulate, sparing them from some of the late consequences that occur if new growth was inhibited. And it provides time between treatments for tumor cells to reoxygenate, thus making them more radiosensitive. (p. 259)

8. **The answer is c.** Effects of radiation may be acute and immediate, seen within the first 6 months, or they may be late, seen after 6 months. Acute effects are due to cell damage in which mitotic activity is altered. If early effects are not reversible, late or permanent tissue changes occur. These late effects are due to the organism's attempt to heal or repair the damage inflicted by ionizing radiation. (p. 262)

9. **The answer is b.** Radiation response is seen mostly in tissues and organs that are within or adjacent to the treatment field; i.e., they are site-specific. Thus, an individual being treated in the abdominal field will not lose scalp hair from radiation (p. 262).

10. **The answer is b.** Many of the acute reactions to high doses of radiation occur as the result of indirect effects on the stromal components (especially the vasculature) that support the parenchyma of irradiated tissues and organs. This explains the damage that can occur to organs in which parenchymal tissue is relatively radioresistant. (p. 260)

11. **The answer is d.** The presence of these toxins may account for the nausea and anorexia, whereas the increased metabolic rate required to dispose of the waste products might be partially responsible for the frequent complaint of fatigue. The extent of these effects depends on the volume of the irradiated area, the anatomic site, and the dose. (p. 265)

12. **The answer is c.** Gently, frequent mouth care with soothing solutions can be helpful. Care should be taken, however, not to dislodge the plaquelike formations of mucositis, causing bleeding. (p. 270)

13. **The answer is d.** Sitz baths are contraindicated if the perineal area is being irradiated. (p. 273)

14. **The answer is d.** Except in cases of whole body irradiation or irradiation to the head, alopecia should not occur. (p. 273)

15. **The answer is b.** In addition to radioactive implantation, some radioactive isotopes are administered orally, intravenously, or by instillation. Liquid sources administered as colloids or solutions are adsorbed or metabolized and present a possibility of contamination of equipment, dressings, and linens, depending on the mode of administration and metabolism. (p. 277)

16. **The answer is b.** Efforts to improve the therapeutic ratio have resulted in the development of certain compounds that act to increase the radiosensitivity of tumor cells or to protect normal cells from radiation effect. Radiosensitizers are compounds that apparently promote fixation of the free radicals produced by radiation damage at the molecular level. (p. 260)

17. **The answer is d.** During a course of radiotherapy, certain treatment-related side effects can be expected to develop, most of which are site specific as well as dependent on volume, dose fractionation, total dose, and individual differences. Many symptoms do not develop until approximately 10–14 days into treatment, and some do not subside until 2 or more weeks after treatments have ended. (p. 269)

# Chapter 14    Chemotherapy: Principles of T'

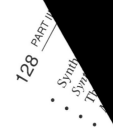

## CANCER CHEMOTHERAPY DRUG DEVELOPMENT

- The National Cancer Institute coordinates the screening of over 10,000 compounds attempt to find new and potentially useful drugs for treating cancer. Less than 1% of sci. pounds proceed to clinical trials.
- Preclinical toxicology studies determine a safe starting dose for use in humans. The lethal dose in 10 . of animals tested ($LD_{10}$) is then used to calculate a starting dose for clinical trials.
- Body surface area (BSA) is the preferred reference point used for making interspecies dose comparisons.

## Phase I Trials

- The primary objective of the first phase of clinical testing is to determine a maximum tolerated dose (MTD).
- Dosing starts at 10% of the $LD_{10}$ determined in mice and is escalated until significant toxicity is seen in 50% or more of the patients treated. This dose is the MTD, and one step below the MTD is used for phase II testing.

## Phase II Trials

- Identifying activity of a new drug in a specified tumor type is the primary objective of phase II clinical trials. The ideal patients for phase II testing are previously untreated; however, most tend to be patients who have shown little or no response to previous chemotherapy. Phase II trials also help determine drug toxicity.

## Phase III Trials

- In phase III testing new drugs are tested as single agents or combined with other drugs and compared with the standard treatment for a specific tumor.
- Traditionally response rates, duration of response, survival, and toxicity are measured; however, quality of life has also become the focus of clinical trials.
- Phase III trials typically require a large number of patients to be treated and observed over a prolonged time period.

## Phase IV Trials

- *Postmarketing* or *phase IV studies* are usually designed to answer questions regarding other uses, such as efficacy in the adjuvant setting. Dosing schedules, as well as new information regarding risks and toxicity, are evaluated.

## SCIENTIFIC BASIS OF CHEMOTHERAPY

### The Cell Cycle

- The cell cycle is made of five phases: $G_1$, S, $G_2$, M, and $G_0$.
- The *growth fraction* is the portion of cells actively cycling compared to the entire population.

esis of RNA and proteins occurs predominantly in the $G_1$ phase.

*hesis*, or *S phase*, is when DNA is being replicated and is a relatively short period.

e $G_2$ phase is typically brief, occurring after DNA synthesis and just before cell division.

*Mitosis*, or *cell division*, ensues during the *M phase*, resulting in two identical daughter cells. The time from mitosis to mitosis is described as the *cycling time*.

Cells that have left the cycle to enter $G_0$ are considered in a *resting* or *dormant phase*.

## Tumor Cell Kinetics

- A kinetic model states that tumor growth is often exponential, doubling times vary widely between tumors, and chemotherapy-sensitive tumors tend to grow faster than slow-growing tumors that are less responsive.
- The factors that affect doubling time are cell cycle time; growth fraction; cell loss by either cell death (apoptosis) or differentiation or metastasis.

## The Effects of Chemotherapy on Tumor Cells

### Cell kill hypothesis

- The cell kill hypothesis is a basic principle often used to describe the effects of cancer chemotherapy on normal and tumor cells. The hypothesis describes a first-order kinetic process in which a percentage rather than a specific number of cells are killed.

### Gompertzian curve

- A Gompertzian growth curve probably best describes the growth of human tumors and the responses observed with the administration of antineoplastic drugs.
- The Gompertzian curve is also useful in describing the observed tumor response to chemotherapy.

## CHEMOTHERAPY DRUG SELECTION AND FACTORS AFFECTING RESPONSE TO CHEMOTHERAPY

### Patient Factors

- Patient factors include toxicity response, organ dysfunction, previous or concomitant treatment, and age.

### Drug Factors

- Antineoplastic activity, pharmacokinetics, dose, and schedule are important drug factors that can influence chemotherapy response and toxicity. The relative cytotoxicity of any antineoplastic drug is dependent on the origin of the tumor and the presence of intrinsic drug resistance.

### Tumor Factors

- Tumor growth, location, histology, and size significantly influence the response to chemotherapy.
- The ability of chemotherapy to reach large solid tumors may be hindered by inadequate blood flow. Surgical excision or debulking of tumors can increase the responsiveness of these tumors.

## LACK OF RESPONSE TO CHEMOTHERAPY AND STRATEGIES TO OVERCOME TREATMENT FAILURE

### Theoretical Basis for Chemotherapy Resistance

- Currently the most popular explanation for chemotherapy treatment failures is the development of drug resistance. The best chance for curing cancer would be to apply effective drugs early to reduce

the total number of cancer cells while preventing resistant cells from developing, thus supporting the established concepts of combination chemotherapy.
- Disease that recurs within six months usually is considered resistant to initial chemotherapy. However, recurrence more than six months following treatment may be successfully treated with the same or similar chemotherapy regimen.
- These assumptions are not always applicable to human tumors.

## Cytotoxic Drug Resistance

- Cytotoxic drug resistance may be expressed as a temporary or permanent insensitivity.
- Temporary resistance is usually observed only in vivo with drugs known to be active against a specific cancer.
- Permanent or phenotypic drug resistance, an inheritable resistance mechanism, is the result of a genetic mutation or preexisting trait. Point mutations usually occur in a single cell and are independent of drug concentration.
- Gene amplification is influenced by drug concentration and occurs with repeated exposure over an extended period of time.
- Expression of the *mdr-1* gene is thought to be responsible for the development of multidrug resistance (MDR).

### Biological basis of phenotypic drug resistance

- If mutations occur early in the growth of a population of tumor cells, a high fraction of resistant cells would result. A mutation occurring later would produce only a small fraction of resistant clones.
- Cytotoxic therapy directed at minimal tumor burden has a much greater likelihood of being successful. The chance of a cell being resistant to two or more antineoplastic drugs simultaneously is less than that of being resistant to single agents when used alone.

### Mechanisms of drug resistance

- Resistance may result from alterations in drug metabolism or alterations in cytotoxic targets.
- Cancer cells can overcome the effects of cytotoxic drugs either by increasing the amount of target enzymes or by modifying the enzyme so as to interfere with binding to antagonistic drugs.
- The ability of cells to repair DNA lesions is an important resistance mechanism seen with alkylating agents and cisplatin.
- Intracellular drug concentrations may be significantly reduced as a result of decreased influx carrier proteins, enhanced efflux pump functioning, or both.

### Multidrug-resistance phenotype

- Tumor cells that exhibit resistance to a group of drugs that are structurally dissimilar, with unrelated cytotoxic mechanisms, or both, are expressing an MDR phenotype.
- The classic form of MDR is associated with overexpression of *mdr-1* gene, which encodes for an energy-dependent cell membrane efflux pump, P-glycoprotein (P-gp). Cytotoxic drugs that have entered the cell probably bind to a carrier protein before reaching their cellular targets and are transported out of the cell via the pump.
- Some cell lines have increased expression of a protein that likely functions as a drug transporter similar to P-gp. This multidrug resistance-associated protein (MRP) gene confers resistance to structurally unrelated natural products.

## Strategies for reversing MDR

- The two most widely investigated modulators are verapamil and cyclosporine A.
- Drugs used as modulators of MDR are often given in doses at or above their therapeutic range, often producing significant toxicity.

## Other mechanisms of MDR

- MDR in cells cross-resistant to topoisomerase poison is associated with P-gp-mediated MDR, but the pattern of resistance is different and cells retain sensitivity to vinca alkaloids, which facilitate elimination of the drug from the tumor cell.
- MDR may also be demonstrated in cells with increased detoxifying systems.

# Chemotherapy as a Treatment for Cancer

## Primary and adjuvant chemotherapy

- *Induction* is used to describe chemotherapy given to patients with leukemia or other advanced disease that is highly sensitive to drugs.
- *Neoadjuvant chemotherapy* describes chemotherapy given prior to alternative treatments in patients who present with primarily local disease.

## Therapeutic strategies

### Combination chemotherapy

- Administering a combination of clinically effective anticancer drugs is the standard chemotherapeutic approach for most malignancies.
- The objectives of combination chemotherapy are achieving maximal tumor cell kill without excessive toxicity; providing cytotoxic drugs that are active against potentially resistant heterogeneous tumor populations; and avoiding selection of resistant cell lines.
- Chemotherapy cycles for drugs with significant myelosuppression are approximately three to four weeks.

### Dose intensity

- Dose intensity is expressed as the amount of drug delivered per unit of time, or simply $mg/m^2/week$.
- The effect of a new regimen on treatment outcome can be expressed as the relative dose intensity (RDI).
- High-dose chemotherapy regimens with hematopoietic support are quickly becoming an acceptable treatment alternative.

### Chemoprotective agents

- Chemoprotective and rescue agents have been developed for use in preventing or reversing drug-induced toxicity for some anticancer agents.

### High-dose chemotherapy with peripheral blood stem cell transplant

- High-dose chemotherapy with autologous rescue is being used more frequently in cancers that respond to increasing doses of marrow-ablative therapy.
- The introduction of the hematopoietic growth factors (HGFs), such as G-CSF and GM-CSF, has been among the major advancements in supportive care measures.
- Peripheral blood stem cells (PBSCs) are committed progenitor cells harvested from peripheral blood, which have the capacity of restoring hematopoiesis.

- Compared with patients receiving autologous bone marrow alone, patients who receive PBSCs either alone or with bone marrow transplantation typically have fewer days of neutropenia and thrombocytopenia.
- A major disadvantage of PBSC transplantation is nausea, vomiting, and hypertension associated with infusion. Another concern is the potential to reinfuse mobilized tumor cells, as well as hematopoietic stem cells.

### Chemotherapy as a radiation sensitizer

- The primary goal of combined-modality treatment is to overcome radiation resistance and improve locoregional control of disease.
- Chemoradiotherapy with fluorouracil has demonstrated improved overall survival. Cisplatin has also been investigated as a radiation enhancer.
- The results of current trials suggest that a maximal benefit of combined therapy is seen in patients with less advanced disease.

### Chronopharmacology and cancer chemotherapy

- Chronopharmacology is described as the temporal variation in the handling of drugs by the body. This new and emerging science examines the variance of chemical and physical processes of a biological system with respect to time.

## PHARMACOLOGY OF CHEMOTHERAPEUTIC DRUGS

## Pharmacokinetics of Antineoplastic Drugs

### Principles of pharmacokinetics

- *Pharmacokinetics* is the study of the movement of drugs in the body.
- The half-life of a drug is the time required for the serum concentration of the drug to decrease by one-half. The drug's half-life determines the time required to reach steady-state concentrations in the serum and the appropriate dosing interval.
- The interval necessary for most of the drug to be removed from the body is equal to three half-lives of the drug.
- Clearance is the most important pharmacokinetic parameter because it determines the steady-state concentration and is independent of half-life. Clearance is determined by blood flow to an organ, and the organ's efficacy in extracting the drug from the blood.
- The volume of distribution ($V_D$) relates the amount of drug in the body to the serum concentration.
- Half-life is dependent on clearance and $V_D$; therefore, variability in half-life may be the result of changes in clearance, $V_D$, or both.
- The basic principles of clinical pharmacokinetics may be divided into four major areas: absorption, distribution, metabolism, and excretion.

### Absorption

- Absorption from the gastrointestinal tract should be sufficient to ensure adequate bioavailability of the drug.

### Distribution

- Distribution of drugs in the body is determined primarily by their ability to penetrate different tissues and their affinity for binding to plasma proteins.

### Metabolism

- The metabolic activation and inactivation or catabolism of drugs is carried out primarily by the liver. Some of these enzymatic processes are also performed in normal and tumor cells.
- Many chemotherapy drugs require activation intracellularly or systemically before they are able to exert their cytotoxic effect.

### Elimination

- Significant decreases in renal function can decrease the clearance of these compounds from the body and cause excessive toxicity.
- The biliary tract is the primary route of elimination for vinca alkaloids, and urinary excretion is minimal.

## Pharmacokinetic principles applied to chemotherapeutic drugs

- Efflux from the cell is a major limitation of antineoplastic drug efficacy.
- The area under the serum concentration-time curve (AUC) is a measure of systemic drug exposure.
- Methods of dose prediction based on target AUCs and a measure of drug elimination may provide a more optimal treatment intensity.

# Drug Interactions in the Patient Receiving Chemotherapy

- Direct interactions involve changes in the pharmacokinetics of the primary drug such as oral absorption, distribution, metabolism, and excretion.
- Drugs may also interact by indirectly altering the eliminating function of the organs of the body.
- Chemotherapeutic drugs often share similar toxicities with other drugs. Therefore, additive toxicities may occur.

# Antineoplastic Drugs

- Cancer chemotherapeutic drugs have traditionally been classified by their mechanism of action, chemical structure, or biological source.
- Although drugs within a class share some characteristics, there are often major differences in their indications, toxicities, and pharmaceutical properties.

## Alkylating and alkylating-like agents

### Classic alkylators

- Alkylators are non-cell cycle phase-specific and are most active in the resting cell ($G_0$).
- Dose-limiting toxicities of most alkylators are myelosuppression, which may be severe, and rapid-onset nausea and vomiting.
- Nitrogen mustard, cyclophosphamide, melphalan, chlorambucil and thiotepa are examples of alkylators.
- Ifosfamide administration is associated with a much higher incidence of urotoxicity than cyclophosphamide. Cystitis can be prevented by the co-administration of mesna, a compound that inactivates urotoxic metabolites in the bladder.
- Thiotepa has some unique skin toxicities, including an acute erythroderma and dry desquamation of the palms and soles; and chronic darkening or bronzing of the skin when used in high-dose regimens.
- Nitrosoureas are distinct from other alkylators in that they are highly lipid-soluble and readily cross the blood-brain barrier.

### Platinum-containing compounds

- Although cisplatin and other platinum analogues behave similarly to alkylators, their cytotoxicity is probably the result of a combination of mechanisms of action, including inhibition of DNA and protein sythesis, alteration in cell membrane transport, and suppression of mitochondrial function.
- Patients who previously received cisplatin may be at increased risk for toxicity with carboplatin and should be evaluated for decreased renal function.
- Although both platinum analogues possess similar antitumor activity, there are significant differences in their dosing, administration, and side effect profiles.
- The dose-limiting toxicity of cisplatin is nephrotoxicity. Acute renal failure may occur within 24 hours of drug administration. Patients most at risk are those who receive inadequate hydration. Nephrotoxicity may usually be avoided by adequately hydrating the patient and administering diuretics.
- Emesis is often more severe and prolonged with cisplatin.

### Other alkylating-like drugs

- Other drugs with alkylating-like activity include dacarbazine, procarbazine, and altretamine (hexamethylmelamine). Dacarbazine does not appear to be cell cycle-phase specific and kills cells in all phases of the cycle.
- The most significant adverse events are nausea and vomiting, which may decrease with repeated courses. Other toxicities include a flu-like syndrome, myelosuppression, and photosensitivity.
- Procarbazine is a major therapeutic agent in the treatment of Hodgkin's disease and brain tumors. Hexamethylmelamine's mechanism of action is uncertain but probably of an alkylating type.

## Antitumor antibiotics

### Anthracycline antibiotics

- Anthracyclines have multiple mechanisms of cytotoxicity including intercalation, DNA binding, free radical formation and inhibition of topoisomerase II enzymes.
- Anthracyclines are metabolized to both active and inactive compounds by the liver. The anthracycline dose should be reduced in patients with hepatic dysfunction.
- The more common and often therapy-limiting cardiotoxicity is the development of cardiomyopathy leading to congestive heart failure. Dexrazoxane is a chemoprotective agent designed to protect heart muscle and may be given to patients at risk for CHF from doxorubicin. Mitoxantrone may be associated with less nausea, vomiting, and alopecia. Cardiac toxicity in patients treated with mitoxantrone appears to be less than that seen with doxorubicin. However, there may be no difference in the incidence of cardiomyopathy at doses equipotent to doxorubicin. Liposomal encapsulation of doxorubicin and daunorubicin has provided two new anticancer agents with therapeutic and toxicity profiles different from the free form of these drugs.
- Liposomal daunorubicin and liposomal doxorubicin are currently established treatments for Kaposi's sarcoma in patients with acquired immunodeficiency syndrome (AIDS). There are also significant data suggesting activity in breast cancer.

### Other antitumor antibiotics

- Tumor cells are most sensitive to bleomycin in the premitotic, or $G_2$, phase, or in the mitotic phase of the cell cycle. Bleomycin has been used to synchronize cells into the $G_2$ and S phases so that other antineoplastic agents that act in those phases may have an increased cell kill potential. Bleomycin is also useful in combination chemotherapy regimens because of its lack of significant myelosuppressive effects.

- Pulmonary toxicity of bleomycin may initially present as cough, dyspnea, and pleuritic chest pain.
- Dactinomycin (actinomycin D) also binds to DNA by intercalation and induces single-strand breaks similar to those seen with doxorubicin. The drug is currently limited to use in pediatric tumors and gestational trophoblastic neoplasms. Mitomycin C produces a delayed and cumulative myelosuppression as well as a hemolytic-aremic syndrome resulting in renal failure.

## Antimetabolites

### Antifolates

- The antineoplastic effect of this group of drugs is related to their ability to inhibit nucleic acid synthesis or to falsely be incorporated into the DNA double helix. Antifolate drugs methotrexate and trimetrexate inhibit the enzyme dihydrofolate reductase (DHFR), which catalyzes the reduction of dihydrofolate (folic acid) to tetrohydrofolate (folinic acid). Most cells can function with relatively small amounts of DHFR to maintain sufficient reduced folate pools. Therefore, a high intracellular concentration of antifolate drugs should be maintained to ensure complete enzyme inhibition. This may be accomplished by administering large amounts of methotrexate.
- Leucovorin circumvents methotrexate-induced enzyme blockade and "rescues" normal cells by providing them with the reduced folates they need. Methotrexate-associated toxicities, besides myelosuppression and mucositis, include nephrotoxicity, hepatotoxicity, and pulmonary fibrosis.

### Pyrimidine analogues

- The administration of 5-FU and leucovorin concurrently enhances depletion of dTTP or false incorporation of other metabolites into DNA and RNA. It also increases the cytotoxic effect of 5-FU.
- When 5-FU or floxuridine is administered directly into the hepatic artery or portal vein, hepatic metastases are directly exposed to the drug with minimal systemic exposure because of the drug's significant first-pass clearance.
- Myelosuppression is more prominent when 5-FU is given by rapid bolus injection, whereas mucositis and gastrointestinal toxicity are more common with prolonged infusions over four to five days.
- Cytarabine may be used alone or in addition to methotrexate for meningeal leukemia.
- Toxicity of cytarabine includes myelosuppression and gastrointestinal epithelial injury.

### Purine analogues

- Thiopurines 6-mercaptopurine (6-MP) and 6-thioguanine (6-TG) are converted to their respective monophosphates, which inhibit purine synthesis and cause an accumulation of nucleic acid precursors. These precursors in turn facilitate the conversion of 6-MP and 6-TG to their active nucleotide forms.

## Plant derivatives

- Many of the drugs in this group are naturally occurring alkaloids that were isolated from plant material. Others are the result of synthetic and semisynthetic processes used to manufacture analogues of compounds originally extracted from plants.

## Vinca alkaloids

- Vincristine has a broad spectrum of activity, including leukemia, lymphoma, breast cancer, lung cancer, and multiple myeloma, while vinblastine is used primarily in germ cell tumors and advanced Hodgkin's disease.
- Vinorelbine is active in breast cancer and non-small-cell lung cancer and is both myelotoxic and neurotoxic.
- Vinca alkaloids belong to a group of compounds now known as the *tubulin interactive agents*. They exert their cytotoxic effects primarily by interfering with normal microtubule formation and function, which is critical for the mitosis phase of the cell cycle and ultimately cell division.
- Peripheral neurotoxicity initially presents as sensory impairment and paresthesias. Patients may later develop neuritic pain and motor dysfunction. Loss of deep tendon reflexes, foot and wrist drop, ataxia, and paralysis may occur with continued vinca alkaloid therapy.

## Taxanes

- The taxanes, paclitaxel, and docetaxel bind to microtubules and inhibit microtubular assembly. They are metabolized in the liver.
- The taxanes cause myelosuppression, neurotoxicity, hypersensitivity, alopecia, and transient arthralgias, and myalgias.
- Hypersensitivity reactions can be significant but are prevented by premedicating the patient with steroids, antihistamines, and $H_2$ blockers.
- Skin reactions, including pruritus, macular or papular lesions, erythema, and desquamation, are seen in 50%–70% of patients treated with docetaxel.

## Epipodophyllotoxins

- Etoposide and teniposide are glycosidic derivatives of podophyllotoxin that possess significant activity in many human tumors such as germ cell tumors and lung cancer.
- The toxicities of both agents are similar, with myelosuppression, hypersensitivity, and infusion-related blood pressure changes being the most significant.

## Camptothecin derivatives

- Topotecan and irinotecan were recently approved by the FDA as single-agent therapy for refractory ovarian cancer and relapsed colon cancer, respectively.
- Myelosuppression is the major dose-limiting toxicity of topotecan, while diarrhea is the primary dose-limiting toxicity for irinotecan when administered on a once-weekly schedule.

## Miscellaneous agents

- L-asparaginase induces a rapid and complete depletion from the blood of the amino acid L-asparagine. This biochemical process is cytotoxic to tumor cells highly dependent on exogenous sources of the amino acid.
- The drug's only antineoplastic use is as part of the induction and consolidation therapy for acute lymphocytic leukemia in both children and adults.
- Hydroxyurea inhibits ribonucleotide reductase. Its major indication is in rapidly controlling blood counts in acute leukemia and other myeloproliferative diseases.

## Hormonal Therapy

- Manipulation of the hormonal environment of the cancer cell is therapeutic when the cancer cell is dependent on the hormone for cell division.
- Steroids and steroid analogues constitute the majority of drugs used for hormonal therapy.

## Retinoids

- Retinoids, a class of compounds structurally related to vitamin A (retinol), have been found to influence proliferation and differentiation of normal and tumor cells. Isotretinoin is under extensive evaluation, often in combination with alfa-interferon, for the prevention of new and recurrent squamous cell tumors.
- Tretinoin has recently been approved for use in induction and maintenance regimens for acute promyelocytic leukemia.

## PRACTICE QUESTIONS

1   Vanessa works in a lab conducting preclinical toxicology studies to determine safe starting doses for potential anticancer agents for use in humans. She has begun phase I trials for Drug E to determine a maximum tolerated dose. Vanessa's study is using patients with advanced cancer as subjects. Dosing starts at 10% of the $LD_{10}$. This:
   a.   will be escalated until significant toxicity is seen in 10% or more of the patients treated.
   b.   will help in determining the MTD when the dose is raised high enough to produce toxicity in at least 50% of the patients treated.
   c.   is one step below the MTD.
   d.   is used for phase II testing.

2.   A phase IV clinical trial is designed to address:
   a.   the use of drugs, usually in combination, where cure is the goal of therapy.
   b.   to answer questions regarding various doses and schedules.
   c.   to offer new information regarding risks and toxicities.
   d.   all of the above.

3.   A Gompertzian growth curve:
   a.   may best describe the growth of human tumors.
   b.   demonstrates the responses observed with the administration of antineoplastic drugs.
   c.   a and b.
   d.   neither of the above.

4.   Terrence has a large solid tumor of a cell type that is generally minimally responsive to chemotherapy. What might the physician do prior to chemotherapy to increase tumor responsiveness?
   a.   Surgical excision to recruit more cells into the proliferative phase
   b.   Debulking the tumor to decrease the tumor's growth fraction
   c.   Injecting agents so that the tumor does not close off the patient's blood supply
   d.   All of the above

5.   A physician hopes to direct cytotoxic therapy at a minimal tumor burden. If mutations occur early in the growth of a patient's population of tumor cells:
   a.   only a small fraction of the clones will be resistant.
   b.   a high fraction of resistant cells will result.
   c.   they will produce only a small fraction of resistant clones when compared with a mutation occurring later.
   d.   a and c

6.   Chemotherapy drug resistance occurs primarily because the cancer cell has the ability to do which of the following?
   a.   increase the number of target enzymes
   b.   repair DNA lesions
   c.   modify target enzymes so as to interfere with binding to antagonistic drugs
   d.   all of the above

7.   Neoadjuvant chemotherapy is:
   a.   is given to patients with leukemia or other advanced diseases that are highly sensitive to drugs.
   b.   given prior to alternative treatments in patients who present with primarily local disease.
   c.   is given to patients with cancers for which no effective alternative treatment exists.
   d.   a and c.

8. In the process of teaching a patient who is to receive peripheral blood stem cell transplant, it is important to include which of the following statements?
   a. PBSCs have the potential to reinfuse mobilized tumor cells, as well as hematopoietic stem cells.
   b. PBSCs have the capacity to restore hematopoiesis.
   ✓ c. PBSCs usually enable the patient to have fewer days of neutropenia.
   d. all of the above.

9. The half-life of a drug:
   a. refers to the volume of distribution or the amount of drug in the body versus its serum concentration.
   b. represents the interval necessary for most of the drug to be removed from the body.
   c. determines the time required to reach steady-state concentrations in the seum.\
   d. a and c.

10. The metabolic activation and inactivation or catabolism of drugs is carried out primarily by the:
    a. liver.
    b. spleen.
    c. gastrointestinal system.
    d. kidneys.

11. Dexrazoxane is:
    a. a chemoprotective agent designed to protect heart muscle from doxorubicin effects.
    b. a platinum analogue with properties similar to alkylators.
    c. a classic alkylator that attacks electron-rich nucleophilic sites on DNA.
    d. an antifolate that inhibits nucleic acid synthesis.

12. Mrs. Carsen is receiving high-dose methotrexate. She is to take leucovorin every 6 hours for 8 doses. The purpose of the leucovorin is:
    a. to rescue normal cells from toxicity.
    b. to augment the effect of methotrexate.
    c. to prevent long-term side effects.
    d. to treat diarrhea.

13. Lynn is about to be treated with a vinca alkaloid for her multiple myeloma. As part of her patient education plan, you will tell her that vinca alkaloids are:
    a. tubulin interactive agents.
    b. interfere with normal microtubule formation and function.
    c. reserved for those patients who may experience peripheral neurotoxicity with other agents.
    d. a and b.

## ANSWER EXPLANATIONS

1. **The answer is b.** In phase I trials, dosing starts at 10% of the $LD_{10}$ determined in mice and is escalated until significant toxicity is seen in 50% or more of the patients treated. This dose is the MTD, and one step below the MTD is used for phase II testing. (p. 285)

2. **The answer is d.** Postmarketing or phase IV studies are usually designed to answer questions regarding other uses, doses, and schedules, as well as new information regarding risks and toxicity of a new treatment. (p. 286)

3. **The answer is c.** A Gompertzian growth curve probably best describes the growth of human tumors and the responses observed with the administration of chemotherapy. (p. 288)

4. **The answer is a.** Larger tumors have small growth fractions and are therefore less responsive to the cytotoxic effects of antineoplastic drugs. The ability of chemotherapy to reach large solid tumors may be hindered by inadequate blood flow. Surgical excision or debulking of tumors can increase the responsiveness of these tumors by recruiting more cells into the proliferative phase. (p. 289)

5. **The answer is b.** If mutations occur early in the growth of a population of tumor cells, a high fraction of resistant cells would result. A mutation occurring later would produce only a small fraction of resistant clones. (p. 291)

6. **The answer is d.** Cancer cells can overcome the effects of cytotoxic drugs either by increasing the number of target enzymes or by modifying the enzyme so as to interfere with binding to antagonistic drugs. The ability of cells to repair DNA lesions is an important resistance mechanism seen with alkylating agents and cisplatin. (p. 292)

7. **The answer is b.** Neoadjuvant chemotherapy is given prior to alternative treatments in patients who present with primarily local disease. Induction chemotherapy is given to patients with leukemia or other advanced disease that is highly sensitive to drugs and for whom no effective alternative exists. (p. 294)

8. **The answer is d.** PBSCs are committed progenitor cells harvested from peripheral blood. They have the capacity of restoring hematopoiesis. Compared with patients receiving autologous bone marrow alone, patients who receive PBSCs either alone or with bone marrow transplantation typically have fewer days of neutropenia and thrombocytopenia. Another concern is the potential to reinfuse mobilized tumor cells, as well as hematopoietic stem cells. (p. 296)

9. **The answer is c.** The half-life of a drug is the time required for the serum concentration of the drug to decrease by one-half. The drug's half-life determines the time required to reach steady-state concentrations in the serum and the appropriate dosing interval. The interval necessary for most of the drug to be removed from the body is equal to three half-lives of the drug. (p. 297)

10. **The answer is a.** The metabolic activation and inactivation or catabolism of drugs is carried out primarily by the liver. (p. 298)

11. **The answer is a.** Dexrazoxane protects the heart muscle from possible CHF effects in the administration of doxorubicin. (p. 305)

12. **The answer is a.** Leucovorin circumvents methotrexate-induced enzyme blockade and "rescues" normal cells by providing them with the reduced folates they need for nucleic acid and protein synthesis. (p. 306)

13. **The answer is d.** Vinca alkaloids belong to a group of compounds now known as the tubulin interactive agents. They exert their cytotoxic effects primarily by interfering with normal microtubule formation and function, which is critical for the mitosis phase of the cell cycle and ultimately cell division. Vinca alkaloids are known for their peripheral neurotoxicity. (p. 308)

# Chapter 15 Chemotherapy: Principles of Administration

## CHEMOTHERAPY ADMINISTRATION
### Professional Qualifications
- Basic qualifications for nurses administering antineoplastic agents include:
  - current licensure as a registered nurse
  - certification in CPR
  - intravenous therapy skills
  - educational preparation and demonstration of knowledge in all areas related to antineoplastic drugs
  - skill in drug administration
  - ongoing acquisition of updated information and verification of continuing knowledge and skills
  - policies and procedures to govern specific actions

### Handling Cytotoxic Drugs
- Antineoplastic agents are mutagenic, teratogenic, and carcinogenic.
- Direct exposure to cytotoxic agents can occur during admixture, administration, or handling.
- Exposure to cytotoxic agents occurs through inhalation, ingestion, or absorption.
- The use of personal protective equipment greatly minimizes risk of exposure.
- OSHA recommends that pregnant employees be informed of potential risks and, if necessary, reassigned to other duties.
- OSHA minimum standards to be met include (1) knowledge of the latest scientific information; (2) established policies and procedures; and (3) ongoing monitoring to ensure compliance and continuous quality improvement.

### Patient and Family Education
- Assessment of the patient should include the individual's response to the diagnosis, communication style, ability to read/comprehend information, family status, lifestyle, and treatment outcome expectations.
- More complex instruction is required when a patient is entering a research protocol.
- Follow-up includes assessment of the patient's understanding of the information imparted and determination that the outcome has been achieved.

### Professional Issues
- Nurses who administer chemotherapy agents must be thoroughly trained in the pharmacology of the drugs, including distribution and elimination patterns and proper techniques of drug preparation, administration, and drug interactions.
- The nurse has primary responsibility for prevention, early detection, and management of acute reactions associated with chemotherapy, including hypersensitivity, anaphylaxis, hypotension, extravasation, nausea, and vomiting.
- Measures to minimize errors in drug delivery include the following:
  - Chemotherapy orders are written by the physician most knowledgable of the patient's needs and most responsible for the patient's care

- Drug names are written clearly and in full without abbreviations.
- Once written, orders are not transcribed or rewritten prior to reconstitution or administration.
- Avoid extraneous decimal points and zeros so that, for example, vincristine 1.0 mg is never mistaken for vincristine 10 mg.
- Drugs are dispensed in individual, sealed bags or trays.
- The drug and dosage are double-checked by someone other than the person admixing the drug.
- When a drug error occurs or an extravasation of a vesicant is suspected or certain, the nurse must document the event thoroughly.
- Often patients have been offered a vascular access device and then refuse the device. This should be documented.
- Chemotherapy is never (with rare exception) an emergency treatment in which a delay of two or three days to place an access device would be detrimental to the patient's condition.
- It is far better for the patient that the nurse refuse to attempt another venipuncture rather than to forge ahead with even more risk of extravasation.

## ROUTES OF DRUG ADMINISTRATION
### Dose Calculation

- In situations where a dose reduction is necessary and the patient's weight is significantly greater than their ideal, a simple method of calculating their dose is to take the average of the ideal and actual weight.
- The dose of drug to be administered is generally based on the individual's body surface area.
- It is often proposed that individual doses be calculated based on a person's physiological age rather than their chronological age.
- The Calvert formula makes it possible to individualize the carboplatin dose in order to obtain a maximally effective dose with tolerable side effects.
  - It is important to note that when using area under the curve(AUC) dosing for carboplatin, the dose is expressed in mg, *not* mg/m$^2$.
  - AUC dosing correlates more closely with drug toxicity than do doses based on body surface area.
  - Glomerular filtration rate (GFR) is essentially equivalent to the creatinine clearance, which can be estimated from the patient's age, serum creatinine, and weight.

### Pretreatment Considerations

- Standards of practice dictate that a physician be physically available where chemotherapy is administered.
- It is still considered appropriate to administer a test dose of bleomycin prior to administering the full dose because the first dose of bleomycin has been known to cause rare but severe allergic reactions, especially in patients with lymphoma.
- Another consideration involves prevention of hypersensitivity reactions (HSR) with paclitaxel or docetaxel.
  - Docetaxel is associated with less risk of HSR.
- In the case of etoposide, the primary reaction is hypotension.
- The last pretreatment consideration involves the sequencing of various drugs to either enhance cytotoxicity or minimize toxicity to normal tissues.

### Topical

- Topical application of antineoplastic agents is most commonly done for cutaneous T-cell lymphoma, basal cell carcinoma, Kaposi's sarcoma, and squamous cell carcinoma. The agents used include nitrogen mustard for cutaneous T-cell lymphoma and fluorouracil for the two mentioned carcinomas.

- When using nitrogen mustard, have sodium thiosulfate available and apply it to areas of the skin that may be inadvertently exposed (after removal of the drug).

## Oral

- The patient needs to understand how critical it is that the prescribed regimen be followed exactly. As is the case with high-dose methotrexate and leucovorin rescue, failure to take the leucovorin as scheduled can result in severe toxicity, or even death.
- Multiple courses of oral antineoplastics should not be given at one time because of the risk of overdose.

## Intramuscular and Subcutaneous

- The development of the biological agents has increased the number of drugs given IM or SQ.
- Since some of the drugs can sting or burn, IM injections are usually given into large muscles, with the Z-track method being optional.

## Intravenous

- When giving a vesicant, it is always better to have a blood return throughout the injection, so a smaller-gauge needle is not preferable in that situation. For patients with small veins, choose an angiocath that is thin-walled with an over-the-needle cannula.
- When selecting a vein, start distally and gradually proceed proximal. Another rule might be to select the best vein, provided that vein is not the antecubital vein. Placing a needle in the antecubital area restricts patient mobility and increases the risk of dislodgment. Any extravasation that occurs is difficult to detect because the area is dense and a lot of fluid can infiltrate before it is detected.
- The reasons to give the vesicant before any other agent are that (1) the venous integrity is greatest earlier on in the procedure, and (2) the nurse's assessment skills and the patient's level of awareness and sensitivity are most acute at the initiation of the infusion. The possibility that the vein will be irritated by other drugs (decadron) or by movement is eliminated.
- It is faulty reasoning to assume that if the vein takes the nonvesicants without any problem, the vesicant will infuse without difficulty. The risk of infiltration of *any* IV increases over time.
- Patients who in the past have experienced severe anxiety and pain with venipuncture claim they feel nothing when Emla cream is in place for at least two hours before the needle goes in.
  - Caution: Emla should not be used in patients who are also receiving a vesicant agent peripherally because they will not be able to feel the pain if the vesicant should infiltrate.

## Vesicant Extravasation Issues

- Several of the most commonly administered chemotherapy drugs are vesicants, meaning they cause tissue necrosis if they infiltrate or extravasate out of the blood vessel and into the soft tissue.
- By definition, an *extravasation* is the infiltration of a vesicant chemotherapeutic agent. A *vesicant* is a drug that, if infiltrated, is capable of causing pain, ulceration, necrosis, and sloughing of damaged tissue.
- When infiltration of a vesicant occurs, underlying tissue is damaged. The damage can be severe enough to result in physical deformity or a functional deficit, such as loss of joint mobility, loss of vascularity, or loss of tendon function.
- The following symptoms could indicate extravasation:
  - swelling (most common)
  - stinging, burning, or pain at the injection site (not *always* present)
  - redness (not often seen initially)
  - lack of blood return (Lack of a blood return *alone* is not always indicative of an extravasation. An extravasation can occur even if a blood return is present.)

- The most benign, inconsequential local reaction to chemotherapy is venous flare. This reaction occurs most commonly in patients receiving doxorubicin and is characterized by a localized erythema, venous streaking, and pruritis along the injected vein. This localized allergic reaction is distinguishable from an extravasation by the absence of pain or swelling and the presence of a blood return.
- Certain nonvesicant chemotherapy agents cause intravascular irritation, often accompanied by pain during infusion, but do not cause ulceration if infiltrated. Antineoplastic agents that can cause skin discoloration, irritation, induration and some discomfort if infiltrated—but do not generally cause ulceration—are called *irritants* (e.g., docetaxel, pacletaxel, BCNU, DTIC).

### Prevention and assessment

- Vesicant agents are given only by nurses/physicians who are certified in chemotherapy administration.
- Vesticants are never given by continuous infusion via a peripheral vein.
- The one obvious sign of drug infiltration is a bleb formation at the injection site that is readily apparent in a superficial vein, or swelling that occurs in more deeply accessed veins.
- An extravasation may go unnoticed, especially when the vein lies deeply in an obese limb. In this situation a large amount of drug can infiltrate, especially if the drug is injected very slowly.
- Any antiemetics, sedatives, or analgesics that may affect the patient's ability to readily report any change in sensation at the injection site should be withheld until after the vesicant has been safely administered.
- A blood return should be assessed every 1–2 ml of drug administration. The presence of a blood return is valuable to determine venous access but does not always ensure an intact vein.
- Vascular access devices have become a common method of drug delivery and are an important option for patients who require chemotherapy over a long period of time and/or have poor venous access.
  - When giving vesicant agents through a port, whether by simple injection or long-term infusion, use a 90-degree bent huber point needle.
  - The ideal catheter for infusion of vesicant agents in the outpatient/home environment is the tunneled externally based catheter or PICC line.

### Management

- If a vesicant agent extravasates, the nurse should follow the institutional guidelines for management of an extravasation. Management depends upon the drug infiltrated.
  - Prompt detection of an extravasation will usually result in minimal tissue damage.
  - The degree of tissue damage is in proportion to the amount and concentration of drug infiltration.
  - If the patient is receiving a drug that has a true antidote, the antidote is prepared and administered as soon as possible according to institutional policy and procedure. For example, sodium thiosulfate is the antidote for mechlorethemine; hyaluronidase is the antidote for vincristine and vinblastine.
  - The physician is notified immediately of an extravasation, and the documentation record is completed.
  - The patient receives written instructions on site care, such as application of ice and follow-up with physician.
  - If an extravasation occurs from a central line, the infusion is stopped immediately.
  - Extravasation from a central venous catheter may be substantial before detected because the infusion is not monitored *constantly* and is generally administered using a mechanical pump. Also, the vesicant may sting or burn less because it is more diluted than when given by intravenous injection.

## Intra-arterial

- Intra-arterial drug administration involves cannulation of the artery that provides a tumor's blood supply and subsequent administration of the drug directly through the arterial catheter to the tumor bed.
- The primary utilization of this route is the hepatic artery for the management of metastasis of colon cancer to the liver.
- The implantable pump offers the patient the greatest level of freedom when receiving intra-arterial chemotherapy; potential disadvantages are infection and the cost.

## Intraperitoneal

- The semipermeable nature of the peritoneal space allows high concentrations of drugs at the tumor sites throughout the peritoneal space, but with lower concentrations entering the bloodstream.
- It is possible to minimize systemic side effects by simultaneously infusing an agent intravenously to counteract drug side effects through the venous system.
- There are three methods of accessing the peritoneal space: (1) intermittent placement of temporary indwelling catheters; (2) placement of a Tenckhoff external catheter; and (3) placement of an implantable peritoneal port.
  - Intermittent placement might be used if the therapy is planned for a short time.
  - Tenckhoff catheters are placed when several months of therapy are planned, especially when the treatment goal is cure of minimal or microscopic residual disease.
  - The implanted port is internal and requires no care.

## Intrapleural

- When effusion is caused by malignant cells, the preferred treatment is sclerosis with an antineoplastic agent such as nitrogen mustard or bleomycin.

## Intravesical

- Direct instillation of chemotherapy into the bladder has been a very effective and simple method of controlling superficial bladder cancer and carcinoma in situ. Agents such as thiotepa, doxorubicin, mitomycin C, and bacillus Calmette-Guerin (BCG) have all been shown to be effective, especially BCG.
  - A unique side effect of BCG is a "creepy-crawling" feeling. Patients report feeling as if their skin is creeping or little things are crawling on them. Administration of a mild sedative can be considered if this side effect occurs.

## Intrathecal or Intraventricular

- Metastatic cancer involving the CNS, specifically the meninges, is seen most commonly in leukemia, breast cancer, and lymphoma.
- Preservative-free chemotherapy is injected directly into the CSF as prophylaxis or to manage existing disease. The two primary methods of instillation are intrathecal and intraventricular.
  - Central instillation of the drug into the ventricle can be achieved via an Ommaya reservoir, which is surgically implanted through the cranium.
  - Intraventricular drugs are capable of entering the systemic bloodstream.
  - Few drugs may be safely given into the CSF. Two examples include methotrexate and cytarabine.

## VASCULAR ACCESS DEVICES

- Intermittent peripheral venous access is preferred for patients with good veins on limited intermittent therapies not involving vesicant infusions.

## General Management

### Nontunneled central venous catheters

- Short-term use of nontunneled CVC, such as a standard subclavian line, is common practice in urgent situations. It is primarily intended to provide immediate access until the emergency can be resolved; it is also available as a multilumen catheter.
- Peripherally inserted central catheters (PICCs) are ideal for short-term access (weeks to months) in patients with adequate antecubital veins, self-care capabilities, and the need for a wide variety of intravenous therapies.

### Tunneled central venous catheters

- Unique features of the TCVC include a Dacron cuff around which granulation tissue forms, actually helping to hold the catheter in place.
- One unique variation of a TCVC is the Groshong catheter, which features a closed-end radiopaque tip. Flow through the catheter is achieved via a patented slit valve.
- There are several major advantages of the TCVC, including its elimination of needle sticks for those people who have a needle phobia, and the ease with which it is removed when no longer needed for care. TCVC is the ideal catheter for TPN administration and for the patient with multiple/frequent vascular access needs, such as the bone marrow transplant patient.
- TCVC is also the only long-term device that offers a triple-access option.
- One unique care issue related to TCVCs is the possibility of the fracture, puncture, or cutting of the external portion of the catheter.

### Implantable ports

- The implantable port, when it is not in use, requires almost no care or maintenance. A *port* is a hollow housing containing a compressed latex septum over a portal chamber connected via a small tube to a silicone or polyurethane catheter inserted into a blood vessel.

#### Port routes

- There are five major types of ports: venous, arterial, peritoneal, intrapleural, and epidural. The arterial and epidural ports have specially designed catheters with very small lumens, since the flow rate through these devices is often low.
- The peritoneal catheter has a very large lumen and multiple fluid outlet holes in the catheter to allow rapid infusion of fluids.

#### Port usage

- The venous port is an ideal choice for patients who are (1) unable or unwilling to care properly for an external device, (2) receiving intermittent therapies, (3) concerned about body image, or (4) physically active. Its major disadvantage is that it requires a needle to pass through the skin and into the port for usage. The procedure of accessing the port could introduce infective organisms, cause a hematoma, or result in extravasation. There is also a very remote chance that the device could extrude through the skin.
- TPN can cause drug crystals or sludge to build up inside the portal housing and occlude the device.
- There is a concern when administering continuous-infusion vesicants because the needle could become dislodged from the septum and remain under the skin, causing a port pocket extravasation.

### Peripheral implantable port

- The P.A.S.-Port allows the peripheral insertion of a port in the forearm instead of the chest area. The peripheral port is best suited for the patient in whom placement of a port in the chest would be difficult—for example, the woman with cancer with extensive skin involvement or the woman who has had bilateral breast reconstruction.

## Complication Management

### Intraluminal catheter occlusion

- The complete inability to withdraw blood or infuse fluid in a VAD is most commonly the result of a blood clot within the catheter. It can also be caused by incompatible drugs or lipids that have crystallized or precipitated and have obstructed the catheter.
- Management of an occluded catheter, when a blood clot is suspected, involves the instillation of urokinase.

### Extraluminal catheter occlusion

- Catheter sluggishness or partial occlusion can be due to two extraluminal phenomena: fibrin sheath formation and thrombosis. The catheter position can also affect flow.
  - Venous thrombosis can be caused by a variety of factors, including endothelial injury, hyper-coagulability, multiple catheters, catheter stiffness, catheter size, and catheter placement.
  - Prevention of thrombus formation around these catheters may be minimized by administering low-dose warfarin (1 mg/daily).
  - Management of venous thrombosis usually involves anticoagulants or thrombolytic agents.

### Infection

- Infections are more common in patients with neutropenia, those with multilumen catheters, and those receiving TPN or chemotherapy.
- Infections in the catheter tunnel or port pocket usually involve a variety of different organisms and are manifested by redness, edema, tenderness or discomfort, exudate, skin warmth, and/or fever.
- Systemic infections can be thrombus-related or caused by intraluminal catheter colonization with a wide variety of infective organisms.
- The VitaCuff impregnated with silver ions provides an antimicrobial barrier within the catheter tunnel. It has been reported to decrease the incidence of catheter infections.
- Another preventive measure successful in decreasing catheter infection rates is the "locking" of the device with a heparinized vancomycin solution.

### Other complications

- Occlusions and device malfunctions can occur for a variety of other reasons. Catheters can be kinked, compressed, malpositioned, severed, punctured, split, or separated. The port access needle can be embedded in the septum, be inaccurately placed, or become dislodged.

# PRACTICE QUESTIONS

1. Exposure to cytotoxic agents occurs primarily by which of the following routes?
   a. inhalation
   b. ingestion
   c. absorption
   d. all of the above

2. Topical application of nitrogen mustard to malignant lesions requires which of the following precautions?
   a. Sodium thiosulfate should be applied to neutralize the nitrogen mustard if it comes in contact with normal tissues.
   b. Prednisone should be applied to areas inadvertently exposed.
   c. Personal protective equipment (PPE) is to be used by the person applying the mustard.
   d. a and c.

3. Which of the following nursing measures are useful to promote safe administration of oral antineoplastic agents?
   a. administering oral methotrexate after radiation therapy
   b. avoiding overdose by dispensing only one course of oral chemotherapy at a time
   c. giving the patient a written schedule of when to take leucovorin following high-dose methotrexate
   d. b and c

4. Ms. Charles needs a peripheral IV infection of doxorubicin, a known vesicant. When giving a vesicant:
   a. it is always better to have a blood return throughout the injection.
   b. a smaller-gauge needle is preferable.
   c. to patients with small veins, choose an angiocath that is thin-walled with an over-the-needle cannula.
   d. a and c.

5. Which of the following statements regarding administration of a vesicant antineoplastic agent is *incorrect*?
   a. An extravasation can be occurring despite an adequate blood return.
   b. If a vein takes a nonvesicant without any problem, the vesicant will infuse without difficulty.
   c. The risk of infiltration of any IV increases over time.
   d. When administering a vesicant agent, it is wiser to administer any antiemetic or antianxiolytic agent *after* the vesicant.

6. When selecting the best vein for Ms. Charles' treatment, you decide to:
   a. start proximally and gradually proceed distally.
   b. start distally and gradually proceed proximally.
   c. start with the antecubital vein, when possible.
   d. a and c.

7. After the administration of doxorubicin, you notice that swelling has occurred at the site. The patient complains of some burning, and you notice redness at the site. In addition, you notice that there is a lack of blood return. These clues alert you to the fact that the patient may be experiencing:
   a. venous flare.
   b. erythema.
   c. extravasation.
   d. all of the above.

8. Next you suspect that the patient in the previous question is experiencing drug infiltration. You suspect this mostly because of the presence of:
   a. a bleb formation or swelling at the site.
   b. the patient's inability to readily report any change in sensation.
   c. venous flare.
   d. loss of blood return.

9. Intra-arterial drug administration is used primarily to treat which of the following?
   a. metastasis of colon cancer to the liver
   b. metastasis of breast cancer to other lymph areas
   c. hepatocellular carcinoma
   d. a and c

10. Mrs. Krohn is being treated for ovarian cancer and is about to undergo several months of intraperitoneal infusion of chemotherapy drugs. The hope is that this will provide a cure of minimal residual disease. The method you will most likely choose for accessing the peritoneal space is:
    a. intermittent placement of an indwelling catheter.
    b. placement of a Tenckhoff external catheter.
    c. placement of an implantable peritoneal port.
    d. any of the above.

11. Mr. Hurston has leukemia. He has recently had an Ommaya reservoir placed to receive intrathecal methotrexate. As you prepare to administer the drug, it is important to remember which of the following?
    a. Methotrexate is the only drug that can be safely administered into the Ommaya reservoir.
    b. The Ommaya reservoir is flushed with 20 cc of saline prior to removal.
    c. Only preservative-free methotrexate is used.
    d. No systemic toxicity is expected from the methotrexate.

12. Ms. Vielland is about to be given a TCVC. As part of her patient education plan, you tell her that TCVCs:
    a. eliminate the need for needle sticks.
    b. are ideal for short-term access.
    c. though difficult to remove, provide great flexibility in terms of use.
    d. a and c.

13. Which of the following is *not* a clear indication for placement of a P.A.S. port?
    a. intermittent 5FU injection
    b. continuous infusion of vesicant drug
    c. a woman with ulcerating breast lesions
    d. radiation changes on the anterior chest

14. While checking the patency of a patient's VAD, you notice catheter sluggishness and a partial occlusion. The most likely cause of these findings includes which of the following?
    a.  endothelial injury
    b.  catheter stiffness
    c.  the catheter's placement on the left side of the body
    d.  any of the above

---

# ANSWER EXPLANATIONS

1.  **The answer is d.** Direct exposure to cytotoxic agents can occur during admixture, administration, or handling. Exposure occurs through inhalation, ingestion, or absorption. (p. 319)

2.  **The answer is d.** When using nitrogen mustard, have sodium thiosulfate available to neutralize the nitrogen mustard; after removal of the drug, apply the sodium thiosulfate to areas of the skin that may be inadvertently exposed. PPE is always used when handling chemotherapeutic drugs (p. 330)

3.  **The answer is d.** With therapy such as leucovorin following methotrexate, noncompliance could be fatal. Therefore, give the patient a written schedule to follow, and avoid overdose by giving only one course of oral drug at a time. (p. 330)

4.  **The answer is d.** When giving a vesicant, it is always better to have a blood return throughout the injection, so a smaller-gauge needle is not preferable in that situation. For patients with small veins, choose an angiocath that is thin-walled with an over-the-needle cannula. (p. 331)

5.  **The answer is b.** It is faulty reasoning to assume that if a vein takes a nonvesicant without any problem, the vesicant will infuse without difficulty. The risk of infiltration of *any* IV increases over time. Often other drugs can cause venous irritation and even spasm that can result in a loss of blood return— a major assessment criteria for safe administration of chemotherapy. (p. 331)

6.  **The answer is b.** When selecting the vein, start distally and gradually proceed proximally. Another rule might be to select the best vein, provided that vein is not the antecubital vein. Placing a needle in the antecubital area restricts patient mobility and increases the risk of dislodgment. Any extravasation that occurs is difficult to detect because the area is dense and a lot of fluid can infiltrate before it is detected. (p. 331)

7.  **The answer is c.** Symptoms that could indicate extravasation include swelling; stinging, burning, or pain at the injection site (not always present); redness (not often seen initially); and lack of blood return. Lack of a blood return alone is not always indicative of an extravasation. An extravasation can occur even if a blood return is present. This patient is presenting the classic signs of extravasation, and the possibility of a flare reaction is inappropriate. (p. 333)

8.  **The answer is a.** The one obvious sign of drug infiltration is a bleb formation at the injection site that is readily apparent in a superficial vein, or swelling that occurs in more deeply accessed veins. (p. 334)

9.  **The answer is d.** The primary use of intra-arterial drug administration in the hepatic artery is for the management of potential or actual metastasis of colon cancer to the liver. (p. 339)

10.  **The answer is b.** Tenckhoff catheters are placed when several months of therapy are planned, especially when the treatment goal is cure of minimal or microscopic residual disease. (p. 341)

11.  **The answer is c.** Intrathecal or intraventricular administration is most commonly used in leukemia as prophylaxis or to manage CNS involvement. Only preservative-free drug is used. (p. 343)

12. **The answer is a.** TCVCs eliminate needle sticks and are easy to remove when they are no longer needed for care. They also allow for a great deal of flexibility in terms of use. They also are the only long-term devices that offer triple access. (p. 350)

13. **The answer is a.** Everything else is an indication for a P.A.S.-Port. (pp. 352–353)

14. **The answer is d.** Venous thrombosis can be caused by a variety of factors, including endothelial injury, hypercoagulability, multiple catheters, catheter stiffness, catheter size, and catheter placement—particularly on the left side or in a smaller vein. (p. 356)

# Chapter 16    Chemotherapy: Toxicity Management

## INTRODUCTION

- The incidence and severity of toxicities are related to the drug dosage, administration, schedule, specific mechanism of action, concomittant illness, and specific measures employed to prevent or minimize toxicities.
- The toxicities of the drug will determine the maximum amount of drug that can be administered safely.

## PRETREATMENT EVALUATION: RISK ANALYSIS

- Individuals with a weakened physical condition and poor nutritional status tolerate chemotherapy poorly.
- Patients who have had multiple courses of chemotherapy, radiation, or immunotherapy are at risk.
- Preexisting organ impairment can affect absorption, distribution, metabolism, or excretion of chemotherapy, increasing toxicity.
- Advancing age alone has not been found to be a significant risk for chemotherapy toxicity.

## SELF-CARE

- The change from inpatient to outpatient administration of chemotherapy necessitates a shift in responsibility for managing treatment of side effects from health care providers to patients and their families.
- Hospitalization and death may be the consequences of side effects that are not managed effectively. Side effects that seem to be the most distressing to patients include fatigue, nausea, vomiting, alopecia, anorexia, and mouth sores.

## PATIENT EDUCATION AND FOLLOW-UP

- Goals of chemotherapy teaching include:
  - helping the patient adjust
  - explaining treatment
  - imparting the sequence of administration
  - controlling side effects
  - encouraging self-care behaviors that minimize the side effects
  - listing side effects to be reported

## CHEMOTHERAPY TOXICITIES
### Grading of Toxicities

- To assess toxicity, the following information should be included in relation to chemotherapy administration:
  - which toxicities occurred
  - toxicity severity
  - time of onset
  - duration of the effect
  - interventions incorporated to minimize the effect

## Systemic Toxicities

### Bone marrow suppression

- Myelosuppression is not only the most common dose-limiting side effect of chemotherapy but also potentially the most lethal.
- Chemotherapy-induced anemia occurs rarely, because the bone marrow begins to recover before the number of circulating RBCs decreases significantly.
  - Erythropoietin can be administered in an attempt to correct anemia induced by chemotherapy.
    - The most common side effect from erythropoietin is hypertension; therefore the patient's blood pressure should be monitored biweekly.
- Currently the standard of practice is to administer platelets prophylactically if the platelet count falls below 20,000 ul.
- Neutropenia typically develops 8–12 days after chemotherapy, with recovery in three to four weeks.
  - Neutropenia can occur when total WBC count is within a normal range. Consequently, quantitating the ANC is essential to achieving a correct assessment of neutrophil status.
  - Monocyte count should also be monitored since an increase in monocytes precedes and predicts resolution of neutropenia.
- Chemotherapy-induced damage to the alimentary canal and respiratory tract mucosa facilitates the entry of infecting organisms; therefore pneumonia and sinusitis are commonly seen.
- Once appropriate cultures are obtained, antibiotics are used to treat chemotherapy-induced infections either (1) until cultures indicate eradication of the causative organism, (2) for a minimum of seven days, or (3) until the neutrophil count is greater than 500/mm$^3$.
- Among all the problems identified with myelosuppression, infection is the most serious. Colony-stimulating factors (CSFs) are used to accelerate neutrophil recovery and to shorten duration of febrile neutropenia.

### Fatigue

- Fatigue is a common effect of cancer and its treatment and often interferes with activities of daily living.
- Changes in skeletal muscle protein stores, metabolite concentration, or the accumulation of various metabolites may contribute to fatigue.
- Fatigue may be chronic and overwhelming, especially with advanced disease.

### Gastrointestinal tract

#### Anorexia

- Anorexia or declining food intake implies alterations in food perception, taste, and smell that result from the effects of chemotherapy and advanced cancer.
- Visceral and lean body mass depletion are common along with muscle atrophy and hypoalbunimia.
- Anorexia can lead to compromised immune status and cachexia.

#### Diarrhea

- Diarrhea results from the destruction of the actively dividing epithelial cells of the GI tract.
- Although 5-fluorouracil is the most common drug to cause diarrhea, other agents include methotrexate, docetaxel, actinomycin D, doxorubicin, and irinotecan.
- Stool cultures are done to rule out an infectious process. Clotridium difficile occurs in patients who have had prior antibiotic exposure.
- Ocreotide acetate is indicated for patients who have excessive diarrhea.

### Constipation

- Vincristine, vinblastine, and navelbine are the most common chemotherapy agents to cause constipation, as a result of autonomic nerve dysfunction manifested as colicky abdominal pain and ileus.

### Nausea/vomiting

- Emesis is a complicated process that occurs because of stimulation of the vomiting center (VC) by visceral and vague afferent pathways from the GI tract, CTZ, vestibular apparatus, and the cerebral cortex.
- Although nausea, retching, and vomiting commonly occur together, they are considered separate conditions.
    - *Nausea* is described as a subjective conscious recognition of the desire to vomit and is manifested by an unpleasant wavelike sensation in the epigastric area, at the back of the throat, or throughout the abdomen.
    - *Retching* is a rhythmic and spasmodic movement involving the diaphragm and abdominal muscles controlled by the respiratory center in the brainstem near the VC. Negative intrathoracic pressure and positive abdominal pressure result in unproductive retching. When the negative pressure becomes positive, vomiting occurs.
    - *Vomiting* is a somatic process performed by the respiratory muscles causing the forceful oral expulsion of gastric, duodenal, or jejunal contents through the mouth.
- Nausea and vomiting can be classified as acute, delayed, and anticipatory.
    - *Acute* nausea and vomiting occur a few minutes to one to two hours after treatment, resolving within 24 hours.
    - *Delayed* nausea and vomiting persist or develop 24 hours after chemotherapy.
    - *Anticipatory* nausea and vomiting occur in 25% of patients as a result of classic operant conditioning from stimuli associated with chemotherapy, usually 12 hours prior to administration.
- Factors that affect the degree and severity of nausea and vomiting include the following:
    - Drug—for example, nitrogen mustard, cyclophosphamide, and Actinomycin D cause severe emesis
    - Dose, rate, and route of drug administration
    - Susceptibility to motion sickness
    - Poor previous emetic control
- The best approach to prevention and management of nausea and vomiting caused by chemotherapy appears to be the combination of a serotonin antagonist and a steroid.
- Behavioral interventions such as progressive muscle relaxation, hypnosis, and systemic desensitization can be used to minimize nausea.

## Organ Toxicities

- In general, organ toxicities are predictable based on the cumulative dose, the presence of concomitant organ dysfunction, the age of the patient, and the manner in which the drug is given.

## Cardiotoxicity

- Cardiotoxicity is described as an acute or chronic process. The acute form consists of transient electrocardiogram (ECG) changes and are not an indication to stop the drug.
- Chronic effects occur weeks or months after administration, involving nonreversible cardiomyopathy presenting as a classic biventricular congestive heart failure (CHF) with a characteristic low-voltage QRS complex.

- Patients typically complain of a nonproductive cough, dyspnea, and pedal edema.
- Anthracyclines are known to cause cardiotoxicity by directly damaging the cardiac myocyte cell.
- Dexrazoxane given with the anthracyclines protects cardiac cells from toxicity.
- Acute pericarditis has been reported with high-dose cyclophosphamide therapy used in the bone marrow transplant (BMT) population with subsequent pericardial effusion and cardiac tamponade.
- Myocardial ischemia has been reported with 5-fluorouracil infusion in patients with or without preexisting heart disease.
- For long-term follow-up it has been recommended to include a minimum of an echocardiogram yearly for high-risk patients and every 2 to 3 years for others, plus a cardiac scan every 5 years if the patient remains asymptomatic.
- The degree of cardiac injury determines the limitations on activities of daily living the individual will experience.

## Neurotoxicity

- Chemotherapy-induced neurotoxicity can arise as direct or an indirect damage to the central nervous system (CNS), peripheral nervous system, cranial nerves, or any combination of the three. The majority of patients experience temporary neurotoxicity.
- Significant neurotoxicity usually requires holding the treatment until the symptom resolves and reinstituting with a 50% dose reduction or discontinuing the drug.
- CNS damage primarily involves the cerebellum, which produces altered reflexes, unsteady gait, ataxia, and confusion.
- Damage to the autonomic nervous system (ANS) causes ileus, impotence, or urinary retention.
- Vincristine is well known for potential peripheral neuropathy. Neuropathy related to cisplatin is usually reversible.
- Neurotoxicity has been reported in 5%–30% of patients treated with ifosfamide.
- High-dose methotrexate occasionally causes encephalopathy after several courses, which usually is transient and reversible.
- 5-FU may cause an acute cerebellar dysfunction, usually more common in the elderly.
- High-dose cytarabine can cause encephalopathy, leukoencephalopathy, and sometimes peripheral neuropathy.
- One of the principal nonhematologic toxicities of paclitaxel and docetaxel is sensory neuropathy. Arthralgias and myalgias occur usually within 4 to 5 days of treatment.

## Pulmonary toxicity

- Pulmonary toxicity usually is irreversible and progressive as a result of chemotherapy administration.
- Pulmonary toxicity usually presents clinically as dyspnea, unproductive cough, bilateral basilar rales, and tachypnea.
- Bleomycin is known to cause pulmonary toxicity.
- Cytarabine exerts a direct toxic effect on the pneumocytes and capillary endothelial cells to diminish the integrity of cell membranes and increase capillary permeability.
- Mitomycin C damage to the lung presents as diffuse alveolar damage with capillary leak and pulmonary edema.
- Cyclophosphamide causes pulmonary toxicity in less than 1% of patients and is associated with high doses.
- Carmustine inhibits lung glutathione disulfide reductase, which mediates the resultant cellular injury.
- Methotrexate can also produce an acute or a chronic process related to endothelial injury.

## Hepatotoxicity

- The initial site of damage seems to be the parenchymal cells. Obstruction to hepatic blood flow results in fatty changes, hepatocellular necrosis, cholestasis, hepatitis, and veno-occlusive disease (VOD).
  - Signs of chemotherapy-induced VOD have been described as (1) unexplained thrombocytopenia refractory to platelets, (2) sudden weight gain, (3) sudden decrease in hemoglobin, (4) increase in liver enzymes, (5) intractable ascites, and (6) being associated with dactinomycin.
- Hepatotoxicity presents as elevations of hepatic enzymes, hepatomegaly, jaundice, and abdominal pain.
- Drugs contributing to hepatic toxicity, to widely varying degrees, include methotrexate; cytarabine; 5-FU with combination levamisole; gemcitabine; fluorodeoxyuridine; 6-mercaptopurine; and amsacrine.
- During chemotherapy administration, the nurse monitors liver function tests closely. If liver function is impaired, certain drugs that are broken down in the liver are given with caution. These include Taxol, Taxotere, vincristine, Adriamycin, and vinblastine.
- Third spacing (the shift of fluid from the vascular space to the interstitial space) can occur as a result of hepatotoxicity. Signs of fluid shift are decreased blood pressure, increased pulse rate, low central venous pressure, decreased urine output, increased specific gravity.
- Albumin is administered to replace the plasma protein and hopefully assist with absorption of the fluid. Fluid restriction minimizes third spacing.

## Hemorrhagic cystitis

- Hemorrhagic cystitis is a bladder toxicity resulting from cyclophosphamide and ifosfamide therapy. Hemorrhagic cystitis ranges from microscopic hematuria to frank bleeding, necessitating invasive local intervention with instillation of sclerosing agents.
- When hemorrhagic cystitis develops, drug therapy probably should be discontinued.
- Ifosfamide has a slower rate of metabolic activation, allowing larger dosages to be administered as compared to cyclophosphamide. MESNA, a uroprotectant, is administered before ifosfamide and then intermittently up to 24 hours afterward to protect the bladder.
- Protection of the bladder focuses on hyperhydration, frequent voiding, and diuresis. If hemorrhagic cystitis occurs, the treatment includes bladder irrigations through a three-way Foley catheter to clear developing clots.
- Cystoscopy may be necessary to cauterize bleeders. As a last resort, a cystectomy may be necessary.
- During administration of chemotherapy agents, the nurse should monitor the urine for blood. Strict intake and output measures are imperative.

## Nephrotoxicity

- Prevention of nephrotoxicity primarily involves aggressive hydration, urinary alkalization, diuresis, and careful monitoring of laboratory values.
- Cisplatin can cause mild-to-severe nephrotoxicity, with specific damage to the proximal and distal tubules.
- The use of mannitol in facilitating and inducing diuresis is a means of ensuring adequate urine flow.
- Daily magnesium supplementation is indicated during cisplatin therapy, and electrolyte levels should be monitored frequently. Clinically significant hypomagnesemia occurs with a magnesium less than 1 mg/dl.

- Amifostine is an organic thiophosphate used to reduce the cumulative renal toxicity associated with repeated administration of cisplatin. Side effects include hypotension and nausea/vomiting.
- Standard doses of methotrexate are not associated with renal toxicity unless the patient has preexisting renal dysfunction. High doses can cause an obstructive nephropathy.
- Other drugs associated with some degree of renal dysfunction include streptozocin, lomustine and carmustine, and mitomycin C.
- *Acute tumor lysis syndrome (ATLS)* is a complication of cancer therapy that occurs most commonly in patients with tumors that have a high proliferation index and are highly sensitive to chemotherapy. ATLS is characterized by the development of acute hyperuricemia, hyperkalemia, hyperphosphatemia, and hypocalcemia with or without acute renal failure.
- If a patient is at high risk for ATLS with chemotherapy, allopurinol is generally given as a prophylactic measure.

## Gonadal toxicity

- The likelihood that chemotherapy will affect a patient's fertility depends in part on the patient's gender, age, and the specific drugs.
  - Women over the age of 30 are less likely to regain ovarian function because they have fewer oocytes.
  - Cycle-nonspecific drugs such as alkylating agents are the most detrimental to fertility.
  - Alkylating agents are most commonly associated with compromised fertility, and combination regimens have a greater effect than single agents.
  - The testes of adult men are particularly vulnerable to chemotherapeutic agents. The incidence and length of time for recovery of spermatogenesis depend on the patient's age and the total drug dose.
- Chemotherapy affects fertility by injuring the germinal epithelium of the gonad. It is clear that prepubertal ovaries are profoundly affected histologically after chemotherapy.
- Over time, the more serious consequences of premature estrogen deprivation, such as osteoporosis and vaginal atrophy, can develop; however, if not contraindicated, these can be effectively treated with hormonal replacement.
- Depending on the woman's age as well as the type and total dose of chemotherapy, ovarian function may resume after a period of time.
- In general, patients surviving cancer may be advised to wait at least two years after completion of therapy before attempting parenthood. This allows plenty of time for the elimination of chromosome breaks and damaged germ cells.
- In general, most chemotherapy agents are excreted from the body in the first 72 hours following administration. Patients need to be instructed to use condoms and to avoid oral sex during this period.

## SECONDARY/THERAPY-RELATED CANCERS

- *Second malignancy* refers to a new neoplasm that has developed after treatment of the initial or primary cancer. It implies that the new neoplasm is related in some way to treatment that was not only cytotoxic but also carcinogenic.
- Long-term survivors of Hodgkin's disease who have received both chemotherapy and radiation have the highest incidence of secondary malignancies.
- The alkylating agents, nitrosoureas, and procarbazine are the agents most implicated in chemotherapy-related malignancies.
- Melphalan is probably the most potent leukemogenic agent.
- The schedule of chemotherapy administration may have some bearing on the development of leukemia.

# PRACTICE QUESTIONS

1. Kate is being treated for Hodgkin's disease and is being monitored weekly for myelosuppression. This is appropriate because neutropenia:
   a. is the most common dose-limiting side effect of chemotherapy.
   b. is potentially the most lethal side effect of chemotherapy.
   c. is most severe with antimetabolites and vinca alkaloids.
   d. a and b.

2. Your patient suffers from borderline anemia and is about to receive 5-FU and mitomycin for treatment of colon cancer. Your teaching plan is based on which of the following facts regarding anemia?
   a. It rarely occurs because the bone marrow recovers so quickly.
   b. It is treated prophylactically with the administration of platelets if their count falls too low.
   c. It can be treated with erythropoietin injections 1–3 times a week.
   d. a and c

3. Mrs. Carsen develops a chemotherapy-induced infection and is started on an antibiotic because of fever. You explain that she will take the antibiotic:
   a. until cultures indicate eradication of the causative organism.
   b. for a minimum of seven days.
   c. until the neutrophil count is greater than 500/mm$^3$.
   d. any of the above

4. Which of the following drugs is *least* likely to cause diarrhea?
   a. 5-fluorouracil
   b. methotrexate
   c. doxorubicin
   d. vincristine

5. Mr. Jones is receiving cisplatin therapy for testes cancer and requires a serotonin antagonist and a steroid daily during his treatment. The rationale for this combination is based on which of the following?
   a. Cisplatin is often associated with cumulative and delayed nausea.
   b. The steroid is used to boost the immune system.
   c. The steroid enhances the antiemetic effect of the serotonin antagonist.
   d. a and c

6. Chronic cardiotoxic effects can occur months after treatment with certain chemotherapeutic agents. Patients are routinely monitored for:
   a. nonproductive cough, dyspnea, pedal edema.
   b. biventricular CHF.
   c. low-voltage QRS complex.
   d. all of the above.

7. Davis is taking vincristine. You are able to discern from his conversation that although he is familiar with some of vincristine's adverse effects, he seems unfamiliar with its neurotoxic effects. Thus, you apprise him that vincristine is well known for potential:
   a. encephalopathy.
   b. peripheral neuropathy.
   c. acute cerebellar dysfunction.
   d. leukoencephalopathy.

8. Mr. Johns is undergoing chemotherapy for high-grade testes cancer. He complains of being jittery and his lab tests reveal low magnesium, albumin, and calcium. He is most likely experiencing which of the following complication of chemotherapy?
   a. anorexia and weakness due to chemotherapy
   b. low magnesium due to cisplatin therapy
   c. low calcium due to uremia syndrome
   d. a paraneoplastic syndrome

9. Davis has received prior irradiation to his chest; therefore, his doctor would be particularly cautious prescribing which of the following?
   a. bleomycin
   b. cytarabine
   c. mitomycin C
   d. all of the above

10. A patient receiving mytomycin and 5-FU develops a 15-lb weight gain, decreased hemoglobin, thrombocytopenia, ascites, encephalopathy, and elevated bilirubin and SGOT lab values. You recognize these as classic symptoms of:
    a. liver failure.
    b. severe dehydration.
    c. veno-occlusive disease.
    d. intractable ascites.

11. Mrs. Collins has breast cancer and is about to begin Taxotere. She has taken her decadron as premedication. As you check her lab tests, you notice her liver function tests are elevated. Which of the following statements is important regarding your course of action?
    a. The Taxotere should be delayed until liver function improves.
    b. Taxotere is eliminated by the kidney, so liver function is not important.
    c. The Taxotere dose may need to be reduced because of elevated liver functions.
    d. The steroid often causes an elevation of liver functions and can be ignored.

12. Melanie is about to undergo treatment with cyclophosphamide and doxorubicin. She is at risk for developing hemorrhagic cystitis. What preventive measures can be taken?
    a. Protection of the bladder focuses on minimal, controlled hydration.
    b. Intravenous acrolein may produce sulfhydryl complexes and subsequent detoxification.
    c. She is encouraged to drink 8–10 glasses of fluid a day to prevent hemorrhagic cystitis.
    d. She should receive amifostine therapy daily.

13. Which of the following agents has been found to decrease the renal toxicity associated with cisplatin therapy?
    a. MESNA
    b. cyclosporin A
    c. amifostine
    d. Zinecard

14. Mr. Johns is receiving amifostine with his cisplatin therapy. Which of the following statements is *incorrect* regarding amifostine therapy?
    a. The purpose of amifostine is to rescue normal cells from toxicity therapy, preventing renal damage.
    b. Side effects of amifostine include hypotension, nausea, and vomiting.
    c. Amifostine reduces the incidence of hypomagnesemia.
    d. Amifostine is indicated for prevention of renal damage with cisplatin.

15. Your patient is about to receive chemotherapy for lymphoma. The doctor has placed the patient on allopurinol to prevent acute tumor lysis syndrome. Which of the following is *not* a symptom/sign of this complication of chemotherapy?
    a. acute hyperuricemia
    b. hypercalcemia
    c. hyperphosphatemia
    d. all of the above.

16. Which of the following patients is most likely to have their fertility affected by chemotherapy?
    a. 7-year-old Kevin
    b. 60-year-old Dan
    c. Elaine, who is over 30
    d. Pamela, who is 5

17. Which of the following patients is *most* likely to develop a secondary malignancy?
    a. Allison, whose throat cancer is in remission
    b. Fred, a long-term survivor of Hodgkin's disease
    c. Erin, a long-term survivor of breast cancer
    d. Ike, whose colon cancer is being treated with both chemotherapy and radiation

18. Which of the following agents is most likely to cause chemotherapy-related malignancies?
    a. nitrosoureas
    b. procarbazine
    c. melphalan
    d. all of the above

## ANSWER EXPLANATIONS

1. **The answer is d.** Myelosuppression is not only the most common dose-limiting side effect of chemotherapy but also potentially the most lethal. Antimetabolites, vinca alkaloids, and antitumor antibiotics are most damaging to cells that are in a specific phase of the cell cycle; thus, myelosuppression is less severe with these agents. (pp. 391–392)

2. **The answer is d.** Chemotherapy-induced anemia occurs rarely because the bone marrow begins to recover before the number of circulating RBCs decreases significantly. Erythropoietin can be administered to correct anemia induced by chemotherapy. The most common side effect from the erythropoietin is hypertension, and the prophylactic administration of platelets (if their count falls below 20,000 ul) is for the hypertension—*not* the anemia. (p. 393)

3. **The answer is d.** Antibiotics are used to treat chemotherapy-induced infections either (1) until cultures indicate eradication of the causative organism, (2) for a minimum of seven days, or (3) until the neutrophil count is greater than 500/mm$^3$. (p. 394)

4. **The answer is d.** Drugs that most commonly cause diarrhea are 5-fluorouracil and methotrexate. Others include docetaxel, actinomycin D, doxorubicin, and irinotecan. Vincristine is least likely to cause diarrhea and most likely to cause constipation. (p. 396)

5. **The answer is d.** Cisplatin causes delayed nausea, and a serotonin antagonist plus a steroid is the most effective treatment. (p. 400)

6. **The answer is d.** Chronic cardiotoxic effects present a nonproductive cough, dyspnea, and pedal edema and involve nonreversible cardiomyopathy presenting as a classic biventricular CHF with a characteristic low-voltage QRS complex. (p. 404)

7. **The answer is b.** Vincristine is well known for potential peripheral neuropathy. (p. 406)

8. **The answer is b.** Cisplatin frequently causes hypomagnesemia, which manifests as shaking. Daily magnesium supplementation is indicated during cisplatin therapy, and electrolyte levels should be monitored frequently. (p. 406)

9. **The answer is d.** Agents associated with pulmonary toxicity include, among others, bleomycin, cytarabine, mitomycin C, cyclophosphamide, carmustine, and methotrexate. Prior irradiation to the chest enhances risk for toxicity. (pp. 409–410)

10. **The answer is c.** Signs of chemotherapy-induced VOD have been described as (1) unexplained thrombocytopenia refractory to platelets, (2) sudden weight gain, (3) sudden decrease in hemoglobin, (4) increase in liver enzymes, (5) intractable ascites, and (6) encephalopathy. (p. 410)

11. **The answer is c.** Taxotere is metabolized by the liver, and elevated liver functions can interfere with metabolism, causing enhanced toxicity of Taxotere. Dose will need to be reduced. (p. 412)

12. **The answer is c.** To help prevent hemorrhagic cystitis during therapy with ifosfamide, in particular, MESNA, a uroprotectant, can be administered before ifosfamide and then intermittently up to 24 hours afterward to protect the bladder. (p. 413)

13. **The answer is c.** Amifostine is used to reduce the cumulative renal toxicity associated with repeated administration of cisplatin. (p. 414)

14. **The answer is a.** Amifostine is used to reduce cumulative renal toxicity associated with cisplatin therapy. (p. 414)

15. **The answer is b.** Acute tumor lysis syndrome (ATLS) is a complication of cancer therapy that occurs most commonly in patients with tumors that have a high proliferation index and are highly sensitive to chemotherapy. ATLS is characterized by the development of acute hyperuricemia, hyperkalemia, hyperphosphatemia, and hypocalcemia with or without acute renal failure. (p. 415)

16. **The answer is c.** Women over the age of 30 are less likely to regain ovarian function because they have fewer oocytes. (p. 417)

17. **The answer is b.** Long-term survivors of Hodgkin's disease who have received both chemotherapy and radiation have the highest incidence of secondary malignancies. (p. 419)

18. **The answer is d.** The alkylating agents, nitrosoureas, and procarbine are the agents most implicated in chemotherapy-related malignancies. Melphalan is probably the most potent leukemogenic agent. (p. 419)

# Chapter 17    Biotherapy

---

## FOUNDATION CONCEPTS FOR BIOTHERAPY
### Immune Defense Against Malignancy: An Overview
#### Immune surveillance

- Immune surveillance is a theory first proposed to explain the role of the immune system in defending against neoplastic cells.
- Tumor cells express abnormal tumor antigens on their surfaces that can be recognized and subsequently destroyed by immune cells.
- The immune system is believed to destroy many circulating malignant cells before they can become established sites of tumor.

#### Effector mechanisms of immune function

- The primary defense against transformed cells is cell-mediated immunity carried out by T-lymphocytes and aided by B cells and humoral immunity.
- The key components of the immune response are shown in Figure 17-1 on text page 428.

##### Monocyte/macrophage

- The macrophage is a primary initiator to an inflammatory immune response. It originates in the bone marrow and circulates as a monocyte. It becomes a macrophage when it enters tissue at a site of infection.
- The macrophage is first a phagocytic cell capable of engulfing microbes and altered cells, and processing them in lysosomes with cytolytic enzymes. The macrophage then presents a portion of the processed antigen along with the MHC class II surface molecules as an anitgen-presenting cell (APC) to initiate both humoral- and cell-mediated immune functions.
- The macrophage is also a secretory cell, manufacturing key pyrogenic cytokines such as interleukin 1, tumor necrosis factor, and interleukin 6.

##### T helper lymphocyte ($T_H$ or T4)

- The $T_H$ cell is the coordinator of the immune response and cell-mediated immunity. When activated, the $T_H$ cell manufactures cytokines.

##### Cytotoxic T-lymphocytes (CTL)

- CTL or T8 cells are lymphocytes with MHC class I surface molecules. They need to recognize MHC class I receptors to initiate their cytotoxic response. They damage the target cell wall, and the cell dies.

##### Natural killer (NK) cells

- These cells are able to function without MHC recognition. When activated primarily through cytokines, NK cells are capable of killing transformed cells.

### B-lymphocyte

- This cell is identified by the surface immunoglobulin that it displays. When activated with antigen and cytokines—primarily IL-2, IL-4, and IL-6—the B-lymphocyte differentiates into a plasma cell and manufactures immunoglobulin or antibody specific to the initiating antigen. Later, the plasma cell can evolve into a memory cell, capable of a more rapid response on future exposures with the same antigen.

### Antibody (Ab)

- Ab is a specific protein product of plasma cells that is also known as immunoglobulin. There are five classes of immunoglobulin, with IgG and IgM being the most frequently generated classes of immunoglobulin. Ab is not a cytotoxic substance itself, but is essentially an adaptor that enhances the capability of immune effector cell functions. When antibody links to an antigenic target, the resulting Ab/Ag complex greatly increases the phagocytic capability of the macrophages and can initiate the serum complement protein cascade on the surface of a foreign cell, resulting in lysing of the cell.

### Antibody-dependent cell-mediated cytotoxicity (ADCC)

- ADCC is the cell-killing process enabled by antibody.

### Cytokines

- These are glycoprotein products of immune cells such as lymphocytes and macrophages that coordinate and initiate effector defense functions. They are not cytotoxic agents themselves, with the exception of tumor necrosis factor alpha (TNF-$\alpha$) and lymphotoxin. The characteristics of the primary host defense cytokines are shown in Table 17-1 on text page 430.
- Cytokines generally share the following characteristics:
  - They mediate and regulate immune defense functions.
  - They have brief half-lives and usually function over short distances.
  - They are produced by many different cell types and also act upon diverse cell targets.
  - They act upon diverse cell targets.
  - They can influence the stimulation of other cytokines or antagonize the actions of other cytokines.
  - They act as regulators of cell growth or as mediators of defense functions.

## Origins of Biotherapy

### Biologic response modifiers (BRMs)

- Biologic response modifiers (BRMs) can be classified as (1) agents that restore, augment, or modulate host antitumor immune mechanisms; (2) cells or cellular products that have direct antitumor effects; and (3) biological agents that have other antitumor effects.
- Biotherapy is defined as the use of agents derived from biological sources or that affect biological responses.

## Recombinant DNA Technology

- Recombinant DNA, or the combining of genes from different sources to produce an organism with new qualities, is an important basic principle to biotherapy.
- Table 17-2, text page 431, provides definitions of terms used in biotechnology. This advance in molecular biology has enabled the current generation of biological agents to be available for use in cancer therapy.

- Table 17-3, text page 432, identifies major classifications of biopharmaceuticals presently available or in clinical trial.
- The process of recombinant DNA is illustrated in Figure 17-3, text page 432.

## HEMATOPOIETIC GROWTH FACTORS

- Hematopoietic growth factors (HGFs) are used as supportive therapy to myelosuppressive chemotherapy or bone marrow transplantation (BMT). HGFs influence the development of bone marrow-derived cells to their mature form.

### The Hematopoietic Microenvironment

- The bone marrow is a complex organ composed of hematopoietic stem cells (HSC), progenitor and maturing cells of various lineages, as well as a supportive matrix for developing cells.
- From one originating stem cell, the bone marrow is capable of producing approximately 10 distinct cells that function in body defense (neutrophil, eosinophil, basophil, mast cell, monocyte/macrophage, B- and T-lymphocyte, natural killer cell), oxygen-carrying capability (erythrocyte), and clotting (platelet). See Figure 17-4, text page 434.

### Hematopoietic Progenitor Cells and HGFs
#### Multipotential precursor cells

- The hematopoietic stem cell (HSC), also called a totipotent stem cell, is a self-renewing, originating cell that divides asynchronously.
- HPCs are multipotential precursor cells, also referred to as stem cells, that are responsive to growth factors. They are cells capable of repopulating the marrow after myelosuppressive therapy and maintaining hematopoiesis.

#### Stem cell factor

- The major HGF that influences the multipotential precursor cells, or CFU blast, to develop into myeloid or lymphoid lineages is stem cell factor (SCF). SCF is also known as steel factor or kit ligand.
- In combination with other HGFs such as G-CSF, GM-CSF, IL-3, or EPO, SCF increases the number and size of cell colonies, suggesting that it influences early progenitor activity.
- SCF may have clinical application in expanding the hematopoietic progenitor population that is responsive to a specific lineage factor such as EPO. It may also have a role in restoring chemotherapy-induced myelosuppression by accelerating bone marrow restoration in BMT or restoring bone marrow function in aplastic anemia or myelodysplastic syndrome.
- The most frequent side effects are injection site reactions and mild to severe symptoms of hypersensitivity reactions with urticaria, dyspnea, and throat tightness.

#### Interleukin 3

- This cytokine is also known as multi-CSF or IL-3. Its major role is to promote growth and differentiation of multipotential committed progenitor cells such as the CFU-GEMM for the myeloid cell lineages and the lymphoid progenitor cells.
- Typical side effects include flu-like symptoms, headache, bone pain, neck stiffness, and infection site redness.

## Erythrocyte lineage

- The RBC or erythrocyte is the mature cell of a specialized cell lineage that is demonstrated in Figure 17-4, text page 434.

### Erythropoietin

- EPO is a hormone normally synthesized by peritubular cells in the kidney and secondarily by hepatocytes. EPO production is increased by hypoxia and decreased by inflammatory cytokines.
- There are two identical recombinant products of epoetin alfa or EPO available for use. Procrit® (Ortho Biotech) is licensed for use in anemia associated with cancer chemotherapy, and Epogen® (Amgen) is approved for anemia of chronic renal failure, AIDS, and nonmyeloid malignancies. Both products are given by SQ injection and cause a rise in the red blood cell count within a few days to weeks.

## Platelet cell lineage

- The platelet cell is another highly-specialized cell of the bone marrow that develops from the multipotential myeloid progenitor cell.

### Interleukin 1

- It is believed that IL-1 stimulates multipotential progenitor cells that later result in increased numbers of cells from multicell lineages including platelets.
- IL-1A is known to have a myeloprotective effect when given prior to radiation or high-dose chemotherapy.

### Interleukin 6

- IL-6 is believed to have a role in thrombopoiesis as a cofactor in stimulating the CFU-MK progenitor cell. It is synergistic to other growth factors.
- Typical side effects with SQ administration include fever, chills, malaise, and a rise in hepatic enzymes particularly in patients with hepatic disease.

### Thrombopoietin (TPO) or MGDF

- This growth factor was isolated and described as the factor that stimulates the proliferation of CFU-MK cells and the differentiation of megakaryocytes into platelets.
- Clinical studies are currently underway to investigate its toxicity as well as its therapeutic effects for maintaining platelet counts during chemotherapy and BMT.

## Monocyte/macrophage and neutrophil cell lineages

- The monocyte/macrophage and neutrophil lineages develop from the common multipotential progenitor cell, the CFU-GEMM, into the CFU-GM under the influence of SCF and IL-3.

### GM-CSF

- This colony stimulating factor or growth factor has effects on myeloid precursor cells as well as on maturing monocytes and macrophages. It also enhances the antibody-dependent cytotoxicity of mature cells. Sargramostim is a recombinant form of GM-CSF approved for use in decreasing myelosuppressive effects of allogeneic or autologous BMT.

- Side effects include fever, lethargy, myalgia, bone pain, anorexia, injection site redness, and rash. There is a "first dose reaction" characterized by flushing, tachycardia, hypotension, dyspnea, nausea, and vomiting.

### M-CSF

- M-CSF is a lineage-specific CSF that stimulates the differentiation and maturation of promonocytes into monocytes and macrophages. It also acts on mature cells to enhance their phagocytosis of bacteria, fungi, and potential tumor cells.
- Patients at the highest doses experience malaise, nausea, headache, and various ocular symptoms such as iritis, periorbital edema, and photophobia. M-CSF may also play an important role as an antifungal agent in cancer patients.

### G-CSF

- G-CSF is the prime growth factor in the late development of neutrophils. Filgrastim is a recombinant form of G-CSF that is currently approved by the FDA for use in decreasing neutropenia related to chemotherapy, HIV infection, myelodysplastic syndrome, or BMT.
- The most frequent side effect of filgastrim is bone pain.

## Second Generation HGFs: Fusion Proteins

- A second generation of HGFs, the fusion protein called PIXY 321, is a synthetic molecule combining IL-3 and GM-CSF made by genetic engineering techniques. The coding regions of these cytokines are combined to make a product ten times more potent a stimulator of BFU-E and CFU-GEMM than either substance alone.
- Side effects are typical for other growth factors: malaise, headache, fever, myalgia, bone pain, nausea, and injection site redness and induration. No capillary leak or weight gain was observed.
- PIXY 321 may be the first in a series of genetically engineered molecules to combine several growth factors with the potential to maximize their desired therapeutic effects while decreasing toxic effects.

## ANTICANCER CYTOKINE THERAPY

### Interferon (IFN)

- Interferon was the first cytokine to be explored as an anticancer biological agent. Now interferons are being used as part of biological therapy in low-dose regimens and in combination with other cytokines and chemotherapy regimens.
- See Table 17-4, text page 437, for a description of the interferons presently approved by the FDA for clinical use.

### Types

- There are three major types of interferon (IFN) in the body: alpha, beta, and gamma.
- Alpha and beta are type I IFN and are located on chromosome 9.
- Gamma IFN is the only type II IFN, and its gene is located on chromosome 12.

### Side effects

- The effects a patient experiences when receiving IFN depends on the IFN type, dose level, and schedule. The higher the dose, the more severe the side effects. Table 17-5, text page 437, lists the side effects that the patient typically experiences. Patients receiving alfa-interferon experience the worst flu-like symptoms on the first dose. With continued administration, they develop tachyphylaxis or the lessening of intensity and disappearance of symptoms.

### Clinical application of alfa-interferon

- Alfa-interferon has been approved for use in a high-dose regimen for AIDS-related Kaposi's sarcoma and has shown activity in chronic myelogenous leukemia (CML), alfa malignant melanoma, renal cell carcinoma, non-Hodgkin's lymphoma, multiple myeloma, and squamous cell cancer of the skin.

## Interleukins (ILs)

- Interleukins (ILs) are cytokines that act primarily between lymphocytes and other immune cells and body organs that have a role in the inflammatory immune response.
- Interleukins are not directly cytotoxic to tumor cells. They act as messengers to initiate, coordinate, and sometimes amplify potent immune defense activities. They require a functional, intact immune system to achieve their therapeutic effects.
- Immunosuppressive agents such as corticosteroids can block the therapeutic actions of these interleukins and other cytokines when they are used as an anticancer therapy. This has implications for health care professionals in the selection of medications for the management of symptoms commonly associated with cytokine therapy.
- A number of recombinant interleukins are currently being evaluated for their anticancer therapeutic potential, including recombinant interleukin-2 (aldesleukin), interleukin-1 (IL-1), interleukin-4 (IL-4), IL-6, and IL-12.

## Combination Therapy

- In developing an effective anticancer regimen using cytokines, the major dilemma is how to combine them to their best advantage. The important variables of agent, dose, route, sequencing of agents, and duration of treatment are only a few that may influence significantly the therapeutic outcome for the patient. Two combinations with promising results are as follows: (1) rIL-2 and alfa-interferon and (2) rIL-2 and rIL-1.
- Another form of combination therapy is combining a cytokine or group of cytokines with chemotherapy.

## Tumor Necrosis Factors (TNFs)

- TNFs are a group of glycoproteins produced by immune cells in response to a pathogen.
- TNF-$\beta$ or lymphotoxin is a cytotoxin capable of killing any nearby cells.
- TNF is one of the few cytokines that has direct, tumoricidal capability.

## ACTIVATED CELL THERAPY (ADOPTIVE IMMUNOTHERAPY)

- There are two types of activated cells: lymphokine activated killer (LAK) cells and tumor-infiltrating lymphocytes (TIL).

## Lymphokine Activated Killer Cells (LAK)

- LAK are nonspecific killer cells that can lyse tumor cells without MHC recognition and specificity.
- LAK therapy begins with the administration of high-dose rIL-2 to stimulate cell production. These cells are then removed by a series of plasmaphereses and are cultured in rIL-2 for several days. They are returned to the patient along with additional rIL-2 doses as tolerated.
- The side effects of the therapy are caused by the rIL-2 administered with the cells: fever, chills, hypotension, oliguria, weight gain, mental status change, and pruritis. Only pulmonary congestion and dyspnea are attributable to LAK cells themselves.

- One of the first patients with melanoma to be given IL-2/LAK therapy had a durable complete remission. However, long-term evaluation of IL-2/LAK therapy has shown that only 5%–10% of patients with melanoma or renal cell carcinoma have responded to therapy. The addition of LAK cells has not demonstrated an advantage in response rates over patients receiving high-dose rIL-2 alone.

## Tumor-Infiltrating Lymphocytes (TIL)

- TIL are a second type of activated cell used in cell transfer therapy. TIL are derived from tumor sites and are cytotoxic to autologous (patient's own), but not allogeneic (others of the same type) tumors.
- The toxicity of TIL therapy reflects the same side effects of high-dose rIL-2. Side effects directly related to TIL infusions are pulmonary symptoms such as dyspnea, pulmonary congestion, and hypoxia.
- TIL therapy is being investigated in patients with renal cell cancer and ovarian cancer in which TIL are administered by intraperitoneal infusions. TIL has also been grown from colon, breast, and lung cancers.

## MONOCLONAL ANTIBODIES

- Monoclonal antibodies (Mab) are the product of a single clone of cells sensitized to a specific antigenic protein present on the surface of a target tumor.

## Manufacture of Antibodies and the Hybridoma Technique

- In the 1970s, the hybridoma technique established the ability to make highly specific antibodies in large quantities and made it possible to develop monoclonal antibodies into a potential cancer therapy. However, it also introduced one of this therapy's biggest problems—the use of foreign immunogenic protein. See Figure 17-5, text page 442, for a diagram of how these cells are produced.

## Mab in Cancer Therapy

- Monoclonal antibodies have three essential roles in cancer therapy: diagnostic and screening functions, purging autologous bone marrow of malignant cells ex vivo, and as a cancer therapy capable of killing tumor cells with high specificity.
- Some of the categories of Mab antigen targets include oncofetal antigens, differentiation antigens, tissue-specific antigen, growth factor and oncogene products, and anti-idiotype.

## Design of Monoclonal Antibodies

- The repetitive use of antibodies containing foreign protein is strongly immunogenic in immunocompetent patients.

### Antibody conjugates

- Carrier or conjugated Mabs are capable of cell killing and do not require the host's immune competence. Conjugated Mabs have three major divisions:
  1. Immunotoxins—An immunotoxin (IT) is a Mab or growth factor that is joined to a plant or bacterial cell poison.
  2. Antibody-drug conjugates—Mabs have been linked to chemotherapeutic agents with the goal of increasing drug concentration at the tumor site.
  3. Radioimmunoconjugates—Mab or Mab fragments have been used as carriers of radiation to tumor sites.

## Problems in Mab Therapy

- A primary factor that diminishes the effectiveness of Mabs therapy is the host's immune response to foreign protein. Other problems encountered in Mab therapy center on the characteristics of the tumor target. Unbound circulating antigen from the tumor can bind Mabs and prevent them from reaching their target. Also, tumors modulate or change surface antigens, making it difficult for the Mab to link to the target. Often tumors are bulky, hypoxic, and poorly vascularized, making it difficult for circulating Mabs to gain access. For these reasons, Mabs can have low uptake rates, particularly in solid tumors.

## Side Effects of Mab Therapy

- Acute side effects that occur during Mab infusion are most commonly fever, chills, malaise, myalgia, nausea, and vomiting. Not all Mab therapy causes side effects and the intensity of the symptoms is variable. Dyspnea, cough, and chest pain can occur during a Mab infusion and may be related to the rate of infusion. The symptoms often resolve if the rate is slowed.
- The primary potential toxicity with Mab therapy is an allergic reaction to the foreign protein. A small number of patients may experience symptoms such as bronchspasm, urticaria, pruritis, flushing, restlessness, and hypotension. Skin testing by the administration of small test doses does not always identify those patients who will react.
- Another potential reaction to Mab therapy is serum sickness. This may occur two to four weeks after therapy and results from circulating immune complexes. Serum sickness is characterized by urticaria, pruritis, malaise, and other flu-like symptoms, arthralgia, and generalized adenopathy.
- Side effects of conjugated Mabs vary with the agent used.

## HUMAN GENE THERAPY (HGT)

- HGT is the insertion of a functioning gene into the cells of a patient to correct a genetic disorder or introduce a new function to the cell. HGT is part of a larger technology known as gene transfer or the transfer of genetic material into human cells.
- At this time, HGT is limited to somatic cell therapy; that is, a genetic change in an individual's cells is limited to the individual's lifetime.
- Germline therapy alters the human genome for future generations by placing the gene into the egg or sperm cells. This form of therapy, although feasible, is not presently used in clinical trials and is the subject of intense ethical, social, and legal debates.

## Retroviral Gene Transfer

- Viruses have a special ability to enter a cell's genome and convert the cell's machinery to manufacture virions. In gene transfer techniques, the virus is used as a vector or carrier to deliver the desired gene to a target cell. The virus is disabled from replication by removing its reproductive genes.

## Direct Gene Transfer

- There is growing interest in developing methods of transferring genes to a target cell without the use and associated problems of a viral vector.

## Safety Concerns

- The primary concern with HGT involves the safety of using viral vectors. Other concerns about gene transfer center on the ability to control the expression of the transduced gene.

## Nursing Considerations

- There are two concerns with gene therapy of particular interest to nurses. The first concerns symptoms or side effects the patient will experience from HGT.
- The second concern is safety for the health care provider when handling gene therapy agents, particularly when retroviruses are employed for cell transduction.

## The Future of Gene Therapy

- Problems that must be solved include improving the efficiency of gene delivery methods to the target cells and improving their expression.

## OTHER IMMUNOMODULATING AGENTS

- An immunomodulating agent can be broadly defined as a substance that stimulates host defense mechanisms or indirectly augments aspects of immunity that are beneficial in cancer therapy.
- Nonspecific immunostimulation is based on the theory that the host's responsiveness to a tumor can be increased through overall stimulation of host defense mechanisms using nontumor-related antigenic agents such as microorganisms.
- Some immunomodulating agents provide active specific immunotherapy directed to a specific tumor target.
- Nonspecific immunomodulating agents require that the host be capable of developing an immune response.

## Bacillus Calmette-Guerin (BCG)

- This is a nonspecific immunostimulant originally derived from attenuated *mycobacterium bovis*. BCG strains vary according to the number of organisms per unit of dose administered.
- BCG has been administered intradermally, subcutaneously, by scarification, or via intracavitary infusion. BCG produces both localized side effects of swelling, pain, inflammation, and ulceration of the injection site as well as systemic flu-like symptoms of fever, chills, malaise, and arthragia. Patients can have hypersensitivity reactions to BCG preparations if they have had previous exposure to BCG or a positive PPD. A small number of patients receiving BCG may develop a disseminated BCG infection.
- Special precautions are used with the patient receiving BCG, particularly intralesional therapy. They include the following:
  - Assess the patient's potential for a hypersensitivity reaction to BCG before and during therapy. Patients with prior exposure to this agent will have a more rapid response that can be severe and can lead to anaphylaxis. Changes in the BCG dosage may be required.
  - Premedication of patients with acetaminophen and diphenhydramine to decrease the severity of systemic flu-like symptoms.
  - Patients are monitored for prolonged flu-like symptoms and organ dysfunction (liver, kidney, and pulmonary abnormalities) that suggest potential BCG infection.
  - All BCG syringes and other materials that have come in contact with BCG should be disposed of as hazardous waste to prevent environmental contamination.
- BCG is used as an intralesional injection for superficial metastatic malignant melanoma lesions and as a bladder instillation for maintenance therapy of superficial bladder tumors after transurethral resection.
- The side effects of intravesical BCG therapy include hematuria and dysuria from the inflammatory mucosal reaction to BCG, fever, and rarely, disseminated BCG infection. A long-term outcome of BCG bladder instillations can be a contracted bladder.

## Levamisole

- This drug, also known as Ergamisol, is a nonspecific chemical immunomodulator.
- A large national study using an adjuvant regimen of oral levamisole with intravenous 5-fluorouracil found a significant survival advantage in a subset of patients with Dukes C colon carcinoma.
- Levamisole appears most effective as adjuvant therapy administered with other cytoreductive therapies such as surgery or chemotherapy.
- Side effects of levamisole therapy include mild nausea, liver dysfunction, leukopenia, skin rash, flu-like symptoms, and rarely, neurological effects such as cerebellar dysfunction and mental confusion. Patients who consume alcohol during levamisole administration may experience increased side effects including flushing, throbbing headaches, and respiratory distress.

## Retinoids

- Retinoids are a group of compounds that are natural derivatives of retinol or vitamin A. They include all *trans* retinoic acid (ATRA), 13-*cis* retinoic acid (13-*cis* RA or isotretinoin), and 9-*cis* retinoic acid (9-*cis* RA).
- In cancer, retinoids act as immunomodulators by inducing cellular differentiation and suppressing proliferation. Cancers that may be responsive to retinoids include leukemias, melanoma, neuroblastoma, and various epithelial cancers.
- A serious side effect of retinol therapy in APL is the retinoic acid syndrome. Patients receiving reinoids can exhibit fever, respiratory distress, interstitial pulmonary infiltrates, pleural effusions, and weight gain. Retinoic acid syndrome can be fatal if not promptly recognized and treated, usually with high-dose corticosteroids. It occurs in approximately 25% of patients and can appear within 2 to 21 days of onset of therapy. Symptoms do not abate or reverse when the drug is discontinued.

## Cancer Vaccines

- A vaccine is an immunostimulant that utilizes live, inactivated, or killed organisms or portions of an organism. In cancer, the term *vaccine* is actually a misnomer because the patient already has the disease and the intent is to stimulate the patient's *own* immune system to recognize and destroy the tumor.
- Cancer or tumor vaccines are also known as active specific immunotherapy (ASI). They differ from other immunomodulating therapies in that they stimulate an immune response directed to a specific target versus creating a generalized immune response. ASI requires, however, that the patient be immunocompetent and not have a large tumor burden that may interfere with immunity.
- The source of tumor cells varies. Autologous vaccines are made from the patient's own tumor; allogeneic or polyvalent vaccines contain the same tumor-type cells from several patients.
- Patients typically experience fever, chills, and injection site reactions. These site reactions resolve over several weeks.

## NURSING MANAGEMENT OF THE PATIENT RECEIVING BIOTHERAPY

- In biotherapy, patients frequently experience fever and chills, headache, malaise, and arthralgia. Some patients experience injection site redness, induration, and pain. A few patients may develop generalized swelling, rash, weight gain, hypotension, and, occasionally, respiratory changes. Not all biological agents have the same profile of toxicities.

### Effects of Dose and Schedule

- Biological agents may stimulate the desired biological activity at a dose level far less than the maximum tolerated dose (MTD). This dose is called the optimal biological dose (OBD). Thus, the evaluation of a new biological agent is more complex than evaluation of a new drug.

- Different symptoms predominate with variations in t[...] schedule.

## Preparation, Administration, and Safe Han[...]
- Biopharmaceuticals are protein-based agents [...] the lyophilized product is reconstituted, the vial sh[...] dried powder. Excessive foaming that can denatu[...]
- Some biopharmaceuticals are not compati[...]ng.
- At present, there are no known safety haz[...]oclonal antibodies, or cell therapies. However, the[...]nt inadvertent exposure to immunogenic substances[...]

## Side Effects and Key Nursing Strategies

### Flu-like syndromes (FLS)
- FLS is a constellation of nonspecific symptoms that [...] when one develops an influenza infection. The major symptoms include chills and poss[...]s, moderate to high fever, myalgias, arthralgias, and malaise.
- Pyrogenic pathogens, toxins, or drugs stimulate the release of endogenous pyrogenic cytokines that act on thermal brain centers via prostaglandin release to create an upward reset of the body's temperature set-point. Feedback mechanisms now read the body temperature as cold and initiate heat-producing actions such as involuntary muscular contractions or rigors.
- It is important to control rigors as soon as they occur to prevent undue cardiovascular stress.
- *Tachyphylaxis*, or the development of tolerance to a symptom with repeated frequent doses, commonly occurs with interferon therapy.
- Monoclonal antibody (Mab) therapy has its own FLS pattern of symptoms.

#### Nursing management
- Guidelines for the nursing management of FLS in a patient receiving biologic therapy are as follows:
  - Evaluate the risk for FLS symptoms.
  - Premedicate the patient.
  - Keep the patient warm.
  - For rigors: Administer meperidine parenterally as appropriate.
  - For arthralgia, myalgia, or headache: Continue the use of acetaminophen and indomethacin as appropriate.
  - For uncontrolled, high fevers: Use cooling blanket or tepid bath.
  - Consider alternate times of administration.
  - Consider other sources of fever.

### Fatigue
- Fatigue is a symptom commonly experienced by cancer patients and especially those receiving radiation therapy and chemotherapy. It is also a common side effect of many types of biotherapy.
  - Biotherapy-related fatigue is a chronic fatigue characterized by generalized weariness, weakness, exhaustion, and feelings of tiredness. It can be accompanied by other symptoms such as fever, myalgia, and headache.

### Interferon

- Daily schedules of interferon at doses of 20 million units or greater can result in profound toxicity including fatigue.

### Interleukins

- Fatigue is a common side effect with nearly all interleukins, particularly in long-term outpatient regimens.

### Monoclonal antibodies, colony stimulating factors

- Fatigue is not a common side effect of either Mabs or CSFs.

### Nursing management

- Evaluate the patient self-report of fatigue for perception of amount of fatigue, peak severity, patterns of activity and sleep, impact on self-care activities, and nutritional balance. Teach patient and family the relationship of fatigue to therapy. Plan with patient how to maintain activity and prevent prolonged bedrest.

## Cardiovascular-respiratory changes

- Cardiovascular changes are associated most frequently with high-dose IL-2, and usually occur in association with the capillary leak syndrome (CLS). These changes include supraventricular arrhythmias such as atrial fibrillation and supraventricular tachycardia, symptoms of ischemia, and decreased cardiac contractility.
- Cytokines such as rIL-1, rIL-2, and TNF typically cause hypotension, decrease in central venous pressure, and oliguria.
- Respiratory changes may arise from hypersensitivity reactions or in high-dose IL-2 therapy.

### Nursing management

- Watch the patient's cardiovascular and respiratory status at frequent intervals during high-dose IL-2 therapy.
- Teach patient to report chest pain, palpitations, or changes in respiration that occur during therapy.

## Capillary Leak Syndrome (CLS)

- The capillary or vascular leak syndrome (CLS) is unique to biological agents. It is the extravasation of fluids and albumin into body tissues, associated with a decreased peripheral vascular resistance, hypotension, and intravascular volume. Compensatory mechanisms of oliguria, increased creatinine levels, tachycardia, and weight gain also occur as fluids are administered to maintain the blood pressure. Major organ dysfunction such as mental status changes, nausea and diarrhea, and pulmonary edema occur with a rapid weight gain, sometimes up to 10% of pretreatment body weight.
- CLS can occur rapidly or increase gradually over hours. It is most frequently associated with high-dose IL-2 therapy but has been reported in varying degrees with other cytokines and high-dose GM-CSF.

### Nursing management

- Assess regularly the patient's blood pressure, pulse, respiratory status, urine output, and body weight during therapy. Have the patient remove all restrictive jewelry, particularly rings, before treatment begins.

- For hypotension and oliguria, administer fluid boluses per physician order. Low-dose dopamine may be administered by peripheral vein to increase urine output.
- Instruct patient to stand gradually and allow blood pressure to adjust to the upright position. Request patient to report symptoms of dizziness.

## Dermatologic changes

- Administration of biological agents can stimulate immunoreactive cells in the skin that release cytokines and vasoactive substances contributing to redness, swelling, and itching.
- Allergic reactions, particularly to a foreign protein such as Mab, can occur. These symptoms include acute development of an erythematous rash on the face and upper body, welling, hives, and pruritis.
- IL-2 therapy can create similar reactions, but over a longer period of time.
- Erythema starting on the face and upper body progresses to severe dryness and flaking; pruritis can be intense. In severe cases, skin erosions and the sloughing of the palms, soles, and nails can occur with gradual healing after therapy ends. Hair thinning may occur, but alopecial is rare. Patients with preexisting psoriasis can experience a worsening of their disease with IL-2 therapy, possibly due to T cell activation.
- When cytokines such as IL-2 and GM-CSF are given subcutaneously, inflammatory reactions at the infection site often occur. Swelling and pain resolve within days, but a firm nodule may remain at the site for months.

### Nursing management

- Apply hypoallergenic emollient lotions and creams on the skin frequently. Use bath oil and hypoallergenic soaps for bathing.
- For pruritis: For severe itching, administer antipruritic medications such as hydroxygine HCL, or diphenhydramine. Use Lorazepan with severe itching as needed. Use colloidal oatmeal baths (Aveeno®).
- For subcutaneous site inflammation: Rotate sites and do not reuse until firmness resolves. Use local anesthetics and possibly cooling for inflammation.

## Gastrointestinal symptoms

- Anorexia, nausea, vomiting, and diarrhea can occur primarily with cytokine therapy, but also with Mab therapy.
- The most severe nausea, vomiting, and diarrhea occur with IL-2 therapy, particularly high-dose regimens.

### Nursing management

- The interventions for nausea, vomiting, and diarrhea previously used with chemotherapy may be applicable for use in IL-2 therapy. One exception is that steroids should not be used as an antiemetic because of their effects on immune function.
- Evaluate: Know the potential that the type of therapy has for moderate to severe nausea, vomiting, or diarrhea.
- For nausea and vomiting: Medicate patients either with antiemetics on an "as needed" basis, or administer on a regular schedule, depending on severity of symptoms.
- For diarrhea: Use antidiarrheal medications as needed, starting with the least potent. Observe patient for symptoms of bowel stasis, distension, and signs of an acute abdomen.
- Monitor: Assess patients for symptoms of fluid and electrolyte imbalances.

### Neurological effects

- Patients receiving alfa-interferon or IL-2 can experience simple memory changes, increased anxiety, nightmares, and other sleep disturbances. One symptom frequently encountered but poorly described is the loss of concentration or inability to pay attention.
- More severe symptoms of disorientation, somnolence, and even coma can occur. These symptoms are reversible with supportive care. Neurological changes are infrequent in cytokine therapy and are rare in Mab or other biological therapy. Although rare, neurotoxicity can be severe, particularly in high-dose alfa-interferon or rIL-2 therapy.

#### Nursing management

- Assessment: Assess patient prior to start of therapy for baseline neurological functioning. Elderly patients are at increased risk.
- Patient education: Teach patient and his or her family members early signs of mental status changes that should be reported to the patient's health team.
- Monitor: Protect patient from harm and observe frequently when mental status changes occur.
- Decrease stress: Reduce environmental demands that increase attentional fatigue.

### Anaphylactic reactions

- Anaphylactoid reactions have most commonly occurred with Mab therapy.
- High-dose IL-2 administration has been associated with the development of increased sensitivity to other agents.

#### Nursing management

- Review emergency procedures: Have essential drugs, steroids, epinephrine, and antihistamines available when administering Mab or other biological agents to patients with a history of hypersensitivity reactions.
- Patient education: Instruct patient and family about the symptoms of hypersensitivity. Request that they call their physician if symptoms occur or seek immediate medical assistance if symptoms develop rapidly.

## THE FUTURE OF BIOTHERAPY

- The incorporation of gene transfer technology into biotherapy provides promising new ventures that may bring a cure, effective treatment, or even the prevention of cancer into reality.

# PRACTICE QUESTIONS

1. The macrophage:
   a. manufactures interleukin 3, 4, 6, and alpha- and gamma-interferon to aid in its ultimate function of target cell wall damage.
   b. is a glycoprotein product that initiates effector defense functions.
   c. is a primary initiator to an inflammatory immune response.
   d. a and c.

2. Which of the following substances is *not* a cytokine?
   a. α-interferon
   b. interleukin-2
   c. levamisole
   d. tumor necrosis factor (TNF)

3. How do most biologic response modifiers (BRMs) work?
   a. They control the growth of cells.
   b. They modulate the immune system.
   c. They control the maturation of cells.
   d. They target tumor cells through an antibody-antigen response.

4. Biologic response modifiers are:
   a. agents that restore, augment, or modulate host antitumor immune mechanisms.
   b. cells or cellular products that have direct antitumor effects.
   c. biological agents that have other biological antitumor effects.
   d. all of the above.

5. Stem cell factor (SCF):
   a. also known as IL-3, promotes differentiation of multipotential committed progenitor cells.
   b. is the major hematopoietic growth factor that influences the multipotential precursor cells to develop into myeloid or lymphoid lineages.
   c. is a hormone normally synthesized by peritubular cells in the kidney.
   d. all of the above.

6. Thrombopoietin:
   a. is the factor that stimulates the proliferation of CFU-MK cells.
   b. stimulates multipotential progenitor cells that later result in increased numbers of cells from multicell lineages including platelets.
   c. stimulates the differentiation of megakaryocytes into platelets.
   d. a and c.

7. Among the therapeutic cellular activities of interferons (INFs) are all of the following *except*:
   a. antiviral activity—protecting a virally infected cell attack by another virus.
   b. immunomodulatory activity—interacting with T-lymphocytes that stimulate the cellular immune response.
   c. antiproliferative activity—directly inhibiting DNA and protein synthesis in tumor cells.
   d. immunoregulatory activity—mediating the proliferation and activation of hematopoietic factors.

8. IFN therapy has been most effective in the treatment of what kinds of malignancies?
   a. solid tumors, especially colon and cervical cancers
   b. basal cell and other skin carcinomas
   c. hematologic diseases, including hairy cell leukemia
   d. metastatic foci when a low tumor burden exists

9. Most of the toxicities that occur with the administration of the various types of IRN appear to be related to:
   a. dose.
   b. route of administration.
   c. schedule
   d. IFN type.

10. Adoptive immunotherapy is an experimental approach in which the tumor-bearing host passively receives both IL-2 and cells that possess antitumor activity. What types of cells are administered along with IL-2?
    a. tumor-infiltrating lymphocytes (TILs)
    b. NK cells
    c. LAK cells
    d. helper T cells

11. The monoclonal antibodies (Mabs) used in antibody therapy are produced from a single clone of hybrid cells (a hybridoma). These cells are a hybrid of:
    a. mouse lymphocytes and mouse malignant myeloma cells.
    b. human lymphocytes and mouse malignant myeloma cells.
    c. mouse lymphocytes and human malignant myeloma cells.
    d. human lymphocytes and human malignant myeloma cells.

12. A clinical trial is evaluating the effectiveness of certain Mabs directed to the antigen binding sites of antitumor antibodies in patients with B cell lymphoma and melanoma. The study is probably using _____ Mabs.
    a. anti-idiotype
    b. tissue-specific antigen
    c. oncofetal antigen
    d. differentiation antigen

13. The most common side effects seen with Mab administration appear within 2 to 8 hours and can best be described as:
    a. flu-like symptoms, including fever and chills.
    b. serum sickness, including generalized adenopathies.
    c. anaphylaxis, including a generalized flush and/or urticaria.
    d. hematologic distress, including neutropenia and thrombocytopenia.

14. One of the primary factors that can diminish the effectiveness of Mab therapy is:
    a. immunosuppression.
    b. the characteristics of bound antigen.
    c. the host's immune response to foreign protein.
    d. myelosuppression.

15. The primary toxicity with Mab therapy is:
    a. vascular leak syndrome.
    b. pulmonary edema with weight gain.
    c. an allergic reaction to the foreign protein.
    d. hypoalbuminemia with increased liver enzymes.

16. Mr. Calvin has a superficial cancer of the bladder and receives a transurethral resection. For maintenance therapy, he is given:
    a. levamisole.
    b. BCG.
    c. retinol.
    d. ASI.

17. A patient of yours is to receive a tumor vaccine. You explain that:
    a. the term *vaccine* is actually a misnomer.
    b. a cancer vaccine is an immunostimulant that utilizes live, inactivated, killed, or portions of an organism to increase immunity to a specific cancer.
    c. tumor vaccines are also known as active specific immunotherapy (ASI).
    d. a and c.

18. The drug regimen least likely to cause fatigue is:
    a. high, daily schedules of interferon.
    b. interleukins given in long-term outpatient regimens.
    c. Mab or CSF therapy.
    d. none of the above (all cause fatigue).

19. Which of the following patients is most likely to have an anaphylactoid reaction in response to therapy?
    a. Eddie, who is undergoing Mab therapy.
    b. Ginny, who is undergoing interleukin therapy.
    c. Meredith, who is taking IL-2.
    d. a and b.

## ANSWER EXPLANATIONS

1. **The answer is c.** The macrophage is a primary initiator to an inflammatory immune response. It originates in the bone marrow, circulates as a monocyte, and becomes a macrophage when it enters a tissue at a site of infection. The macrophage is also a secretory cell manufacturing key pyrogenic cytokines such as interleukin 1, tumor necrosis factor, and interleukin 6. (p. 427)

2. **The answer is c.** Cytokines (which include lymphokines) are substances released from activated immune system cells that affect the behavior of other cells. They may alter the growth and metastasis of cancer cells by augmenting the responsiveness of T cells to tumor-associated antigens, enhancing the effectiveness of B cell activity, or decreasing suppressive functions of the immune system, thereby enhancing immune responsiveness. Included among the cytokines are the interferons and interleukins, tumor necrosis factor (TNF), and colony stimulating factors (CSFs). (p. 428)

3. **The answer is b.** A BRM is any soluble substance that is capable of altering (modifying) the immune system with either a stimulatory or a suppressive effect. It may act by restoring, augmenting, or modulating the host's immunologic mechanisms, by having direct antitumor activity, or by having some other biologic effects including interfering with tumor cells' ability to survive or metastasize. (p. 431)

4.  **The answer is d.** Biologic response modifiers can be classified as agents that restore, augment, or modulate host antitumor immune mechanisms; cells or cellular products that have direct antitumor effects; and biological agents that have other biological antitumor effects. (p. 431)

5.  **The answer is b.** The major hematopoietic growth factor that influences the multipotential precursor cells, or CFU blast, to develop into myeloid or lymphoid lineages is stem cell factor (SCF). SCF is also known as steel factor or kit ligand. (p. 433)

6.  **The answer is d.** Thrombopoietin is the factor that stimulates the proliferation of CFU-MK cells and the differentiation of megakaryocytes into platelets. (p. 435)

7.  **The answer is d.** The IFNs are a family of naturally occurring complex proteins that belong to the cytokine family. Each of the three major types in humans—$\alpha$-IFN, $\beta$-IFN, and $\gamma$-IFN—originates from a different cell and has distinct biologic and chemical properties. All three types of IRN exhibit the cellular effects listed in choices **a-c.** (pp. 436–437)

8.  **The answer is c.** Hematologic diseases have responded best to IFN therapy, with measurable responses occurring in the lymphoproliferative malignancies (such as hairy cell leukemia, non-Hodgkin's lymphoma, and multiple myeloma) and in chronic myelogenous and AIDS-associated Kaposi's sarcoma. (pp. 437–438)

9.  **The answer is a.** It appears that most IFN toxicities, as well as toxicities from most other BRMs, are dose-related. Low doses of IFN are well tolerated, whereas high doses often require cessation of therapy. A common reaction to any type of IFN is the occurrence of fever, chills, fatigue, and malaise, referred to collectively as flu-like syndrome. (p. 437)

10. **The answer is c.** Adoptive immunotherapy involves incubating lymphocytes with IL-2 to generate LAK cells, and then infusing the LAK cells in conjunction with additional doses of IL-2. LAK cells are capable of selectively lysing tumor cells that are resistant to NK cells without affecting normal cells. (p. 441)

11. **The answer is a.** In the production of Mabs, an animal (usually a mouse) is injected with the desired antigen (human tumor cells). The mouse's lymphocytes recognize the antigen as foreign and produce antibodies. The immunized lymphocytes are removed from the mouse and fused with mouse malignant myeloma cells to form a hybrid capable of unlimited cell division. The end result after purification is a monoclonal antibody directed against specific tumor-associated antigens. (p. 442)

12. **The answer is a.** Anti-idiotype Mabs are directed to the antigen binding sites of antitumor antibodies, and have been used in clinical trials with B cell lymphoma and melanoma. (p. 443)

13. **The answer is a.** Anaphylaxis occurs infrequently and suddenly and is predicted by the presence of generalized flush and/or urticaria followed by pallor and/or cyanosis. Serum sickness, which includes a variety of symptoms, may occur 2 to 4 weeks after Mab therapy. Dillman reports that the most common side effects of Mab administration—fever, chills, rigors, and diaphoresis—occur within 2 to 8 hours. (p. 444)

14. **The answer is c.** A primary factor that diminishes the effectiveness of Mab therapy is the host's immune response to foreign protein. Other characteristics in Mab therapy center on the characteristics of the tumor target. (p. 444)

15. **The answer is c.** The primary toxicity with Mab therapy is an allergic reaction to the foreign protein. Another potential reaction to Mab therapy is serum sickness. Patients receiving IT therapy occasionally experience vascular leak syndrome with pulmonary edema and weight gain, hypoalbuminemia, and increased liver enzymes. (p. 444)

16. **The answer is b.** Bacillus Calmette-Guerin (BCG) is a nonspecific immunostimulant used as an intralesional infection for superficial metastatic malignant melanoma lesions and as a bladder instillation for maintenance therapy of superficial bladder tumors after transurethral resection. (p. 448)

17.  **The answer is d.** A vaccine is an immunostimulant that utilizes live, inactivated, killed, or portions of an organism. In cancer, the term vaccine is actually a misnomer as the patient already has the disease and the intent is to stimulate the patient's own immune system to recognize and destroy the tumor. Cancer or tumor vaccines are also known as active specific immunotherapy (ASI). (p. 449)

18.  **The answer is c.** Daily schedules of interferon at doses of 20 million units or greater can result in profound toxicity including fatigue. Fatigue is a common side effect with nearly all interleukins, particularly in long-term outpatient regimens. Fatigue is not a common side effect of either Mabs or CSFs. (p. 451)

19.  **The answer is a.** Anaphylactoid reactions have most commonly occurred with Mab therapy. Although anaphylaxis is not described with interferons and most interleukins, high-dose IL-2 administration has been associated with the development of increased sensitivity to other agents. (p. 454)

# Chapter 18    Allogeneic Bone Marrow Transplantation

## INTRODUCTION

- Bone marrow transplant (BMT) has evolved during the past 30 years from an experimental procedure to an established and effective treatment for increasing numbers of selected patients.

## HISTORICAL PERSPECTIVES

- Historically, total-body irradiation (TBI) plus cyclophosphamide has been the most common pre-transplantation conditioning regimen. Currently, the use of fractionated (versus single dose) TBI and antileukemic drugs with TBI has increased markedly.
- The increased use of busulfan and cyclophosphamide without TBI for pretransplant conditioning is another important trend.
- In the early 1980s cyclosporine emerged as an important treatment and was used with corticosteroids to prevent GVHD.
- As BMT technology moved into the 1990s, the role of recombinant colony stimulating factors (CSFs) dominated clinical research.
- The use of blood cells rather than marrow for allogeneic transplantation is becoming an important area of study. Blood cell transplantation may replace marrow transplantation in the next millennium.

## CONCEPTS OF BONE MARROW TRANSPLANTATION

- The dose of most chemotherapeutic agents is limited by subsequent dose-related marrow toxicity.
- The availability of donor marrow make it possible to administer chemoradiotherapy in supralethal doses in an effort to kill malignant cells.
- The patient is then rescued with donor marrow to prevent iatrogenic death.
- Complications that follow BMT are the result of the (1) high-dose chemotherapy and irradiation conditioning regimens; (2) graft-versus-host disease and its management; (3) adverse effects of medication; and (4) relapse.
- See Table 18-1, text page 462, for the sequence and time of events in the process of allogeneic bone marrow transplantation.

## TYPES OF BONE MARROW TRANSPLANTATION

- The selection of marrow transplantation to treat hematologic or nonhematologic disorders depends on the availability of an appropriate donor source.
- Allogeneic donor sources are related family members or unrelated matched volunteers. If the recipient's twin is the donor, the transplant is called a syngeneic (twin) transplant.
- Umbilical stem cell transplantation is emerging as a promising treatment. Numerous ethical issues surround umbilical stem cell transplantation.

### Syngeneic

- A higher incidence of leukemic relapse has been reported in syngeneic than in allogeneic marrow recipients because of the demonstrated antileukemic effect of graft-versus-host disease.

## Allogeneic

- Allogeneic marrow transplantation depends on the availability of an HLA-matched donor.

### Diseases treated with allogeneic BMT

- Allogeneic transplantations are done most commonly for acute and chronic leukemia, lymphomas, multiple myeloma, severe aplastic anemia, genetic disease, immunologic deficiencies, and inborn errors of metabolism.
- See Table 18-2, text page 464.

## Donors

### Tissue typing

#### Human leukocyte antigen/mixed lymphocyte culture

- Until recent years, most allogeneic transplantations were from HLA-identical siblings, but selected family members or unrelated phenotypically identical donors have been used successfully as marrow donors.

#### ABO typing

- Major ABO-incompatible marrow grafting can be performed without significant hemolytic transfusion reactions.
- Blood group typing, however, must be done on all patients and potential donors.

### Marrow collection

- Donor marrow is harvested in the operating room under sterile conditions. The marrow is obtained from the posterior iliac crests in 2-ml aspirates, up to a total of 10 to 15 mg/kg recipient body weight. If necessary, the anterior iliac crests and the sternum can be used.

#### T-Cell depletion

- Ex vivo T-cell depletion of donor marrow has proven to be the most successful method to prevent life-threatening GVHD.
- The purpose of T-cell depletion is to remove T-cells thought to be responsible for GVHD before the donor marrow is reinfused.
- There are three methods of T-cell depletion: physical, immunologic, and pharmacological.

#### Unrelated donors

- The use of unrelated volunteer donors has increased.
- Improvements in genetic tissue typing hold promise for improving the reliability and speed of current screening methods.

## PROCESS OF BONE MARROW TRANSPLANT

### Pretransplant Evaluation and Preparation of the Patient

- See Table 18-3, text page 467.
- A patient and family conference is held (1) to obtain informed consent, (2) to discuss expected risk and transplant-related morbidity and mortality, and (3) to discuss expected outcomes with the patient.
- All patients have multilumen indwelling central catheters inserted before admission.
- Gonadal failure caused by the high-dose chemotherapy and total-body irradiation used in preparative regimens is a concern for BMT patients.

## Preparation of the Donor and Nursing Care

- Donors need to be comprehensively evaluated prior to surgery, especially for the ability to tolerate general or spinal anesthesia.
- As with the patient, donors and their families can be effectively supported through education.
- Physical and psychological follow-up care for the donor is essential.

## THE BONE MARROW TRANSPLANT

### Admission to the Hospital

- Patients transplanted in protective isolation undergo decontamination of their gastrointestinal tracts, skin, and body cavities.

### Pretransplant Conditioning Regimens

- The methods used to prepare patients for grafting differ according to the underlying disease. Patients receive high-dose chemotherapy alone or with supralethal doses of irradiation to eradicate malignant cells and to prevent graft rejection by the patient's own immune system.
- The array of drugs for high-dose chemotherapy in preparation for marrow transplantation is limited secondary to major organ toxicity.
- Total-body irradiation is delivered in varying doses from cobalt or linear accelerator units.
- Prevailing practice favors fractionated doses to reduce toxicities.

### Marrow Infusion

- The marrow is infused through a central lumen catheter over the course of several hours. Marrow cells pass through the lung and home to the marrow cavity.
- Within two to four weeks, the marrow graft becomes functional, and peripheral platelets, leukocytes, and red cells increase in number.

## COMPLICATIONS OF BONE MARROW TRANSPLANTATION

- Complications are the result of (1) high-dose chemotherapy and irradiation for conditioning regimens, (2) graft-versus-host disease, or (3) problems associated with the original disease and the adverse effects of medications.
- The major complications following autologous BMT are similar, except for GVHD.

### Interrelationships of BMT Complications

- The chemoradiation therapy would be fatal if the patients were not rescued with marrow infusion.
- Major complications after transplantation usually result from the chemoradiation or from the marrow transplantation, not from the original disease.
- Complications often occur simultaneously. Clinical manifestations of different complications can be identical; one complication can cause or exacerbate another.
- The treatment of one complication can cause or exacerbate another complication.
- Prophylaxis or treatment for one complication may have to be modified because of another complication.

### Acute Complications

- See Table 18-4, text pages 471–473, which presents possible acute complications of bone marrow transplantation.

## Gastrointestinal toxicity

- Gastrointestinal toxicity may be exhibited by severe mucositis throughout the gastrointestinal tract.
- Nausea and vomiting following chemotherapy and TBI is a consistent problem.
- Diarrhea is one of the most obsequious symptoms associated with BMT and can continue up to 100 days after BMT.

## Hematologic complications

- Transplant recipients are at high risk for pancytopenia and must be supported with blood component therapy and in some cases with CSFs until the donor marrow becomes fully engrafted and functional.
- Blood products must be irradiated to destroy T-lymphocytes that can cause GVHD in the marrow recipient.
- See Table 18-5, text page 474, for prevention and management of hemorrhage in the recipient bone marrow transplant.
- Prevention of hemorrhagic cystitis involves continuous bladder irrigation and/or aggressive intravenous (IV) therapy to flush cyclophosphamide metabolites from the bladder.

## Acute graft-versus-host disease

- GVHD is an immunologic disease that is a direct consequence of allogeneic marrow transplantation.
- This disease remains a major impediment to successful marrow grafting and occurs in 30%–50% of HLA-identical recipients and up to 75% of unrelated donor transplants.
- Acute GVHD targets the skin, liver, and gut.
- Clinical manifestations of acute GVHD typically begin with a maculopapular erythema that may be pruritic and may cover about 25% of the body. The disease can progress to a generalized erythroderma with frank desquamation and blistering similar to second-degree burns. Liver involvement may appear.
- Skin and liver biopsy and clinical, laboratory, and x-ray data help establish the differential diagnosis imperative to treatment.
- Immunosuppressive medications are aimed at removing or inactivating T-lymphocytes that attack target organs. Cyclosporine and methotrexate inhibit T-lymphocytes that are believed to be responsible for acute GVHD and are the first line of therapy. Used in combination, they are more effective than either agent alone.
- Several studies demonstrate encouraging results for patients with acute GVHD using Psoralen and ultraviolet A irradiation (PUVA).

## Renal complications

- The abrupt onset of anuria may be an early indication of acute tubular necrosis or acute renal failure. Acute tubular necrosis is damage to the epithelial cells of the lining of the renal tubules from nephotoxic or ischemic injury.
- Nursing assessment for acute tubular necrosis focuses on early recognition of symptoms of either prerenal or intrarenal failure.

## Veno-occlusive disease (VOD) of the liver

- Veno-occlusive disease is almost exclusive to BMT and is the most common nonrelapse life-threatening complication of preparative-regimen-related toxicity for bone marrow transplantation.
- Liver damage caused by chemoradiotherapy involves two histopathological processes: (1) venule occlusion and (2) hepatocyte necrosis.
- Marrow recipients who require renal dialysis also have VOD because of liver-kidney hemodynamic interaction.
- Continuous and careful monitoring of the fluid status of the patient is a nursing responsibility.

## Pulmonary complications

- Pulmonary complications are a major cause of morbidity and mortality. They occur as a result of chemoradiotherapy toxicity or bacterial, viral, or fungal infection in severely immunosuppressed patients.
- Interstitial pneumonia occurs in the interstitial spaces of the lungs in approximately 35% of allogeneic marrow recipients and is the most frequent cause of death during the first 100 days after transplant.
- CMV pneumonia is the leading cause of infectious pneumonia after BMT.
- Patients who are seropositive and whose donors are seropositive may benefit from the use of antiviral agents such as acyclovir, or from passive antibody prophylaxis with immunoglobulin.
- Idiopathic pneumonia is believed to be a result of high-dose irradiation.
- Other pneumonias that occur may be caused by a virus, bacterium, or fungus.
- Respiratory syncytial virus (RSV) pneumonia has been identified in the BMT recipient. RSV is a common cause of winter outbreaks of acute respiratory disease.

## Neurological complications

- Neurological and neuromuscular complications occur in 59%–70% of marrow recipients. The underlying causes are pretransplant chemoradiotherapy, central nervous system infection, and immunosuppressive agents.

## Cardiac complications

- Cardiomegaly, congestive heart failure, and fluid retention can develop and can be managed with fluid balance to avoid iatrogenic pulmonary edema.

## Infection

- Profound immunosuppression caused by myeloablative therapy used in conditioning regimens and postBMT immunosuppression can result in infections, which remain a major impediment to successful marrow grafting.
- The most common sites of infections are the gastrointestinal tract, oropharynx, lung, skin, and indwelling catheter sites.

### Preengraftment (days 0–30)

- The herpes simplex virus (HSV) types I and II, Epstein-Barr virus, cytomegalovirus, and varicella zoster virus are the major viruses that occur in the first 30 days after BMT.
- Neutropenia with concomitant damage to mucosal surfaces contributes to gram-negative bacteremia immediately after transplantation.
- Profound immunosuppression with resulting neutropenia (concomitant with denuding of the mucosa in the gastrointestinal tract) places marrow recipients at risk for *Candida* infection.

- *Aspergillus* is a major infectious problem during days 0–30. The portal of entry for *Aspergillus* infection is the respiratory tract.

### Early engraftment (days 30–90)

- Cytomegalovirus infection is the most significant infection during this phase.
- Bacterial infections are less frequent.
- Fungal infections are problematic during this recovery phase, and marrow recipients with GVHD are at higher risk for infections than recipients without GVHD.

- Fever is the cardinal symptom of infection.
- Cultures are necessary to identify and treat pathogenic organisms.
- See Table 18-7, text page 480, for nursing and medical management of infection in the bone marrow transplant recipient.
- Antimicrobial therapy has proven to be successful.

## DISCHARGE FROM THE HOSPITAL

- Hospital discharge after allogeneic BMT averages 20–25 days. The use of CSFs has decreased the length of hospital stays for autologous recipients.
- Some institutions are offering outpatient TBI as well as dose-intensive chemotherapy.
- See Table 18-8, text page 482, for patient and caregiver guidelines upon discharge from the hospital.

## Discharge Criteria

- The following are representative discharge criteria:
  - 24-hour outpatient medical care
  - oral intake
  - nausea, vomiting, and pain controlled without IV medications
  - diarrhea controlled at <500 ml/day
  - platelet count supportable at 5000–15,000 mm$^3$
  - granulocytes >500 mm$^3$ for 24 hours
  - hematocrit >25%
  - tolerating PO medications for 24 hours
  - family support at home

## CLINICAL MANAGEMENT OF THE BMT OUTPATIENT

- Chronic complications of BMT may appear around 80 days after BMT, including acute and chronic GVHD, herpes, varicella zoster, cytomegalovirus, *Pneumocystis carinii* pneumonia, and sexually transmitted diseases.
- Most allogeneic recipients experience at least three months of severe immune deficiency.
- An evaluation determining the allogeneic recipient's stability and risk factors for discharge home is usually initiated approximately 80 days after BMT.
- Relapse or treatment failure remains a limiting factor in BMT.
- Community-based physicians and nurses can expect to see a patient at least weekly for the first month alone.
- Patients typically return to the BMT center for annual evaluations for up to three years following BMT.

## LATE COMPLICATIONS OF BMT

- Late complications, like the acute complications, are a direct result of high-dose conditioning regimens, GVHD and its long-term immunosuppressive management, and other transplant-related insults. Late complications are those developing 100 days or more after transplant.
- See Tables 18-12 and 18-13, text pages 487–491.

### Chronic Graft-Versus-Host Disease (Allogeneic BMT)

- Risk factors for chronic GVHD include mismatched donors/recipients, female to male transplants, positive herpes simplex and CMV virus, over 18 years of age, prior grade 2-3 acute GVHD, and CML recipients who received methotrexate and cyclosporine as chronic GVHD prophylaxis.
- Chronic GVHD is a multisystem disorder.

#### Onset and classification

- *Progressive onset*, a direct extension of acute GVHD, has the poorest prognosis.
- *Quiescent* onset develops after clinical resolution of acute GVHD, and these patients have a fair prognosis.
- Patients with *de novo* onset have had no prior acute disease and have the best prognosis.

#### Clinical manifestations of chronic GVHD

- See Table 18-3, text page 491.
- The skin is affected in more than 70%–80% of patients.
- Manifestations include erythema, alopecia, and nail ridging; fibrosis can result in joint contracture, skin ulcerations, and poor wound healing.
- Closure of portals of entry for infection may require skin allografting.
- Liver disorders are observed in about 50% of patients.
- Chronic liver GVHD symptoms may include right upper quadrant pain, hepatomegaly, and jaundice.
- Oral mucosal involvement will develop in approximately 70% of patients with extensive chronic GVHD and may include xerostomia, in combination with decreased or absent salivary lubrication, and IgA secretion, as well as stomatitis and herpes simplex virus.
- Ocular involvement symptoms include burning, itching, and complaints of a "gritty" feeling in the eye with a possible inability to close the eyelid and lack of ability to form tears.
- Sinusitis is common with symptoms of fever or headache.
- Gastrointestinal tract symptoms include dysphagia, painful swallowing, diarrhea, abdominal pain, and retrosternal pain caused by esophageal thinning.
- Vaginal inflammation, stricture formation, and adhesions have occurred one to three years after transplantation, causing painful intercourse leading to sexual dysfunction.
- Problems in other organ systems will develop in 20% of patients with extensive chronic GVHD, particularly musculoskeletal and renal involvement.

#### Treatment

- Classic treatment of chronic GVHD is long-term administration of cyclosporine using a slow taper starting at week 7 following the transplant, followed by an abrupt taper. If acute GVHD flare-up occurs, the initial treatment is to reinstitute full-dose cyclosporine therapy. If resolution does not occur after several weeks, prednisone may be added and followed by a rapid taper.
- GVHD is accompanied by a graft-versus-leukemic effect noted by a lower rate of relapse in patients with GVHD.

## Late Infectious Complications

- Nearly one-third to one-half of long-term allogeneic BMT survivors develop recurrent varicella zoster virus (VZV). Reactivation occurs most often in marrow recipients with chronic GVHD; however, autologous BMT patients also are at risk.
- Aggressive antiviral therapy with intravenous acyclovir is the standard therapy for VZV.
- All marrow recipients are at risk for infection from encapsulated bacteria.
- Immunizations against a number of infectious diseases play an important role in these patients.
- Family members of BMT recipients should not be given the Sabin oral polio vaccine during the first years following BMT because of possible virus shedding with subsequent infection in the recipient.

## Pulmonary Complications

- Twenty percent of patients with chronic GVHD will have restrictive lung disease, 10% will have obstructive lung disease, and 10% will be at risk for bronchiolitis obliterans.

## Gonadal Dysfunction

- Most transplant patients conditioned with TBI will demonstrate gonadal dysfunction. The adverse effects of single agent high-dose chemotherapy on gonadal function depends on the patient's age at the time of BMT.
- Girls and boys who are prepubertal at the time of BMT develop normally.
- Younger women can expect return of menstrual periods, but only a few have borne children.
- Women treated with TBI have gonadal dysfunction, including sterility and early menopause.
- Most men conditioned with TBI preserve Leydig cell function and testosterone and luteinizing hormone production, but spermatogenesis usually is absent.
- Most prepubertal girls who receive TBI have primary ovarian failure, do not achieve menarche, and do not develop secondary sexual characteristics. A few prepubertal boys conditioned with TBI develop secondary sexual characteristics, but most have delayed onset of puberty. The children most profoundly affected are prepubertal boys who receive testicular irradiation prior to marrow conditioning.

### Growth in children

- Children who undergo conditioning with high-dose cyclophosphamide alone have normal growth and development. In contrast, children receiving cyclophosphamide and busulfan face the possibility of growth and development problems.
- All children have decreased growth rates after TBI, and those who have chronic GVHD are the most significantly affected.
- As the pediatric BMT survivor approaches adolescence and young adulthood, sexual and reproductive counseling needs to be part of routine long-term follow-up care.

## Thyroid Dysfunction

- Thyroid dysfunction occurs in 30%–60% of patients prepared for BMT with a regimen that includes single-dose TBI.

## Ophthalmologic Effects

- Ophthalmologic effects include chronic GVHD and posterior capsular cataracts.
- Lens shielding during TBI should be considered as a preventative measure.

## Graft Failure

- Graft failure occurs rarely in an HLA-matched marrow transplantation. However, graft failure in patients who have had transplantation with HLA-mismatched or T-cell-depleted marrow typically occurs early, or months after transplantation.
- *Primary graft failure* is the absence of hematologic recovery in patients surviving more than 21 days postBMT.
- *Transient engraftment* is defined as complete or partial recovery of hematopoiesis, in the absence of moderate to severe GVHD, followed by recurrent pancytopenia.

## Avascular Necrosis

- Avascular or aseptic necrosis of the bone is a direct result of bone softening associated with steroid therapy.

## Dental Effects

- Dental effects related to pretransplant conditioning or to chronic GVHD can lead to dental decay.
- Temporomandibular dysfunction or myofascial pain dysfunction may also be a problem.

## Genitourinary Effects

- Total-body irradiation, drug toxicity related to antimicrobial therapy, and cyclosporine are causative factors in possible chronic renal failure.

## Radiation Nephritis

- Radiation nephritis from radiation damage and multiagent preparative regimens occurs approximately five months postBMT.
- Hemolytic uremic syndrome (HUS) associated with renal failure is also a delayed and fatal complication after BMT.

## Neurological Complications

- Neurological complications in the BMT recipient are associated with intrathecal methotrexate, central nervous system (CNS) irradiation, and immunosuppressive agents.

## Second Malignancy

- Second malignancies occur at the rate of up to almost four times that of the normal population.

## RELAPSE

- Relapse remains a major problem. Most patients in whom relapse occurs have disease in host cells.

## PSYCHOSOCIAL ISSUES

### Patients

- Once discharged from the hospital, marrow recipients often experience a normal reactive depression because of neuropsychological deficits, body image changes, malaise, sexual dysfunction, and a slower than anticipated return to normal activities. These symptoms might progress to clinical depression if not recognized and treated promptly.
- Unusual psychological reactions include suicidal ideation, depression greater than expected from the normal grief reaction, disruptive anxiety, pathological regression, and organic delirium.

## Donors

- Donors experience a variety of psychological reactions before and after their marrow donation.

## Family/Caregivers

- Families need to confront the long-term issues of caring for a recovering family member until the physical sequelae of treatment have vanished.

## Staff

- There is the potential for staff stress related to caring for BMT patients whose conditions may change rapidly.
- Nurses are challenged by family interactions as well as patient concerns, and they become part of a psychosocial team caring for acutely ill patients who may die.
- *Staff support programs* can be developed that will help maintain emotional health, clinical excellence, and staff retention.

## Quality of Life

- Researchers have attempted to measure quality of life in four domains: physical, social, psychological, and spiritual.

## Ethical Issues

- Rights of children, informed consent, allocation of resources, prolonged life support in the face of irreversible organ failure, and the competitive selection of marrow recipients involve complex moral and ethical considerations.
- Worldwide banking of placental blood for transplant raises questions.

## FUTURE APPLICATIONS

- Fetal liver stem cell transplants have been reported in the treatment of selected patients with severe combined immunodeficiency disease syndrome (SCIDS).
- Successful allogeneic stem cell transplants for children and adults using umbilical cord blood are being reported.
- Gene transfer holds promise for future applications of BMT. It involves replacement of defective genetic material with healthy genes in marrow transplantation candidates with genetic diseases.

## PRACTICE QUESTIONS

1. In future allogeneic transplantations, the use of bone marrow may be replaced by the use of:
   a. blood cells.
   b. chemotherapy.
   c. irradiation.
   d. syngeneic transplants.

2. A higher incidence of leukemic relapse has been reported in _____ marrow recipients because of the demonstrated antileukemic effect of graft-versus-host disease.
   a. allogeneic
   b. umbilical cell
   c. fetal liver cell
   d. syngeneic

3. Four patients with whom you have been working have asked about the possibility of marrow transplantation. The only patient for whom BMT may be a treatment choice is:
   a. Sibyl, who does not have SCIDS.
   b. Derek, who has sickle cell anemia.
   c. Francis, who has an HLA-matched sibling.
   d. Molly, whose mother may be a match.

4. Which is true regarding donor marrow?
   a. Major ABO-incompatible marrow grafting can be performed without significant hemolytic transfusion reactions.
   b. Donor marrow is obtained from the posterior iliac crests and the sternum (if necessary), but never from the anterior iliac crests.
   c. Ex vivo T-cell depletion of donor marrow has proven to be a controversial method of preventing life-threatening GVHD and is rarely used anymore.
   d. The purpose of T-cell depletion is to remove those T-cells thought to be responsible for GVHD after the donor marrow has been infused.

**Questions 5–7 concern Mr. Jackson, who is admitted for marrow infusion.**

5. Mr. Jackson is admitted for marrow infusion. He will receive allogeneic BMT and is about to undergo total-body irradiation. You tell him that TBI:
   a. offers optimal tumor cell kill but without penetrating the CNS.
   b. is given before marrow infusion to prevent graft rejection by the patient's own immune system.
   c. is usually given in single doses to reduce toxicities.
   d. should not be given as a booster in any form to patients with bulky disease because of the risk of major organ toxicity.

6. Mr. Jackson acquires chronic GVHD some time after his discharge, which frustrates you because he has had no prior acute disease. Mr. Jackson has _____ onset.
   a. progressive
   b. quiescent
   c. de novo
   d. acute

7. Mr. Jackson's wife and children come with him for subsequent follow-up examinations. Although things are going very well, you instruct his family not to take _____ during the first years following Mr. Jackson's BMT because of possible shedding with subsequent infection in Mr. Jackson.
   a. amoxicillin and ampicillin
   b. Sabin oral polio vaccine
   c. chemotherapeutic agents
   d. the "flu shot"

**Questions 8–15 concern Ms. Daniels, who is experiencing complications after allogeneic BMT.**

8. Ms. Daniels experiences complications after allogeneic BMT. Which of the following is *least* likely to be true?
   a. Ms. Daniels' complications may be the result of chemoradiation used in preparation for the transplantation.
   b. The complications could be a result of the marrow transplantation itself.
   c. Ms. Daniels' complications are probably from the original disease.
   d. Treating one complication may exacerbate another.

9. Ms. Daniels is about to receive a blood product. You must ensure that the blood has been specially treated to prevent GVHD. This means you will check to be sure that the blood product has been:
   a. exposed to alloimmunization and platelet refractoriness.
   b. infiltrated with saline solution.
   c. treated via plasmapheresis.
   d. irradiated.

10. It is determined that Ms. Daniels will most likely need pharmacologic intervention in prophylaxis or treatment of GVHD. What is the first-line therapy?
    a. methotrexate
    b. cyclosporine
    c. PUVA
    d. a cyclosporine and methotrexate combination

11. After transplantation, Ms. Daniels is monitored for complications. Naturally, you will monitor her for possible relapse and any related complications. Besides relapse, what reaction is the most common life-threatening complication experienced by BMT patients in response to preparative-regimen-related toxicity?
    a. renal complication
    b. veno-occlusive disease
    c. congestive heart failure
    d. interstitial pneumonia

12. Ms. Daniels develops certain pulmonary complications. You are mindful that, because of prolonged periods of immunosuppression caused by her medication, she is at greater risk for developing:
    a. interstitial pneumonia.
    b. CMV pneumonia.
    c. idiopathic pneumonia.
    d. RSV pneumonia.

13. Ms. Daniels has been through profound immunosuppression that has resulted in neutropenia, along with a denuding of the mucosa in the GI tract. This combination puts her at particular risk for:
    a. *Candida* infection.
    b. *Aspergillus* infection.
    c. Epstein-Barr virus infection.
    d. *Pneumocystis carinii* pneumonia.

14. If Ms. Daniels were to acquire chronic GVHD as a late complication of BMT, which factor would be *most* likely to be a causative risk factor?
    a. mismatched donor and recipient
    b. male-to-female transplant
    c. age under 18
    d. failure to receive methotrexate and cyclosporine as chronic GVHD prophylaxis in CML

15. After a long period of time, Ms. Daniels develops recurrent varicella zoster virus (VZV). What will be the most likely treatment approach?
    a. cyclosporine
    b. methotrexate
    c. acyclovir
    d. cyclosporine and methotrexate in combination

16. Mr. Howard's physician consults with you, saying that Mr. Howard is experiencing transient engraftment. This refers to:
    a. the absence of hematologic recovery 21 days post-BMT.
    b. partial recovery of hematopoiesis in the absence of moderate to severe GVHD, followed by recurrent pancytopenia.
    c. absence of host T-cells in the presence of graft failure.
    d. CMV infection in the presence of T-cells and graft failure.

## ANSWER EXPLANATIONS

1. **The answer is a.** The use of blood cells rather than marrow for allogeneic transplantation is becoming an important area of study. Blood cell transplantation may replace marrow transplantation in the next millennium. The availability of bone marrow makes it possible to administer chemoradiotherapy in supralethal doses—so it is unlikely that either of these will replace BMT. Syngeneic transplants do not indicate an alternative treatment but rather represent a specific source—that of a twin. (pp. 461–462)

2. **The answer is d.** A higher incidence of leukemic relapse has been reported in syngeneic than in allogeneic marrow recipients because of the demonstrated antileukemic effect of graft-versus-host disease. (p. 462)

3. **The answer is c.** Currently, marrow transplantation is a treatment choice only in the presence of an HLA-matched sibling. BMT for sickle cell anemia is under investigation; however, considerable controversy still exists and the risks must be balanced against expected morbidity and mortality. (p. 463)

4. **The answer is a.** Major ABO-incompatible marrow grafting can be performed without significant hemolytic transfusion reactions. Donor marrow is obtained from the posterior iliac crests, as well as from the anterior iliac crests and the sternum, if necessary. Ex vivo T-cell depletion of donor marrow has proven to be the most effective method of preventing life-threatening GVHD, and the pur-

pose of T-cell depletion is to remove those T-cells thought to be responsible for GVHD *before* the donor marrow has been infused. (pp. 464–465)

5. **The answer is b.** TBI is given before marrow infusion to prevent graft rejection by the patient's own immune system. It offers optimal tumor cell kill because it penetrates the CNS and other privileged sites. It is usually given in fractionated doses to reduce toxicities, and it can be given as a booster to patients with bulky disease. (pp. 468–469)

6. **The answer is c.** Patients with de novo onset have had no prior acute disease and have the best prognosis. Progressive onset, a direct extension of acute GVHD, has the poorest prognosis. Quiescent onset develops after clinical resolution of acute GVHD, and these patients have a fair prognosis. (p. 486)

7. **The answer is b.** Family members of BMT recipients should not be given the Sabin oral polio vaccine during the first years because of possible virus shedding with subsequent infection in the recipient. If the vaccine is given, the patient needs to be isolated from that family member for 8 to 12 weeks. (p. 495)

8. **The answer is c.** Major complications after transplantation usually result from the chemoradiation or from the marrow transplantation, not from the original disease. The treatment of one complication can cause or exacerbate another complication. (p. 470)

9. **The answer is d.** Blood products must be irradiated to destroy T-lymphocytes that can cause GVHD in the marrow recipient. Patients whose platelets become refractory to random platelet transfusions can receive HLA-matched platelets from family or community donors, and platelets that have undergone plasmapheresis from marrow donors yield optimal increments. Alloimmunization and platelet refractoriness contribute to a 1% case fatality rate from hemorrhage complications. (p. 474)

10. **The answer is d.** Immunosuppressive therapy is aimed at removing or inactivating T-lymphocytes that attack target organs. Cyclosporine and methotrexate inhibit T-lymphocytes that are believed to be responsible for acute GVHD and are the first line therapy. Used in combination, they are more effective than either agent alone. Several studies demonstrate encouraging results for patients with acute GVHD using Psoralen and ultraviolet A irradiation (PUVA). (p. 475)

11. **The answer is b.** Veno-occlusive disease is almost exclusive to BMT, and is the most common non-relapse life-threatening complication of preparative-regimen-related toxicity for bone marrow transplantation. (p. 476)

12. **The answer is b.** CMV pneumonia is the leading cause of infectious pneumonia after BMT. The incidence of CMV pneumonia may be higher in the allograft versus autograph recipients—specifically because of prolonged periods of immunosuppression caused by medication. (p. 477)

13. **The answer is a.** Profound immunosuppression with resulting neutropenia concomitant with denuding of the mucosa in the GI tract places marrow recipients at risk for *Candida* infection. (p. 479)

14. **The answer is a.** Risk factors for late chronic GVHD include, among others, mismatched donor and recipient, female-to-male transplants, positive herpes simplex and CMV virus, over 18 years of age, prior grade 2–3 acute GVHD, and CML recipients who received methotrexate and cyclosporine as chronic GVHD prophylaxis. (p. 486)

15. **The answer is c.** Aggressive antiviral therapy with intravenous acyclovir is the standard therapy. (p. 494)

16. **The answer is b.** Transient engraftment is defined as complete or partial recovery of hematopoiesis, in the absence of moderate to severe GVHD, followed by recurrent pancytopenia. CMV infection is only one cause of pancytopenia. (p. 497)

## Chapter 19    Autologous Bone Marrow and Blood Cell Transplantation

### OVERVIEW OF BONE MARROW TRANSPLANTATION

#### Allogeneic Bone Marrow Transplantation

- The primary purpose of allogeneic BMT is to treat patients with defective bone marrow in nonmalignant disease or diseased marrow.
- The biggest drawback is the availability of an appropriate marrow donor.
- Histocompatibility is another limitation of allogeneic BMT.

#### Autologous Bone Marrow Transplantation (ABMT)

- There is a steep dose-response relationship in some malignancies, with response rates improving with dose escalation of chemotherapy and radiation therapy.
- The limiting toxicity, myelosuppression, can be overcome by "rescue" with the patient's own pluripotent stem cells (PPSCs).
- Improvements in the technology for cell storage, harvesting, and purging have led to increasing use of autologous BMT.

#### Blood Cell Transplantation

- It was learned that cells for autologous transplant could also be obtained from peripheral blood.
- Peripheral blood stem cell transplant (PBSCT) or peripheral blood progenitor cell transplant (PBPCT) involves obtaining and infusing an unspecified number of true pluripotent stem cells with or without committed progenitor and precursor cells. The current terminology for this process is *blood cell transplant* (BCT).
- Currently the CD34 assay is the best technique available to identify the cells that have been proved to be correlated with successful engraftment. There are advantages to using peripheral PPSCs and progenitor cells obtained from peripheral blood.
    - One advantage is the more rapid recovery of neutrophils and platelets when progenitor cells are used. Another advantage is that no anesthesia is required for BCT, so there is less risk of complications and fewer medical contraindications than with bone marrow harvest.
    - Also, individuals who cannot have bone marrow harvested may be able to undergo BCT.

#### Standards Development

- Refer to Table 19-1, text page 510.
- BCT apheresis can be performed safely in hospital outpatient clinics as well as in for-profit outpatient settings.

### INDICATIONS

#### Indications for ABMT

- The use of ABMT is well established in patients with leukemia, lymphoma, and some solid tumors. The advantages for ABMT over allogeneic BMT are the absence of GVHD and fewer toxicities.
- The advantages of BCT over ABMT are yet to be proved.

### Leukemia

- ABMT is indicated for patients with AML who do not have an allogeneic donor.
- The advantage of ABMT over allogeneic BMT in leukemia is less toxicity since there is no veno-occlusive disease or GVHD. However, there is a potential risk of tumor contamination in the autologous marrow, and there is no benefit of the graft-versus-leukemia (GVL) effect. ABMT is used in individuals with acute lymphocytic leukemia who have relapsed or are at high risk for recurrence of disease. Allogeneic BMT is the treatment of choice for cure in individuals with chronic myelogenous leukemia (CML). Patients in the chronic phase of CML do not benefit from ABMT.

### Lymphoma

- Individuals with early or relapsed Hodgkin's disease may be treated with ABMT. ABMT is curative for low-grade non-Hodgkin's lymphoma.
- Individuals with intermediate- to high-grade lymphoma who do not achieve remission with first-line therapy are generally referred for transplant as well.

### Solid tumors

- Disease-free survival of patients with advanced breast cancer receiving ABMT is similar to survival rates in those receiving standard chemotherapy.
- Individuals with germ cell tumors who are refractory to treatment or who relapse quickly respond well to ABMT.
- Women with ovarian cancer with residual disease are candidates for ABMT.

## Indications for BCT

### Leukemia

- Hematopoietic repopulation is earlier after BCT than after either purged or unpurged ABMT.
- BCT is considered only for those patients with CML who have no options for related or unrelated allogeneic BMT.

### Lymphoma

- Poor-risk lymphoma patients who received either ABMT or conventional chemotherapy may benefit from BCT.

### Multiple myeloma

- BCT has been used to treat small numbers of individuals with multiple myeloma.

## PROCESS OF AUTOLOGOUS TRANSPLANTATION

- The process of autologous transplant is the same for ABMT and BCT except for the procedure used to obtain the cells needed to recover hematopoiesis.

## Cells for Autologous Transplant

### Harvest for autologous BMT

- The process of obtaining bone marrow for ABMT is the same as for allogeneic BMT, but the volume harvested may be greater if there is a need for purging or other manipulation.
- The bone marrow is harvested when the patient is in remission and recovered from other treatment. A double- or triple-lumen silicone catheter is placed centrally to use for reinfusion of bone marrow cells, administration of conditioning chemotherapy and hydration, and supportive therapy.

### BCT mobilization

- The purpose of mobilization for BCT is to release an increased number of PPSCs and progenitor cells into the peripheral bloodstream.
- Chemotherapy is used for mobilization either alone or in combination with hematopoietic growth factors (HGFs). HGFs stimulate enhanced proliferation and maturation of neutrophils.
- A single apheresis can obtain the desired number of cells, but two to three procedures usually are needed.

### BCT apheresis

- Blood cell separators collect the PPSCs and progenitor cells since each cell type has a different density.
- The patient undergoing BCT requires a catheter that is stiffer than the traditional CVC used for ABMT because of the need for high volume and pressure during pheresis.
- Apheresis begins when the desired white blood cell (WBC) count is achieved.
- When chemotherapy is used for mobilization, adequate WBC count is >10,000 cells/mm$^3$ and there is clear evidence of rising counts.
- If growth factor is used to stimulate neutrophil production, a count of 20,000 cells/mm$^3$ indicates that the patient is ready.
- A large volume of the anticoagulant sodium citrate is used to keep the blood from clotting. The citrate binds to ionized serum calcium, causing hypocalcemia.
- TUMS® are usually given at the beginning of apheresis and throughout. However, intravenous (IV) calcium gluconate may be needed if the hypocalcemia becomes severe.
- Hypovolemia may also be a problem, especially for patients with a history of cardiac problems.
- Thrombocytopenia is problematic with some types of equipment.

## Cell Processing/Storage

- The CFU-GM assay provides a real number of circulating progenitor cells.
- One of the main reasons to use cells derived from blood rather than from bone marrow is to avoid tumor contamination from bone marrow and to separate the malignant cells in a positive selection process.
- The outcome after either ABMT or BCT in individuals with AML is similar. Therefore, the shortened nadir period produced by BCT may be the only advantage of one procedure over the other.
- Purging of autologous bone marrow and peripheral blood cells is another strategy to decrease the risk of tumor contamination.

## Conditioning Therapy

- Conditioning therapy is given to remove any remaining malignant cells. In the process, the bone marrow is depleted and the immune response is altered and numerous side effects are possible.
- Commonly used conditioning regimens include cyclophosphamide and total-body irradiation (TBI). The use of busulfan and cyclosphosphamide without TBI is also effective. Numerous regimens exist.

## Reinfusion

- The reinfusion procedure usually takes less than an hour.
- Antiemetic prophylaxis is recommended. IV hydration for two hours prior to reinfusion is recommended to ensure optimal renal function. Hemoglobulinuria develops due to red blood cell lysis.
- The patient experiences nausea and vomiting, chilling, cramping, and a bad taste from the DMSO.

## POSTTRANSPLANT CARE

- Refer to Table 19-4, text page 518, for a comparison of frequency of complications after bone marrow or blood cell transplantation.

### Infection

- A predictable period of myelosuppression follows BMT. Engraftment after ABMT for hematologic malignancy occurs beginning at day 21, with full recovery by day 30.
- By decreasing the length of the nadir and with aggressive use of prophylaxis, there is less risk of infection with ABMT and BCT than with allogeneic BMT. Recipients of allogeneic BMT remain immunosuppressed for six months to two years, depending upon the presence and degree of GVHD.
- Standard prophylaxis and empiric therapy are used to manage infection in patients undergoing ABMT and BCT. Empiric antibiotic therapy is initiated at the onset of fever in the presence of neutropenia.

### Bleeding

- Bleeding may occur secondary to thrombocytopenia during the preengraftment period. Patients may require platelet transfusions.

### Anemia

- Fatigue and decreased oxygenation occur due to anemia. Red blood cell infusions are given to keep the hematocrit above 25%.

### Gastrointestinal Toxicity

- Gastrointestinal toxicity is common with the chemotherapeutic drugs used for all types of transplant.

### Urinary System Toxicity

- Hemorrhagic cystitis can be a severe side effect of high-dose cyclophosphamide.

### Outpatient Care

- Safe and effective care for ABMT and BCT requires significant allocation of resources.
- The neutropenic patient must be seen and evaluated daily.

## PRACTICE QUESTIONS

1. Blood cell transplant (BCT) involves:
   a. obtaining and infusing an unspecified number of true PPSCs.
   b. infusion with committed progenitor cells.
   c. infusion without precursor cells.
   d. all of the above.

2. A patient is originally considered for bone marrow transplant. However, the physician selects blood cell transplantation as the treatment of choice, using peripheral PPSCs and progenitor cells obtained from peripheral blood. This procedure:
   a. delays recovery of neutrophils and platelets when progenitor cells are used.
   b. enables neutrophils and platelets to recover rapidly.
   c. involves collecting committed progenitors that are not as far along the differentiation pathway as the PPSCs harvested from the bone marrow.
   d. b and c.

3. Mrs. Adams has diseased marrow as a result of leukemia. Her physician plans a bone marrow transplant and chooses autologous rather than allogeneic BMT. Mrs. Adams tells you, "I've never heard of using a person's own bone marrow cells. Why would anyone do that when I'm the one with the disease?" You explain that autologous bone marrow transplantation:
   a. eliminates the risk of GVHD and other toxicities, such as myelosuppression.
   b. is less toxic, although there is an increased risk of veno-occlusive disease.
   c. reduces the risk of tumor contamination seen in allogeneic BMTs.
   d. reduces the risk of the GVL effect (GVL effect can increase the risk of relapse).

**Questions 4–11 concern Mr. Prang, who is to receive a blood cell transplant.**

4. Mr. Prang is to receive blood cell transplant (BCT). BCT is:
   a. inappropriate for individuals with multiple myeloma and poor-risk lymphoma patients who have received either ABMT or conventional chemotherapy.
   b. considered only for those patients with CML who have no options for related or unrelated allogeneic BMT.
   c. causes delayed hematopoietic repopulation compared to either purged or unpurged ABMT.
   d. all of the above.

5. As you prepare Mr. Prang for mobilization for BCT, you are aware that which of the following is/are true?
   a. The purpose of mobilization for BCT is to inhibit the release of excess numbers of PPSCs and progenitor cells into the peripheral bloodstream.
   b. Chemotherapy can be used for mobilization either alone or in combination with HGFs; however, chemotherapy alone yields more predictable results.
   c. Chemotherapy alone for mobilization is useful in patients with residual malignancy, but fever and pancytopenia can interfere with the schedule for apheresis.
   d. all of the above.

6.  Mr. Prang asks you to explain the function of HGFs in his treatment. Which of the following could be part of your response?
    a.  HGFs cannot act alone to stimulate enhanced proliferation and maturation of neutrophils.
    b.  HGFs provide a much more controlled response for mobilization.
    c.  While HGFs can enhance chemotherapy, chemotherapy alone yields more predictable results.
    d.  all of the above.

7.  Which of the following factors should influence the choice of catheter used in the BCT process for Mr. Prang?
    a.  The patient undergoing BCT requires a catheter that is stiffer than the traditional CVC used for ABMT.
    b.  The stiff catheters used in ABMT are not necessary in BCT pheresis because there is a less rapid withdrawal of blood in BCT.
    c.  High volume and pressure are needed during pheresis.
    d.  a and c.

8.  What side effects may Mr. Prang experience as a direct result of pheresis?
    a.  Fever—especially localized fever—from rapid movement and return of large volumes of blood to the body.
    b.  Hypercalcemia from high volumes of IV calcium gluconate
    c.  Hypovolemia may be a problem, especially for patients with a history of cardiac problems.
    d.  a and c.

9.  After treatment, Mr. Prang learns that he is to undergo conditioning therapy. As part of your education plan for Mr. Prang, you will mention that in conditioning therapy:
    a.  any remaining malignant cells are removed.
    b.  the bone marrow is depleted.
    c.  the immune response is altered.
    d.  all of the above.

10.  Mr. Prang is at high risk for developing hemorrhagic cystitis in response to conditioning therapy. You would propose to help prevent this development with the use of:
    a.  hydration.
    b.  Foley catheter.
    c.  the uroprotectant mesna.
    d.  all of the above.

11.  In addition to Mr. Prang, you have been working with Mrs. Adams, who has been treated with ABMT, and Ms. Creighton, who is receiving allogeneic BMT. Now, in posttransplant care, you are aware that, by decreasing the length of the nadir and with aggressive use of prophylaxis:
    a.  Ms. Creighton will be at less risk of infection than Mr. Prang.
    b.  Mrs. Adams will be at less risk of infection than Ms. Creighton.
    c.  Mr. Prang will still be at greatest risk for infection than the other two.
    d.  a and c.

## ANSWER EXPLANATIONS

1.  **The answer is d.** Peripheral blood stem cell transplant (PBSCT) or peripheral progenitor cell transplant (PBPCT) involves obtaining and infusing an unspecified number of true PPSCs with or without committed progenitor and precursor cells. The current terminology for this process is blood cell transplant (BCT). (p. 508)

2.  **The answer is b.** One advantage to using peripheral PPSCs and progenitor cells obtained from peripheral blood is the more rapid recovery of neutrophils and platelets when progenitor cells are used. This is because the committed progenitors collected for BCT are farther along the differentiation pathway than the PPSCs harvested from the bone marrow. Another advantage is that no anesthesia is required for BCT so there is less risk of complications and fewer medical contraindications than with bone marrow harvest. (p. 508)

3.  **The answer is a.** The advantages of ABMT over allogeneic BMT are the absence of GVHD and fewer toxicities. ABMT is less toxic since there is no veno-occlusive disease or GVHD. However, there is a potential risk of tumor contamination in the autologous marrow, and there is no benefit of the GVL effect, which can reduce the risk of relapse. (p. 511)

4.  **The answer is b.** BCT is considered only for those patients with CML who have no options for related or unrelated allogeneic BMT. Poor-risk lymphoma patients who received either ABMT or conventional chemotherapy may benefit from BCT. BCT has been used to treat small numbers of individuals with multiple myeloma. Hematopoietic repopulation is earlier after BCT than after either purged or unpurged ABMT. Platelet recovery is more rapid with BCT as well, although it seems to be more directly related to the dose of cells collected. (pp. 511–12)

5.  **The answer is c.** The purpose of mobilization for BCT is to release an increased number of PPSCs and progenitor cells into the peripheral bloodstream. Chemotherapy is used for mobilization either alone or in combination with HGFs. The results using chemotherapy are variable and less predictable than with HGFs. Chemotherapy alone for mobilization is useful in patients with residual malignancy, but fever and pancytopenia can interfere with the schedule for apheresis. (p. 514)

6.  **The answer is b.** HGFs provide a much more controlled response for mobilization. HGFs stimulate enhanced proliferation and maturation of neutrophils. (p. 515)

7.  **The answer is d.** The patient undergoing BCT requires a catheter that is stiffer than the traditional CVC used for ABMT because of the need for high volume and pressure during pheresis. (p. 515)

8.  **The answer is c.** Chilling can occur due to the large volume of blood being returned to the patient. A large volume of the anticoagulant sodium citrate can cause hypocalcemia. IV calcium gluconate may be needed if the hypocalcemia becomes severe. Hypovolemia may be a problem, especially for patients with a history of cardiac problems. Thrombocytopenia is problematic with some types of equipment. (p. 515)

9.  **The answer is d.** Conditioning therapy is given to remove any remaining malignant cells. In the process, the bone marrow is depleted and the immune response is altered. (p. 516)

10. **The answer is d.** Prevention of hemorrhagic cystitis is the key to success with aggressive use of hydration, Foley catheter, and administration of the uroprotectant mesna. (p. 516)

11. **The answer is b.** By decreasing the length of the nadir and with aggressive use of prophylaxis, there is less risk of infection with ABMT and BCT than with allogeneic BMT. Recipients of allogeneic BMT remain immunosuppressed for six months to two years, depending upon the presence and degree of GVHD. (p. 518)

# Chapter 20    Pain

## INTRODUCTION AND BACKGROUND

### Definitions of Pain

- The need for a standard definition of pain prompted the International Association for the Study of Pain (IASP) to form a subcommittee charged with developing a definition acceptable to both clinicians and researchers. The major result of their labors, published in 1979, was the following: "Pain is an unpleasant sensory and emotional experience associated with actual or potential tissue damage, or described in terms of such damage."
- Chronic pain and acute pain are distinctly different phenomena.
- Acute pain rarely has a strong psychopathological or environmental component, as does chronic pain.

### Theories and Mechanisms of Pain

- There are several current theories of pain. Most notable of these is the *gate control theory of pain*, proposed by Melzack and Wall in 1965.
- The perception of and response to pain are due to four distinct processes that operate simultaneously and are all required for pain to occur.
- *Transduction* begins when a noxious stimulus affects a peripheral sensory nerve ending, depolarizing it and setting off electrical activity that initiates the whole phenomenon of pain perception.
- *Transmission* consists of the series of subsequent neural events that carry the electrical impulses throughout the nervous system, from peripheral to central.
- *Modulation* is a neural activity that controls pain transmission neurons, those originating in the periphery and/or the central nervous system (CNS).
- *Perception*, is less an actual physiological/anatomic process than it is the vague subjective correlate of pain that encompasses complex behavioral, psychological, and emotional factors that are little understood.

### Cancer Pain as a Multidimensional Phenomenon

- A multidimensional model of care related to pain has been hypothesized: (1) *physiological*, (2) *sensory*, (3) *affective*, (4) *cognitive*, (5) *behavioral*, and (6) *sociocultural*.
- In addition to these five dimensions of the multidimensional model of cancer-related pain, there is a sixth important area—the sociocultural dimension.

#### The physiological dimension

- Foley described three types of pain observed in patients with cancer: (1) pain associated with direct tumor involvement, (2) pain associated with cancer therapy, and (3) pain unrelated to either the tumor or its treatment.
- Table 20-2 on text page 532 lists the major causes of tumor- and treatment-related cancer pain.
- Three specific pain syndromes occur in patients with cancer and are caused by tumor: somatic, visceral, and neuropathic pain. These syndromes are characterized by pain of different qualities, located in different anatomic parts of the body, and caused by different mechanisms (Figure 20-2,

text page 533). Many cancer patients with pain will have one or more of these three syndromes simultaneously.

- Each syndrome responds differently to therapeutic modalities.
- Related to etiology of pain are two other characteristics. *Duration* of pain refers to whether pain is acute or chronic. The second characteristic related to etiology of pain is the *pattern* that pain displays: (1) brief, momentary, or transient; (2) rhythmic, periodic, or intermittent; and (3) continuous, steady, or constant.

## Sensory dimension

- Three specific components of this dimension are location, intensity, and quality.
- The first component, *location* of pain, is important. Many cancer patients have been reported to have pain at two or more locations. Given the patterns of metastasis or sites of involvement seen in many solid tumors and some hematologic malignancies, this finding is not surprising.
- *Intensity* of pain, or how strong it feels, is the second important component of the sensory dimension. Intensity is a perceived, and therefore a subjective, phenomenon, subject to individual sensation threshold.
- The *quality* of pain refers to how it actually feels.

## Affective dimension

- The affective dimension consists of depression, anxiety, or other psychological factors or personality traits associated with pain.
- Specific personality factors probably are not related to the experience of cancer pain; there is little evidence that affective disorders such as depression and anxiety are *strongly* related to pain.

## Cognitive dimension

- The cognitive dimension of cancer pain encompasses the manner in which the pain influences a person's thought processes or the manner in which the person views her- or himself.
- Level and quality of cognition in relation to pharmacological therapy may influence the ability of individuals to report pain. Knowledge can affect responses both to pain and to interventions. Educational intervention of nurse counseling and printed materials resulted in a higher likelihood of cancer patients with pain taking the proper dose of analgesic on the proper schedule.

## Behavioral dimension

- The behavioral dimension of pain includes a variety of observable behaviors related to pain such as nonverbal and verbal communication and strategies or activities that patients engage in to control pain.
- The most commonly cited pain reduction methods involved medications, rest or lying down, heat, and distraction.

## Sociocultural dimension

- The sociocultural dimension of cancer pain consists of a variety of demographic, ethnic, cultural, spiritual, and related factors that influence a person's perception of and response to pain.

## Implications of the multidimensional model

- The six dimensions are highly appropriate for assessment and management of cancer pain; each contributes in its own way to various aspects of these two critical processes.

## SCOPE OF THE CANCER PAIN PROBLEM

- Pain often is managed inadequately.

## Prevalence

- Prevalence of pain by clinical setting, regardless of cancer diagnosis, indicates that patients in hospice and specialty units report a higher prevalence of pain than patients in other settings.
- Patients with advanced disease report more severe pain than those who are in the early stages of their illness.
- Examination of pain prevalence data by cancer diagnosis shows the likelihood of pain becoming a significant problem with the progression of disease, particularly in common solid tumors such as lung and breast cancer.

## Significance

- Quality of life is significantly affected by cancer pain.
- Quality of life also serves as a foundation for reexamining the current issue of suicidal ideation or actual suicide in persons with progressive cancer accompanied by severe pain.
- Families' experience of pain included three themes: helplessness, coping by denial of their own feelings, and a wish for the patient's death.
- Caregivers in the home hospice setting reported lower burden, better mood, less distress, and more feelings of being supported in their attempts to care for their loved one.
- Ethical concerns related to the use of high technology in medicine are important issues, particularly with respect to costs, access, social justice, informed consent, and autonomy.
- Because fear of regulatory scrutiny has been identified as a barrier in cancer pain management, state and national laws and regulations are also problematic.

## Professional Issues

### Organizational efforts

- Organizations and agencies involved with cancer treatment and pain management have directed their efforts toward improving pain management. The ONS position paper highlighted the fact that control of cancer pain is largely inadequate.

### Obstacles to successful management

- A number of obstacles to pain management can be attributed to health care professionals, patients and family, and the health care system. These obstacles are identified in Table 20-3 on text page 540.
- Inaccurate knowledge about pharmacological principles represents a major problem area.
- Issues surrounding addiction and potential toxicities of potent opioids are reasons for suboptimal pain control. Although some evidence strongly suggests that addiction is not a problem for individuals who require opioids, nurses, physicians, and medical students fear iatrogenically induced addiction.
- Factors that prohibit patients from receiving reasonable pain control include the following: lack of basic assessment skills, failure to acknowledge and document the existence of pain, and inaccurate or nonexistent documentation when the problem is known to exist.
- Patients' reluctance to report pain to their health care providers and concerns about analgesics are major problems.

- Perceptual differences between patients and professionals about severity of existing pain have been documented.
- Complete relief of pain traditionally has not been viewed as a treatment objective.
- The role of government agencies and existing legal statutes have contributed to inadequate prescribing by physicians because of fear of regulatory scrutiny.

### Improvements in management

- Improvement of pain management can be accomplished through formal performance improvement programs.
- Major programmatic efforts have made the cancer pain problem much more visible, leading to heightened efforts to improve the care of patients with cancer pain.

### Delivery of pain management services

- Practitioners who take care of oncology patients should possess basic skills in assessment and management.
- Some practitioners may feel more comfortable in referring a patient to a "specialist" for pain management or a multidisciplinary pain team that can provide services.
- Utilization of resources, costs, and outcomes in today's health care climate needs careful consideration.

## PRINCIPLES OF ASSESSMENT AND MANAGEMENT

- The ONS position paper delineated the nurse's role as (1) describing pain, (2) identifying aggravating and relieving factors, (3) determining the meaning of pain, (4) determining its cause, (5) determining individuals' definitions of optimal pain relief, (6) deriving nursing diagnoses, (7) assisting in selecting interventions, and (8) evaluating efficacy of interventions.
- Their focus is on individual definitions of optimal pain relief, psychosocial and physical problems amenable to nursing interventions, and evaluation of the overall response to treatment.

## Multidisciplinary Approach

- The multidimensional conceptualization of cancer pain requires the involvement of multiple health care disciplines in assessment and management.

## Nursing's Scope of Practice and Responsibilities

- Oncology nurses are best prepared to assume a leadership role in the assessment and management of cancer pain.
- At the generalist level, the nurse needs a cancer pain-specific knowledge base that enables appropriate assessment, development of a care plan based on the nursing process, evaluation of the plan, and consultation with others when needed.
  - At the advanced level, the nurse (an individual with a master's degree) should have substantially more theoretical knowledge and clinical expertise in cancer pain that allows assessment, diagnosis, analysis of complex problems, and the use of relevant research and theory to problem-solve.
- The ONS position paper deals with the ethical and practice responsibilities of nurses in managing pain (Table 20-4, text page 542).

## Assessment and Diagnosis

### Rationale and basic principles

- Systematic nursing assessment of pain is important: it establishes a baseline from which to plan and begin interventions, it assists in the selection of interventions, and it makes possible evaluation of the interventions. Key clinical parameters that require assessment in each dimension are highlighted in Table 20-5, text page 544.

### Assessment tools

- Pain assessment tools can be classified by the number of dimensions of pain they assess.
- Ten-centimeter visual analogue scales (VAS) or verbal descriptor scales (VDS) measuring pain intensity are examples of commonly used unidimensional tools. VASs and VADs measure only one parameter of one dimension of pain and thus are limited in their representation of the total pain experience.
- Other unidimensional tools consist of body diagrams to assess location of pain and rating scales to assess behavioral indicators of pain. Multidimensional tools focus on two or more dimensions of the pain experience (see Tables 20-5 and 20-6, text pages 544–545).
- Multidimensional methods for assessing pain have been developed to assist nurses in making both baseline and ongoing assessments, taking the form of comprehensive questionnaires and flow sheets.
- Patients with cancer often suffer not only from pain but from numerous other symptoms.
- The Memorial Symptom Assessment Scale (MSAS) is designed to collect information about the prevalence, characteristics, and distress of 32 common symptoms, including pain.
- Several instruments for measuring pain in children ages 3 years and older have been developed and tested (see Table 20-6, text page 544).
- The tool selected should be able to assess the relevant parameters of the dimension(s) of interest.
- Baseline assessments will require a more detailed and comprehensive tool, while ongoing assessments can use brief, simple tools.

### Nursing diagnoses and documentation

- The outcome of a thorough baseline assessment of the cancer patient with pain should be identification of problems or nursing diagnoses that structure the design and implementation of the management plan.
- Of critical importance is the need for nurses to document their assessments and diagnoses in a manner appropriate for their clinical settings.
- The use of standardized pain assessment and documentation appears to have a positive impact on pain intensity and to facilitate management of pain.

## Incorporation into Practice

- The ONS position paper places the *coordination* of pain management squarely on the oncology nurse.
- The AHCPR cancer pain guidelines provide a useful framework for incorporating sound pain assessment and management principles into clinical practice.

## Special Populations

- Several populations require special consideration in the areas of pain assessment and management.

### Children

- The developmental level of children is directly related to how they perceive, interpret, and respond to pain, regardless of etiology.
- There is significant evidence to indicate that neonates, including premature ones, do feel pain.
- Children who are verbally fluent may deny they have pain when in fact they *do* have it.
- The child who sleeps, plays, or is otherwise distracted may still have a good deal of pain.
- Children do *not* tolerate pain better than adults do.
- Opioids may be used safely in children provided there is an understanding of the pharmacokinetics and the children are properly observed.
- Pain is *not* a harmless entity in children, without side effects or life-threatening potential.
- The issue of undertreatment of children with pain is important.
- Pain that is acute and related to operative procedures may be treated in the same manner as adult postoperative pain.
- It is important to note that children metabolize opioids more quickly than adults do, so their doses may need to be scheduled more frequently. Since needles and shots are uniformly hated by children, the intravenous route immediately postoperatively followed by the oral route when possible is the preferred strategy.
- The treatment of acute, procedure-related pain is somewhat different.
- Interventions range from pharmacological approaches to cognitive and behavioral techniques.
- Sedatives should be used with caution, for they do not decrease pain and anxiety.
- The management of pain due to terminal cancer is a challenging area, since the goal is pain relief without undue sedation.

### The elderly

- The problem of cancer pain in elderly cancer patients has been grossly neglected.
- While it may be true that people develop more chronic diseases as they age the experience of pain does not need to be an expectation.
- The elderly experience greater alterations in the musculoskeletal system and are more vulnerable to acute and soft-tissue pain.
- Chronic problems may confuse the pain problem for individuals who also have cancer-related pain.
- The elderly may experience significant sensory and cognitive impairment.
- A very important piece of assessment data to obtain in the elderly is any change from baseline behaviors, usual routines, and social interactions.
- Another unique problem is the issue of the sensitivity of elderly patients to both perception of pain and sensitivity to pharmacological interventions.
- Physiological responses to medication in light of changes in absorption, distribution, metabolism, and excretion of drugs are a major concern.
- Since the elderly have more chronic diseases and take more medications for these illnesses, the risk of adverse drug reactions may be higher solely because of increased drug intake.
- The elderly have fewer opioids prescribed for them than younger patients.
- If the elderly perceive pain less often, indicating a lower prevalence of pain, then less frequent prescribing of analgesics is appropriate. If, however, the elderly experience pain similar to the younger population of patients, and choose not to report the pain, *or* respond more slowly to painful stimuli, indicating a higher prevalence of pain, then underprescribing creates needless suffering.
- Some general recommendations for management of pain in the elderly are listed in column one, text page 550.

### Substance abuse history

- For the patient in a methadone maintenance program or with a long-standing prior history, health care providers need to be concerned about recidivism.
- The patient should be asked to share any concerns about using opioids for pain relief.
- With all patients having any previous or current substance abuse history, it is important that an adversarial relationship not begin or escalate between patient and staff.
- The substance abuse patient's report of pain should not be questioned or doubted. Appropriate medications should not be withheld as a form of punishment, and pain relief should not become a bargaining tool.
- Sometimes a contract may be useful for establishing realistic goals between the health care provider and the patient.
- Regularly scheduled meetings to review the goals of care may avoid unnecessary conflict.

### Critical care

- Patients who receive aggressive treatment for their malignancy or patients who experience serious symptoms from their disease may require intensive critical care monitoring.

### Culturally diverse populations

- In the American system of health care, provision frequently is not made for even acknowledging the individual's ethnocultural perspective, let alone understanding or using it in planning health care interventions.
- Respect for cultures other than one's own, and for the fact that people have specific beliefs and behaviors that emanate from their cultural background, is known as cultural sensitivity.
- Developing rapport is the foundation of successful nursing interventions.
- A key principle is the use of negotiation to achieve feasible treatment plans and to enlist the patient's and family's participation in reaching treatment goals.
- In patients who are culturally different from their caregivers, as well as those who are similar, the area of spirituality is important.

### Palliative and terminal care

- The nurse must practice the art of creating a nursing environment that allows a peaceful death.
- The focus of terminal care is on relief of pain and other symptoms and on psychological support of both the patient and the family.
- Withdrawal from those who are dying is a common reaction, yet remaining with the individual is one of the most important aspects of terminal care.
- There is no reason why terminally ill people with worsening or new symptoms of pain should be evaluated, diagnosed, and treated any differently than nonterminally ill individuals with cancer pain.

## INTERVENTIONS

- Methods for managing cancer pain can be categorized into three major approaches: (1) treatment of the underlying pathology or organic etiology of the pain; (2) changing the individual's perception or sensation of pain; (3) diminishing the emotional or reactive component of pain.

## Treatment of Underlying Pathology

- Chemotherapy, radiotherapy, and surgery are the major modalities used to treat cancer when cure is the intent, but they can also be useful when palliation is the goal.

## Chemotherapy

- The effect of chemotherapy on pain relief has not been well documented.
- Hormonal therapy may afford significant relief of pain, sometimes even for prolonged periods of time.

## Radiotherapy

- Radiation has long been used to treat painful bone metastases. It is standard treatment for relieving pain from epidural cord compression, and it may be helpful in relieving pain from headaches and increased intracranial pressure due to brain metastases, nerve root infiltration, hepatic metastases, and advanced gynecologic, gastrointestinal, or upper aerodigestive cancers. Relief of pain can begin to occur within 24–48 hours of initiation of radiotherapy.

## Surgery

- Surgery as a modality for treating cancer pain can take many forms, but the primary goal is palliative.
- Table 20-7 (text page 554) shows clinical conditions and tumors that may benefit from various types of palliative surgery for relief of pain.

## Change in Perception/Sensation of Pain

- Pharmacological therapy—consisting of nonopioids, opioids, and adjuvant drugs—is a major responsibility of nurses.

### Pharmacological therapy

- The pharmacological management of cancer pain accounts for the major source of pain treatment.

#### Nonopioids

- Nonopioids are presented as two distinct categories—nonsteroidal antiinflammatory drugs (NSAIDs) and acetaminophen.
- The indication for using nonopioids in patients with cancer pain is when pain is mild to moderate in intensity.
- In cancer-related pain, NSAIDs can be useful for (1) metastatic bone pain; (2) pain from mechanical compression of tendons, muscles, pleura, and peritoneum; and (3) nonobstructive visceral pain.
- The major potential toxicities from NSAIDs are gastrointestinal disorders.
- The elderly may have a significantly increased risk for developing peptic ulcer disease, especially with high doses.
- Table 20-9 (text page 556) indicates many of the common drugs and doses. Table 20-10 (text page 557) lists considerations in the use of nonopioids.
- The benefits of nonopioids in patients who have pain of severe intensity and who require high doses of opioids have not been established.

#### Opioids

- Opioids are classified into three groups:
  1. *Morphinelike opioid agonists.*
  2. *Opioid antagonists.*
  3. *Opioid agonist-antagonists.* It is generally accepted by cancer pain experts that opioid agonist-antagonist drugs have very limited usefulness in cancer pain management because of their propensity to induce opioid withdrawal.

- Table 20-11 (text page 557) contains information about the relative potencies of commonly used analgesics for mild to moderate pain and for severe pain.
- All opioid analgesics share common effects as a result of their action. Table 20-12 (text page 558) shows the CNS, respiratory, cardiovascular, gastrointestinal, genitourinary, and dermatologic effects of these drugs. The four most common side effects are sedation, respiratory depression, nausea and vomiting, and constipation.
- Respiratory depression rarely occurs if opioids are given based on commonly accepted principles.
- If a patient experiences opioid-related nausea and vomiting, there are many options available:
  1. Treat aggressively on initial presentation.
  2. Use antiemetics that act at the CTZ.
  3. Use metoclopramide if gastroparesis is a possible etiology of the nausea and vomiting.
  4. Use an antivertigo drug if symptoms worsen with movement.
  5. Consider drug combinations.
  6. Maximize dose response, especially if symptoms partially improve.
  7. Prescribe antiemetics on an around-the-clock basis for one to two weeks.
- Constipation can become a significant clinical problem for patients taking opioid analgesics if preventive measures are not instituted.
- The use of laxative preparations generally is necessary when patients must take opioids. Table 20-13 (text page 559) lists six categories of laxatives, their mechanisms of action, and commonly available preparations.
- There are inherent properties in opioids than can create potential problems for patients if health care professionals do not understand the distinctions among them.
- Tolerance requires that doses of specific analgesics be adjusted to accommodate the pharmacological phenomenon.
- Physical dependence becomes an issue when patients no longer require opioids for pain control; they must be tapered slowly off of them.
- Addiction is not a problem for patients who require opioids for justifiable medical indications.
- Specific drug selection: Opioid administration guidelines are described in Table 20-14 (text page 559).
- Morphine is the most frequently used opioid analgesic for moderate to severe pain.
- The availability of long-acting morphine has contributed to improvements in patients' quality of life.
- When patients are initially placed on fixed schedules of methadone and levorphanol, they are at risk of developing significant sedation and respiratory depression as the level in their plasma rises.
- Oxycodone has been used in relatively low doses either alone or in combination with aspirin or acetaminophen.

## Adjuvant analgesics

- Adjuvant analgesics are defined as those medications that enhance the action of pain-modulating systems.
- Antidepressants are useful for patients with a neuropathic component to their pain. Their use has been for pain due to tumor infiltration of nerves or from treatment-related injury such as postmastectomy pain syndrome.
- A partial list of antidepressants with starting and usual doses for cancer-related pain is given in Table 20-15, text page 560.
- The major side effects from antidepressants are anticholinergic.
- Anticonvulsants are a primary treatment for the pain caused by trigeminal neuralgia and neurogenic or neuropathic pain described as having a lancinating, stabbing quality.

- Table 20-16 (text page 561) lists common doses and toxicities of four common anticonvulsants.
- Psychostimulants are useful in counteracting the sedation that accompanies opioid analgesics.
- If the sedation is present without any other CNS problems and if pain occurs when the opioid dose is lowered, then psychostimulants may be indicated.
- Steroids are essential for managing the pain from epidural cord compressions, but their use as an adjuvant analgesic is based on limited data.
- The known toxicities from steroids, particularly an increase in appetite and elevation of mood, may be desirable in some patients, especially those with advanced disease.
- Biphosphonates: These powerful inhibitors of bone resorption are used for treating disorders such as Paget's disease and hypercalcemia of malignancy.
- Patients who received pamidronate had significant decreases in bone pain.

### Routes of opioid administration

- There are five overall categories of routes of opioid administration: (1) oral, (2) parenteral (includes IM, subcutaneous [SQ], and IV by intermittent bolus or infusion), (3) transdermal, (4) rectal, and (5) intraspinal.
- The oral route is an effective, comparatively inexpensive, and safe way for patients to receive opioids.
- Changing a patient to another route should be considered if high doses of oral opioids are ineffective or if toxicities occur that cannot be successfully treated.
- The scheduling of oral medications should be on a fixed-interval basis.
- Patients with acute pain, such as postoperative pain, often are the recipients of intermittent IM or SQ injections. For cancer patients, if a patient requires immediate pain relief and does not have peripheral or central venous access, then an occasional IM or SQ injection might be indicated.
- Intravenous bolus is a common alternative to IM or SQ injections.
- Continuous infusions provide the patient with steady blood levels of the opioid and can help avoid the potential side effects and the return of pain associated with intermittent dosing. Guidelines for initiating and managing continuous infusions are given in Table 20-17, text page 563.

### Continuous subcutaneous

- Continuous SQ infusions are alternatives to continuous or bolus IV infusions if venous access is unavailable.
- Continuous SQ infusions are a reasonable alternative for patients who are unable to use the oral route as a result of vomiting or obstruction, lack of control with the oral route, and no venous access.

### Transdermal

- One of the newest opioid delivery systems is transdermal administration. Fentanyl, which is 75–100 times more potent than morphine, is the only opioid available via this route.
- Advantages and disadvantages of transdermal fentanyl are highlighted in Table 20-18 (text page 564).

### Rectal

- With the advent of transdermal fentanyl and sophisticated pump technology, the use of the rectal route may not be as common an alternative to orally administered analgesics.
- The advantages and disadvantages of the rectal route of opioid administration are summarized in Table 20-19, text page 565.

*Intraspinal*

- The identification of opiate receptors in the brain and spinal cord and the results of early animal work involving spinal opioids provided the bases for the use of intraspinal opioid administration for cancer pain.
- Morphine and fentanyl have been the most common agents used for intraspinal opioid administration.
- Advantages and disadvantages of the intraspinal drug delivery system are highlighted in Table 20-20, text page 566.

*Patient-controlled analgesia*

- Patient-controlled analgesia (PCA) has been used in patients who receive analgesics via the parenteral route and the epidural route.
- PCA is designed to allow the patient to self-administer analgesics within preset programming parameters from special infusion pump, thereby avoiding the peaks and troughs of conventional PRN parenteral administration. PCA can be used in either of two ways: (1) bolus dosing only, or (2) bolus dosing with continuous infusion.
- See text pages 566–567 for a detailed discussion of PCA.

## Anesthetic and neurosurgical modalities

- Anesthetic, or nerve-block, procedures for cancer-related pain help modulate a patient's neural responses to noxious stimuli.
- Nondestructive nerve blocks serve two functions: (1) they are used for treatment of intractable pain; (2) they are used for prognostic/diagnostic purposes.
- Neurolytic (destructive) nerve blocks can lead to more prolonged pain relief than nondestructive nerve blocks.
- Destructive neurosurgical procedures most often are used when standard pharmacological and nonpharmacological strategies are no longer effective.
- The nursing responsibilities for patients undergoing anesthetic and neurodestructive procedures include (1) knowledge about the purpose of the procedure and how it is performed; (2) potential complications based on type of block, agent, and location; and (3) potential benefit of the procedure.

## Diminishing the Emotional and Reactive Components of Pain

- The nonpsychiatric, nonpharmacological strategies encompassed in this major treatment approach are those that help individuals cope with their pain in a positive and proactive way.
- Both physicians and nurses have little information about nonpsychiatric, nonpharmacological interventions.
- The role of these techniques is clearly that of an adjuvant to standard pharmacological therapy.
- The benefits of many of the techniques are that they may increase sense of personal control, reduce feelings of helplessness, provide opportunities to become actively involved in care, reduce stress and anxiety, elevate mood, raise pain threshold, and thereby reduce pain.
- *Cognitive* methods are those that attempt directly to modify thought processes in order to attenuate or relieve pain.
- *Behavioral* methods are those that modify physiological reactions to pain or behavioral manifestations of pain.
- Another group of interventions that diminish the emotional and reactive components of pain are those that provide counterirritant cutaneous stimulation; examples include menthol ointments, heat, cold, and massage.

- Most of these interventions are simple and can be initiated when ongoing assessment of pain suggests a need for them.

## Counterirritant cutaneous stimulation

- This group of methods is thought to help relieve pain by somehow physiologically altering the transmission of nociceptive stimuli. Examples include mentholated ointments, heat, cold, massage, and transcutaneous electrical nerve stimulation (TENS).

## Immobilization/mobilization

- Methods such as complete or partial immobilization of the body or parts of the body and positioning of specific body parts may be quite helpful.
- In other circumstances, mild exercise may help decrease pain.

## Distraction

- Distraction is "directing one's attention away from the sensations or emotional reactions produced by a noxious stimulus. Examples include conversation, verbalization to self or others, deep thinking, visualization and imagery, mind-body separation, routines/rituals, breathing exercises, counting, reading, and watching television.

## Relaxation and guided imagery

- Relaxation training helps produce physiological and mental relaxation.
- The two most common methods are progressive muscle relaxation and autogenic relaxation.
- Guided imagery, in which an individual visualizes pleasant places or things, is frequently used in conjunction with relaxation.

## Biofeedback

- There are several biofeedback techniques, electromyography being the most common. The purpose of the technique is to decrease muscle tension and/or sympathetically mediated responses, such as vasoconstriction, that might produce or worsen pain.

## Hypnosis

- Hypnosis is "a state of aroused, attentive focal concentration with a relative suspension of peripheral awareness."
- While an individual is under hypnosis, there are perceptual, motor, and cognitive alterations.

## Comprehensive cognitive/behavioral methods

- Several individuals have proposed comprehensive cognitive and behavioral "treatment" packages for cancer pain.

## Summary and nursing implications

- Many of these techniques require patient and family education, and a willingness to try them as adjuncts to pharmacological therapy.
- Table 20-21 (text page 571) presents the most commonly used nursing interventions for decreasing the emotional and reactive components of pain, along with advantages, disadvantages, and information on specific techniques.

### Education and information

- Accurate and appropriate education and information for patients with cancer-related pain and their caregivers are an essential aspect of comprehensive pain management.

## CONCLUSIONS AND FUTURE DIRECTIONS

- A great deal of information is readily available for nurses and other health professionals to use in achieving the best possible care for individuals with cancer pain. The challenge for the future is to utilize this knowledge to its fullest, to continue experimenting with new ways to treat pain, and to share the information gained with colleagues.

## PRACTICE QUESTIONS

1. Which of the following processes associated with the occurrence of pain is considered vague and subjective in that it encompasses complex behavioral, psychologic, and emotional factors?
   a. transduction
   b. transmission
   c. modulation
   d. perception

2. The dimension of pain that encompasses the meaning that the pain experience has for a person is the:
   a. behavioral dimension.
   b. affective dimension.
   c. sensory dimension.
   d. cognitive dimension.

3. Of the following, which population is statistically likely to have the highest prevalence of pain?
   a. patients in a hospice setting
   b. patients in the general ward
   c. patients in the early stages of illness
   d. pediatric patients

4. Which of the following is *not* a common obstacle to successful pain management?
   a. inaccurate knowledge about pharmacological principles
   b. a lack of basic assessment skills
   c. a lack of available knowledge in the field
   d. legal impediments

5. As a nurse, you know that which of the following is part of your caregiving role?
   a. determining the meaning of your patients' pain.
   b. deriving nursing diagnoses.
   c. assisting in selecting interventions.
   d. all of the above.

6. Assessment of behavioral parameters in cancer pain would include an evaluation of:
   a. the quality of the pain.
   b. associated psychologic problems.
   c. the effect of pain on activities of daily living.
   d. the duration of the pain.

7. One misconception about pain in the elderly person is that:
   a. age effects the absorption, distribution, metabolism, and excretion of analgesic drugs.
   b. an elderly person is better qualified to describe his or her pain than is an informed son or daughter.
   c. the risk of toxic effects of narcotics is higher in the elderly due to interactions of multiple medications.
   d. pain is a common aspect of normal aging.

8. Respect for cultures other than one's own, and for the fact that people have specific beliefs and behaviors that emanate from their cultural background, is known as:
   a. multiculturalism.
   b. cultural sensitivity.
   c. ethnoculturalism.
   d. developing rapport.

9. Nonsteroidal anti-inflammatory drugs (NSAIDs) are most useful for which of the following?
   a. phantom limb pain
   b. nonobstructive visceral pain
   c. postoperative pain
   d. pain due to leukemic infiltrates\

10. The drug used to treat respiratory depression related to narcotics is:
    a. naproxen.
    b. methadone.
    c. meperidine.
    d. naloxone.

11. Which of the following is *not* a common side effect of opioids?
    a. sedation
    b. respiratory depression
    c. increased motility
    d. constipation

12. Antidepressants such as amitriptyline may be used to treat pain that is due to:
    a. tumor infiltration of nerves.
    b. narcotic withdrawal.
    c. brain metastases.
    d. surgery.

13. Mrs. Villegas experiences extreme sedation as a result of her course of opioid analgesics. There are no other CNS problems, and she is in severe pain when the opioid dose is lowered. _____ may be indicated.
    a. antihistamines
    b. steroids
    c. biphosphonates
    d. psychostimulants

14. Steroids are sometimes used in the management of pain related to:
    a. bowel obstruction.
    b. spinal cord compression.
    c. trigeminal neuralgia.
    d. tumor pressing on a vital organ.

15. Scheduling of oral analgesics generally should be:
    a. at fixed intervals.
    b. every two hours.
    c. as needed (prn).
    d. related to a patient's activity level.

16. The transdermal route of narcotic administration was first used with which opioid?
    a. methadone
    b. fentanyl
    c. morphine
    d. levorphanol

17. An example of counterirritant cutaneous stimulation is:
    a. subcutaneous administration of morphine.
    b. minor surgery.
    c. massage.
    d. imagery.

18. Directing one's attention away from the sensations and emotional reactions produced by pain is known as:
    a. distraction.
    b. biofeedback.
    c. autogenic relaxation.
    d. hypnosis.

## ANSWER EXPLANATIONS

1. **The answer is d.** The neural activities that occur in transmission and modulation culminate in the mechanism of pain known as perception. Because perception varies considerably from one individual to the next, it is the mechanism that contributes to the great diversity in response to noxious stimuli/events. This process is the least understood of all those related to pain. (p. 531)

2. **The answer is d.** Of the five dimensions of the cancer pain experience described by Ahles et al., the cognitive dimension relates to the manner in which pain influences a person's thought processes, view of self, and the meaning of the pain. (p. 531)

3. **The answer is a.** Evidence suggests that children experience no more or less pain than adults, and patients in the general ward or in the early stages of their disease have less prevalence of pain than do those in a hospice or terminal care setting. (p. 537)

4. **The answer is c.** A great deal of valuable information is available in the field of pain management, but the lack of basic assessment skills, a lack of coordinated and detailed records, and inaccurate knowledge concerning pharmacological principles all create problems for successfully managing patients' pain. Existing legal statutes and government agencies have contributed to inadequate prescribing by physicians because of fear of regulatory scrutiny. (p. 540)

5. **The answer is d.** All of these are part of the nursing role as defined by the ONS, including as well describing pain, identifying aggravating and relieving factors, determining individual's definitions of optimal pain relief, and evaluating efficacy of interventions. (p. 541)

6. **The answer is c.** An assessment of behavioral parameters of pain should include the effect of the pain on activities of daily living (ADLs), such as eating, mobility, and social interactions, as well as activities/behaviors that increase or decrease the intensity of pain. A behavioral assessment would also consider pain behaviors used, including grimacing or other nonverbal communication and the use of medications or other pain control interventions. (Table 20-5, p. 544)

7. **The answer is d.** Pain is not a normal sequalae of aging. Although it may be true that people develop more chronic conditions as they age, it does not necessarily follow that pain accompanies the aging process and that complaints of pain by an elderly person should be dismissed. Because of

this common misconception, elderly patients may not report pain as a problem, and interventions to control their pain might not be implemented. (p. 549)

8.  **The answer is b.** Cultural sensitivity is having respect for cultures—and the beliefs connected with those cultures—other than your own. (p. 551)

9.  **The answer is b.** Nonsteroidal anti-inflammatory drugs (NSAIDs) act on the peripheral nervous system by preventing the conversion of arachidonic acid to prostaglandin. These medications have a maximum ceiling effect for analgesic potential, and their indication for use in cancer patients should be pain that is mild to moderate in intensity. (p. 555)

10. **The answer is d.** Naloxone is the drug of choice in the treatment of respiratory depression related to opioid overdosing. The amount of naloxone a patient receives should be titrated to changes in respiratory rate. Rapid injections of naloxone should be avoided in opioid-tolerant patients, so as not to precipitate an abstinence syndrome that may include intense pain. (p. 558)

11. **The answer is c.** All of these are common side effects except increased motility—opioids commonly decrease motility. (p. 558)

12. **The answer is a.** Antidepressants (e.g., amitriptyline, desipramine, imipramine) control pain by inhibiting the uptake of neurotransmitters into nerve terminals. They are used in the treatment of many types of nonmalignant pain such as migraine headaches but are also felt to be useful in neuropathic pain that is due to tumor infiltration of nerves, often described as having a continuous, burning quality. (p. 560)

13. **The answer is d.** Psychostimulants may be indicated when the dose of the opioid causes extreme sedation, no other side effects, and the dose cannot be lowered. (p. 561)

14. **The answer is b.** Steroids are extremely efficacious for managing the pain caused by epidural cord compression. Some side effects of steroid use such as mood elevation and increased appetite may also be desirable in some patients. However, the use of these drugs as adjuvant analgesics early in the course of a patient's pain problem is not recommended. (p. 562)

15. **The answer is a.** Except in a few circumstances, oral pain medication should be on a fixed-interval basis. While the evidence is not conclusive, most caregivers agree that round-the-clock scheduling is most effective in treating pain. (p. 562)

16. **The answer is b.** Fentanyl, 75 times more potent than morphine, is currently being administered via transdermal patches that are changed at prescribed intervals. This delivery system is an exciting new option for cancer patients who are experiencing pain, but it is not without its side effects, among them a prolonged effect after patch removal secondary to the long half-life of fentanyl. (p. 564)

17. **The answer is c.** Counterirritant cutaneous stimulation (e.g., massage, heat or cold therapy, transcutaneous electrical nerve stimulation) is thought to help relieve pain by somehow physiologically altering the transmission of nociceptive stimuli referred to in Melzack and Wall's gate control theory of pain. It is also felt that the relief achieved may outlast the actual application of the counterirritant. (p. 568)

18. **The answer is a.** Distraction (e.g., conversation, imagery, breathing exercises, watching television) directs one's attention away from the sensations and emotional reactions produced by pain and blocks one's awareness of the pain stimulus and its effects. It can be very helpful in reducing pain, but caregivers must remember that the mere fact that a patient is effectively distracted from the pain does not mean that he or she is pain-free. (p. 569)

# Chapter 21    Infection

## SCOPE OF THE PROBLEM

- The types of infections presenting the greatest problems for cancer patients have changed over the years as a result of emerging resistant and opportunistic organisms.

### Incidence

- Infection is a major cause of increased morbidity and mortality in individuals diagnosed with cancer.

### Etiology and Risk Factors

- Infectious processes may be the result of the underlying malignancy, intensive treatment modalities, prolonged hospitalization, or a combination of these factors. The term *immunocompromised host* refers to a person who has one or more defects in natural defense mechanisms significant enough to predispose to severe, sometimes life-threatening infection.

## PHYSIOLOGICAL ALTERATIONS
### Normal Anatomy, Physiology, and Scientific Principles
#### Integumentary, mucosal, and chemical barriers

- Intact skin constitutes the most important physical barrier against invasion by both exogenous and endogenous organisms.
- When a break in the skin occurs, environmental microbes and those that normally inhabit hair follicles and sebaceous glands may enter the body and cause infection.
- A second major defense against infection in the mucociliary activity found in the mucous membranes.
- Acid pH inhibits or prevents bacterial growth on the skin and in the stomach, bladder, and vagina. Microbicidal elements found in prostatic fluid and in tears also provide a protective effect.

#### Leukocytes

- PMNs which are also referred to as *polys* or *segmented neutrophils (segs)* are short-lived white blood cells (WBCs) that respond quickly to bacterial invasion.
- PMNs are the most numerous of the leukocytes, constituting 55%–70% of circulating WBCs.
- The primary function of PMNs is the destruction and elimination of microorganisms through phagocytosis.
- Without sufficient numbers of PMNs, the body's ability to mount an inflammatory response is compromised.

#### Monocytes and macrophages

- Monocytes and macrophages constitute what was previously referred to as the *reticuloendothelial system.*
- Under normal conditions more than 95% of these cells are mature tissue macrophages, while less than 2% are circulating monocytes.

- Following initial contact with a foreign protein, macrophages process and present antigens to lymphocytes, which stimulate the immune response and cytokine production.

## Lymphocytes

- Lymphocytes provide long-term protection against a variety of microorganisms. They usually constitute 25%–30% of the total WBC count. B lymphocytes produce antibodies, which neutralize, destroy, or facilitate phagocytosis of foreign proteins.
- T lymphocytes initiate activities that result in elimination of microorganisms or other foreign substances.
- T-helper cells normally constitute over 75% of total T-lymphocyte counts. T-helper cells serve as the principal regulators of immune function through secretion of protein mediators (cytokines) that act on other cells involved in the immune and inflammatory responses.

## Cytokines

- Cytokines are small protein hormones synthesized by a variety of leukocytes.
- Cytokines initiate and/or regulate a number of inflammatory and immune responses.
- Cytokines include interferons, interleukins, growth factors, and colony-stimulating factors.

## Pathophysiology

### Alterations in nonspecific defenses

#### Disruptions in protective barriers

- Primary and metastatic tumor growth invades healthy tissue and disrupts normal circulation, resulting in ulceration and necrosis. Chemotherapy and radiation may further alter the integrity of skin and mucosal surfaces.
- Diagnostic and treatment strategies typically include a variety of invasive procedures.
- Infection rates associated with diagnostic and therapeutic interventions are high.
- Host defenses are further compromised by neurological consequences of primary or metastatic disease involving the central nervous system (CNS).

#### Changes in normal flora

- Over 80% of infections developing in individuals with cancer arise from endogenous organisms, nearly half of which are acquired during hospitalization.
- The most significant factor contributing to transmission of infectious agents during hospitalization is poor hand washing by health care personnel.

#### Obstruction

- Obstruction, usually associated with solid tumors or lymphoma, may contribute to risk of infection by interfering with normal clearing and drainage mechanisms.

### Granulocytopenia

- There is a direct relationship between the number of circulating PMNs (segs) and incidence of infection.
- Individuals whose granulocyte count is lower than $1000/mm^3$ are considered to be granulocytopenic and at increased risk of infection. When the granulocyte count is less than $500/mm^3$, risk of infection is significant.
- Because of the short life span of circulating PMNs, their absolute number must be determined on a daily basis for granulocytopenic individuals.

- The absolute neutrophil count is determined by multiplying the percentage of PMNs (segs) and bands times the total number of WBCs. (ANC = total WBC x (%PMNs(segs) + % bands)

### Implanted vascular access devices
- The incidence of catheter-related bacteremia is influenced by specific therapy, degree of use, patient population, catheter insertion technique, and care and maintenance procedures.
- Neutropenia remains the primary risk factor for infection in vascular access catheters.
- Thrombus and fibrin sleeve formation have also been associated with catheter-related infection.
- Urokinase is used in combination with antibiotic therapy to improve treatment outcome for catheter-related infections.

## Immunosuppression

### Infection
- Both lymphocyte and macrophage functions may be abnormally depressed during and after acute infections, thereby extending susceptibility beyond the acute episode.

### Acquired immunodeficiency syndrome
- Acquired immunodeficiency syndrome (AIDS) is characterized by loss of T-helper cells, resulting in progressive loss of immunocompetence, development of opportunistic infections and chronic wasting, impairment of the CNS, and emergence of unusual malignancies.
- Only blood, semen, and vaginal secretions are proven vectors for HIV, with limited evidence to suggest that transmission via breast milk is possible.
- Infection with HIV is not synonymous with AIDS. AIDS is part of a continuum of illnesses related to infection with HIV.

## Tumor-associated abnormalities
- The types of infection that occur in persons diagnosed with cancer are somewhat predictable.
- Abnormal cell-mediated immunity in Hodgkin's disease and acute leukemia is associated with increased incidence of intracellular pathogens.
- Individuals who are asplenic as a result of trauma, staging laparotomy for malignant lymphoma, hypersplenism, or sickle-cell disease have impaired opsonization that can increase susceptibility to infection. The risk of overwhelming sepsis and death in persons with asplenia, especially those with Hodgkin's disease, is at least 50 times greater than in the normal population.
- Although fever may be caused by the underlying cancer, 55%–70% of fevers result from infection, especially during periods of granulocytopenia.
- Lymphomas, hypernephromas, and hepatomas may cause fever unrelated to infection.
- Fever caused by an underlying cancer cannot be distinguished, on the basis of duration or the degree of temperature elevation, from fever caused by infection.
- Fevers in the individual with cancer warrant thorough and prompt evaluation to rule out infection as the cause.

## Nutrition
- The tumor can interfere with the functional capacity of GI structures or organs.
- Chronic obstruction can compromise the blood supply to surrounding tissue, especially if vascular impairment is severe or prolonged.
- Cachexia is a complex metabolic syndrome characterized by significant involuntary weight loss.

- Nutritional research suggests that the failure of certain cachectic cancer patients to increase lean body mass despite adequate nutritional support results from the tumor effects on the host's metabolism.

## Cancer Therapy

### Surgery

- Various factors can increase the incidence of infectious complications in the individual undergoing surgery.
- Preoperative prophylactic antibiotics may be given to provide protection during the perioperative risk period.
- The surgical wound is the most common site of infection during the postoperative period.
- Surgical instrumentation of the genitourinary (GU) and GI tracts is associated with higher incidence of morbidity and mortality.

### Radiation therapy and chemotherapy

- Radiation therapy and chemotherapy interfere with essential metabolic functions of the cell and can cause inflammation and ulceration of normal tissues, predisposing the host to infection.
- The major risks associated with therapeutic radiation and cytotoxic chemotherapy relate to the induction of granulocytopenia and immunosuppression.
- Not all chemotherapeutic agents produce immunologic compromise.
- During radiation therapy leukocytes are the first to decrease, followed by platelets and erythrocytes.
- Depending on the total dose and type of radiation, skin and mucous membrane integrity may be impaired.

## CLINICAL MANIFESTATIONS

## Bacterial Infections

- Changing patterns in bacterial infections are primarily the result of improvements in antibiotic therapy.

### Gram-negative organisms

- Despite current shifts in the patterns of infection, the primary cause of infection in granulocytopenic patients continues to be gram-negative organisms.
- The most significant consequence of gram-negative infection is the potential for endotoxic or systemic shock.
- Without early detection and prompt initiation of treatment, endotoxic shock leads to hypotension, tissue ischemia, multisystem failure, and death.

### Gram-positive organisms

- *S aureus* and *Staphlococcus epidermidis* are responsible for most gram-positive infections occurring during periods of granulocytopenia.
- Although less common, infection with gram-positive organisms may result in shock produced by secretion of noxious proteins called exotoxins.

### Treatment

- Empirical antibiotic therapy is treatment initiated before infecting organisms have been identified.

- Selection of antibiotic agents must be individualized to consider the probable cause of infection and likely site of origin, as well as institutional patterns of infection and antibiotic resistance. In general the empirical antibiotic regimen should cover a broad spectrum of pathogens without significant risk for emergence of resistant organisms or drug-related toxicity.

## Mycobacterial Infections

- Although mycobacterial infections are uncommon in individuals with cancer, they tend to be associated with defects in cellular immunity.
- Latent infections with *M tuberculosis* may be reactivated.
- MAC has been observed in those with hairy-cell leukemia and in those undergoing intensive chemotherapy for non-Hodgkin's lymphoma.

### Treatment

- While isoniazid is the treatment of choice for tuberculosis, it is not effective therapy for MAC. Combination therapy has been more successful in treating MAC.

## Fungal Infections

- Fungal infections have become an increasingly important cause of morbidity and mortality in individuals with cancer, particularly hematologic and lymphoreticular neoplasms.
- Factors predisposing to fungal infection include severe prolonged granulocytopenia, implanted vascular access catheters, administration of parenteral nutrition or corticosteroids, prolonged use of broad-spectrum antibiotics, and damage to oropharyngeal or GI mucosa due to disease or treatment.

### *Candida*

- *Candida* is the most common cause of invasive fungal infection.
- Broad-spectrum antibiotics alter the function of normal bacterial flora and therefore are associated with increased risk of fungal overgrowth and infection.
- Dermatologic infections with *Candida* occur most frequently in skin folds.
- Oral candidiasis (thrush) is a common yeast infection that can disseminate throughout the GI tract. Disseminated candidiasis often involves the lungs, kidneys, bones, joints, and CNS.

### *Aspergillus*

- *Aspergillus* causes serious infections in individuals with cancer.
- The fungus enters the host through the upper airway and typically causes pneumonia or sinus infection.
- Aspergillosis is characterized by blood vessel invasion, which can lead to thrombosis and infarction of pulmonary arteries and veins.
- The infection is difficult to diagnose, often necessitating aggressive treatment before the diagnosis is confirmed. Without prompt and aggressive therapy with amphotericin, *Aspergillus* pneumonia is almost always fatal in granulocytopenic patients.

### *Cryptococcus*

- *Cryptococcus neoformans* is generally acquired by inhalation.
- The infection appears most often in individuals with advanced Hodgkin's disease and other lymphomas. It commonly occurs as an insidious meningoencephalitis. Headache, vomiting, and diplopia without fever are typical symptoms.

- Intrathecal administration of antifungal agents may be required for individuals whose cerebrospinal fluid does not clear with IV therapy.

### Histoplasma

- Histoplasmosis generally occurs as a pulmonary infection, usually in individuals with lymphoreticular neoplasms.
- The infection commonly disseminates, causing adenopathy and hepatosplenomegaly.
- Disseminated histoplasmosis can occur in individuals whose cancer is in remission, as well as in those with active disease.

## Phycomycetes

- The Phycomycetes are opportunistic fungi widespread in dust and air. The lungs, nasal sinuses, and GI tract are the three major sites of infection.

### Coccidioides

- *Coccidioides* is found in the soil of the southwestern United States and typically enters the body through inhalation.
- Immunocompromised individuals are susceptible to the development of serious pulmonary infection.

## Treatment

- Two major problems in treatment of fungal infections are the difficulty associated with culturing organisms from infected tissues and the limited number of effective agents available to manage severe fungal infections.
- Amphotericin B is the drug of choice for treatment of systemic fungal infections. However, it is associated with significant side effects and toxicities, including nephrotoxicity, fever, chills, rigors, nausea, vomiting, hypotension, bronchospasm, and occasionally seizures.
- Premedication with acetaminophen and the addition of hydrocortisone sodium succinate to the IV solution generally reduce the reactions associated with the drug.
- Flucytosine (5-FC) is another antifungal agent used for treatment of *Candida* and *Cryptococcus* infections. The major limitation to its use is the rapid onset of drug resistance.
- Side effects include nausea, vomiting, diarrhea, myelosuppression, skin rash, nephrotoxicity, and hepatotoxicity.
- The antifungal agent fluconazole is well absorbed and is able to penetrate into cerebrospinal fluid, the eye, and peritoneal fluid.
- Side effects include exfoliative skin disorders, hepatotoxicity, and, less frequently, GI disturbances and headaches.
- Ketoconazole is used to treat disseminated and pulmonary coccidioidomycosis, candidiasis, and histoplasmosis. The most frequent side effects are nausea, vomiting, and diarrhea.
- The oral agent itraconazole may be used in the treatment of aspergillosis in persons who are intolerant of or resistant to amphotericin.
- Itraconazole should be taken with food to increase absorption.
- Miconazole is a parenteral antifungal agent primarily considered to be second-line therapy.
- For treatment of fungal meningitis, IV miconazole must be supplemented with intrathecal administration to achieve therapeutic drug levels.
- Side effects include hypersensitivity reactions, phlebitis, and GI disturbances.

## Viral Infections

- Viruses are replicated by host cell mechanisms after invasion by a single virus.
- Most viral infections in granulocytopenic patients are caused by herpes viruses.
- HSV, varicella zoster virus (VZV), and CMV.

### Herpes simplex

- HSV can cause serious infection in persons with cancer, from either primary exposure to or reactivation of a latent virus.
- Major sites of infection are the oropharynx, esophagus, eyes, skin, urogenital tract, and perianal area.

### Varicella zoster

- Infection with VZV ("chickenpox") can cause serious vesicular eruption in individuals with cancer, especially children, and results in a mortality rate of up to 18%.
- Following primary VZV infection, reactivation ("shingles") can occur because the virus remains dormant in the spinal ganglia.
- Since skin lesions (vesicles) can become confluent, meticulous skin care is required to prevent secondary bacterial infection.
- The major complication of VZV infection is visceral dissemination, resulting in pneumonitis, hepatitis, and meningoencephalitis.
- Varicella is highly contagious, and the risk of spread to other seronegative immunocompromised individuals is substantial, especially in adults with Hodgkin's disease and children with leukemia.
- Management of individuals with cancer who are seronegative and who have been exposed to VZV includes interruption of cancer therapy and administration of varicella zoster-immune globulin (VZIG).

### Cytomegalovirus

- CMV is a common cause of interstitial pneumonitis in individuals with impaired cellular immunity or following BMT. CMV pneumonia characteristically occurs within three months of transplant and is often fatal.
- CMV retinitis is the most common opportunistic ocular infection noted in immunocompromised persons, especially those with AIDS.

### Hepatitis virus

- Hepatitis in individuals with cancer can occur as a primary infection with one of the hepatitis viruses or as a secondary infection with other viruses.
- Although transfusions of blood products constitute the primary route of transmission, nonparenteral transmission occurs through sexual intercourse and contact with contaminated saliva, urine, and feces.
- Risk of infection to health care providers is high and warrants strict adherence to universal precautions.

### Treatment

- Acyclovir is an antiviral agent preferentially taken up by cells infected with HSV and VZV.
- Treatment with acyclovir decreases viral shedding from infected cells, accelerates healing of lesions, and decreases pain and itching.
- Side effects are minimal and consist primarily of nausea, vomiting, diarrhea, and anorexia.

- Vidarabine is an IV antiviral agent primarily used as second-line therapy for VZV and HSV infections.
- Toxicities include bone marrow suppression, GI disturbances, and neurological effects such as tremor, confusion, alterations in mentation and behavior, and ataxia.
- Ganciclovir is used in treatment of CMV infection. It is a virostatic agent and suppresses viral replication.
- Foscarnet is another virostatic agent that suppresses CMV replication.

## Protozoa and Parasites

- Protozoal infections are associated with defects in cell-mediated immunity.
- Protozoal infections are often difficult to treat and quickly become life-threatening.

### Pneumocystis carinii

- *Pneumocyctis carinii* causes infection in malnourished infants, children with primary immunodeficiency disorders, persons with AIDS, and those with cancer undergoing immunosuppressive therapy.
- Clinical manifestations of infection include fever, nonproductive cough, tachypnea with intercostal retraction, and potentially life-threatening respiratory compromise.

### Toxoplasma

- Persons at greatest risk of infection with *Toxoplasma gondii* include those with AIDS and those receiving immunosuppressive therapy for hematologic malignancies or prevention of organ transplant rejection.
- CNS involvement occurs in over 50% of infected individuals.

### Cryptosporidium

- Although a common cause of enteritis in individuals with AIDS, cryptosporidiosis has only occasionally been observed in other immunocompromised patients.

### Treatment

- Untreated *P carinii* is fatal. Even with therapy, mortality is high. The treatment of choice for *P carinii* is trimethoprim-sulfamethoxazole.
- In individuals with known history of sulfonamide sensitivity, dapsone-trimethoprim or atovaquone may be prescribed.
- Pentamidine is effective in treating *P carinii* unresponsive to trimethoprim-sulfamethoxazole.
- Prophylactic treatment of high-risk patients is most often accomplished with trimethoprim-sulfamethoxazole.
- Treatment with pyrimethamine plus sulfamethoxazole has been effective against *T gondii* in immunocompromised patients.
- To date, there is no known treatment for cryptosporidiosis other than supportive therapy with antidiarrheal agents and replacement of fluid and electrolytes.

## THERAPEUTIC APPROACHES AND NURSING CARE
## Prevention

- Nursing care focuses on prevention of infection, measures to optimize the person's health status, and aggressive therapeutic interventions when infection occurs.

- When an infection develops, prompt initiation of medical and nursing interventions is imperative to prevent life-threatening complications.

### Reducing environmental pathogens

- The single most important intervention to prevent infection is meticulous hand washing by every person who enters the room or comes in contact with the individual at risk for infection. Neutropenic patients are advised of their risk and are encouraged to remind staff, family, and visitors about hand-washing precautions.
- When hospitalized, the patient is given a private room.
- Ideally, staff members caring for a patient with an active infection are not also assigned to a neutropenic patient.
- When the ANC is less than 1000, live plants, cut flowers, and fresh fruit should not be brought into the patient's room.
- During granulocytopenic episodes, invasive procedures are kept to a minimum, with adherence to strict aseptic technique when they are performed. Indwelling urinary catheters are also avoided whenever possible.

### Optimizing health status

- Adequate nutritional intake during periods of increased risk requires a high-calorie, high-protein diet. If severe neutropenia is anticipated, a low-bacteria cooked-food diet may be prescribed.
- A low-bacteria diet excludes fresh fruit, raw vegetables, fresh eggs, cold cuts, and many dairy products.
- Fluid intake is monitored to assure adequate hydration.
- Strategies to maintain skin and mucous membrane integrity include: meticulous personal hygiene; mild soap and water-soluble lubricant; shaving with an electric razor; fingernails and toenails kept short.
- The optimal plan for oral hygiene includes use of a soft to medium toothbrush, toothpaste, and dental floss.
- Enemas, rectal temperatures, and suppositories are likely to traumatize fragile rectal mucosa and are avoided as much as possible in the high-risk patient.
- Activities consistent with current health status are encouraged to maintain optimal circulatory and pulmonary function.

## Management

### Early detection

- When the inflammatory response is diminished or absent, classic signs and symptoms of infection—fever, erythema, edema, pain, and purulence—may not be present, making early identification difficult.
- The most reliable indicator of infection is a low-grade fever. A temperature elevation of 1° that persists for 24 hours may be the only early evidence of infection.

#### Respiratory system

- The high incidence of pneumonia in immunocompromised patients mandates thorough assessment of the respiratory system.
- Neutropenic individuals may experience only slight temperature elevation and mild dyspnea if pneumonia is present.

### Oropharynx

- The oral mucosa is often traumatized by chemotherapeutic agents, especially the antimetabolites and antibiotics.
- The oral cavity is regularly inspected for white plaques, gingival edema, erythema, bleeding, and ulceration.

### Gastrointestinal system

- Disruption of intestinal mucosa by anticancer therapy facilitates bacterial invasion and increases the potential for sepsis. If a granulocytopenic patient receiving broad-spectrum antibiotics complains of dysphagia and/or retrosternal burning, *Candida* or HSV esophagitis must be considered.
- The perirectal area should be routinely inspected for signs of inflammation, infection, hemorrhoids, and fissures.

### Central nervous system

- The development of any neurological abnormality warrants immediate attention.
- CNS infections present with a variety of symptoms including headache, fever, visual impairment, personality changes, focal neurological signs, nuchal rigidity, altered mental status, and seizures.

### Urinary tract

- Classic symptoms of UTI are typically absent in neutropenic patients.
- Observation of the clinical characteristics of the urine, specifically if cloudy and foul-smelling, is usually helpful.

### Skin

- Skin integrity should be regularly assessed.

### Cardiovascular system

- Symptoms of cardiovascular infection are generally nonspecific: fever, chills, malaise, and night sweats.

## Nursing care during episodes of infection

- Infection in the neutropenic patient is always considered a potentially life-threatening emergency.
- Fatality rates in untreated individuals during the first 48 hours of infection can exceed 50%.
- Cultures are obtained from all potential sites of infection.
- Empirical broad-spectrum antibiotic therapy is promptly initiated and the patient's response closely monitored for efficacy of antimicrobial treatment.
- If little or no improvement is apparent following three to five days of antibiotic treatment, cultures are repeated.
- Other supportive nursing care strategies include restoring circulatory fluid volume, maintaining adequate oxygenation and promoting optimal nutritional status.

## Treatment of infection

- Persons with cancer who are not immunocompromised or granulocytopenic can be treated with appropriate antibiotic therapy for the specific infectious agent identified.

- However, empirical treatment with a broad-spectrum antibiotic is initiated if a serious infection develops rapidly.
- Patients who have fever during periods of granulocytopenia will have a thorough physical examination, chest radiograph, appropriate laboratory studies, and cultures of all potential sources of infection.
- Progression to systemic infection and septic shock is usually rapid.

### Empirical antibiotics

- Empirical antibiotic therapy in the patient with fever and granulocytopenia reduces the number of infections that could become severe. (See Table 21-4, text page 598, for common infection sites.)
- The particular empirical antibiotic regimen selected should meet the following criteria: provide broad-spectrum coverage for major pathogenic organisms; be synergistic and contain one bactericidal agent; and have minimal organ toxicity, satisfactory absorption by the route administered, consistent distribution to infected tissues, and adequate excretion.

### Isolation precautions and protected environments

- Routine protective isolation does not appear to reduce the risk of infection any more than consistent and frequent hand washing during patient care.
- Efforts to exclude all microorganisms through the use of patient isolator units (usually laminar air flow rooms), nonabsorbable prophylactic antibiotics, and sterilization of the patient's food and water may prevent or delay the onset of some infection.
- Laminar air flow rooms are protected environments developed to protect the compromised host from exogenous and endogenous sources of infection.
- Patients undergo cutaneous and GI decontamination with oral nonabsorbable antibiotics before entry into the room. All objects brought into the room are sterilized by steam or gas, and food is semisterile.
- Although laminar air flow rooms reduce incidence of infection and improve short-term survival, they have not affected long-term survival.

### Granulocyte replacement

- Granulocyte colony-stimulating factor (G-CSF) and GM-CSF are hormonelike glycoproteins that promote the proliferation and maturation of phagocytes.
- Studies have shown that the duration of granulocytopenia following chemotherapy administration is markedly decreased when G-CSF or GM-CSF is used.

## Approach to the patient with gram-negative sepsis

- Shock develops in approximately 27%–46% of patients with gram-negative bacteremia.
- Mortality approaches 80% unless vigorous treatment is begun promptly.
- The first sign of impending shock in the immunocompromised host may be limited to a low-grade fever, shaking chills, and/or mild hypotension.

### Early (warm) shock

- The early phase consists of vasodilation, decreased peripheral vascular resistance, normal to increased cardiac output, and mild hypotension.
- The patient may appear flushed with warm extremities and adequate urinary output.
- If myocardial function and fluid replacement are adequate, the syndrome may not progress provided immediate and appropriate antibiotic therapy is instituted.

- The duration of this early phase may vary from 30 minutes to 16 hours.

### Late (cold) shock

- The late phase of septic shock is characterized by a profound reduction in cardiac output, increased peripheral vascular resistance, oliguria, and metabolic acidosis. These factors create a cycle of vasoconstriction, ischemia, and vasodilation that result in irreversible damage to the heart, vascular system, kidneys, liver, and vasomotor center of the brain.

### Treatment of septic shock

- The treatment of septic shock is based on two objectives: reversing the shock and treating the underlying sepsis.
- Individuals in shock require adequate oxygenation, effective circulation and tissue perfusion, nutritional support, and immediate, appropriate broad-spectrum antibiotic therapy.
- Persistent hypotension despite fluid replacement may be managed through administration of vasoactive agents.
- Care is taken to meet the psychosocial needs of patients with septic shock and their significant others.
- Nursing responsibilities include providing honest information, education, and assurance to both patients and family members.

## Approach to the HIV-infected patient with cancer

- These individuals are at increased risk for opportunistic infection not only because of HIV-related impairment of cellular immunity but also because of granulocytopenia secondary to cancer treatment and/or antimicrobial therapy.
- Antimicrobial therapy is usually continued indefinitely, since discontinuing treatment commonly results in recurrent symptoms of infection.

## Continuity of Care

- Education about risk of infection begins at the time of diagnosis. The patient and family are instructed about blood counts, anticipated time until the nadir is reached, and self-care activities to minimize risk of infection.
- The patient and caregiver must understand the necessity of communicating to the health care team any deviations from normal health status.
- If antibiotic therapy will be administered at home, patients and family members are informed of potential side effects, particularly those that are to be reported promptly to the health care team.
- Referral to a home health agency should always be considered for an individual who is at risk for infection, especially if caregiver support is inadequate, if home environmental concerns are present, or if reinforcement of instruction is indicated.

## CONCLUSION

- Individuals with cancer are especially prone to develop infections as a result of impaired host defense mechanisms.
- Infection in the immunocompromised person with cancer can quickly progress to life-threatening sepsis. Diligent nursing care directed toward prevention, early detection, and aggressive treatment is of primary importance for patient survival during high-risk periods.

## PRACTICE QUESTIONS

1. The body's first line of defense against bacteria, which is commonly altered by cancer or the cancer process, is:
   a. granulocytes.
   b. the skin.
   c. macrophages.
   d. the acid pH of fluid.

2. The type of white blood cell that constitutes 55%–70% of circulating white blood cells and that responds quickly to bacterial invasion is the:
   a. polymorphonuclear neutrophil.
   b. monocyte.
   c. macrophage.
   d. lymphocyte.

3. What is the name given to the microbes that normally live in the body and lead to over 80% of infections in cancer patients?
   a. Exogenous organisms
   b. Intracellular organisms
   c. Extracellular organisms
   d. Endogenous organisms

4. Which of the following variables do *not* influence the incidence of sepsis?
   a. Type of radiotherapy and chemotherapy
   b. Length of myelosuppressive therapy
   c. Absolute granulocyte count less than 500/mm$^3$
   d. Duration of granulocytopenia

5. The complication of infection with gram-negative organisms that can quickly lead to death is:
   a. dehydration.
   b. gastrointestinal bleeding.
   c. endotoxic shock.
   d. anaphylaxis.

6. Meticulous skin care is required when caring for the patient with reactivated varicella zoster virus, in order to:
   a. minimize spread to other areas of the body.
   b. prevent a secondary bacterial infection.
   c. promote drainage of the vesicles.
   d. provide the primary source of pain relief.

7. *Pneumocystis carinii* is potentially fatal and requires treatment with:
   a. foscarnet.
   b. ganciclovir
   c. trimethoprim-sulfamethoxazole.
   d. an aminoglycoside.

## Erythrocyte physiology and function

- The red blood cell (RBC) is a thin, biconcave disk-shaped cell with a thin membrane. The shape of the cell allows for oxygen transport and easy movement throughout the body.
- The normal RBC count in men is approximately 5.2 million cells/mm$^3$, and in women 4.7 million cells/mm$^3$.
- The reticulocyte count is a useful indicator of bone marrow function with regard to RBC production.
- The development of the erythrocyte is induced by erythropoietin (EPO). EPO is produced primarily in the kidneys in response to hypoxia or hyperoxia.
- The average life span of a red blood cell is 120 days.
- The major function of the RBC is the transport of hemoglobin, which carries oxygen to all tissues. The RBC also eliminates carbon dioxide, provides for hemoglobin synthesis and maintenance, and acts as a buffering agent in the blood.

## Platelet physiology and function

- Platelets, or thrombocytes, are formed when the mature, granular megakaryocyte sheds its cytoplasm.
- The normal platelet count in men and women is approximately 150,000–400,000 cells/mm$^3$.
- Under normal circumstances, any reduction in the platelet count causes an increased production of megakaryocytes and platelets in the bone marrow.
- The life span of the platelet is about ten days.
- Circulating platelets perform several functions. First and most important is that of *hemostasis*. A second platelet function is to facilitate the action of the clotting factors of the intrinsic system. Finally, platelets are necessary for *fibrinolysis*, or lysis of the fibrin clot, and vessel repair.

## Hemostasis

- Hemostasis is the process by which the fluid component of blood becomes a solid clot.
- When blood vessel injury occurs, vasoconstriction initially provides a minimal degree of control of the bleeding. Platelets are attracted to and adhere to the underlying layer of collagen of the exposed subendothelial tissue. Platelets then release a number of components.
- ADP causes platelets to swell and become "sticky," thus increasing the adherence of platelets to one another.
- The end result of ADP-mediated platelet accumulation is the formation of a large platelet aggregate, or a hemostatic plug.
- This primary hemostatic mechanism produces only a temporary cessation of bleeding.

## Coagulation

- Blood coagulation may be considered a mechanism for rapid replacement of an unstable platelet plug with a stable fibrin clot.
- Coagulation is initiated by tissue factor, a transmembrane glycoprotein present on the surface of many cell types that is not normally in contact with the circulation. This factor is exposed to blood upon vascular damage.
- The clot is soluble until it becomes polymerized by factor XIIIa (fibrin-stabilizing factor), which converts it into a stable (insoluble) clot.
- The fibrin clot must be remodeled and removed to restore normal tissue structure and function, as well as to restore normal blood flow.

### Fibrinolysis

- Fibrinolysis, or clot breakdown, is initiated by enzymes that are present in most body fluids and tissues.
- The breakdown of fibrinogen and fibrin results in polypeptides called *fibrin degradation products* (FDPs), which are powerful anticoagulant substances that have a destructive effect on fibrin in the platelet plug. They also are able to impair platelet aggregation, reduce prothrombin, and interfere with polymerization of fibrin. When these products are increased in the circulation there is a predisposition to bleeding.
- These processes constitute a threat to the organism if they extend beyond the site of injury to the general circulation.

## CLINICAL MANIFESTATIONS

### Causes of Bleeding in Cancer

#### Tumor effects

- Bleeding is a common presenting symptom of cancer, generally occurring as a result of tumor extension and local tissue invasion, erosion and blood vessel rupture. Blood loss and the resultant iron-deficiency anemia are frequently the initial signs of lung, gynecologic, genitourinary, or colorectal carcinomas.
- Other structural causes of bleeding that frequently occur in the individual with cancer include cavitational and ulcerative effects of local infections at sites of vessels; destructive effects of radiotherapy on normal structures in the radiation field; and denuded remains of vessels at the site of radical cancer surgery.
- In individuals with multiple myeloma, hemorrhage has been noted to be more common in those individuals with markedly increased serum proteins or viscosity, in patients who produce kappa rather than lambda light chains, and when abnormal platelet function was present.
- Invasion and replacement of bone marrow by tumor may affect hematopoiesis. This process, called *myelophthisis*, can result in anemia and is due to the decrease in production of normal marrow elements in response to the physical "crowding out" of normal cells, competition for cellular nutrients, and the production by the invading cells' metabolic end products that are toxic to normal cells.
- Marrow infiltration may represent metastatic disease or a primary disease process such as acute leukemia in which the leukemia cells "pack" the marrow.
- Clinically the individual may present with symptoms ranging from minor incidents of vaginal bleeding to gross blood loss.
- More gradual bleeding involving smaller circulatory structures is usually less obvious and therefore more difficult to diagnose. Melena due to colorectal carcinoma can persist undetected until manifested by iron deficiency anemia.
- The most definitive diagnostic test for iron deficiency anemia is a bone marrow biopsy, which demonstrates absent stainable iron stores.
- The homeostatic mechanisms in the body provide such remarkable compensatory adaptation that iron deficiency anemia may be quite serious before the person actually develops significant symptoms.
- Fatigue, weakness, irritability, dyspnea, and tachycardia are typical clinical symptoms experienced by individuals with anemia.
- If wound breakdown is in the neck area and carotid exposure occurs, wound debridement followed by a skin or skin-muscle flap carrying its own blood supply generally is done.
- If acute bleeding occurs, direct methods to halt the hemorrhage are instituted immediately. Direct, steady pressure is applied at the site of bleeding. Mechanical pressure can be used if the site of bleeding is not directly exposed. Iced saline gastric lavages or enemas may help control gastrointestinal (GI) bleeding.

- Control of life-threatening hemorrhage is generally achieved by a combination of packed red cells with crystalloids or albumin, as opposed to whole blood, in correcting a volume deficit.
- Minor vascular bleeding due to capillary destruction is best controlled by treating the underlying malignancy. If iron deficiency anemia has occurred, oral or parenteral iron supplements are indicated.
- If the hemoglobin level drops below 8 g/dl, blood replacement may be considered.

## Platelet abnormalities

- Abnormalities of platelet production, function, survival, and metabolism frequently occur in individuals with cancer.

### Quantitative abnormalities

#### Thrombocythemia

- Thrombocythemia, also known as *essential* or *primary thrombocythemia*, is a clonal disorder of the multipotential hematopoietic stem cell.
- The major complications related to thrombocythemia are bleeding and thrombotic complications. The most common sites of bleeding and potential hemorrhage associated with thrombocythemia are the mucosa and the GI tract, although bleeding at other sites such as the genitourinary tract and the skin can occur.
- Care of patients with thrombocythemia may include no treatment for asymptomatic patients to a variety of platelet-reducing modalities.
- Drugs considered for the prevention of thrombotic complications include aspirin and dipyridamole.

#### Thrombocytosis

- Thrombocytosis, also known as *secondary* or *reactive thrombocytosis*, is used to describe the platelet count elevation in patients with a variety of other diseases. Thrombocytosis occurs in about 30%–40% of patients with malignant neoplasms.
- The patient with secondary thrombocytosis is usually asymptomatic, but thrombocytosis may cause thrombosis in a small proportion of cases.
- Thrombosis may result in symptoms associated with venous thrombosis, pulmonary embolism, transient cerebral ischemia, peripheral vascular ischemia, myocardial infarction and angina, or portal mesenteric vein occlusion.
- Patients with thrombocytosis who are asymptomatic do not require treatment. Symptomatic thrombocytosis can be treated with platelet pheresis. Aspirin and dipyridamole can be used.

#### Thrombocytopenia

- Thrombocytopenia, a reduction in the number of circulating platelets, is the most frequent platelet abnormality associated with cancer.

#### Platelet production

- The most common cause of thrombocytopenia in patients with cancer is a disorder of production involving decreased megakaryocytopoiesis.
- Chemotherapy is the treatment most often associated with hematologic toxicity and bone marrow suppression.
- Radiation therapy can also cause hematologic toxicity, particularly when large areas of bone marrow are treated. The most significant factor that determines the risk of bone marrow depression related to radiation therapy is the volume of productive bone marrow in the radiation field.

### Platelet distribution

- Thrombocytopenia due to an abnormal distribution of platelets can occur in cancer patients with hypersplenism. An enlarged spleen may sequester up to 90% of the platelet population.
- The thrombocytopenia related to hypersplenism is generally mild (platelet count 40,000–100,000 cells/mm$^3$).
- If the primary cause of thrombocytopenia is platelet sequestration, the bone marrow will contain normal to increased numbers of megakaryocytes.

### Platelet destruction

- Thrombocytopenia can also be due to rapid platelet destruction, characterized by a dramatically shortened platelet life span and an abundance of megakaryocytes in the bone marrow.
- The first situation in which rapid platelet destruction occurs is immune thrombocytopenia, or idiopathic thrombocytopenic purpura (ITP).
- Patients may be classified as having ITP that is mild (platelet counts > 80,000 cells/mm$^3$), moderate (platelet counts > 50,000 cells/mm$^3$), or severe (platelet counts < 30,000 cells/mm$^3$). This disorder occurs most frequently in individuals with lymphoproliferative diseases.
- ITP is rarely described with solid tumors.
- The second type of rapid platelet destruction is seen in conditions of increased platelet consumption.

### Platelet dilution

- Dilution is another cause of thrombocytopenia. It is thought that rapid reconstitution of the intravascular volume by the use of stored platelet-poor blood dilutes thrombocytes that are already present.
  - The platelets in the whole blood lose considerable effectiveness after 24 hours at usual storage temperatures of 4° C.
  - Stored blood is deficient in factors V, VIII, and XI.
- The platelet count is considered the single most significant factor for predicting bleeding in the individual with cancer.
- The risk of spontaneous hemorrhage is considered to be greater than 50% when the platelet count is less than 20,000 cells/mm$^3$.
- Although thrombocytopenia may be the immediate cause of bleeding in individuals with platelet disorders, therapy must address the underlying cause of the decreased platelet level.
- Platelet transfusions are often given to maintain a safe level of circulating thrombocytes until tumor regression occurs and marrow function returns.
- Platelet sequestration within a spleen enlarged due to malignancy is treated most effectively by aggressive tumor therapy. Chemotherapy and radiotherapy usually are most effective.
- Individuals who are found to have asymptomatic, mild or moderate ITP may be followed closely with no treatment. Individuals who experience severe thrombocytopenia are generally treated with prednisone therapy.
- Platelet transfusions are seldom indicated for patients with ITP because the survival time of transfused platelets is shortened.
- Splenectomy may be done early on in the course of severe thrombocytopenia that is unresponsive to prednisone, or it may be done after several months if a remission from the disease cannot be attained.

## Qualitative abnormalities

### Platelet malfunction

- At times patients with cancer may bleed despite normal platelet counts and/or coagulation factors. Alterations in platelet function may be responsible for the bleeding seen in these situations.
- The major abnormality noted in these diseases is a decrease in the procoagulant activity of the platelets, which is a measure of platelet factor III.
- Also noted in these diseases are platelets that are larger or smaller than normal, abnormally shaped platelets, a variation in the number of storage pool granules, and qualitative defect in platelet function as a result of the M protein coating the platelet and interfering with platelet aggregation.
- Numerous drugs are known to affect platelet function.
- For all of the drugs known to affect platelet function, the effect of the drug is measured by an abnormality of platelet function or bleeding time.
- Only aspirin has been demonstrated to cause a significant increased risk of bleeding.
- The mechanisms of action of nonsteroidal anti-inflammatory drugs appear to be similar to that for aspirin—that of inhibition of platelet cyclooxygenase.
- Beta-lactam antibiotics, including the penicillins and cephalosporins, characteristically cause a prolonged bleeding time and abnormal platelet aggregation.
- The frequency of clinically significant hemorrhage due solely to the effect of antibiotics on platelet function is rare, but risk of bleeding may be increased in patients with coexisting hemostatic defects.
- Patients taking psychotropic drugs may have impaired platelet aggregation and secretion responses to ADP, epinephrine, and collagen.
- Mithramycin, when administered to a total dose of 6–21 mg, has been associated with decreased platelet aggregation, increased bleeding time, and mucocutaneous bleeding. BCNU and carmustine are both known to inhibit platelet aggregation and secretion but are not linked to clinically significant bleeding.
- A prolonged bleeding time due to aspirin may be corrected by infusion of desmopressin.
- The clinical risk for bleeding associated with nonsteroidal anti-inflammatory drugs is much less than that for aspirin.

## Hypocoagulation

- Malignancy, or the metabolic alterations that frequently accompany it, may precipitate an imbalance in the coagulation factors.
- Successful tumor therapy should bring about a normalization of coagulation values.
- The most significant factor leading to a state of hypocoagulability is liver disease, which may be due to tumor invasion, chemotherapy, infection, or surgical resection.
- Regardless of the etiology, liver disease has been reported to cause a prolonged bleeding time, reduced platelet aggregation, and procoagulant activity.
- A deficiency of vitamin K may also cause a hypocoagulation syndrome.
- Frozen plasma has deficient levels of factors V and VIII, which can lead to an altered state of coagulation.
- Isolated factor deficiencies are also reported in neoplastic disease.
- Although any type of coagulation abnormality can lead to bleeding, conditions of decreased coagulability less frequently cause serious bleeding when they do occur.
- Effective tumor therapy generally is the best means of controlling hypocoagulability abnormalities.

- The treatment of specific inhibitors of coagulation factors depends on the severity of the abnormality. Life-threatening bleeding requires therapy, but lesser symptoms may require observation only.
- Albumin is safer than plasma, since it carries no risk of hepatitis transmission. It may, however, precipitate congestive heart failure in patients with compromised cardiovascular function.
- Generally, SQ vitamin K is administered to correct the protein defects when this vitamin is deficient.
- Isolated factor deficiencies are generally treated by specific plasma components.

## Hypercoagulation

- Disseminated intravascular coagulation (DIC) is the most common serious hypercoagulable state in individuals with cancer.
- Ultimately the body becomes unable to respond to vascular or tissue injury through stable clot formation, and thus hemorrhage ensues.
- This syndrome is always secondary to an underlying disease process, such as malignancy, septicemia, obstetric complications, or similar systemic stressors.
- The syndrome often remains undetected until severe hemorrhage occurs and frequently is discovered only at the time of autopsy. Currently, the overall incidence of DIC in patients with cancer is estimated to be approximately 10%.
- The most common cause of DIC is infection.
- APL has a high correlation with DIC.
- The solid tumors most often associated with DIC are the mucin-producing adenocarcinomas.
- Disseminated intravascular coagulation is always secondary to an underlying disease process.
- The bleeding manifestations of DIC are caused by the combination of the consumption of platelets and certain clotting factors, plasmin's fibrinolytic properties, and the anticoagulant properties of the fibrin degradation products.
- The patient generally is not critically ill from chronic DIC. Chronic DIC may produce minimal or no clinical manifestations.
- Chronic DIC is more likely to cause thrombosis than bleeding.
- Acute DIC (also called *uncompensated*) occurs rapidly over hours to days.
- Signs of acute DIC include petechiae; hematuria; acral cyanosis; bleeding or oozing from the gums, nose, or venipuncture sites; or oozing from surgical wounds.
- Thrombus formation often occurs simultaneously with bleeding in DIC.
- When thrombosis occurs, the signs and symptoms include focal ischemia, acral cyanosis, superficial gangrene, altered sensorium, ulceration of the GI tract, and dyspnea, which can lead to acute respiratory distress syndrome.
- There is no specific laboratory finding that is absolutely diagnostic of DIC.
- A classic triad of tests is generally done to help support the diagnosis of DIC: prothrombin time (PT), platelet count, and the plasma fibrinogen level.
- Treatment of the underlying malignancy is vital in the patient with a hypercoagulability abnormality, for the tumor is the ultimate stimulus. All other therapy, although effective on a short-term basis, will provide only an interval of symptomatic relief.
- Early detection of the signs and symptoms of DIC may allow for prompt diagnosis and treatment.
- The fluid status of the patient with DIC is often tenuous.
- Replacement fluids may include red blood cells, platelets, fresh-frozen plasma, and albumin, in addition to IV solutions.
- Albumin may be the component of choice for volume expansion.
- A compromised respiratory status might result from bleeding.

- Prevention of further complications of DIC includes removal of any tight or restrictive clothing. If edema is present, it is measured daily. Elastic support stockings may help to minimize stasis and promote venous return. Platelets can be given if the platelet count drops below 30,000/mm$^3$.
- Though both are controversial, heparin may be used in chronic DIC of malignancy, and EACA (Amicar) can be used when fibrinolysis of DIC has been resolved but uncontrolled bleeding persists.
- Compression to the knee vessels is minimized by avoiding placing anything under the knees while in bed, avoiding crossing of the knees or legs, and avoiding dangling the patient's legs over the side of the bed.

## ASSESSMENT
### Patient/Family History

- Key aspects of a comprehensive history for the individual at risk for bleeding include the following: bleeding tendencies; family history of any bleeding abnormalities; drugs and chemicals taken that might interfere with the coagulation mechanism; general performance status that helps to identify the effects of the disease or the presence of complications; current blood component therapy; nutritional status; and presence of any signs or symptoms of anemia.

### Physical Examination

- Observation is the most important measure in early detection of bleeding. Diagnostic signals can be subtle, including skin petechiae noticed while bathing the person, traces of blood as the person brushes her or his teeth, and oozing from venipuncture sites or sites of injections.
- Common sites of hemorrhage include the gums, nose, bladder, GI tract, and brain.

### Screening Tests

- Several screening tests provide information regarding hemostatic function.

#### Bleeding time

- This test measures the time it takes for a small skin incision to stop bleeding.
- The time varies from one to nine minutes.

#### Platelet count

- This test measures the actual number of circulating platelets per cubic millimeter of blood. Normal counts are considered to be 150,000–400,000/mm$^3$.

#### Whole blood clot retraction test

- This test, which measures the speed and extent of blood clot retraction in a test tube, is done to determine the degree of platelet adequacy. A normal clot shrinks to one-half its normal size in 1–2 hours and shrinks completely in 24 hours.

#### Prothrombin time

- The test is measured against the time needed for a normal sample of blood to clot.

#### Partial thromboplastin time (activated)

- The aPTT is determined by adding phospholipid reagents to plasma in the presence of calcium chloride. Normal aPTT is 30–40 seconds.

### Fibrin degradation products test

- This test is determined by adding peripheral venous blood to serum containing antifibrinogen degradation fragments. The measurement of FDPs provides an indication of the activity of the fibrinolytic system.

## THERAPEUTIC APPROACHES AND NURSING CARE

- Potential threats of injury in the environment are identified and then reduced or eliminated.
- Diligent measures to maintain skin integrity are instituted.
- All unnecessary procedures are avoided in the thrombocytopenic patient, including intramuscular or SQ injections, rectal temperatures or suppositories, and indwelling catheters.
- Severe uterine hemorrhage can be a complication in thrombocytopenic women who are menstruating. Menses can be suppressed by pharmacological agents.
- Forceful coughing, sneezing, or nose blowing can lead to bleeding.
- The patient with epistaxis is placed in high Fowler's position.
- Hygiene is a problem in the patient who has active bleeding.
- Physical and emotional rest are essential when the patient is actively bleeding.

## Blood Component Therapy

- The technological advances in blood transfusion therapy have led to a decrease in the morbidity and mortality of cancer and its treatment.
- Whole blood is removed from a donor and is then "fractionated" into the various components.

### Red blood cell therapy

- The decision to transfuse generally is based on an overall clinical picture, including any underlying cardiac or pulmonary condition or any concurrent conditions that might impair the patient's tolerance for anemia.
- An attempt is generally made to keep the patient's hemoglobin level higher than 8 g/100 ml.
- Physiological signs of anemia should be relieved when the hemoglobin is raised to 10 or 11 g/100 ml.
- If the patient is not actively bleeding, 1 unit of packed red cells should increase the peripheral hematocrit level by 3% and the hemoglobin by 1 g/dl.
- The advantage of packed red blood cells is that they provide more than 70% of the hematocrit of whole blood with only one-third of the plasma.
- Leukocytes in red blood cell transfusions can cause reactions if the recipient has antileukocyte antibodies.

### Platelet therapy

- Generally the decision to transfuse is indicated when there is actual bleeding associated with thrombocytopenia, when the platelet count is > 20,000/mm$^3$ yet bleeding is present, and in patients with abnormally functioning platelets who are bleeding.
- Theoretically, one unit of platelets should increase the recipient's peripheral blood platelet level by 10,000–12,000 cells/mm$^3$.
- In the absence of normal platelet production, platelet transfusions generally are required every three days.
- Platelets can be given in fresh whole blood, platelet-rich plasma, or platelet concentrates.
- Platelets are stored at room temperature and are stored up to 5 days.
- Patients with fever or sepsis require frequent transfusions to maintain an adequate platelet count.

- Patients with fever due to infection can be premedicated with antipyretics prior to platelet transfusion in an attempt to minimize platelet destruction.
- Platelet survival is greatly decreased when alloimmunization to the platelet transfusion develops.
- A 24-hour postplatelet transfusion count helps to determine if other factors are responsible for a poor platelet recovery, such as infection, fever, or another cause for accelerated platelet consumption.
- To be most effective, platelets must be fresh and metabolically active. Maximum effectiveness remains for up to six hours after being obtained.

### Plasma therapy

- The most common use of plasma and plasma components in cancer is with coagulation disorders associated with this disease. Plasma component therapy is also administered for severe bleeding, shock, bleeding associated with infections, and management of acute DIC.
- Replacement plasma is usually calculated in units, with 1 unit of plasma equaling the activity present in 1 ml of normal human male plasma.

## Transfusion Complications

- The major hazards include hemolytic and nonhemolytic transfusion reactions, transmission of diseases, and complications associated with IV therapy and transfusions.
- If significant red cell contamination has occurred, the donor and recipient are matched by A,B,O antigens. If matching is not done when spillage occurs, hemolytic reactions are likely.
- A serious transfusion complication in patients who are significantly immunosuppressed is the risk of developing graft-versus-host (GVH) disease.
- To prevent proliferation of lymphocytes, it is generally recommended that all blood products given to the severely immunocompromised host be exposed to pretransfusion irradiation with 15 cGy.

### Leukocyte-depleted blood products

- Leukocytes remaining in donor blood collected for transfusion are responsible for many of the complications related to transfusion therapy, including immunologic effects, nonhemolytic febrile reactions, and transmission of viral infections.

## Home Transfusion Therapy for the Cancer Patient

- Services that are now provided in the home include complex IV therapy, including blood transfusion therapy.
- There are no specific legal constraints against transfusing patients at home, as long as the procedure is performed by licensed and qualified medical personnel.
- The patient is at greater risk for complications than would be the case in a hospital setting (lack of sophisticated emergency equipment).

### Selection criteria

- The seven basic criteria for inclusion in a home transfusion therapy program include the following:
  1. Physical limitations of the patient that make transportation difficult
  2. Stable cardiopulmonary status
  3. Patients who do not have an acute need for blood or who do not require more than 2 units in a 24-hour period
  4. Absence of reactions to the most recent transfusion
  5. A cooperative patient

6. Presence of a responsible adult during and after transfusion
7. A telephone available for medical needs or the need to call an ambulance
8. A diagnosis supporting the need for transfusion therapy
- The person administering the transfusion should be a registered nurse with current venipuncture and IV therapy skills.

## Preadministration considerations

- Ideally, the pretransfusion blood sample collection is done the day before the scheduled transfusion, and by the nurse who will administer the blood.
  - Once the informed consent has been signed by the patient, a means of identification is placed on the patient and must remain in place until after the transfusion.
  - Documentation records include physician's written orders for the blood transfusion, a signed informed consent, laboratory results, nursing progress records, and a "Home Transfusion Flow Sheet."
  - Once the transfusion is complete, the nurse will discontinue the transfusion bag yet maintain a patent IV line. The nurse remains with the patient for at least 30 minutes after transfusion to observe the patient and to monitor vital signs.
  - Follow-up of the transfused patient should be done within 24 hours of the transfusion.

# PRACTICE QUESTIONS

1. Colony stimulating factors (CSFs) act on the stem cells to mediate which of the following steps in hematopoiesis?
   a. Cellular proliferation only
   b. Cellular differentiation only
   c. Stem cell maturation only
   d. All of the above

2. The typical response of the body to a reduction in the platelet count, such as that caused by bleeding, is a(n):
   a. increase in the fibrinolytic activity of remaining platelets.
   b. release of ADP into the bloodstream, which increases the oxygen-carrying capacity of available platelets.
   c. sequestering of red blood cells in the spleen.
   d. increased production of megakaryocytes in the bone marrow.

3. Circulating platelets perform several vital functions, including all of the following *except*:
   a. fibrinolysis, or the lysis of fibrin clots and vessel repair.
   b. the release of plasminogen activators required for clot formation.
   c. furnishing a phospholipid surface for the biochemical phase of hemostasis.
   d. the formation of a mechanical hemostatic plug at the site of vessel injury.

4. Which of the following pairings of substances and functions in hemostasis is incorrect?
   a. fibrin: the actual substance of a clot
   b. thrombin: acts on fibrinogen to form fibrin
   c. plasmin: breaks up clots
   d. factor Xa: acts on plasminogen to form plasmin

5. Bleeding as a symptom of cancer is most often due either to the mechanical pressure of tumors on organs or to:
   a. interference with vasculature.
   b. damage to the spleen.
   c. hypocoagulability of the blood.
   d. infection.

6. Acute bleeding that occurs as a result of tumor-induced structural damage to vasculature is best managed by prevention. If acute bleeding does occur, however, and the site is not directly exposed, the best management approach is often:
   a. radiotherapy combined with chemotherapy.
   b. oral or parenteral iron supplements to reduce anemia.
   c. mechanical pressure, e.g., nasal packing during epistaxis.
   d. direct and steady pressure at the site of bleeding.

7. The single most significant factor for predicting bleeding in the individual with cancer is:
   a. tumor site.
   b. platelet count.
   c. abnormal platelet function.
   d. an imbalance in coagulation factors.

8. Thrombocytopenia in cancer patients can be caused by any of the following factors *except*:
   a. an abnormal distribution of platelets that results in increased platelet sequestration.
   b. rapid platelet destruction characterized by a shortened platelet life span.
   c. overstimulation of normal coagulation causing rapid platelet thrombosis.
   d. decreased production of platelets in the bone marrow due to tumor involvement.

9. Patients with cancers may at times have bleeding despite normal platelet counts and coagulation factors. An example is bleeding caused by:
   a. platelet sequestration.
   b. disseminated intravascular coagulation (DIC).
   c. decreased platelet adhesiveness.
   d. hypocoagulability.

10. Malignancy or the metabolic alterations that accompany malignancy may lead to an imbalance in coagulation factors, leading to decreased hemostasis (hypocoagulability). The most significant factor that leads to a state of hypocoagulability is:
    a. liver disease.
    b. a deficiency of vitamin K.
    c. thrombocytosis.
    d. DIC.

11. The symptoms of disseminated intravascular coagulation (DIC) seem paradoxical because:
    a. both platelet function and platelet numbers are implicated in DIC.
    b. patients may experience fever at the same time their bodies are hypothermic.
    c. DIC may be both the cause and effect of malignancy.
    d. thrombosis and hemorrhage may occur simultaneously.

12. Therapy for disseminated intravascular coagulation (DIC) often involves the administration of several substances. Which of the following is *not* a common treatment for DIC?
    a. Heparin
    b. Epsilon-amino caproic acid (EACA or Amicar)
    c. Vitamin K
    d. Platelet replacement

13. The most important measure in the early detection of bleeding is:
    a. accurate screening, beginning with a platelet count.
    b. observation for subtle diagnostic signals such as skin petechiae.
    c. a family history, focusing on possible congenital bleeding disorders.
    d. diagnostic testing of the complete cardiovascular system.

14. Ms. Edwards, a cancer patient, is being assessed for abnormal bleeding. She is to receive a prothrombin time test. The prothrombin time is a screening test of hemostatic function that is performed when tissue thromboplastin and ionized calcium are added to citrated plasma. Clotting time is then recorded and compared with the clotting time of a normal blood sample. This test is a measure of:
    a. the ability of platelets to aggregate.
    b. the concentration of functional factor in plasma.
    c. platelet plug formation.
    d. diminished or absent coagulation factors.

15. Ms. Edwards is found to be at definite risk for bleeding. Her nursing care should incorporate all of the following measures *except*:

    a. avoidance of trauma.

    b. use of intramuscular rather than intravenous injections.

    c. avoidance of unnecessary procedures, including rectal temperatures or suppositories.

    d. suppression or monitoring of menses.

16. Under which of the following circumstances would administration of platelet concentrate from a single donor or HLA-matched donor be preferable to that of a random donor platelet concentrate?

    a. When the patient is severely immunosuppressed

    b. When cost is a major factor

    c. When a patient's red blood cell antigens (ABO) are not known

    d. When time is a major factor

17. Mrs. Ryan has metastatic cancer and presents with fever, increased pulse rate, and flushing during her transfusion. As you are checking her vital signs, she experiences anaphylaxis. Mrs. Ryan's reaction is most likely due to:

    a. ABO incompatibility.

    b. recipient antibodies against immunoglobulin in the plasma.

    c. antileukocyte antibodies directed against the donor blood.

    d. development of alloantibodies to transfused blood.

# ANSWER EXPLANATIONS

1. **The answer is d.** CSFs mediate all of these steps. (p. 607)

2. **The answer is d.** Megakaryocytes mature in the bone marrow and fragment to form platelets, which are then released into the bloodstream. Under normal circumstances any reduction in platelet count—from bleeding, malignancy, chemotherapy or radiotherapy, or other causes—will cause an increase in the production of megakaryocytes and platelets in the bone marrow. This activity is controlled by a regulatory hormone called thrombopoietin. (p. 607)

3. **The answer is b.** Plasminogen activators are enzymes that are present in most body fluids and tissues. They are responsible for the conversion of plasminogen to plasmin in the presence of thrombin. It is plasmin that is responsible for the lysis (and not the formation) of fibrin clots. (p. 607)

4. **The answer is d.** Factor Xa, along with cofactor Va, catalyzes the conversion of prothrombin to thrombin, the most powerful of the coagulation enzymes. It is thrombin that catalyzes the conversion of plasminogen to plasmin during fibrinolysis. (p. 608)

5. **The answer is a.** All of the other choices can be factors in bleeding, but erosion and rupture of vessels precipitated by tumor invasion or pressure is the other major cause of bleeding in persons with cancer. Any tumor involvement of vasculature tissue or any tumor lying in close proximity to major vessels is seen as a threat of bleeding. Bleeding may also be the result of radiotherapy or radical cancer surgery and various platelet and coagulation abnormalities. (p. 609)

6. **The answer is c.** If acute bleeding does occur, direct methods to halt the hemorrhage should be instituted immediately. Choices **a** and **b** are preventive methods; choice **d**, while immediate and direct, applies to an exposed bleeding site. Another example of the use of mechanical pressure to stop acute bleeding is the insertion of an occlusion balloon catheter into the bronchus. (p. 611)

7. **The answer is b.** Although all of the other choices are factors in bleeding as well, platelet count is the single most important factor in predicting bleeding in the individual with cancer. Patients with platelet

counts below 20,000 cells/mm³ have a greater than 50% chance of bleeding. Low platelet count (thrombocytopenia) is also the most frequent platelet abnormality associated with cancer. (p. 614)

8. **The answer is c.** The other choices all result in lowered platelet count. Choice **a** is often associated with splenomegaly, an enlarged spleen; **b** is frequently due to an autoimmune response in which antibodies are formed against the person's own platelets; **d** may also be the consequence of cancer therapy on bone marrow. A fourth cause of thrombocytopenia is platelet dilution often caused by the use of stored platelet-poor blood. (p. 612)

9. **The answer is c.** Choices **b** and **d** are coagulation abnormalities; choice **a** is a quantitative abnormality. Qualitative abnormalities such as choice **c** refer principally to alterations in platelet function, which may include a decreased procoagulant activity of platelets, decreased platelet adhesiveness and decreased aggregation in response to ADP, thrombocytosis associated with myeloproliferative disorders, and the coating of platelets by fibrin degradation products as a result of the increased activation of coagulation factors. (p. 616)

10. **The answer is a.** Liver disease may result from a variety of causes, including tumor invasion, chemotherapy, infection, or surgical resection. Regardless, it may either interfere with the synthesis of plasma coagulation factors or interfere with their functioning, decreasing hemostasis. Other causes of hypocoagulability include vitamin K deficiency, the use of large amounts of frozen plasma, the presence of coagulation protein antagonists, and coagulation factor deficiencies. (p. 618)

11. **The answer is d.** DIC always results from an underlying disease process that triggers abnormal activation of thrombin formation. Thrombin is both a powerful coagulant and an agent of fibrinolysis. Thus small clots may be formed in the microcirculation of many organs at the same time clots and clotting factors are being consumed. The result is hemorrhage as the body is unable to respond to vascular or tissue injury. (p. 619)

12. **The answer is c.** Vitamin K might be administered to a patient experiencing hypocoagulability, but not the hypercoagulability caused by DIC. All of the other therapies may provide short-term relief of DIC symptoms. Treatment of the underlying malignancy is vital in treating the patient with DIC, inasmuch as the tumor is the ultimate stimulus. (p. 622)

13. **The answer is b.** Because diagnostic signals may be subtle (including skin petechiae that may be noticed while bathing the person, traces of blood during tooth brushing, etc.), it is important for the nurse to be keenly observant. A family history and various screening tests may be valuable in assessment, but they do not substitute for observation. (p. 623)

14. **The answer is d.** This screening test is called prothrombin time (PT). Choice **a** is the platelet aggregation test; **b** is the specific factor assays test; **c** is the bleeding time test. (p. 624)

15. **The answer is b.** If the patient requires parenteral administration of medication, the intravenous route is used whenever possible. Intramuscular and subcutaneous injections place the patient at risk for the development of hematomas. Injections, if unavoidable, are administered with a needle of the smallest possible gauge. (p. 625)

16. **The answer is a.** A random donor platelet concentrate may expose the recipient to multiple tissue antigens leading to platelet refractoriness. A single donor platelet concentrate is taken from one donor or one HLA-matched donor; patients are therefore not exposed to multiple antigens. This may be important with patients who are severely immunosuppressed, such as those who have undergone bone marrow transplantation. (pp. 626–627)

17. **The answer is a.** These are signs of ABO incompatibility, which is an acute hemolytic transfusion reaction. Choice **b** is a mild allergic reaction; choice **c** is a febrile, nonhemolytic reaction. Choice **d** characterizes a delayed hemolytic reaction. (p. 631, Table 22-12)

# Chapter 23    Fatigue

## SCOPE OF THE PROBLEM

- Fatigue is the most common side effect of cancer treatment. People with cancer may also experience fatigue as a symptom of the disease or as a result of physical deconditioning.
- Major impediments to addressing CRF in clinical practice include a misconception on the part of health care providers that CRF is transient and relieved by rest like the acute fatigue experienced in day-to-day life.
- *Acute fatigue* is a relatively temporary state that is relieved by rest, although one night of undisturbed sleep may not provide complete relief.
- When fatigue persists over time, it is known as *chronic fatigue*. Chronic fatigue is not readily relieved by rest, is often viewed by the person experiencing it as an "exaggerated" response to activity compared with their previous experience, and is extremely debilitating.
- Individuals with cancer may experience both acute and chronic fatigue.

## DEFINITION OF FATIGUE

- Fatigue has been defined in terms of both objective performance and subjective experience. Early fatigue research focused on individuals' jobs or athletic performance.
- In this approach to understanding fatigue, an objective indicator of the point at which performance declines, such as exercise endurance or accuracy of completion of a mental task, is used to define fatigue.
- In the subjective experience approach, fatigue is conceptualized as a feeling state. In contrast to weakness, defined as the *inability* either to initiate or to maintain specific muscular activities, subjectively defined fatigue has a voluntary component.
- The subjective view of fatigue is the most relevant to cancer care. The actions individuals take in response to fatigue will be based on their perceptions rather than on the results of a performance test or an evaluation of their level of fatigue made by another person.

## PATHOPHYSIOLOGY OF FATIGUE

### Theories of Causation

- Although causes of fatigue have been explored in numerous studies, no clear support has emerged for any of the major hypotheses. Several of these are discussed below.

#### Accumulation hypothesis

- The accumulation hypothesis proposes that a buildup of waste products in the body produces fatigue.
- Although it is common for fatigue in cancer patients receiving radiation treatment or chemotherapy to be attributed to the presence of by-products of cell death, to date no research has been conducted to test this hypothesis.

### Depletion hypothesis

- The depletion hypothesis was based on the idea that muscular activity is impaired when certain substances—such as carbohydrates, fats, proteins, adenosine triphosphate (ATP), and adrenal hormones—are not readily available.
- The limited research in this area does not provide adequate support for this line of reasoning.

### Biochemical and physiochemical phenomena

- Changes in the production, distribution, use, balance, and movement of substances such as muscle proteins, glucose, electrolytes, and hormones may be important factors influencing the experience of fatigue.
- Many of the drugs used to treat cancer or to manage side effects of treatment also can produce biochemical and physiochemical changes related to those believed to produce fatigue.

### Central nervous system control

- In Grandjean's neurophysiological model of fatigue, the level of fatigue is determined by the balance between two opposing systems: the activating system and the inhibiting system. The *reticular activating system* controls alertness of wakefulness by stimulating the cerebral cortex and responding to both sensory stimulation and feedback from the cerebral cortex. The *inhibitory system* depresses the activity of the reticular activating system.
- The neurophysiological model of fatigue may explain the occurrence of fatigue in conditions of low stimulation, such as immobility produced by bedrest, even when there is little expenditure of energy.
- Reports of declines in the ability to concentrate and to process information are consistent with the neurophysiological model of fatigue.

### Adaptation and energy reserves

- Every individual has a certain amount of superficial energy available for adaptation; fatigue occurs when that energy supply is depleted. Rest allows time for energy to be replenished from the individual's deep reserves so that adaptation can continue.
- The idea that fatigue is relieved by sufficient rest is consistent with the experience of healthy people experiencing acute fatigue but does not fit the chronic fatigue model applied to CRF.
- The quality of sleep and rest may also be important. Research on sleep patterns during illness tends to focus on environmental disruptions such as hospital noise and contact for the delivery of care. The role of side effects and symptoms as well as illness management activities in sleep disruption has not been addressed.

### Energy balance hypotheses

- According to the psychobiological-entropy hypothesis, decreased activity decreases the production of energy needed to support activity. A trajectory that can be viewed as a downward spiral is then established in which the response to lower energy resources is to further decrease activity, which again decreases energy resources.
- The deconditioning model proposes that muscle loss occurs rapidly in the face of immobility. As a result, the amount of energy expended in completing simple activities, such as getting out of bed, increases while capacity for work decreases.
  - The work on deconditioning and immobility is based in the objective model of fatigue and has not been linked to subjective fatigue.

- Energy storage is typified by advice to save or conserve energy. The assumption is that the individual has a finite amount of energy to invest in activity and that conservation will allow the saved energy to be devoted to another activity.

## CANCER AND FATIGUE: PATHOPHYSIOLOGY AND PATHOPSYCHOLOGY
### Treatment Effects
#### Surgery
- Fatigue is a consistent finding in patients who are recovering from surgery and is generally assumed to have multiple causes.

#### Radiation treatment
- Fatigue is the only common *systemic* side effect of local radiation treatment and has been reported to be the most severe side effect of radiation during the last week of treatment.
- Several studies of patients receiving radiation treatment document various levels of prevalence of fatigue and suggest that factors such as age, diagnosis, and pretreatment condition may influence the severity of fatigue experienced during treatment.

#### Chemotherapy
- Despite variation among treatment regimens, fatigue is the most frequently reported side effect of chemotherapy.
- In addition, fatigue was positively related to emotional distress.

#### Biologic response modifiers
- Fatigue is described as the most important dose-limiting side effect of interferons.
- It appears that this cancer treatment modality is likely to produce fatigue that is more severe than that associated with surgery, radiation treatment, and the most commonly used chemotherapy regimens.
- Since fatigue is a dose-limiting side effect of biologic response modifiers, a high priority for nursing care of individuals receiving this form of treatment is preventing and ameliorating fatigue.

#### Combined-modality treatment
- Research is needed to determine whether fatigue produced by sequential or combined-modality treatment exceeds that produced by the most toxic treatment alone. Such research will help to determine the extent to which fatigue will be a problem for patients on these regimens.

### Other Etiologic Factors
#### Physical factors
- Physical problems (such as pain, pruritis, urinary frequency, diarrhea, nausea, and vomiting) may interfere with patients' ability to rest or sleep. Nutritional deficits, changes in nutrient metabolism, and alteration in fluid and electrolyte balance are produced by a number of factors that may be related to treatment.
- Bone marrow depression can produce anemia, bleeding, and increased susceptibility to infection.
- Some physical conditions increase energy expenditure.

### Psychosocial factors

- The impact of the severity of fatigue and associated changes in activity depends upon the individual's perception of what limitations are acceptable to the self and the family as well as the expected duration of the limitations. These value judgments will differ substantially from person to person.

## NURSING CARE OF THE CANCER PATIENT AT RISK FOR FATIGUE

- The goal of nursing care for the patient with cancer is to minimize the negative impact of fatigue on quality of life.

## Assessment

- Among those who were assessing patients' level of fatigue, the average frequency of assessment was "sometimes."
- A survey of supportive care programs in National Cancer Institute–designated cancer centers revealed that none of the responding centers had clinical programs that addressed fatigue.

### Level of fatigue

- Since the patient's perception of fatigue will influence decisions about activities, participation in treatment, and overall quality of life, so-called objective ratings of fatigue made by health care professionals are much less relevant to the patient's situation than assessments made by the patient.
- The definition of fatigue shifts as the person with cancer experiences it. This change takes the form of a new definition of the level at which one is fatigued, which is higher than that used prior to experiencing CRF.
- Level of fatigue should be assessed at multiple points in time.
- To assist patients in planning ways to deal with fatigue, the nurse must obtain information about both the daily pattern of fatigue and variations in fatigue in relation to the treatment cycle.

### Usual activities

- Information about the type and intensity of the individual's usual activities can be obtained by asking the patient to describe a typical day. Individuals who report fatigue should be asked to describe what they do about it and to indicate the extent to which their self-care activities are effective in relieving their fatigue.
- To assist the person in planning ways of modifying daily activities, the nurse determines who might be available to assume some of the individual's usual responsibilities and gains an understanding of the meaning and value of each of the individual's activities.
- Individuals experiencing fatigue over time may gradually downgrade their perception of the level of activity that is "usual." They may not become aware of the impact of fatigue on their usual activities until months after treatment ends.

### Additional assessment data

- The assessment includes information about potential causes of fatigue. Chronic diseases may contribute to fatigue.

## Interventions

- The interventions suggested for CRF include providing preparatory information, energy conservation and activity management, increasing sleep or rest, and exercise. See Table 23-1, text page 649, for interventions for cancer treatment-related fatigue.

## Preparatory information

- The rationale for providing preparatory information is that it provides patients with an accurate mental image of the impending experience.
- This is the standard used by patients in processing information and assigning meaning.
- Accurate information about impending experiences does not increase the number of patients who report specific side effects of treatment.

## Rest and sleep

- Rest is the most frequently recommended intervention for cancer patients who experience fatigue.
- However, increased sleep or rest may not improve fatigue for all individuals.
- Symptoms or treatment side effects that interfere with sleep and rest should be controlled to the extent possible.
- Timing medication administration, fluid administration, and self-monitoring activities so that the schedule does not interfere with the individual's desired rest time may also be helpful in maintaining sleep.

## Energy conservation and activity management

- Rearranging activities to allow for rest periods or to shorten the time that high-energy output is required is another approach to dealing with limitations imposed by fatigue.

## Exercise

- Research involving women receiving adjuvant chemotherapy for breast cancer indicates that exercise may relieve fatigue.
- Women assigned to a combined structured walking and support group intervention had less fatigue, higher levels of psychosocial adjustment, and better physical performance than a control group.
- Considerations in recommending exercise should include adherence to published recommendations for safety. Mobility problems, neurological deficits, dizziness, and medications such as catabolic steroids are examples of factors that increase risk of injury in the use of exercise for cancer patients.

## Posttreatment fatigue

- When fatigue is experienced as a side effect of treatment, it does not disappear immediately once treatment ends.
- Individuals with advanced cancer may complete treatment and subsequently experience worsening of their fatigue.

## CONCLUSION

- Although a number of hypotheses have been proposed to explain the causes of fatigue experienced as a symptom of cancer or as a side effect of cancer treatment, none has been adequately tested.
- To plan nursing care for the patient who is experiencing fatigue, the patient's pattern of usual activities and the relative importance or value of each activity must also be understood.

## PRACTICE QUESTIONS

1. Subjectively defined fatigue has a/an _____ component, which differentiates it from weakness.
   a. involuntary
   b. voluntary
   c. initiation
   d. duration

2. Mary says that she has been feeling tired for several weeks now. She finds it difficult to concentrate, and she does not have the energy to perform simple chores around the house. She still walks her dog and swims twice a week at the YMCA, but she feels very drained afterwards. She's tried getting more sleep, but that does not seem to be helping. Mary is probably experiencing:
   a. acute fatigue.
   b. chronic fatigue.
   c. weakness.
   d. depression.

**Questions 3 and 4 concern Mark's fatigue.**

3. You see a colleague assessing his patient, Mark, for fatigue. He asks Mark about the activities he usually performs, and he gives him several tests for concentration. When you ask your colleague about it later, he says that he is trying to gather a thorough assessment of Mark's fatigue. You suggest:
   a. an exercise endurance test.
   b. asking Mark's family for more information.
   c. asking Mark to describe his fatigue.
   d. choosing an objective indicator.

4. You learn later that one of the probable causes for Mark's fatigue is bone marrow suppression that is at the level of classic anemia. Mark is receiving transfusions to treat the anemia. Which is most likely to occur as a result?
   a. Mark's hemoglobin will improve and his hematocrit will not, resulting in an improvement in the anemic condition but not the fatigue.
   b. Mark's hemoglobin and hematocrit will improve, resulting in an improvement in both the anemic condition and the fatigue.
   c. Mark's hematocrit will improve and his hemoglobin will not, resulting in an improvement in the anemic condition but not the fatigue.
   d. Mark's hematocrit will remain the same and his hemoglobin will improve, resulting in an improvement in both his fatigue and his anemia.

**Questions 5–8 concern Karen, who is experiencing some symptoms of anemia and chronic CRF.**

5. You have a patient, Karen, who is experiencing some symptoms of anemia and chronic CRF. Her anemia is not as severe as Mark's. You ask your colleague, who has studied a great deal of outside information on the topic, what is likely to happen. He tells to you to expect that her anemic symptoms will be treated:
   a. with similar expected results for both the anemia and the fatigue.
   b. with better expected results for both the anemia and the fatigue.
   c. with worse expected results for both the anemia and the fatigue.
   d. with no expectations based on Mark's case.

6. Karen tells you that it seems as if because she is doing less, she has less energy to do things at all. She is getting more rest, letting her children help her with the heavier household chores, and she takes either Friday or Monday off each week at work. She used to go biking twice a week, but now that she's "so tired from fighting this disease," she has almost no energy even for this very enjoyable and important activity. Karen's description is consistent with:
   a. the psychobiological-entropy model.
   b. the depletion model.
   c  the adaptation model.
   d. the accumulation model.

7. You are faced with a dilemma concerning treatment and assessment of Karen's CRF. While you know that giving Karen preparatory information regarding fatigue as it relates to her adjuvant chemotherapy will help her have an idea of what to expect, you are worried that this information will lead to increased report of side effects of her treatment. When you investigate this issue prior to making a decision on the matter, you find that:
   a. preparatory information provides a standard against which patients process information and assign meaning; it tends to encourage self-diagnosis.
   b. preparatory information provides a standard against which patients process information and assign meaning; it does not increase the number of patients who report specific side effects.
   c. preparatory information tends to confuse and often frighten patients who are worried about decreases in quality of life.
   d. none of the above.

8. Karen tells you that she has been reading as much information as possible on her disease and on a variety of the side effects that accompany it, including fatigue. In her reading, she found some information that indicated that exercise actually helped some patients suffering from fatigue. She is very excited about this and asks you if such an option is possible for her. You know from earlier conversations that she has always enjoyed bicycling, but that she sometimes gets dizzy. She is currently taking a number of medications including catabolic steroids. You tell her that:
   a. exercise would be ideal for her, but her dizziness makes bicycling dangerous.
   b. exercise would be ideal for her, and the catabolic steroids she is taking will help her system adapt.
   c. exercise has not been proven to help those with CRF who are receiving adjuvant chemotherapy.
   d. exercise has not been proven to help women suffering from breast cancer, as Karen is.

9. The _____ model of fatigue attempts to explain the causes of fatigue in terms of two opposing systems—the activating and inhibiting systems. This model may best explain the occurrence of fatigue in conditions of low stimulation even when there is little expenditure of energy.
   a. energy balance
   b. adaptation and energy reserves
   c. neurophysiological
   d. depletion

10. Why are the possible cumulative effects of multiple surgical procedures important to those studying CRF?
   a. Fatigue is a consistent finding in patients who are recovering from surgery.
   b. It is not unusual for patients to undergo several surgical procedures for diagnosis and treatment of cancer.
   c. Both a and b are true.
   d. Neither a nor b is true.

11. Based on modality of treatment, which of your patients would you expect to have the most severe fatigue?
    a. Joe, who is being treated with biologic response modifiers
    b. Karen, who is undergoing chemotherapy
    c. Martha, who has just had surgery
    d. Thomas, who is undergoing radiation treatment

12. Which statement is true of individuals who have suffered from CRF once they have completed treatment?
    a. Fatigue will disappear almost immediately upon the conclusion of treatment.
    b. Fatigue may gradually fade after the treatment is finished.
    c. Fatigue absolutely should improve upon the completion of treatment.
    d. The use of assistive devices and systematic planning of activities should be unnecessary upon completion of treatment.

## ANSWER EXPLANATIONS

1. **The answer is b.** In contrast to weakness, fatigue has a voluntary component. Individuals with fatigue may push themselves to engage in highly valued activities in spite of their fatigue. Individuals suffering from weakness are unable to initiate or maintain specific muscular activities. (p. 641)

2. **The answer is b.** Chronic fatigue, as opposed to acute fatigue, persists over time and is not readily relieved by rest. Weakness would have left Mary unable to walk her dog and swim, and depression would have been indicated if Mary had expressed a general sadness which resulted in her low levels of activity. (p. 641)

3. **The answer is c.** Choosing an objective indicator, giving Mark an endurance test, and asking Mark's family for information are all choices for gathering objective information—which your colleague says he wants. However, these things should be regarded as responses to fatigue rather than fatigue itself, and fatigue should be measured subjectively, according to the patient's perception of the problem. (p. 641)

4. **The answer is b.** Mark's hematocrit and hemoglobin values are expected to improve, resulting in an improvement in both the anemic condition and, in a case like this, the fatigue. (p. 642)

5. **The answer is d.** Studies focused on reversing severe anemia caused by bone marrow suppression may not generalize to most patients receiving cancer treatments. Karen's much less severe anemia could be caused by many different factors and may be treated in a number of different ways, all of which may or may not improve the condition and her fatigue. (p. 642)

6. **The answer is a.** Karen is describing her fatigue in terms of the psychobiological-entropy model of fatigue, which suggests that the less activity the subject engages in, the less energy the subject will produce. This model would tend to encourage a balance of rest and activity. (p. 643)

7. **The answer is b.** Preparatory information is essential in providing the patient with a standard in processing information and assigning meaning. (p. 648)

8. **The answer is a.** Exercise is indicated in women suffering from breast cancer who are receiving adjuvant chemotherapy; research has shown that, in this case, it may indeed relieve fatigue. However, because Karen suffers from dizziness, exercise may not be the answer for her. Certainly bicycling would be very dangerous under the circumstances. (p. 650)

9. **The answer is c.** The neurophysiological model of fatigue explains fatigue as the interaction of two opposing systems—the activating system and the inhibiting system. (p. 643)

10. **The answer is c.** Because cancer patients often undergo multiple surgical procedures and because fatigue is a consistent side effect found in patients recovering from surgery, the cumulative effects of these procedures on patients suffering from CRF are very important. (p. 644)

11. **The answer is a.** Biologic response modifiers tend to produce fatigue that is more severe than that associated with surgery, radiation therapy and the most commonly used chemotherapy regimens. (p. 646)

12. **The answer is b.** Fatigue may persist for months after the conclusion of treatment, and may in fact worsen for those patients with advanced cancer. Assistive devices may still be necessary and appropriate. (p. 651)

# Chapter 24      Nutritional Disturbances

## INTRODUCTION

- In optimal nutrition, nutrient intake provides adequate energy and protection from disease.
- When intake of nutrients is less than adequate or more than required, nutritional stores are reduced below or increased above normal. Nutritional lesions of varying magnitudes result, depending on the type and extent of the deficiency or excess.
- Undernutrition is seen as the more common problem in both pediatric and adult cancer populations. However, the evidence that both under- and overnutrition negatively affect morbidity, survival, and quality of life emphasizes the need for oncology nurses to evaluate the nutritional status of all individuals under their care.

## SCOPE OF THE PROBLEM

### Definitions

- *Obesity* is defined as weighing more than 20% over ideal body weight.
- Among individuals with cancer, increased weight may reflect tumor mass or fluid retention while masking loss of lean body mass.
- Terms used to describe nonmalignant nutritional deficiencies, and occasionally malignant starvation, are *kwashiorkor* (protein malnutrition with an adequate caloric intake) and *marasmus* (simple starvation with protein-calorie malnutrition). *Cachexia*, a general term meaning ill health, can occur in nonneoplastic diseases, such as sepsis, cardiac failure, and starvation.
  - Cancer cachexia is characterized by anorexia, weight loss, skeletal muscle atrophy, and asthenia (loss of strength).
  - Primary cachexia results from tumor-produced metabolic abnormalities or host response. Secondary cachexia results from mechanical effects of the tumor or treatment. Primary cachexia resolves with successful cancer treatment. Secondary cachexia can be treated with a variety of approaches and is often more amenable to treatment than the primary form.
- Other terms include *hypogeusia* (decreased taste sensitivity), *dysgeusia* (perverted taste perception), *odynophagia* or *dysphagia* (painful swallowing), *hyposmia* (diminished ability to smell), and *inanition* (progressive deterioration with muscle wasting and energy loss).

### Incidence

- Neither the incidence nor the prevalence of malnutrition is accurately documented in the cancer population.
  - The absence of these basic statistics arises from several factors: (1) nutritional status is not assessed when cancer is diagnosed, especially in the obese; (2) because assessment of nutritional status frequently is delayed, the opportunity to find minimal nutrient deficiencies in early stages is often lost; and (3) there is no consensus on what indicators of nutritional status should be used.
- Severe undernutrition was reported to be the single most common cause of death among individuals with cancer in the early twentieth century.
- Overnutrition is most common in the breast cancer population.

- 40% to 70% of women with breast cancer receiving adjuvant chemotherapy gain weight. There is evidence that women who are obese may have poorer survival than women who are not.

## Risk Factors

- Identification of the risk factors for nutritional problems in cancer is based on assessment of the person's existing nutritional status and an appreciation of cancer malnutrition etiology.
- Even with a satisfactory nutritional status, all individuals with cancer face two major risk factors for undernutrition: having the disease and being treated for it.

### External and internal factors

- External factors include transportation, access to food shopping, availability of different nutrients, adequacy of housing and food preparation facilities, programs that supplement food, age, body image, past history of food fads or eating disorders, social support, educational level, alcohol or tobacco intake, and the presence of comorbid diseases.

### Cancer-related factors

- The type of cancer affects the probability of malnutrition.
- Individuals with breast cancer or leukemia are at low risk, while those with cancer of the upper aerodigestive tract and gastrointestinal tract are at special risk for undernutrition.
  - These differences may arise from (1) mechanical difficulties imposed by the location of tumors in the digestive area or (2) host responses to the cancer or (3) the cancer itself causing changes in metabolism and energy needs.

### Treatment-related factors

- All cancer therapies can cause nutritional deficiency.
- The magnitude of the treatment-related risk depends on the area of treatment, type of treatment, number of therapeutic modalities used, dosages of therapy used, and length of treatment.

#### Surgery

- The effects of surgery on an individual's nutritional status depend on the extent of the procedure as well as the site of operation.
- Complications associated with surgery also are related to the nutritional status of the individual prior to the operation.
  - Malnourished individuals have higher incidences of morbidity and mortality than do those who are adequately nourished. This is of particular relevance to individuals with cancers of the aerodigestive or gastrointestinal tract.
- Surgery can increase energy requirements by 28 kcal/kg/day or 1.5 times normal dietary requirements.

#### Radiation

- Radiation therapy can alter nutritional status by both systemic and local effects.
  - Radiation alters function in the treatment area and poses particular problems for patients with aerodigestive or gastrointestinal cancers, including anorexia, diarrhea, bleeding, nausea, vomiting, weight loss, mucositis, esophagitis, gastritis, xerostomia, and changes in taste. Local desquamation reactions can temporarily increase energy needs.
  - Fatigue and appetite changes commonly occur among individuals receiving radiation therapy, which can alter the person's desire and ability to procure, prepare, and ingest food.

Delayed effects of radiation, such as intestinal strictures, fibrosis or obstruction, fistulas, and pulmonary and hepatic fibrosis, cause mechanical problems in gut function and oxygenation. These in turn interrupt the person's ability to absorb and ingest food and may necessitate long-term management.

### Chemotherapy

- Direct effects include alteration of the intestinal absorptive surface, excitation of the Chemoreceptor Trigger Zone and True Vomiting Center, and interference with specific metabolic and enzymatic reactions.
- Indirect effects of chemotherapy on nutrition include interference with nutrient intake related to anorexia, fatigue, constipation, taste changes, and food aversions.

### Biotherapy/immunotherapy

- Biotherapy-induced fevers produce a direct increase in energy and fluid needs. Indirect influences, such as fatigue and flu-like symptoms, can make food procurement and preparation difficult.

## NORMAL NUTRITIONAL PHYSIOLOGY

- Nutritional status is a function of an energy exchange system made up of four compartments: the *reference compartment*, *set point*, *controller*, and *body storage*.
  - The reference compartment is the repository of the standards governing nutrient intake. The standards have physiological, psychological, and cultural determinants. These standards are monitored by the set point. The standards are maintained by the controller, largely through balancing energy intake and expenditure.
  - The result of the controller activity is the body storage, or body composition. The body storage provides feedback to the set point regarding its status via physiological, psychological, and cultural perceptions.

## PATHOPHYSIOLOGY

- Cancer, host response, and cancer treatment alter normal physiology.

### Cancer-Induced Changes in the Reference Compartment
#### Changes in appetite

- There is some evidence that loss of appetite is related to circulating factors produced by the cancer and/or the host.
- Cytokines have been proposed as one class of circulating anorectic agents. There is also support for an effect of serotonin and bombesin on appetite suppression, especially among individuals with carcinoid or lung cancers.
  - Animal studies support the importance of serotonin and ammonia as anorectics in cancer; studies in humans have been limited. Increased circulating lipids and lactic acid caused by tumor metabolism can also decrease appetite.
- Loss of appetite also may be precipitated by cancer-induced psychological distress.
- Increased appetite has been reported among women with breast cancer. Grindel suggests that increased as well as decreased appetite may occur as a function of psychological distress.

### Changes in taste and smell

- Altered taste and smell sensors, with loss of taste and olfactory cues, change the normal references that are part of appetite and intake.
  - Changes may be caused by direct tumor invasion; cancer-induced deficiencies in zinc, copper, nickel, vitamin A, and niacin; or cancer-associated circulating factors. Circulating factors are hypothesized sources of taste changes occurring early in the disease process.
  - Physiological increases in the recognition thresholds for sweet, sour, and salt and decreases in the recognition levels for bitter are common. These threshold changes can lead to meat and other food aversions.
  - Psychological factors may also contribute to food aversions.

### Changes in electrolyte balance

- Alterations in micronutrient availability occur in paraneoplastic syndromes. Cancer can cause hyper- and hypocalcemia, hyponatremia, and hypo- and hyperphosphatemia.

## Cancer-Induced Changes in the Controller
### Changes in energy expenditure

- Patients with cancer can have increased energy needs initiated by cancer-induced sepsis, fistulas, or lesions. These energy demands can produce malnutrition in some patients, but they are not responsible for cachexia.

### Changes in nutrient metabolism

- Cancer is associated with abnormalities in carbohydrate, protein, and lipid metabolism.
- Like diabetics, the individual with cancer has delayed glucose clearance, reduced glucose uptake in skeletal muscles, and an inability to produce glycogen in muscle. Unlike diabetics, individuals with cancer have normal plasma insulin levels. It is not known whether cancer patients also have normal insulin secretion.
- Increased hepatic glucose production has been reported in both undernourished and normal-weight cancer patients.
- In normal starvation, hepatic glucose production falls; this does not occur in cancer cachexia.
- Individuals with cancer may develop altered protein metabolism.
- In addition to the shunting of needed proteins to the cancer, there can be increased muscle break-down and hepatic protein activity. Despite the increased hepatic activity, protein synthesis does not match protein catabolism. The net result is increased whole-body protein turnover.
- Abnormal lipid metabolism noted in cancer includes increased lipid mobilization and turnover, elevated triglyceride levels, decreased lipogenesis, altered glycerol transport, and decreased lipoprotein lipase activity.

### Changes in the gastrointestinal tract

- Controller function is heavily dependent on an intact gastrointestinal system. Cancer can produce direct negative effects on the digestive system.
- The type and magnitude of the nutritional deficit depend on the tumor site and size.

### Changes in body storage

- The most striking change in body composition is seen in cachexia. The total body fat and skeletal muscle components can drop as much as 85% and 75%, respectively. Reduction in intracellular water and mineral supplies also occurs, although not to the same degree.

## Treatment-Induced Changes in the Reference Compartment

### Changes in appetite

- Depressed appetite can be caused by some biotherapeutic agents, notably tumor necrosis factor.
- Appetite loss can follow stimulation of the Chemoreceptor Trigger Zone and True Vomiting Center.
- Psychological responses to having and being treated for cancer can alter mood and change appetite.
- Medications prescribed for treatment also affect mood and appetite.
  - Corticosteroids, prescribed in both pediatric and adult populations, can increase appetite. Foltz suggests that chemotherapy reduces production of estradiol, a regulatory hormone for appetite, leading to increased appetite.
- Chemotherapy and radiation produce indirect effects on appetite through the induction of nausea, vomiting, and food aversions.
- Taste changes can follow head and neck surgery, radiation, and chemotherapy.

## Treatment-Induced Changes in the Controller

### Changes in energy expenditure

- Some biotherapeutic agents elicit shaking chills and fever, which increase energy demands.
- Antifungal agents administered to immunocompromised patients cause fever and chill responses.
- Nutritional needs increase as the body responds to repair damage induced by surgery, radiation, or chemotherapy.

### Changes in the gastrointestinal tract

- Surgical resection removes or bypasses areas of the aerodigestive or gastrointestinal tract. Chemotherapy and radiation cause direct injury to the intestinal villi, reducing the absorptive surface. These are major threats to the proper absorption of both macro- and micronutrients. Side effects of treatment include anorexia, nausea, vomiting, lactose intolerance, diarrhea, and constipation.
- Graft-versus-host disease—a complication of bone marrow transplantation—and radiation enteritis can lead to long-term patient dependence on parenteral nutritional support.

## CLINICAL MANIFESTATIONS

- The most common clinical manifestation identified with cancer is cancer cachexia, which is characterized by skeletal muscle wasting, weight loss, and reduced function.

## ASSESSMENT AND GRADING

- Nutritional assessment consists of four elements: anthropometrics, laboratory findings, clinical examination, and dietary evaluation.

## Anthropometrics

- *Anthropometrics,* the measurement of the weight, size, and proportions of the body, commonly includes height, weight, and skinfold thickness.
  - Weight, in combination with height, is an indirect measure of body composition.
  - The Metropolitan Life Insurance Company Height-Weight Table is a frequently used measure of nutritional status.
  - Weight and height can also be used to calculate the body mass index (BMI).

- The BMI has limited use in individuals with increased lean muscle mass or with large frames.
- The formula for BMI calculation is as follows: Weight in kilograms / height in meters squared.
- Another important function of the anthropometric measures of height and weight is their use in calculating an individual's caloric needs. Resting metabolic rate nomograms have been developed for this purpose. Formulas are also commonly used:
  - For women: = 655 + (9.6 x weight in kg) + (1.7 x height in cm) – (4.7 x age in years).
  - For men: 66 + (1.37 x weight in kg) + (5 x height in cm) – (6.8 x age in years)
- These equations indicate the number of calories expended while the individual is at rest, or the *resting energy expenditure* (REE). This number is corrected for the level of required energy. The level varies according to activity, treatment, and morbid condition.
- Despite the overall importance, practicality, and clinical relevance of weight and height measures in nutritional assessment, the reliability of both measures is questionable.
- Anthropometric measures of skinfold thickness and various body part circumferences assess fat and muscle compartments.
  - The basis for using skinfold measures lies in the fact that almost half of the body fat is located in subcutaneous tissue and is accessible for relatively straightforward measurement.
  - There are seven commonly identified skinfold measures. Thirty minutes or more may be necessary to complete measurement of all seven sites. However, the accuracy of body composition estimates is lower when fewer than five sites are used.
  - Use of skinfold thickness in people with a significant shift of fluid to the intracellular compartment will be misleading.

## Laboratory Tests

- A number of laboratory tests are commonly used to evaluate nutritional status.
- Several disease- and treatment-related variables exist that can cause abnormal values consistent with malnutrition.
- The tests are often not sensitive to nutritional deficiencies.

## Physical Examination

- The fact that physical changes such as glossitis, muscle wasting, or diarrhea exist in many cancer patients secondary to their disease or treatment does not minimize their usefulness as indicators of problems in energy intake, absorption, or need.
- Management of symptoms of nutritional disturbances in cancer can include medication, oral care, and specific nutritional counseling as opposed to the simple dietary supplementation with vitamins and protein-rich foods used to treat symptoms caused by inadequate intake of nutrients.
- Careful clinical examination is as sensitive in assessing nutritional status as are more expensive and labor-intensive assessment methods.

## Dietary Information

### Diet history

- In a full diet history, information that reflects both diet and general health is included.
- Dietary information is obtained using a number of approaches: 24-hour recall surveys, food frequency measures, diet diaries, calorie counts, or monthly purchase records.
- Questions about changes in weight over time provide a basis for estimating the magnitude and rapidity of any changes.
  - Percent weight change = (usual weight – actual weight) ÷ usual weight x 100.
  - Weight loss of 5% compared with usual weight is considered a sign of undernutrition. Greater than 25% loss reflects severe undernutrition.

- It is important to assess the length of time over which the weight loss occurred. A percent weight change of 2% in one week is much more ominous than the same degree of weight change over six months.
- A full diet history includes sociodemographic items, food preferences, religious restrictions, food allergies, past history of dieting, current drug therapy, activity, and measures of current intakes.

### 24-hour recall

- In a 24-hour dietary recall, the patient is asked to list all foods and beverages ingested, the time of consumption, preparation method, and an estimate of the amount consumed in the previous 24 hours.
- The reliability of the recall is also somewhat dependent on the interviewer's skill, as well as the patient's memory, accuracy of portion estimate, and willingness to list all foods and beverages ingested.
- The previous 24-hour intake may not be representative of usual intakes, especially among individuals who may be learning about or receiving care for cancer.

### Food frequency

- A food frequency record usually consists of a checklist of common foods, a portion estimate, and a frequency estimate. This method provides a broader picture of consumption than does the 24-hour recall and can be completed relatively rapidly.
- The accuracy of the data depends on the memory and truthfulness of the patient.

### Diet diary

- A diet diary is a list of all foods and beverages consumed for a period of three to seven days. The patient typically is asked to list time of consumption, food or beverage consumed, and a portion estimate.
- A diary's usefulness depends on the honesty of the person reporting and continued cooperation during the period of collection.

### Calorie count

- A calorie count is a useful method of estimating intakes while the patient is hospitalized.
- The accuracy of the count is dependent on the person observing and recording the intake.
- A calorie count of intake while hospitalized may not reflect the patient's intake outside the hospital.

## Functional Assessment

- Skeletal muscle strength is a sensitive indicator of both positive and negative changes in food intake.
- Muscle strength measures can be used to indicate both the degree of nutritional deficit and the effectiveness of nutritional intervention.

## Nutritional Screening Methods

- The Nutritional Screening Initiative has developed a screening history that provides a numerical score converted into categories of zero, moderate, and high nutritional risk.
- The Subjective Global Assessment (SGA) evaluates weight change, dietary intake changes, gastrointestinal symptoms lasting more than two weeks, and activity levels.
- The patient's diagnosis and the results from a focused physical examination are included.
  - The clinician subjectively categorizes the patient as well-nourished, having moderate or suspected malnutrition, or being severely malnourished.

- The SGA has been favorably compared with strictly objective measures in predicting infection susceptibility.
- A modified assessment includes more cancer-specific symptoms and a refinement of the activity level estimation.
- A number of formulas integrate several objective measures into assessment of nutritional risk: the Nutritional Index (NI), the Prognostic Nutritional Index (PNI), the Hospital Prognostic Index (HPI), and the Nutrition Risk Index (NRI). These indexes are especially helpful in identifying which individuals undergoing head and neck or gastrointestinal surgery might benefit from nutritional intervention prior to and following operation.

## Nutrition-Related Symptom Assessment

- Assessment of symptoms that interfere with intake is part of an oncological nutritional assessment. These symptoms include anorexia, nausea, vomiting, diarrhea, constipation, mouth sores, dry mouth, pain when eating or swallowing, other pain, taste change, fatigue, difficulty in swallowing, indigestion, early satiety, cramping, and bloating.

## Summary

- The nurse is in the best position to determine the risk for malnutrition and to pursue further assessment.

## THERAPEUTIC APPROACHES AND NURSING CARE
### Introduction

- Both deficiency and oversufficiency malnutrition have been associated with increased morbidity and mortality rates among individuals with cancer. This finding suggests that nutritional intervention should reduce morbidity and mortality in the cancer population. Although this is true for some people, it is not true for others.
  - Positive outcomes can be expected for most individuals when the cancer is curable, the problems are due to treatment, or the deficit is mechanical.
  - However, for other individuals, methods that reverse the nutritional deficits caused by the cancer and the host-cancer interaction are ineffective. This reality makes the prescription of nutritional intervention complex.
- The nutritional prescription for any individual with cancer is best made with input from several disciplines. A nutritional team with expertise in cancer-associated malnutrition is optimal.
  - When such specialization is not present, an approach to nutritional intervention can be determined with collaboration of nurses, physicians, dietitians, and, when needed, pharmacists, speech therapists, and social workers. The patient and family or significant others are an integral part of the effort.

## Nutritional Interventions

- The level of intervention is dictated by the patient's baseline nutritional state, disease status, risks for malnutrition from treatment, anticipated response to therapy, and resources.
- Intervention must also be based on realistic goals.
- For patients in whom response to treatment is expected or for whom morbidity will be reduced, intervention is a sound practice.
- Often, family members concentrate on the patient's lack of appetite and weight loss, which can put undue stress on the patient and the family relationship.
- Advising both the patient and the family that emphasis on eating does not improve survival may allow them to put their energies elsewhere.

## Nutritional Prescription

### Alteration in single dietary components

- In cancer patients nutrient deficits arise from a combination of chemotherapy-related effects on bone marrow, anemia of chronic disease or from medications for comorbid conditions and/or antibiotic use.
- Other deficiencies that are more specific to cancer include hypomagnesemia related to platinum chemotherapy; hyponatremia and hypercalcemia, resulting from paraneoplastic syndromes; and zinc deficiency. Medication commonly is used to control these problems; however, dietary manipulation may be a supplemental treatment requiring education of the patient about foods high in potassium or zinc.
- A target for specific intervention is dietary fat intake.
  - Fat-intervention trials indicate that with verbal counseling, individuals can decrease fat intake to desired levels within three months.

### Alteration in total nutrient intake

#### Nutrient interventions

- A major emphasis has been on improving the patient's overall intake and nutritional status to minimize treatment side effects and maximize treatment delivery. Verbal counseling, use of supplements, enteral feedings, parenteral nutrition, and combinations of nutritional interventions have been used for this purpose.
- Enteral feeding maintains the normal stimulation of enzymatic and mucosal activity in the gut, which is not accomplished with parenteral nutrition. When oral intake is not sufficient or is contraindicated, and the gastrointestinal tract is functioning, enteral feeding is the intervention of choice. For individuals without a functioning gastrointestinal tract or who need rapid repletion, total parenteral nutrition (TPN) may be the nutritional treatment of choice. TPN reduces morbidity in malnourished patients undergoing surgery. Patients with significant gastrointestinal malfunction, but otherwise with cured, controlled, or indolent disease, may also benefit from parenteral feeding. The largest group of cancer patients receiving home parenteral nutrition are those with severe enteritis following curative radiation treatment.
- Although subsets of patients benefit from nutritional repletion, aggressive nutritional intervention does not alter morbidity or mortality for the majority of individuals with cancer.
- The problems and common solutions associated with enteral and parenteral nutritional interventions are listed in Tables 24-14 and 24-15, text page 675.

#### Pharmacological interventions

- Taking medicine has been rated as one of the most effective self-care techniques in controlling constipation, diarrhea, nausea, vomiting, and mucosal irritation.
- For the most part, cancer-associated nutritional problems are best reversed by successful treatment of the malignancy. In treatment-induced changes, medication and self-care actions are usually helpful.
- Medications commonly used to counter loss of appetite include alcohol, corticosteroids, megestrol acetate, metoclopramide, and delta-9-tetrahydrocannabinol (THC).
- Psychotropic drugs also may assist those patients for whom depression is a factor in diminished appetite.
- The beneficial effect of corticosteroids is seen especially in individuals with asthenia and those with tumor-induced fever.
  - These drugs should be avoided in diabetics and in those who might be at added risk of infection.

- Megestrol acetate has been found to improve appetite, cause weight gain, control nausea, and improve quality of life among individuals with cancer.
  - The drug comes in a liquid form, reducing the mechanical problem of the patient having to swallow a number of tablets.
  - Side effects include edema and hyperglycemia, with some increase in risk of an embolism.
  - Because of this, megestrol acetate should be avoided in individuals with congestive heart failure, pericardial effusions, or a history of thrombotic problems.
  - Diabetics should monitor themselves closely, especially during initiation of treatment.
- Metoclopramide has been used to improve oral intake based on its effect on nausea and on gastric motility.
  - Metoclopramide increases gastric motility and can reduce early satiety and minimize reflux.
  - The drug has also been used to reduce chemotherapy-related nausea.
- THC, like metoclopramide, has been explored largely in terms of its effect on chemotherapy-induced nausea and vomiting.
  - Effectiveness may be greater in individuals who have used the drug before.
  - Side effects are more common in older persons, especially at higher doses, and may be reduced with timing administration of the drug after a meal.

### Nonpharmacological interventions

- Patient education material commonly includes interventions for decreased appetite, nausea, vomiting, constipation, and taste changes. See Table 24-16, text page 677, for nonpharmacological interventions to treat these side effects. There has been little research exploring the effectiveness of most of these actions.

### Questionable cancer nutritional interventions

- An unknown number of individuals with cancer use questionable cancer therapies.
- Nutritional approaches are the most commonly used questionable treatments and include metabolic, macrobiotic, and megavitamin therapy. The oncology nurse must be alert to patient usage of these therapies because some have significant side effects.

## CONCLUSION

- The connection between nutrition and health is especially important in oncology, because nutrition influences carcinogenesis itself as well as the quantity and quality of life once the disease exists.
- The nurse can attend to basic nutritional information during the diagnostic process.
- Given this base, the nurse can work with other care providers to prioritize and define nutritional care.
- Early nutritional intervention, when the tumor burden is relatively small, has the best chance to alter patient outcomes.
- Appropriate nutritional intervention reduces morbidity, length of hospital stay, and possibly mortality in these patients.

## PRACTICE QUESTIONS

**Questions 1–4 deal with Betty, who is receiving adjuvant chemotherapy for breast cancer.**

1. Betty is one of your patients who is receiving adjuvant chemotherapy for her breast cancer. She is near her ideal weight when she begins treatment. Given what you know of patients similar to Betty, which of the following is something you might explain to her during her nutritional assessment?
   a. The majority of women with breast cancer who do not receive chemotherapy lose weight.
   b. The majority of women with breast cancer who receive chemotherapy gain weight.
   c. Gaining weight, or overnutrition, is not known to be harmful for women undergoing treatment.
   d. none of the above

2. A little later in your assessment of Betty, she asks you why you are concerned with undernutrition in her case. You tell Betty that she has _____ of the two major physical risk factors for undernutrition in all cancer patients: _____.
   a. one; having the disease.
   b. both; having the disease and dealing with psychological distress.
   c. both; having the disease and being treated for it.
   d. one; receiving chemotherapy.

3. Because of Betty's questions, you decide to do some research to find out how and why chemotherapy causes an effect on nutrition. In your reading, you learn all but which of the following?
   a. Chemotherapy can indirectly cause food aversions.
   b. Chemotherapy can alter the intestinal absorptive surface.
   c. Chemotherapy does not interfere with specific metabolic reactions.
   d. Chemotherapy may cause excitation of the True Vomiting Center.

4. Betty will be going in for surgery in several weeks. In planning ahead and helping her to get ready for the surgery, you tell her that:
   a. surgery, because of the bed rest required in recovery, will decrease her energy requirements.
   b. nutritional problems resulting from her surgery will probably extend well past the immediate perioperative period.
   c. she should not be too concerned; surgery on her breast cancer should not have any direct involvement in her nutritional needs.
   d. surgery can increase her energy requirements 1.5 times what she normally needs.

**Questions 5–11 deal with Charles, a diabetic patient with lung cancer.**

5. Charles is one of your patients with lung cancer. Because he is diabetic and already well under his ideal weight, one of your major concerns is providing Charles with adequate nutrition and preventing cachexia. You are dismayed to learn that he "lost his appetite" when he recently received his diagnosis and almost entirely stopped eating. Which of the following is probably *not* a factor that would have contributed to the loss of appetite?
   a. circulating cycotines
   b. cancer-induced sepsis
   c. psychological distress
   d. bombesin

6. When you give Charles a complete assessment, you find that he is suffering from anorexia, skeletal muscle atrophy, and asthenia. His hepatic glucose production is at normal levels, perhaps even a bit higher. What is your diagnosis?
   a. primary cachexia
   b. secondary cachexia
   c. starvation
   d. marasmus

7. In a case like Charles's, the total body fat and skeletal muscle components can drop as much as _____ and _____ respectively.
   a. 20%; 30%
   b. 50%; 40%
   c. 85%; 75%
   d. 60%; 80%

8. In trying to determine how much weight Charles has lost over what span of time, you learn that he is 5 feet 10 inches tall and weighed 170 pounds one year ago. Three months ago, he weighed 160 pounds, and now he weighs 132 pounds. What is the percentage of Charles's weight change in the past three months?
   a. 17%
   b. 23%
   c. 22%
   d. 7%

9. You are attempting to choose an instrument to gain a more complete diet history from Charles. He has already told you that he doesn't pay much attention to what he eats, and he has a hard time remembering what he had for lunch (or if he had lunch) yesterday. Charles is very upset about his recent diagnosis, and this has changed his eating habits considerably. However, he is willing to cooperate with you, and he understands the importance of being honest in the things he tells you. Keeping in mind that Charles is in the hospital now, but he will not be for most of his treatment, you choose:
   a. a calorie count.
   b. 24-hour dietary recall.
   c. a food frequency record.
   d. a diet diary.

10. When you speak with Charles's mother, she tells you that she understands that Charles has lost too much weight recently. An obese woman herself, she is tremendously worried about Charles's loss of appetite. You tell her that:
   a. she should encourage Charles to eat as much as possible.
   b. she should try not to worry; Charles's nutritional deficits will go away after his treatment is complete.
   c. she should try not to worry; Charles's eating more is not what determines his survival.
   d. she should provide Charles with a high-protein diet.

11. Charles asks you for an appetite stimulant, and considering his condition, you are quite happy to find something appropriate for him. Keeping in mind that Charles is on an extensive chemotherapy regimen, he is diabetic, and he has not had problems with nausea or vomiting, which of the following drugs is the best possible intervention for him?
    a. corticosteroids
    b. megestrol acetate
    c. metoclopramide
    d. THC

12. One of your patients, Sean, has been participating in professional athletics for several years. At 170 pounds, he weighs far more than he should for his height of 5 feet 6 inches, but he does not appear to be overweight. In trying to determine whether you should counsel Sean to reduce his caloric and fat intake, you decide to use a(n) _____ to determine his percentage of body fat.
    a. body mass index
    b. resting metabolic nomogram
    c. skinfold measure
    d. REE

13. When considering which laboratory tests for evaluating nutritional status would be best to use with patients like Charles, Sean, and Betty, which of the following is *not* a consideration?
    a. Oncology patients may have disease variables that can cause abnormal values.
    b. Several of the tests can harm patients undergoing chemotherapy.
    c. Some tests are not sensitive to nutritional deficiencies.
    d. A number of the tests are fairly expensive.

14. Cancer-associated nutritional problems, rather than treatment-related nutritional problems, are best reversed by:
    a. extensive verbal counseling.
    b. self-care actions.
    c. medications.
    d. successful treatment of the tumor.

15. At what stage does nutritional intervention have the best chance to alter patient outcome?
    a. early, when the tumor burden is small
    b. later, when the malignancy is aggressive
    c. during treatment
    d. after treatment has ended

## ANSWER EXPLANATIONS

1. **The answer is b.** The majority of women who receive adjuvant chemotherapy for breast cancer do gain weight. There is no evidence to support the idea that women with breast cancer who do not receive chemotherapy will lose weight, and there is some evidence to indicate that women who are obese may have a poorer survival rate than women who are not. (p. 657)

2. **The answer is c.** Betty, like all cancer patients, is at risk for undernutrition because she has cancer and because she is being treated for it. Although it is true that cancer has a strong psychological impact on those diagnosed with it, various cancers and treatments also have a direct—though not always understood—physical impact on nutrition. (p. 657)

3.  **The answer is c.** Chemotherapy does interfere with specific metabolic and enzymatic reactions, as well as causing excitation of the True Vomiting Center, alteration of intestinal absorptive surface and, indirectly, food aversions. (p. 659)

4.  **The answer is d.** Surgery can increase energy requirements by 1.5 times the normal dietary requirements. Betty can be somewhat reassured by the fact that her cancer is not in the aerodigestive or gastrointestinal tract because she is likely to have nutritional problems resulting from the surgery only in the immediate perioperative period. (p. 658)

5.  **The answer is b.** Cancer-induced sepsis initiates an increase of energy needs, which might or might not bring about an increase of appetite, but which would *not* contribute to loss of appetite. All of the rest of these factors—bombesin, cytokines, and psychological distress—could produce a loss of appetite. (p. 660)

6.  **The answer is a.** Charles is suffering from primary cachexia. Secondary cachexia is caused by mechanical effects of the tumor or treatment—unlikely in Charles's case because he is suffering from lung cancer. Simple starvation and marasmus are not indicated when hepatic glucose production is at normal levels. (p. 657)

7.  **The answer is c.** In cachexia, body fat can drop as much as 85% and skeletal muscle can drop as much as 75%. (p. 662)

8.  **The answer is a.** The percentage of Charles's weight change can be determined by subtracting his actual weight from his usual weight and dividing the result by the usual weight. This number is multiplied by 100 to get the actual percentage. (p. 667)

9.  **The answer is d.** Because Charles's eating habits have changed considerably and because he is not going to be staying in the hospital for most of his treatment, both the calorie count method and the 24-hour recall method are inappropriate. A food frequency would not be ideal because Charles has a hard time remembering what he ate. A diet diary would provide you with an extended record of Charles's eating habits that would rely on his cooperation and honesty—both of which you feel you can count on. (p. 668)

10. **The answer is c.** Charles's mother should try not to worry over his food intake. Charles is suffering from anorexia and cachexia, and the emphasis on eating does not improve survival rates. (p. 670)

11. **The answer is b.** Corticosteroids are not indicated in Charles's case because he is a diabetic, and both metoclopramide and THC are indicated in cases of a patient experiencing chemotherapy-induced nausea—which Charles is *not* experiencing. Even though diabetics taking megestrol acetate must monitor themselves closely, the drug is indicated in this case because it increases appetite, causes weight gain, and improves quality of life. (p. 676)

12. **The answer is c.** The skinfold measure, if taken in all seven sites, can produce a fairly accurate measure of body composition. However, if less than five of the sites are used, the accuracy is lowered. (p. 664)

13. **The answer is b.** Tests for evaluating the nutritional status of oncology patients might respond to disease- and treatment-related variables by offering abnormal values; they might not be sensitive to nutritional deficiencies, and they might be quite expensive. The commonly used assesment tests are not dangerous to patients undergoing chemotherapy. (p. 665)

14. **The answer is d.** Treatment-induced nutritional problems are often successfully handled by medication and self-care actions. Cancer-associated nutritional problems are best resolved by successful treatment of the malignancy. (p. 675)

15. **The answer is a.** Early nutritional intervention, while the tumor burden is still small, has the best chance to alter patient outcomes. (p. 678)

# Chapter 25     Hypercalcemia

---

## INTRODUCTION

### Incidence

- Primary hyperparathyroidism and malignancy are responsible for 90% of all cases of hypercalcemia. Although the majority of cases of hypercalcemia are associated with hyperparathyrodism, malignancy-associated hypercalcemia remains a challenging clinical problem.
- Hypercalcemia of malignancy is usually progressive, causes unpleasant symptoms, can cause the patient to deteriorate rapidly, and may be the cause of death in some patients.

### Definition

- Hypercalcemia is considered to exist when the serum calcium level exceeds 11.0 mg/dl (2.75 mmol/l).

## PHYSIOLOGY OF CALCIUM HOMEOSTASIS

- The majority of calcium (99%) is found in bone combined with phosphate. The remaining 1% is divided evenly in the plasma between protein-bound and freely ionized forms. It is the freely ionized form that is biologically active.

### Normal Calcium Homeostasis

- Extracellular calcium levels are maintained within a narrow range, primarily through the effects of three systemic hormones: parathyroid hormone (PTH), 1,25-dihydroxyvitamin D (the major biologically active metabolite of vitamin D), and calcitonin.
- The ability to control extracellular calcium levels is influenced primarily by the rate of calcium absorption from the intestine and the kidney's threshold for calcium resorption.
- Renal regulation of calcium is controlled by PTH and 1,25-dihydroxyvitamin D.

#### Calcitonin

- Secreted by thyroid parafollicular cells, calcitonin inhibits bone resorption and thus acts as a counterregulator to PTH.
- Calcitonin can be an important inhibitor of bone resorption in pathological states.

#### Parathyroid hormone

- Secreted by the parathyroid gland, PTH prevents serum calcium concentration from falling below the normal level directly by stimulating bone resorption and calcium liberation from the bony matrix and by calcium resorption in the renal tubules, and indirectly by influencing intestinal calcium absorption.
- The primary role of PTH on the kidney appears to be maintenance of extracellular calcium levels.
- Since phosphate resorption is inversely related to calcium resorption, PTH's actions in the proximal tubule are directed at inhibition of water, sodium, calcium, bicarbonate, and phosphate resorption.
- PTH-mediated resorption of calcium occurs in the ascending limb of Henle's loop and in the distal tubule.

- In the skeleton, PTH plays a mediating role in bone resorption by stimulating the number and activity of bone osteoclasts, leading to the release of calcium and phosphate into the circulation.

### 1,25-dihydroxyvitamin D

- 25-hydroxyvitamin D is the major circulating and storage form of vitamin D.

### Homeostatic responses to increased calcium loads

- With an increased extracellular fluid calcium load, the secretion of PTH is suppressed; this decreases physiological calcium release from bone and inhibits intestinal calcium resorption.
- In addition, decreased PTH results in increased urinary calcium excretion.
- Once compensatory mechanisms are exceeded, renal insufficiency enhances calcium resorption and phosphate wasting in the proximal tubule, further exacerbating the development of hypercalcemia and renal failure.

### The role of bone in calcium homeostasis

- Skeletal bone serves as the body's calcium reservoir.
- In disease states skeletal calcium plays a larger role in extracellular calcium levels.
- There are two mechanisms through which skeletal calcium can enter extracellular fluid: bone remodeling and calcium exchange between the bone surface and extracellular fluid.

### Bone remodeling

- The bone cells primarily concerned with *bone remodeling* are the osteoclasts, osteocytes, and osteoblasts.
- The action of PTH promotes the cellular differentiation of osteocytes, osteoblasts, and their precursors, while 1,25-dihydroxyvitamin D promotes the differentiation and fusion of osteoclasts.
- An elevated serum alkaline phosphatase indicates osteoblastic activity, which can be seen in states of high bone turnover: Paget's disease, prostate cancer with blastic skeletal involvement, or healing of a bone fracture.

## Pathophysiology

- Disruption of normal calcium homeostasis is caused by the action of tumor-produced factors on bone, kidney, and intestine.
- The two primary pathophysiological defects are enhanced osteoclastic bone resorption, and the ability of the kidney to excrete extracellular calcium.
- Our current understanding of MAHC is that there are two primary syndromes: humoral hypercalcemia of malignancy (HHM) and local osteolytic hypercalcemia (LOH).

### Parathyroid hormone-related protein and humoral hypercalcemia of malignancy

- Parathyroid hormone-related protein (PTHrP) is the major mediator of hypercalcemia of malignancy and is responsible for 80%–90% of all cases of MAHC. PTHrP is the primary cause of hypercalcemia in solid tumors without bone metastases.
- The hypercalcemic effect of PTHrP is related to increased bone resorption, increased renal tubular, calcium resorption, and phosphate wasting.

### Other osteolytic factors

- The cause of hypercalcemia in cancer patients with skeletal metastases is thought to be related to three cellular mediators of osteolysis: osteoclasts, tumor-associated macrophages, and cancer cells.

The activities of these cellular mediators are influenced by the presence of one or more of the osteoclast-activating cytokines and growth factors.

### Local osteolytic hypercalcemia

- The bone matrix, which contains growth factors and cytokines, is ideal for the development of bone metastases. The development of bone metastases appears to be dependent on the presence of osteoclast-activating factors such as PTHrP.

### Breast cancer

- In breast cancer patients with hypercalcemia and bone metastases, 70%-80% will have elevated circulating levels of PTHrP and 50% will have raised urinary cyclic AMP levels, indicating an important role for PTHrP-induced hypercalcemia even when bone metastases are present.
- Hypercalcemia occurs in up to 40% of women with breast cancer.
- In hypercalcemia extensive bone metastases are almost always present.
- Osteoclast activation is the major mechanism associated with hypercalcemia.
- Some women with estrogen receptor-positive metastatic breast cancer treated with estrogens or antiestrogens suddenly develop hypercalcemia that may be associated with bone pain within one month of starting estrogens, androgens, or tamoxifen.
- *Tumor flare* is associated with a temporary period of accelerated tumor growth shortly after beginning additive hormonal therapy.
  - Tumor flare is generally self-limiting and is thought to indicate a hormonally responsive tumor.

### Hematologic malignancies

- Hypercalcemia is more common in myeloma than in any other hematologic malignancy and can be either a presenting symptom or an indicator of terminal disease.
- Intractable bone pain is a prominent presenting symptom in 80% of patients.
- Hypercalcemia in myeloma can be expected whenever patients become bedridden and may be caused by or contribute to renal failure.
- In myeloma the cause is increased bone resorption and decreased glomerular filtration.
- Hypercalcemia in myeloma always occurs in the presence of extensive bone destruction occurring adjacent to collections of myeloma cells.
- HTLV-I and HTLV-II-associated adult T-cell lymphoma/leukemias (ATLL) are frequently associated with hypercalcemia, occurring in as many as 50% of patients.

### Other factors

- Local mechanical forces such as weight bearing are important to stimulate osteoblast function and bone formation.
- Passive range-of-motion exercises are not helpful in preventing hypercalcemia. Weight bearing is more important.

## CLINICAL MANIFESTATIONS

## Signs and Symptoms

### Gastrointestinal

- Anorexia, nausea, vomiting, abdominal pain, and constipation are early and common symptoms of hypercalcemia.
- The development of obstipation and ileus are late findings associated with high serum calcium levels and are probably exacerbated by dehydration.

### Neuromuscular

- Initial CNS dysfunction can present as personality changes, impaired concentration, mild confusion, drowsiness, and lethargy.
- Neuromuscular involvement is primarily neuropathic, involving decreased muscle strength, a decrease in respiratory muscular capacity, and hypotonia, usually with severe hypercalcemia.

### Renal

- Hypercalcemia interferes with the action of ADH; subsequent volume contraction decreases the glomerular filtration rate (GFR). Decreased GFR stimulates sodium and water reabsorption in the proximal tubule.

### Cardiovascular

- Hypercalcemia results in bradycardia.
- Significant dysrhythmias may also occur, particularly in patients taking digitalis. Digitalis toxicity may be potentiated.

## Laboratory Assessment

- An elevated serum calcium (corrected for abnormal protein albumin values) is diagnostic for hypercalcemia.
- Calcium is found in the serum in three forms: 45% protein-bound (primarily to albumin), 45% freely ionized, and 10% complexed to ions such as sulfate, phosphate, or citrate. It is the freely ionized form that is biologically active.
- The more common finding in individuals with cancer is hypoalbuminemia, in which more calcium may be ionized as a result of low levels of serum albumin available for binding. When ionized calcium levels are not available, total serum calcium levels can be corrected to more accurately reflect the true serum calcium. (See formula, text page 694.)

## TREATMENT

- Most important initially is improving renal calcium excretion by correcting those factors impairing renal function, usually dehydration and diminished GFR.
- Second, bone resorption must be stopped either by eliminating the primary cause or by inhibiting osteoclast function.
- Unless the primary tumor or skeletal metastases can be controlled, all antihypercalcemia interventions tend to be palliative.
- Most pharmacological interventions are directed at osteoclast inhibition and thus do little to modify the increased renal tubular calcium resorption caused by PTHrP in HHM.
- To correct the two major pathophysiological alterations of hypercalcemia,—impaired renal calcium excretion and increased osteoclastic bone resorption—the cornerstones of therapy are hydration and saline diuresis followed by inhibition of osteoclast function.
- The bisphosphonates, plicamycin, calcitonin, and gallium nitrate are all osteoclast inhibitors.
- Once rehydration has been established, initiation of bisphosphonate therapy is useful in the outpatient setting for treatment of hypercalcemia, prevention of bone pain, skeletal fractures, and maintenance of normocalcemia.

## General Measures

- Initial measures should involve correcting volume contraction and removing factors that may exacerbate hypercalcemia, such as thiazide diuretics, vitamins A and D, and, in some breast cancer patients, hormonal agents.
- Medications whose actions are potentiated by hypercalcemia, such as digoxin, should be adjusted.

## Hydration and Saline Diuresis

- The initial step in hypercalcemic therapy is to expand volume, correct dehydration and renal insufficiency, and promote calciuresis.
- Measurement of fluid intake and output and body weight, as well as frequent assessment for signs of fluid overload, are important.
- Hypokalemia, hypomagnesemia, hypophosphatemia, and hyperosmolar states may occur with high fluid volumes.

## Loop Diuretics

- Mild to moderate hypercalcemia can usually be managed by saline diuresis alone.
- Once rehydration and improvement in renal function have been achieved, inhibition of osteoclastic bone resorption must be attained.
- Although antitumor therapy is the treatment of choice when available, pharmacological inhibition of bone resorption is usually indicated in order to prevent the movement of calcium from bone into extracellular fluid.

## Bisphosphonates

- The bisphosphonates are effective inhibitors of osteoclast bone resorption.
- A second-generation bisphosphonate, pamidronate, is widely used and is efficacious in inhibiting osteolysis-related sequelae of metastatic bone disease.

### Etidronate

- Etidronate has been shown to be more effective than either saline hydration alone or calcitonin after saline hydration.

### Pamidronate

- Pamidronate has been demonstrated to be more effective than etidronate. It is given intravenous over 2–4 hours every 3 weeks.

### Clodronate

- Clodronate has been reported to have an 80% complete response rate with onset of effect by day 3.

### Third-generation bisphosphonates

- Alendronate, neridronate, amifostine, tiludronate, YM175, and BM 21.0955 are all third-generation bisphosphonates with higher potency levels than first- and second-generation bisphosphonates.

## Calcitonin

- Calcitonin produces transient inhibition of bone resorption through its direct effects on osteoclast formation. Calcitonin also acts directly on the kidney to promote urinary calcium excretion and can be used safely in patients with dehydration or renal failure.

- Unfortunately, inhibition of bone resorption is short, and tachyphylaxis or "escape" from therapeutic effect limits its usefulness.

## Glucocorticoids

- Glucocorticoids (prednisone and hydrocortisone) are most effective in hypercalcemia associated with multiple myeloma, other hematologic diseases, and sometimes breast carcinoma.
- Glucocorticoids used alone are not as effective as when used with calcitonin.

## Plicamycin

- Plicamycin (mithramycin) is a cytotoxic drug with antihypercalcemic effects.
- Use of this agent is recommended only when other less toxic regimens have failed.

## Phosphates

- Phosphates prevent intestinal calcium absorption.
- In addition, phosphates inhibit mineral and bone matrix resorption.

## Prostaglandin Inhibitors

- Aspirin, indomethacin, and nonsteroidal antiinflammatory drugs have been tried, but only on occasion is there an antihypercalcemic response.

## Gallium Nitrate

- Gallium nitrate has been found to inhibit bone resorption and restore normocalcemia with few side effects in 75%–85% of patients.
- A major disadvantage to the use of gallium nitrate is the five-day continuous treatment regimen, which makes outpatient treatment inconvenient.

## PRACTICE QUESTIONS

1. Which of the following types of malignancies is *least* likely to be associated with hypercalcemia?
   a. lung cancer
   b. breast cancer
   c. multiple myeloma
   d. colon cancer

2. The pathophysiology of hypercalcemia involves a combination of two factors—bone resorption and:
   a. decreased renal calcium clearance.
   b. increased osteoclast activity.
   c. increased glomerular function.
   d. decreased availability of ionized calcium.

3. Control of extracellular calcium levels within a narrow range is achieved through the action of several agents, including all of the following *except*:
   a. parathyroid hormone (PTH), which controls renal regulation of calcium.
   b. 1,25-dihydroxyvitamin D, which controls intestinal calcium absorption.
   c. calcitonin.
   d. glucocorticoids, which control osteoclast activity.

4. How does the body typically respond to elevated levels of extracellular calcium?
   a. by reducing PTH secretion
   b. by increasing bone resorption
   c. by increasing renal synthesis of 1,25-dihydroxyvitamin D
   d. by decreasing urinary calcium excretion

5. The location and frequency of bone remodeling activity is controlled by several factors, including all of the following *except*:
   a. local factors such as prostaglandins, regulatory proteins, and constituents of the organic matrix.
   b. mechanical factors such as weight bearing.
   c. skeletal calcium, which couples bone resorption and bone formation.
   d. osteotropic hormones, especially PTH and 1,25-dihydroxyvitamin D.

6. Factors that are produced by tumors themselves have been implicated in malignancy-associated hypercalcemia. Probably the most important of these circulating tumor-produced, or humoral, factors is:
   a. prostaglandin.
   b. PTH-like factor.
   c. bisphosphonate.
   d. osteoclast-activating factor.

7. A patient is found to have a large tumor mass associated with high levels of PTH-related protein but normal levels of 1,25-dihydroxyvitamin D and normal intestinal absorption rates. Bone absorption is found to exceed bone formation. The most likely diagnosis is:
   a. primary hyperparathyroidism.
   b. multiple myeloma.
   c. humoral hypercalcemia of malignancy (HHM).
   d. Hodgkin's disease.

8. Which of the following statements about the association between breast cancer and hypercalcemia is correct?
    a. Bone resorption in breast cancer patients is probably due to cancer cells directly rather than to PGE mediation.
    b. Tumor flare is thought to be the result of PGE inhibition by breast cancer cells.
    c. Not all patients with metastases develop hypercalcemia, although most breast cancer patients with hypercalcemia have widespread skeletal metastases.
    d. Hypercalcemia in breast cancer patients is usually responsive to prostaglandin inhibitors.

9. The symptoms of hypercalcemia in cancer patients are best described as:
    a. similar to those of acute renal failure.
    b. easily identified but difficult to treat.
    c. distinct from those of end-stage disease.
    d. numerous, vague, and nonspecific.

10. Among the common early symptoms in hypercalcemic patients are all of the following *except*:
    a. nausea and vomiting.
    b. diarrhea.
    c. hypertension.
    d. polyuria.

11. The most important initial treatment of hypercalcemia is:
    a. improving renal calcium excretion.
    b. treating the primary tumor.
    c. inhibiting osteoclast function.
    d. inhibiting bone resorption.

12. A loop diuretic such as furosemide would be used in the treatment of hypercalcemia in order to:
    a. rehydrate the patient.
    b. correct electrolyte imbalance.
    c. enhance calcium excretion.
    d. increase bone resorption.

13. A patient with multiple myeloma and compromised cardiac and renal function is diagnosed as hypercalcemic. Of the following treatments, the one most likely to be administered is:
    a. saline diuresis.
    b. intravenous injection of inorganic phosphates.
    c. plicamycin.
    d. calcitonin with glucocorticoids.

14. A patient with acute hypercalcemia may need treatment that rapidly decreases extracellular calcium concentration. Of the following agents, the one most likely to be administered under these emergency circumstances is:
    a. plicamycin.
    b. bisphosphonates.
    c. phosphates.
    d. prostaglandin inhibitors.

## ANSWER EXPLANATIONS

1. **The answer is d.** Patients with lung and breast cancer account for the highest percentage of malignancy-induced hypercalcemia. This high frequency is related to the high overall incidence of these two types of cancers. However, multiple myeloma, which is relatively rare, is the underlying cause in 10% of malignancy-associated hypercalcemia cases. (p. 685)

2. **The answer is a.** Hypercalcemia is characterized by excess extracellular calcium. This condition results from bone resorption—the release of skeletal calcium into serum—and from the failure of the kidneys to clear extracellular calcium. As calcium levels rise, symptoms of hypercalcemia appear. (pp. 688 and 690)

3. **The answer is d.** Glucocorticoids, including prednisone and hydrocortisone, are used to treat hypercalcemia. They are not part of the body's normal homeostatic mechanism that regulates serum calcium. PTH and 1,25-dihydroxyvitamin D exert their effects by controlling movement of calcium across bone, kidney, and small intestine. PTH's action on the kidney occurs through the formulation and action of NcAMP, which acts as a second messenger influencing calcium transport. (pp. 686–687, 697)

4. **The answer is a.** The body's homeostatic response to increased calcium loads involves suppression of PTH, which decreases bone resorption and inhibits intestinal calcium absorption. This inhibitory effect occurs as a result of decreased renal synthesis of 1,25-dihydroxyvitamin D and increased urinary calcium excretion. The calcium load is cleared principally by the kidney. (p. 686)

5. **The answer is c.** Bone remodeling, the process of bone formation and resorption, involves three types of bone cells: osteoblasts, osteocytes, and osteoclasts. Incitement of bone remodeling is thought to be directed at the osteocyte. Bone remodeling is said to be coupled; bone resorption is coupled with bone formation. Uncoupling refers to the failure of bone formation to follow the resorption process. Bone remodeling activity is influenced by mechanical factors such as weight bearing, by the activity of osteotropic hormones, and by local factors such as prostaglandins, regulatory proteins, and constituents of the organic matrix. (p. 688)

6. **The answer is b.** Malignancy-associated hypercalcemia is a complex metabolic complication in which bone resorption exceeds both bone formation and the kidney's ability to excrete extracellular calcium. Both humoral and local factors have been implicated in this process. Humoral, or tumor-produced, circulating factors include a PTH-like factor, transforming growth factors (TGF-alpha), and 1,25-dihydroxyvitamin D. Hypercalcemia that develops in patients with solid tumors without bone metastases, including HHM, is thought to be due to PTH-like factor. (p. 690)

7. **The answer is c.** In humoral hypercalcemia of malignancy (HHM), patients secrete high levels of PPTH-related protein but have normal levels of 1,25-dihydroxyvitamin D and normal intestinal absorption rates. Osteoblastic and osteoclastic activities are "uncoupled" so that bone resorption exceeds bone formation. Hypercalcemia and hypercalciuria thus occur. Conversely, in primary hyperparathyroidism a parathyroid adenoma secretes excessive PTH, which stimulates intestinal and renal calcium absorption. Bone remodeling is accelerated, with a "coupled" increase in both osteoclastic and osteoblastic activity. Hypercalcemia occurs as a result of the combined action of PTH and 1,25-dihydroxyvitamin D on the kidney and 1,25-dihydroxyvitamin D on the gut. (p. 690)

8. **The answer is c.** Bone resorption in breast cancer patients is probably due to PGE-mediated osteolysis rather than direct bone resorption. Tumor flare is thought to indicate the release of PGE by a hormonally responsive tumor. Hypercalcemia in breast cancer patients is generally unresponsive to prostaglandin inhibitors. (pp. 691–692)

9. **The answer is d.** Hypercalcemia symptoms are numerous, vague, and nonspecific, and since many cancer patients with hypercalcemia have large tumor burdens and will die in 3 to 6 months, symptoms of hypercalcemia may be confused with those of end-stage disease. (p. 692)

10. **The answer is b.** Constipation, and not diarrhea, is more likely to be observed during the early stages of hypercalcemia. Elevated extracellular calcium levels depress smooth muscle contractility, leading to delayed gastric emptying and decreased gastrointestinal motility. (p. 693)

11. **The answer is a.** Before excessive bone resorption can be treated, impaired renal calcium excretion must be improved, usually by correcting dehydration and removing factors that may exacerbate hypercalcemia, including thiazide diuretics. Oral or intravenous hydration with normal saline may be required. (p. 694)

12. **The answer is c.** Although loop diuretics such as furosemide may be used to enhance calcium excretion, patients treated with high doses of furosemide must be monitored in an intensive care setting to ensure that fluid and electrolyte losses are replaced and that extracellular fluid volume is not depleted. (p. 696)

13. **The answer is d.** Both calcitonin and glucocorticoids have been shown to be effective in treating hypercalcemic patients with multiple myeloma. Both inhibit bone resorption. Glucocorticoids also increase urinary calcium excretion and decrease intestinal calcium absorption. Unlike saline diuresis or plicamycin, both calcitonin and glucocorticoids can be used in patients with renal or cardiac failure who are dehydrated. Another substance, gallium nitrate, appears to be more effective than calcitonin in achieving a sustained decrease in calcium levels. (pp. 697–698)

14. **The answer is c.** Intravenous injection of inorganic phosphates rapidly decreases extracellular calcium concentration by promoting skeletal calcification. Because nephrocalcinosis and other extraskeletal calcification may also occur, however, use of intravenous phosphates is limited to a last resort. Both plicamycin and bisphosphonates have a slow onset of action. Prostaglandin inhibitors such as aspirin, indomethacin, and nonsteroidal antiinflammatory drugs have not proved consistently effective in lowering calcium levels. (p. 698)

# Chapter 26    Paraneoplastic Syndromes

## INTRODUCTION

- Paraneoplastic syndromes (PNSs), can be described as the "remote" or indirect effects of cancer. These rare diseases are the result of the secretion of substances, usually proteins, by the primary tumor or its metastases.
- PNSs most frequently occur with lung cancer, specifically small-cell lung carcinoma.
- Most PNSs appear in the later stages of the disease.
- PNSs rarely occur with childhood malignancies with the exception of Wilms' tumor and neuroblastoma.
- The existence of a PNS frequently predicts a poor prognosis.
- A PNS may be useful as a monitoring tool to evaluate response and as an indication of recurrent disease.
- Response of the PNS to therapy frequently correlates with tumor response.

## ENDOCRINE PARANEOPLASTIC SYNDROMES

### Scope of the Problem

- The endocrine PNSs are the most frequently occurring and the most well-defined.
- The most common and well-known endocrine PNSs are hypercalcemia, paraneoplastic adrenocorticotropic hormone (ACTH) syndrome, and syndrome of inappropriate antidiuresis (SIAD).

### Definitions

- Paraneoplastic or humoral hypercalcemia is defined as an elevated serum calcium level caused by tumor secretion of parathyroid hormone-related protein (PTHrP).
- Paraneoplastic ACTH syndrome is the development of pituitary-independent Cushing's disease caused by the secretion of ACTH.
- The syndrome of inappropriate secretion of antidiuretic hormone (SIADH) is described as tumor production of ADH or arginine vasopressin (AVP) resulting in a syndrome of hyponatremia, urine inappropriately higher in osmolality than the plasma, and high concentrations of urinary sodium despite serum hyponatremia. SIADH is more commonly referred to as SIAD to reflect that vasopressin may not be the only agent to effect sodium excretion.

### Incidence

- Hypercalcemia is the most common metabolic complication of malignancy.
- Although paraneoplastic ACTH syndrome occurs rarely, it is considered the second most frequent paraneoplastic syndrome.
- SIAD is primarily associated with small-cell lung cancer.

### Etiology and Risk Factors

- PTHrP is the primary factor in the development of paraneoplastic hypercalcemia.
- The etiology of paraneoplastic ACTH syndrome is ectopic secretion of ACTH by neoplastic cells. This leads to bilateral adrenal hyperplasia and the symptoms of Cushing's disease.

- ACTH syndrome has been widely reported, with more than 75% of the cases associated with tumors located in the chest and mediastinum.
- The etiology of SIAD as a PNS is related to ectopic production of vasopressin by malignant cells.

## Pathophysiology

- Paraneoplastic or humoral hypercalcemia in solid tumors is most often caused by tumor secretion of parathyroid hormone-related peptide (PTHrP).
- Hypercalcemia associated with multiple myeloma and lymphomas results from local bone destruction rather than the effects of PTHrP.
- Paraneoplastic ACTH syndrome is related to tumor secretion of ACTH.
- SIAD affects the body's fluid and sodium balance. The excess AVP stimulation leads to an expanded extracellular volume, serum hypo-osmality, hyponatremia, and hypertonic urine.

## Clinical Manifestations

- The acute symptoms of hypercalcemia include polyuria, polydipsia, nausea, vomiting, anorexia, constipation, lethargy, weakness, and dehydration.
- Cushing's disease is a disorder of excess ACTH. Patients with paraneoplastic ACTH syndrome are most likely to exhibit hypokalemic alkalosis, glucose intolerance, and muscle weakness.
- Water intoxication accounts for the signs and symptoms seen with SIAD, although most patients are asymptomatic.
- Symptoms may include nausea, weakness, anorexia, fatigue, and muscle cramps. These vague, nonspecific complaints can be easily attributed to the cancer, and often are not identified as early signs of hyponatremia.
- As the hyponatremia worsens, symptoms may progress to include altered mental status, confusion, lethargy, combativeness, or psychotic behavior.

## Assessment

### Diagnostic studies

- Hypercalcemia is defined as a serum calcium level >11.0 mg/dl.
- Diagnosis of paraneoplastic ACTH (pACTH) syndrome is made primarily by lab testing. Plasma cortisol and 24-hour urinary free cortisol levels may be obtained. The simplest test to do is a dexamethasone suppression test.
- Most cases of SIAD are diagnosed inadvertently when hyponatremia is found through routine serum chemistry studies. The diagnosis of SIAD requires the presence of hyponatremia in addition to plasma hypo-osmolality and inappropriately concentrated urine.

## Therapeutic Approaches and Nursing Care

- Treatment of hypercalcemia involves vigorous hydration and the use of drug therapy. Intravenous pamidronate sodium has proved to be the most effective and least toxic therapy for hypercalcemia associated with solid tumors.
- Treatment of pACTH syndrome is primarily focused on treatment of the malignancy. Measures to control the effects of Cushing's disease while waiting for the malignancy to respond include the following:
  - Aminoglutethimide lowers cortisol levels.
  - Ketoconazole impairs corticosteroid production.
  - Mitotane is an oral adrenal cytotoxic agent.
  - Bilateral adrenalectomy is used when medical intervention is ineffective.
- The treatment of SIAD is directed at the underlying malignancy. However, stabilization of the patient, and correction of the hyponatremia is essential.

- Severe hyponatremia requires more aggressive treatment, especially if the patient is experiencing seizures or coma. Hypertonic saline and furosemide are often used.
- Chronic mild to moderate hyponatremia may be managed with certain oral medications.

## NEUROLOGICAL PARANEOPLASTIC SYNDROMES

### Scope of the Problem

- Neurological PNSs do not always correlate with the status of the underlying malignancy.
- Neurological PNSs are thought to occur from an autoimmune reaction to the tumor.
- Two major neurological PNSs are paraneoplastic cerebellar degeneration (PCD) and LEMS.

### Definitions

- Subacute cerebellar degeneration is a group of paraneoplastic neurological disorders known to be caused by antineuronal antibodies characterized by progressive ataxia and severe vision changes.
- LEMS is a paraneoplastic antibody-mediated autoimmune disorder characterized by weakness and easy fatigability of muscles, that primarily affects patients with small-cell lung carcinoma.

### Incidence

- Paraneoplastic cerebellar degeneration (PCD) is a rare disorder, symptoms are severe and easily identifiable.
- The malignancy most often associated with PCD is ovarian cancer.
- LEMS occurs in approximately 6% of patients with small-cell lung cancer and has been incidentally reported in patients with breast, gastric, prostate, ovarian, and rectal cancers.

### Etiology and Risk Factors

- The paraneoplastic cerebellar degeneration disorders arise from the presence of anti-Purkinje cell antibodies associated with specific neoplasms.
- LEMS as a PNS may be the result of autoantibodies attacking the neuromuscular structures involved in muscle nerve contraction.

### Pathophysiology

- PCD is a result of the loss or dysfunction of cerebellar Purkinje cells.

#### Antineural antibodies

- The belief that PCD is an autoimmune disorder is based on the idea that the patient's immune response to the tumor produces antibodies that unfortunately recognize Purkinje cells as being similar to tumor cells, thereby attacking and destroying or disabling them.
- Several antibodies have been identified related to the development of PCD.
- In LEMS, the presence of tumor cells stimulates an autoimmune response that produces IgG antibodies against calcium channels expressed by both the cancer and the neuromuscular junction.
- Resulting in insufficient acetylcholine release into the synaptic cleft and therefore very low-amplitude muscle action potentials.

### Clinical Manifestations

- The onset of PCD usually occurs prior to the diagnosis of cancer. The cerebellar dysfunction is characterized by neurological signs and symptoms that are usually bilateral, symmetrical, and progressive. Initial symptoms are a slight difficulty in walking that rapidly progresses to severe ataxia.
- Patients with PCD frequently have other mild neurological deficits.

- Unfortunately, even if the underlying malignancy is successfully treated, the neurological symptoms rarely improve.
- LEMS is characterized by muscle weakness and easy fatigability, with the muscle groups of the pelvic girdle and thighs primarily affected, the arms and shoulders to a lesser extent.
- Additional symptoms may include double or blurred vision, dysarthria, dysphagia, ptosis, parasthesias, and muscle pain.

## Assessment

### Diagnostic studies

- Routine neurological diagnostic studies include magnetic resonance imaging (MRI) and/or computed tomography (CT) scan of the brain, as well as lumbar puncture.
- The diagnosis of LEMS rests in part upon distinguishing it from myasthenia gravis (MG).

## Therapeutic Approaches and Nursing Care

- PCD rarely responds to treatment.
- Treatment of LEMS is based upon treatment of the underlying malignancy. Frequently the symptoms associated with LEMS improve with tumor response.
- The drugs used to treat LEMS are pharmacological agents that promote ACh release from the nerve terminal such as 3,4-diaminopyridine and guanidine.

## HEMATOLOGIC PARANEOPLASTIC SYNDROMES

## Scope of the Problem

- The most common hematologic problem is anemia of chronic disease or malignancy.

## Definitions

- Anemia in the cancer patient may be due to the effects of chemotherapy or radiation, bleeding, bone marrow invasion by tumor, or a primary hematologic disorder. Anemia as a remote effect of neoplastic disease is much less common and is caused by tumor product impairment of bone marrow function and/or red cell metabolism.
- Cancer patients have a higher risk of thromboembolism (TE) or clot formation due to the hypercoagulable state induced by the malignancy.
- Trousseau's syndrome describes a variety of thromboembolic disorders affecting both veins and arteries, including specific types of peripheral vascular disease and ischemic heart disease.

## Incidence

- The malignancies primarily associated with TE include small-cell lung cancer (SCLC) and non–small-cell lung cancer (NSCLC), as well as colon, pancreas, and—to a lesser extent—breast, prostate, ovarian, and bladder carcinomas. The type of cancer most often implicated is mucin-secreting adenocarcinoma of the gastrointestinal (GI) tract.
- The incidence of TE appears to rise during chemotherapy and hormonal therapy.

## Etiology and Risk Factors

- The etiology of anemia of malignancy involves the tumor secretion of cytokines, such as interleukin-1 (IL-1), affecting red cell metabolism; other factors include protein-calorie malnutrition, bone marrow failure, and chronic hemorrhage.
- The etiology of thromboembolism is the ability of tumor cells to affect systemic activation of coagulation and cause platelet dysfunction.

## Pathophysiology

- A protein called *anemia-inducing substance* reduces the osmotic resistance of red blood cells, increasing their susceptibility to destruction.
- Tumor cells may remotely precipitate paraneoplastic TE by any one of three mechanisms: activation of the coagulation pathway, damage to the endothelial lining of blood vessels, or platelet activation.

## Clinical Manifestations

- Anemia of malignancy is characterized by a low hemoglobin that may or may not be symptomatic.

## Assessment

### Diagnostic studies

- Anemia of malignancy is primarily a diagnosis of exclusion based on laboratory results combined with the clinical picture. It is characterized by a low serum iron and low iron-binding capacity.

## Therapeutic Approaches and Nursing Care

- Anemia of malignancy is usually managed through the use of transfusions whenever the patient becomes symptomatic or the hemoglobin falls below 8.0 g/dl.

## RENAL PARANEOPLASTIC SYNDROMES

## Scope of the Problem

- The majority of renal complications of malignancy are related to the effects of tumor infiltration of the kidneys, renal vein thrombosis, amyloidosis, urethral or ureteral obstruction, and complications of treatment, specifically chemotherapy.
- The only true renal PNSs are nephrotic syndrome produced by glomerular lesions and obstruction of the glomerulus by tumor products.
- Obstruction by tumor products refers to the secretion of substances by malignant cells causing renal dysfunction.

## Definitions

- The presence of paraneoplastic lesions in the renal glomerulus leads to a disease known as *nephrotic syndrome*, which is defined as impaired renal function resulting in massive proteinuria.

## Incidence

- The incidence of nephrotic syndrome as a PNS is difficult to determine.

## Etiology and Risk Factors

- Nephrotic syndrome is most commonly known as a benign disorder either resulting from a primary glomerular disease or occurring secondary to infection, drugs, or systemic diseases.
- The etiology of paraneoplastic nephrotic syndrome is the presence of glomerular lesions.

## Pathophysiology

- The renal lesion present in 80% of patients with Hodgkin's lymphoma is known as *lipoid nephrosis*. Lipoid nephrosis is characterized by the presence of nephrotic syndrome and minimal glomerular changes on histological examination, also called *minimal change disease*.

## Clinical Manifestations

- The cardinal sign of nephrotic syndrome is massive proteinuria, accompanied by hypoalbuminemia, hyperlipidemia, and edema.
- Signs and symptoms include brown, foamy urine, and facial and peripheral edema, which may progress to anasarca or edema of all body tissues.

## Assessment and Grading
### Diagnostic studies

- As with many PNSs, paraneoplastic nephrotic syndrome is a diagnosis of exclusion.

## Therapeutic Approaches and Nursing Care

- The primary treatment of paraneoplastic nephrotic syndrome is focused on the underlying malignancy. Resolution of the nephrotic syndrome is fairly rapid following tumor response to therapy.
- Management of the nephrotic syndrome itself includes the use of steroids and diuretics.

## MISCELLANEOUS PARANEOPLASTIC SYNDROMES
## Cutaneous Paraneoplastic Syndromes

- No one malignancy is predominantly associated with cutaneous PNSs in general, although some are pathognomonic for a certain malignancy. The etiology of most cutaneous PNSs is unknown.
- Cutaneous PNSs are extremely rare.
- A true cutaneous PNS must meet two criteria: (1) the appearance of the dermatosis must follow the development of the malignancy, and (2) the disease course of both the dermatosis and the malignancy must coincide.
- The primary treatment of the cutaneous PNSs is treatment of the underlying malignancy.

## Anorexia-Cachexia Syndrome

- The predominant and most well-known PNSs affecting the GI system are anorexia and cachexia.
  - Anorexia refers to a loss of appetite and subsequent reduction in food intake.
  - Cancer cachexia is a syndrome defined as progressive loss of body fat and lean body mass associated with anorexia, anemia, and profound weakness.
- Anorexia-cachexia does not result from the nutritional demands of the malignancy.
- Anorexia-cachexia differs from other PNSs in that it is not associated with specific malignancies but can occur with any cancer.
- Anorexia-cachexia is a dominant feature of lung cancer, occurring much earlier in the disease course than is seen in breast cancer patients.
- Several cytokines are believed to be responsible for the cancer cachexia syndrome. The major cytokine involved is tumor necrosis factor-alpha (TNF-alpha), also known as cachectin.

## Tumor Fever

- Tumor fever is a PNS primarily associated with lymphomas, as well as with leukemias, myelodysplastic syndromes, renal cell carcinoma, hepatoma, and metastatic liver disease. It is produced by tumor secretion of cytokines, primarily IL-1, IL-6, interferon, and TNF.
- The primary therapy for tumor fever is treatment of the underlying malignancy.

## PRACTICE QUESTIONS

1. Which of the following is *not* true of paraneoplastic syndromes (PNSs)?
   a. Most PNSs appear in the middle stages of the disease course.
   b. PNSs rarely occur with childhood malignancies.
   c. The existence of a PNS frequently predicts a poor prognosis with regard to the malignancy.
   d. Response of the PNS to therapy frequently correlates with tumor response.

2. The most frequently occurring and most well-defined PNSs are the:
   a. renal PNSs.
   b. neurological PNSs.
   c. endocrine PNSs.
   d. hematologic PNSs.

3. Mr. Bradford, a patient with small-cell lung cancer, develops anorexia, weakness, anorexia, and fatigue. At first, these are attributed to the cancer itself. As his condition worsens, though, Mr. Bradford's wife, who is caring for him through a hospice arrangement, calls you in tears, reporting that he has suddenly become combative. You tell her that he must have a serum chemistry as soon as possible because you suspect:
   a. hypercalcemia.
   b. hyponatremia.
   c. pACTH syndrome.
   d. end-stage cancer.

4. Hank, who has small-cell lung cancer, develops hypokalemic alkalosis, glucose intolerance, and muscle weakness. He also has symptoms of Cushing's disease. You conclude that he should be assessed for:
   a. SIADH.
   b. hypercalcemia.
   c. water intoxication.
   d. pACTH.

5. Diagnosis of paraneoplastic ACTH syndrome is made by which of the following?
   a. dexamethasone suppression test
   b. plasma cortisol levels
   c. calcium levels
   d. a and b

6. Mr. Frederick develops confusion, disorientation, and hallucinations with an elevated serum calcium and occasional bradycardia. Therapeutic interventions might include which of the following?
   a. saline diuresis
   b. intravenous pamidronate
   c. aggressive cancer therapy
   d. all of the above

7. pACTH syndrome often presents as Cushing's syndrome (hypertension, edema, and muscle weakness). The primary approach to managing this clinical problem is:
   a. bilateral adrenalectomy.
   b. aminoglutethimide or ketoconazole.
   c. treating the malignancy.
   d. infusion of hypertonic saline and furosemide.

8. LEMS (Lambert-Eaton myasthenic syndrome) is a PNS that is:
   a. caused by anti-Purkinje cell antibodies.
   b. characterized by progressive ataxia and severe vision changes.
   c. a paraneoplastic antibody-mediated autoimmune disorder that can result from autoantibodies attaching the neuromuscular structures involved in muscle nerve contractions.
   d. b and c.

9. Paraneoplastic cerebellar degeneration is a neurological disorder characterized by which of the following?
   a. onset usually occurs prior to the diagnosis of cancer.
   b. cerebellar dysfunction is characterized by neurological signs that are usually unilateral and progressive.
   c. symptoms will resolve when the malignancy is successfully treated.
   d. all of the above.

10. As LEMS progresses, which of the following may occur?
    a. double vision
    b. dysarthria
    c. ptosis
    d. all of the above

11. Treatment of LEMS may include:
    a. 3,4-diaminopyridine.
    b. guanidine.
    c. calcitonin.
    d. a and b.

12. The most common hematologic problem(s) for oncology patients is (are):
    a. latent hemophilia.
    b. anemia of malignancy.
    c. blood dyscrasias.
    d. a and b.

13. Anemia can occur as a remote effect of neoplastic disease. This is caused by:
    a. tearing of interstitial tissue with subsequent slow but long-term blood loss.
    b. tumor product impairment of bone marrow function.
    c. red cell metabolism.
    d. b and c.

14. Thromboembolism (TE) is most frequently seen with which of the following?
    a. small-cell lung cancer.
    b. non–small-cell lung cancer.
    c. mucin-secreting bladder carcinoma.
    d. mucin-secreting adenocarcinoma of the GI tract.

15. The etiology of thromboembolism is:
    a. the tumor secretion of cytokines, such as interleukin-1 (IL-1), affecting red cell metabolism.
    b. the ability of tumor cells to affect systemic activation of coagulation and cause platelet dysfunction.
    c. chronic hemorrhage.
    d. bone marrow failure.

16. Tumor cells may remotely precipitate paraneoplastic thromboembolism by:
    a. activation of the coagulation pathway.
    b. damage to the endothelial lining of blood vessels.
    c. protein-calorie malnutrition.
    d. a and b.

17. Nephrotic syndrome is a PNS characterized by which of the following?
    a. the presence of lesions in the renal glomerulus
    b. a secondary benign disorder resulting from a primary glomerular disease
    c. impaired renal function due to obstruction of the glomerulus by tumor products
    d. all of the above

18. As you take the history of a client with nephrotic syndrome, what signs and symptoms would you expect to see or hear reported?
    a. brown, foamy urine
    b. "gaunt" face and generalized weight loss with anorexia
    c. mild hypotension
    d. a and b

19. The cause of most cutaneous PNS is unknown but may be related to:
    a. abnormal stimulation of epidermal cells.
    b. tumor products.
    c. a hypersensitivity reaction.
    d. b and c.

20. Anorexia-cachexia:
    a. is a syndrome of progressive loss of body fat and lean body mass associated with loss of appetite, anemia, and profound weakness.
    b. results from the nutritional demands of the malignancy.
    c. is usually associated with several specific malignancies but can occur with any cancer.
    d. all of the above.

---

# ANSWER EXPLANATIONS

1. **The answer is a.** Most PNSs appear in the later stages of the disease course. It is true that PNSs rarely occur with childhood malignancies with the exception of Wilms' tumor and neuroblastoma. The existence of a PNS frequently predicts a poor prognosis for the malignancy. Finally, response of the PNS to therapy frequently correlates with tumor response. (p. 703)

2. **The answer is c.** The endocrine PNSs are the most frequently occurring PNSs and the most well-defined in terms of their etiology. (p. 703)

3. **The answer is b.** Brad most likely has hyponatremia secondary to SIAD. SIAD is primarily associated with small-cell lung cancer. Water intoxication accounts for the signs and symptoms seen with SIAD. The early symptoms, such as nausea, weakness, anorexia, fatigue, can be easily attributed to the cancer. However, as the hyponatremia worsens, symptoms may progress to include altered mental status, confusion and combativeness. (pp. 704; 706–707)

4. **The answer is d.** The etiology of paraneoplastic ACTH syndrome is ectopic secretion of ACTH by neoplastic cells. This leads to bilateral adrenal hyperplasia and symptoms such as hypokalemic alkalosis, glucose intolerance, and muscle weakness. ACTH syndrome has been widely reported, with more than 75% of the cases associated with tumors located in the chest and mediastinum. (pp. 704; 706–707)

5.  **The answer is d.** Diagnosis of paraneoplastic ACTH (pACTH) syndrome is made primarily by lab testing. Plasma cortisol and 24-hour urinary free cortisol levels may be obtained. The simplest test to do is a dexamethasone suppression test. Hypercalcemia diagnosis is based on an elevated calcium level, and SIAD requires the presence of hyponatremia in addition to plasma hypo-osmolality and inappropriately concentrated urine. (p. 707)

6.  **The answer is d.** Paraneoplastic hypercalcemia often presents as confusion, disorientation, and hallucinations with bradycardia. Treatment of hypercalcemia includes vigorous hydration and pamidronate. (p. 706)

7.  **The answer is c.** Treatment of pACTH syndrome is primarily focused on treatment of the malignancy. Measures to control the effects of Cushing's disease while waiting for the malignancy to respond include the following: aminoglutethimide, ketoconazole, mitotane, and rarely, bilateral adrenalectomy. (p. 707)

8.  **The answer is c.** LEMS is a paraneoplastic antibody-mediated autoimmune disorder that can result from autoantibodies attaching the neuromuscular structures involved in muscle nerve contractions. The other two descriptions fit PCD. (pp. 708–709)

9.  **The answer is a.** PCD's onset usually occurs prior to the diagnosis of cancer. Cerebellar dysfunction is characterized by neurological signs that are usually bilateral (not unilateral), symmetrical, and progressive. Unfortunately, PCD's symptoms will often not resolve—even when the malignancy is successfully treated. (p. 710)

10. **The answer is d.** Additional symptoms of LEMS may include double or blurred vision, dysarthria, dysphagia, ptosis, parasthesias, and muscle pain. (p. 711)

11. **The answer is d.** Treatment of LEMS symptoms can be treated with agents that promote ACh release from the nerve terminal such as 3,4-diaminopyridine and guanidine. (p. 711)

12. **The answer is b.** The most common hematologic problem for oncology patients is anemia of chronic disease or malignancy. (p. 711)

13. **The answer is d.** Anemia as a remote effect of neoplastic disease is caused by tumor product impairment or bone marrow function and/or red cell metabolism. (p. 712)

14. **The answer is d.** The type of cancer most often implicated in incidence of TE is mucin-secreting adenocarcinoma of the GI tract. Other malignancies primarily associated with TE include SCLC, NSCLC, and colon and pancreatic cancers. To a lesser extent, TE-associated cancers include breast, prostate, ovarian, and bladder carcinomas. (p. 713)

15. **The answer is b.** The etiology of thromboembolism is the ability of tumor cells to affect systemic activation of coagulation and cause platelet dysfunction. Anemia is caused by the other choices given: the tumor secretion of cytokines, such as interleukin-1 (IL-1), affecting red cell metabolism; chronic hemorrhage; and bone marrow failure. (p. 713)

16. **The answer is d.** Tumor cells may remotely precipitate paraneoplastic TE by activation of the coagulation pathway, damage to the endothelial lining of blood vessels, or platelet activation. Choice **c**—protein-calorie malnutrition—is involved in the etiology of anemia of malignancy. (p. 713)

17. **The answer is d.** Nephrotic syndrome is impaired renal function resulting in massive proteinuria due to obstruction. It is caused by the presence of paraneoplastic lesions in the renal glomerulus and is a secondary benign disorder resulting from a primary glomerular disease. (p. 714)

18. **The answer is a.** Signs and symptoms of nephrotic syndrome include massive proteinuria and brown, foamy urine, as well as facial and peripheral edema, which may progress to anasarca or edema of all body tissues. The combined water and electrolyte retention may cause mild to moderate hypertension, not hypotension. (p. 715)

19. **The answer is a.** The etiology of cutaneous PNS is unknown, but theories include secretion of transforming growth factor-alpha, resulting in abnormal stimulation of epidermal cells. (p. 716)

20. **The answer is a.** Anorexia-cachexia is a syndrome of progressive loss of body fat and lean body mass associated with loss of appetite, anemia, and profound weakness. It does not result from the nutritional demands of the malignancy and is not associated with specific malignancies but can occur with any cancer. (p. 716)

# Chapter 27    Malignant Effusions and Edemas

## SCOPE OF THE PROBLEM

- Abnormal leakage from blood and lymph vessels into tissues (edema) or cavities (effusions) occurs with many kinds of malignancy. Effusions and edemas are usually associated with advanced disease but sometimes occur as the presenting symptom.
- *Malignant effusions* occur most commonly in the pleural space of the lung (pleural effusion), the peritoneal cavity in the abdomen (ascites), or the space surrounding the heart (pericardial effusion).
- The brain and the extremities are frequent sites for *malignant edemas*.

## NORMAL FLUID REGULATION

- The distribution pattern of body water is termed *fluid spacing*. *First spacing* describes a normal distribution of fluid in both the extracellular and intracellular compartments.
- *Second spacing* refers to an excess accumulation of interstitial fluid (edema), while third spacing is fluid retention in areas that usually have no fluid or a minimum of fluid (effusion).

## FLUID DISTURBANCES IN CANCER

### Effects of Cancer and Cancer Treatment

- Cancer treatments can affect or be altered by effusions/edemas. Cancer, either a primary tumor or a metastatic lesion, can affect fluid pressure dynamics in several negative ways: by direct extension of the tumor, by seeding of body cavities with malignant cells, by lymphatic or venous obstruction, and/or by causing severe hypoproteinemia. See Table 27-1, text page 723.

### General Considerations: Similarities and Differences

#### Benign versus malignant

- Of the six fluid retention states discussed in this chapter, all except lymphedema are directly due to cancer.
- Lymphedema is a benign iatrogenic problem secondary to radical cancer surgery.

#### Rapid versus slow accumulation

- Cavities and tissues can accommodate surprisingly large volumes of fluids if the abnormal liquid accumulates slowly over time.
- Malignant effusions and edemas usually begin slowly but then increase and expand exponentially.

#### Assessment

- The individual's history and physical exam point to the likely etiology of the effusion/edema.
- The most helpful diagnostic tools for pleural effusion are the chest x-ray and examination of the pleural fluid, while the echocardiogram is the most important tool in pericardial effusions.
- The physical examination helps determine the diagnosis with ascites, lymphedema, and pedal edema.
- Brain lesions causing cerebral edema are usually diagnosed with computerized tomography (CT).

### Transudates versus exudates

- Classification as transudates versus exudates has diagnostic implications and can be a distinguishing characteristic between a malignant or a nonmalignant cause.
  - A *transudate* is a low-protein fluid that has leaked from blood vessels due to mechanical factors.
  - An *exudate* is protein-rich fluid that has leaked from blood vessels with increased permeability. Most malignant effusions are exudates, caused by irritation of the serous membrane by sloughed cancer cells or solid tumor implants.

### Treatment

- For effusions, systemic treatment is usually employed first if the underlying cancer is responsive to chemotherapy. Otherwise, local therapy for malignant effusions is similar: drain the fluid, attempt to obliterate the third space, and prevent reaccumulation. No single clearly superior approach for local control of any of the effusions has been demonstrated by randomized clinical trial.
- The main goals of treatment for malignant effusions and edemas are similar:
  - Short-term goals:
    - Determine underlying cause.
    - Relieve discomfort.
    - Prevent fluid reaccumulation.
  - Long-term goals:
    - Prevent complications.
    - Prolong survival.
    - Enhance quality of life.

### Nursing Care

- Ongoing *assessment* of each cancer patient for signs or symptoms of fluid retention is crucial so that intervention can be instituted early.
- The patient and family will need *emotional support* to counteract the stress and fears associated with advancing disease.
- With the treatment of effusions, important nursing interventions include minimizing discomfort, providing reassurance, and monitoring the patient during and after these procedures for untoward reactions.
- *Patient education* will prepare the patient and family for tests and procedures.
- *Prevention* is important, particularly with lymphedema.
- *Pain evaluation and control* are often in order since the abnormal fluid accumulation can put pressure on nerve endings in surrounding structures.
- *Medications* (steroids, diuretics) may need to be administered and assessment for iatrogenic complications completed.

## LUNG: MALIGNANT PLEURAL EFFUSION
### Incidence

- Fifty percent of all cancer patients will develop pleural effusion at some time during their disease. It may be the first sign of malignancy.
- Lung and breast cancer account for most malignant pleural effusions.

## Physiological Alterations

- Pleural fluid is a filtrate from the parietal pleura.
- In the presence of a massive effusion process, the interpleural space may contain as much as 1500 ml of fluid.
- There are five ways that fluid equilibrium in the pleural space can be disturbed by cancer.
  - Implantation with cancer cells on the pleural surface leads to increased capillary permeability.
  - Obstruction of pleural or pulmonary lymphatic channels can prevent reabsorption of fluid.
  - The pulmonary veins can be obstructed by tumor.
  - The pleural space colloid osmotic pressure may be increased by necrotic malignant cells being shed into the pleural space.
  - The thoracic duct may be perforated.
- Tumor-related pathologies can cause pleural effusion.

## Clinical Manifestations

- The extent of alteration of respiratory function depends on the amount and rate of pleural fluid accumulation as well as the patient's underlying pulmonary status.
- The fluid accumulation restricts lung expansion, reduces lung volume, alters the ventilation and perfusion capacity, and results in abnormal gas exchange and hypoxia.
- Common symptoms and signs are dyspnea; orthopnea; dry, nonproductive cough; and chest pain, chest heaviness.
- Other indicators include labored breathing; tachypnea; dullness to percussion; restricted chest wall expansion; and impaired transmission of breath sounds.

## Assessment

### Radiographic examination

- Chest x-rays are important in visualizing free fluid in the pleural cavity.

### Pleural fluid examination

- Any new pleural effusion must be aspirated to confirm the presence of malignant cells and to rule out nonmalignant causes.
- Pleural fluid cytological analysis yields a definitive diagnosis in most patients with malignant pleural effusion. Thoracoscopy with direct pleural biopsy leads to a diagnosis 100% of the time.
- A bloody effusion is the strongest indicator of malignancy.

## Therapeutic Approaches and Nursing Care

- How the malignant pleural effusion is treated depends on the type of tumor and previous therapy.
- Small, asymptomatic effusions are first treated with systemic chemotherapy or hormonal therapy.
- Patients with chemotherapy-resistant tumors will require alternative treatment approaches.
- If the underlying disease is unresponsive to therapy, palliative measures should be implemented.

### Removal of fluid

- Relief of symptoms is a short-term treatment goal that is usually achieved when the pleural fluid is mechanically drained.
- Long-range treatment goals are directed toward the obliteration of the pleural space so that pleural fluid cannot reaccumulate.

### Thoracentesis

- In thoracentesis the pleural fluid is removed by needle aspiration through the chest wall.
- Effective for diagnosis, palliation, or relief of acute respiratory distress, thoracentesis is of little value for treating recurrent malignant effusions because the fluid usually reaccumulates quickly.

### Thoracostomy tube

- A thoracostomy tube may be inserted to facilitate fluid drainage and then left in place to assess the degree of fluid reaccumulation. Chest tube drainage alone is only partially effective. Measures to prevent fluid reaccumulation are also needed.

## Obliteration of the pleural space

- If the pleural space can be obliterated, then the reaccumulation of pleural fluid may be prevented.

### Chemical agents

- Obliteration is achieved by instilling a chemical agent that causes the visceral and parietal pleura to become permanently adhered together.
- Chemical sclerosing does not prolong the patient's life but may enhance quality of life by relieving symptoms and reducing the time a patient spends in the hospital.
- Nursing management during chest tube insertion and pleural sclerosing includes patient education and reassurance, pain control, positioning, and the management of the chest tube drainage as well as maintaining the drainage system.

### Surgical methods

- If a pleural effusion remains uncontrolled and if a patient has a good life expectancy and a good performance status, pleural stripping is advocated. Success rates approach 90%, but there can be serious complications such as air leak, bleeding, pneumonia, and empyema.
- Pleurectomy has been reported to be effective in some cases. Pleuroperitoneal shunt has been developed for control of malignant effusion.

### Radiation

- Although external beam radiation may be used as local treatment for mediastinal tumors, hemithoracic radiation is not recommended as a first-line management of malignant pleural effusions because of the hazard of pulmonary fibrosis. Radiation is limited to treatment of the underlying disease, not the resultant effusion.

## HEART: MALIGNANT PERICARDIAL EFFUSION
### Incidence

- Autopsy series indicate metastasis to the heart, and pericardium occurs in 8%–20% of cases. However, only 30% of affected patients are symptomatic.

## Pathophysiology

- Pericardial metastasis results from lymphatic or hematogenous spread or from direct invasion by an adjacent primary tumor.
- The majority of pericardial effusions result from obstruction of lymphatic and venous drainage of the heart.

- The effects of pericardial fluid accumulation are largely dependent on the rate of exudation, the physical compliance capacity of the pericardial cavity, ventricular function, myocardial size, and blood volume.

## Clinical Manifestations

- Pericardial effusion interferes with cardiac function because the fluid burden occupies space and reduces the volume of the heart in diastole. Systemic circulatory effects of decreased cardiac output and impaired venous return lead to generalized congestion. The body tries to compensate in several ways:
  1. A tachycardia is created by adrenergic stimulation to offset decreased stroke volume.
  2. Systemic and pulmonary venous pressure increases in an attempt to improve ventricular filling.
  3. The adrenergic stimulation increases the ejection fraction, leading to increased peripheral resistance that will support arterial blood pressure.
- Most persons with pericardial effusions are asymptomatic, so cardiac involvement may be overlooked. The individual may have only nonspecific symptoms at first: dyspnea, cough, and chest pain.
- Signs and symptoms of a developing pericardial effusion are often insidious and include pleural effusion, tachycardia, jugular venous distention, hepatomegaly, peripheral edema, pulsus paradoxus, and hypotension.
- Cardiac tamponade is the most severe symptom complex and is an oncological emergency.
- Nursing management of patients in tamponade includes measures to minimize activity and promote adequate respiration, elevation of the head of the bed, and administration of oxygen and medications to relieve anxiety and pain. Intravascular volume maintenance with intravenous (IV) fluids, vasopressors, and other cardiac medications may be in order while preparation is made for pericardiocentesis or surgical intervention.

## Assessment

### Radiography

- Echocardiography is the fastest, least invasive, and most precise method for visualization and quantification of malignant pericardial effusion.
- Difficult-to-detect lesions may be better visualized by CT.

### Electrocardiography

- Electrocardiograph (ECG) changes with neoplastic pericarditis or effusions include tachycardia, premature contractions, low QRS voltage, and nonspecific ST- and T-wave changes.

### Pericardial fluid examination

- Fluid withdrawn from the pericardial cavity by pericardiocentesis that has a bloody appearance is indicative of malignancy, especially with lung cancer. Such fluid is always exudative.

## Therapeutic Approaches and Nursing Care

- Choice of treatment depends on the physiological impairment caused by the effusion and the degree of tamponade.

### Removal of fluid

#### Pericardiocentesis alone

- Percutaneous pericardiocentesis guided by ECHO is an important diagnostic tool and is useful for initial drainage of fluid from the pericardium.

- Nursing care during the pericardiocentesis includes explaining the procedure, positioning the patient in a semi-Fowler's position, and maintaining asepsis. The nurse must continuously monitor the patient and the ECG during the pericardiocentesis and afterward monitor for complications such as pneumothorax, myocardial laceration, and coronary artery laceration.
- Other procedures for drainage and examination of the pericardial space include subxiphoid pericardiotomy, balloon pericardiotomy, and pericardioperitoneal shunt.

### Obliteration of the pericardial space

#### Pericardiocentesis with sclerosing agent instillation

- Sclerosing agents are instilled into the pericardial cavity via pericardiocentesis, but they are associated with significant toxicity. Sclerosing agents used in pericardial effusions include tetracycline, 5-fluourouail, radioactive gold or phosphorus, quinacrine, and thiotepa.

#### Surgery

- Surgical intervention, including pleuropericardial window via thoracotomy and pericardiectomy, is generally reserved for medically appropriate patients whose malignant effusion is unresponsive to other therapies or who have required repeated pericardiocentesis.
- Nursing measures postoperatively include prevention of infection, atelectasis, pleural effusion, and pneumothorax, as well as ongoing assessment for cardiac arrhythmia due to surgical irritation or the presence of the pericardial catheter.

#### Radiation

- The use of external beam radiation is primarily reserved for pericardial effusion due to lymphomas, which are highly radiosensitive.
- Carcinoma of the lung and breast are also sufficiently radiosensitive.

## ABDOMEN: MALIGNANT PERITONEAL EFFUSION

### Incidence

- Malignant peritoneal effusion (ascites) is most common in women with ovarian cancer. Ascites will be found at presentation in 33% of these women, and over 60% will develop ascites at some time before death.
- Ascites also develops in patients with GI malignancies.
- The appearance of ascites in patients with advanced disease is prognostically grim.

### Physiological Alterations

- The most common cause of ascitic fluid buildup is tumor seeding the peritoneum, resulting in obstruction of the diaphragmatic and/or abdominal lymphatics. This occurs primarily with gynecologic cancers.

### Clinical Manifestations

- Several liters of ascitic fluid can be accommodated in the abdomen. Some people report gaining 50–60 lb of body weight as a result of excess fluid.
- This massive accumulation of fluid leads to negative body image changes, anorexia, early satiety, and difficulty in breathing and walking.

## Assessment

- Peritoneal effusion is diagnosed primarily by physical exam, with malignant characteristics confirmed by paracentesis.
- The following signs are characteristic of effusion: bulging flanks, tympany at the top the abdominal curve, elicitation of a fluid wave, and shifting dullness.
- Abdominal x-rays, ultrasound, and CT are used to diagnose. Paracentesis is the definitive diagnostic test.

## Therapeutic Approaches and Nursing Care

### Diet and diuresis

- Unless the underlying malignancy causing the ascites responds to antineoplastic therapy, the pathophysiology of ascites will remain unaltered and fluid accumulation will continue despite exogenous fluid restriction measures.

### Removal of fluid

Paracentesis

- Fluid removal by paracentesis alone is of little therapeutic benefit. This procedure is usually reserved until a large volume of fluid has accumulated and the patient is profoundly symptomatic because the fluid reaccumulates rapidly.

Obliteration of the intraperitoneal space

- Chemotherapy instillation is designed to provoke an inflammatory response leading to sclerosis of the peritoneal space linings. Although sclerosing therapy is effective in treating malignant pleural effusions, it is less successful with ascites.
- Access to the peritoneal cavity for drug administration is an important technical problem. The peritoneum can be entered on a temporary basis with various catheters, but repeated puncture of the abodominal wall and peritoneum is risky.

Peritoneovenous shunting

- Shunt devices (LeVeen® and Denver®) can be used to recirculate ascitic fluid continuously to the intravascular space.
- A pressure differential between the abdominal cavity and the thoracic vein enables fluid to ascend from the peritoneal cavity into the superior vena cava.
- Peritoneovenous shunting is usually reserved for individuals in whom all other treatment options have failed.
- In some instances postoperative complications might be predicted by a preoperative procedure designed to assess patient tolerance to the proposed permanent shunt. This is termed *peritoneovenous autotransfusion*.
- Nursing care of the patient with a perioneovenous shunt includes teaching the patient and family the purpose and care of the shunt, signs and symptoms of problems with the shunt, and recognition and prevention of infection, as well as alleviating anxiety.

## BRAIN: MALIGNANT CEREBRAL EDEMA

## Incidence

- Cerebral edema results from an increase in brain volume caused by an increase in the fluid content of the brain.

- Malignant cerebral edema is caused by increased permeability of the cerebral capillary endothelial cells. Most cerebral edema accompanies primary or metastatic brain tumors or carcinomatous meningitis.

## Physiological Alterations

- Mechanisms in the formation of malignant cerebral edema are (1) direct injury to the vascular endothelium by the expanding tumor, (2) dysplastic vascular structures within tumor lesions, (3) biochemically mediated alterations of capillary permeability and (4) a less stable blood-brain barrier.

## Clinical Manifestations

- Malignant cerebral edema produces diffuse signs and symptoms reflecting its more global effects on brain functioning, as opposed to the focal signs and symptoms caused by direct destruction of tissue by tumor.
  - Most patients with metastatic brain tumors have regional swelling of tissue, mostly in the cerebrum. In such patients the clinical deficits manifested are more often caused by peritumoral edema than by the tumor mass itself.
  - Subtle early changes in the patient's status are vague and usually observed only by someone who knows the patient well. Family members may notice the patient's lack of persistence in tasks, undue irritability, emotional lability, inertia, faulty insight, forgetfulness, reduced range of mental activity, indifference to common social practices, and lack of initiative and spontaneity.
  - Seizure is the most common symptom of acute onset.
  - Headache, another common early symptom, is due to distortion and traction of pain-sensitive structures by the edema.
  - Other indications of brain edema can be generalized or focal, including the following: mental disturbance, gait disorder, visual disturbance, language disturbance, hemiparesis, and impaired cognition.

## Assessment

- Neurological examination, CT scanning, and magnetic resonance imaging (MRI) are the primary studies used for diagnosing a brain tumor mass. MRI is best for visualizing cerebral edema.

## Therapeutic Approaches and Nursing Care

- Aggressive therapy is warranted to sustain or restore neurological function. The principal treatment regimen is radiation therapy. In addition, patients receive supportive care and steroids to reduce edema.
- In most patients, neurological symptoms resolve or improve with treatment. Improvement is often maintained until the patient succumbs to systemic disease.
- With advanced cerebral edema and the resultant intracranial hypertension, changes in vital signs such as bounding radial pulse, elevated temperature, and respiratory impairment may be seen.
- Decreased level of consciousness, change in pupil size and reaction to light, and altered motor response, in addition to other vital sign changes, should alert the nurse to impending brain herniation, an oncological emergency.

### Steroids and osmotherapy

- The single most important adjunctive treatment to combat the effects of vasogenic cerebral edema is the use of glucocorticoids (dexamethasone, prednisone).
- The aim of steroid therapy is to reduce intracranial pressure and increase cerebral blood flow.

- Once radiotherapy has relieved the neurological symptoms caused by the edema, steroids are slowly tapered to prevent addisonian crisis. Steroid withdrawal can result in headache, lethargy, postural dizziness, or nausea, even if there is no laboratory evidence of adrenal insufficiency.
- Dexamethasone doses as high as 100 mg/day have been used for patients who are refractory at lower doses.

### Radiation therapy

- Ionizing radiation to the underlying tumor is the most effective way to decrease malignant edema as well as tumor bulk. Despite initial response rates or 80%, radiation accomplishes little in terms of survival; median survival after treatment is three to six months.

### Surgery

- Surgical decompression or debulking can rapidly reduce the effect of the mass and remove the source of edema production. Neurosurgical procedures have significant associated risk, such as infection, hemorrhage, and operative mortality. Appropriate patient selection is a critical factor for successful surgical outcome.

## ARMS/LEGS: IATROGENIC SECONDARY LYMPHEDEMA
### Incidence and Physiological Alterations

- Unlike the other effusions and edemas, postsurgical lymphedema of the arm or leg is a benign condition.
  - Arm lymphedema was the frequent postoperative sequela of the most common treatment for all types of breast cancer in the past: radical mastectomy with axillary node dissection followed by radiation. With the less invasive breast cancer treatments today, arm lymphedema occurs less frequently.
  - Even so, lymphedema affects 5%–10% of women who have a modified radical mastectomy.
- Mechanical interruption (surgical technique) and radiation often produce lymphatic obstruction, the most common cause of lymphedema.
- Other factors contributing to the development of lymphedema are obesity, insufficient muscle contraction, inflammation, trauma, formation of fibrosclerotic tissue within the lymph vessel, and scarring secondary to radiation therapy or infection.
- Chronic lymphedema is a late postoperative complication that can occur anywhere from 6 weeks to 20 years after surgery.
- Lymphedema of the leg may develop after groin dissection.
  - The incidence of leg lymphedema after this type of surgery increases gradually over time, and by the fifth postoperative year is estimated to occur in 80% of patients.
  - Improved surgical technique and a preventive regimen of leg elevation and elastic stockings reduce the overall incidence of mild to moderate lymphedema to 20%, with no severe lymphedema occurring.

### Assessment

- Assessment for extremity lymphedema includes monitoring the circumference of the limb, condition of the skin, mobility of the extremity, signs of infection, nutritional status, impairment of circulation, and constriction caused by clothing and other objects.
- Measurements of the arm circumference are taken prior to surgery and at each postoperative visit.

## Therapeutic Approaches and Nursing Care

- The goals of therapy are primarily aimed at prevention, to increase the flow of lymph away from the limb and minimize formation of new lymph fluid.
- Elevation, progressive mild exercise, and massage help mobilize fluid out of the limb. Use of an elastic sleeve is important to reduce the potential of stagnation of lymph fluid.
- Prophylactic measures to prevent new fluid from forming include elastic support sleeves or stockings; sodium restriction; and avoidance of infection, excessive use of the limb, local heat, and trauma to the limb.
- The primary nursing interventions for lymphedema involve measures to prevent complications.
- The secondary phase of nursing management is directed toward the early detection and initial treatment of lymphedema and include: detection of signs and symptoms of lymphedema; management of discomfort; measurement of the arms/legs at regular intervals; elevation of the affected limb; massage therapy; an elastic wrap or sleeve; hand and arm care measures and exercise.
- Tertiary care is associated with the long-term care of the patient with lymphedema and includes exercises, massage therapy, elastic wrap or sleeve to the extremity, pain control, and assessment of the patient for general functioning and ability to perform activities of daily living.

## FEET: MALIGNANT PEDAL EDEMA

- Peripheral, or dependent, edema is common in patients with far-advanced cancer.
- As much as 10 lb of liquid can accumulate in the lower extremeties before it is recognizable as pitting edema.

## Assessment

- Measurement of the ankle is useful to record changes.
- Pitting can be assessed by pressing the thumb into the patient's skin over a bony surface.
- The edema of advanced cancer is bilateral; a unilateral edema would lead to a search for a treatable cause such as thrombophlebitis.

## Therapeutic Approaches and Nursing Care

- First, the patient's nutritional status may be improved with concentrated dietary supplements.
- Protein is particularly important.
  - Water should be restricted if the patient is hyponatremic.
- Second, improve venous blood return by elevating the legs while sitting, wearing support stockings, eliminating clothing that constricts the lower legs, and instituting gentle exercise.
- Third, diuretics may be helpful and can be tried on a short-term basis.

# PRACTICE QUESTIONS

1. Third spacing is:
   a. the normal fluid distribution in the extracellular and intravascular compartments.
   b. an excess of interstitial fluid accumulation.
   c. fluid retention in sites that normally have very little or no fluid.
   d. lack of normal osmotic pressures.

2. Which of the following conditions is benign and iatrogenic in origin and is usually secondary to radical cancer surgery?
   a. pericardial effusion
   b. lymphedema
   c. pleural effusion
   d. anasarca

3. Choose the statement that most accurately describes the degree of subjective symptoms produced by malignant pericardial and pleural effusions.
   a. Symptoms tend to be related more to the rate of fluid accumulation than to the volume collected.
   b. Symptoms tend to be related more to the volume of fluid collected than to the rate of the collection.
   c. Symptoms are related more to the underlying disease and length of time the patient has been diagnosed with cancer.
   d. Symptoms correspond directly to whether the metastatic disease is from microscopic seeding of the cavities or from local extension.

4. Thoracentesis involves fluid removal from:
   a. the pericardial sac.
   b. the pleural cavity.
   c. the abdominal cavity.
   d. the spinal column.

5. The first and most common means of obliteration of the pleural cavity in a patient with chronic, recurrent malignant pleural effusions is:
   a. pleuroperitoneal shunt.
   b. pleural stripping.
   c. sclerosis.
   d. local radiation.

6. Malignant pericardial effusions:
   a. are extremely rare.
   b. are easily detected by tachycardia, low blood pressure, and shortness of breath.
   c. occur in 50% of all patients with cancer, especially the hematologic malignancies.
   d. are not easily detected by routine tests and are found in 8%–20% of autopsies.

7. The patient who is experiencing a pericardial effusion shows signs and symptoms that include:
   a. chest pain, confusion, nausea, and vomiting.
   b. confusion, nausea, vomiting, and hypertension.
   c. hypertension, bradycardia, and increased cardiac output.
   d. decreased cardiac output, dyspnea, cough, and chest pain.

8. The cancer most often associated with malignant ascites is:
   a. ovarian cancer.
   b. pancreatic cancer.
   c. breast cancer.
   d. esophageal cancer.

9. The most common acute sign of malignant cerebral edema is:
   a. headache.
   b. nausea/vomiting.
   c. seizure.
   d. disorientation.

10. Prophylactic measures to prevent new fluid from forming in patients with lymphedema of the arm or leg include all of the following *except*:
    a. elastic support sleeves or stockings.
    b. pain control.
    c. sodium restriction.
    d. avoidance of infection.

## ANSWER EXPLANATIONS

1. **The answer is c.** The distribution pattern of body water is termed *fluid spacing. First spacing* describes a normal distribution of fluid in both the extracellular and the intracellular compartments. *Second spacing* refers to an excess accumulation of interstitial fluid (edema), and *third spacing* is fluid retention in sites that normally have no fluid or a minimum of fluid (effusion). (p. 722)

2. **The answer is b.** Lymphedema is a benign, iatrogenic problem caused by radical cancer surgery. Arm lymphedema often developed after the most common treatment for all types of breast cancer in the past: radical mastectomy with axillary node dissection followed by radiation. It now occurs much less frequently. Lymphedema of the leg may develop after groin dissection that is performed for the treatment of metastatic disease from primary tumors. Mechanical interruption (surgical technique) and radiation often produce lymphatic obstruction, the most common cause of lymphedema. (p. 738)

3. **The answer is a.** Common presenting signs and symptoms of malignant effusions are distressing to most patients. The degree of subjective symptoms produced by a pleural effusion depends less on the amount of fluid involved than on the rapidity with which it has accumulated. If fluid accumulation is gradual, the heart and lungs can accommodate, but rapid accumulation can trigger an oncologic emergency. (pp. 725–726)

4. **The answer is b.** Relief of pleural effusion symptoms such as dyspnea, cough, and dull, aching chest pain is a short-term treatment goal that is usually achieved when the pleural fluid is mechanically drained. Thoracentesis involves pleural fluid removal by needle aspiration through the chest wall. Fluid tends to reaccumulate when it is not possible to control the underlying cancer. Long-range treatment goals are directed toward the obliteration of the pleural space so that pleural fluid cannot reaccumulate. (p. 727)

5. **The answer is c.** Sclerosis with chemical agents is the most common method used to obliterate the pleural space in patients with malignant pleural effusions. Chemical sclerosing does not prolong the patient's life but may enhance quality of life by relieving symptoms and reducing the time a patient spends in the hospital. Shunts and stripping are surgical methods that become options after other approaches have been tried and the pleural effusion remains uncontrolled. Although external beam

radiation may be used as local treatment for mediastinal tumors, hemithoracic radiation is not recommended as a first-line management of malignant pleural effusions because of the hazard of pulmonary fibrosis. (p. 729)

6.  **The answer is d.** Malignant pericardial effusions are not easily detected by routine tests and are found in 8%–20% of autopsies. Only 30% of affected patients are symptomatic. Since pericardial effusion is not easily detected by routine tests, it is often not discovered while the patient is alive. (pp. 729–730)

7.  **The answer is d.** Pericardial effusion interferes with cardiac function because the fluid burden occupies space and reduces the volume of the heart in diastole. Systemic circulatory effects of decreased cardiac output and impaired venous return lead to generalized congestion. The body tries to compensate in several ways: tachycardia, an increase in systemic and pulmonary venous pressure, and increased ejection fraction. (p. 730)

8.  **The answer is a.** Malignant peritoneal effusion (ascites) is most common in patients with ovarian cancer. Ascites is found at presentation in 33% of these patients, and over 60% will develop ascites at some time before death. (p. 733)

9.  **The answer is c.** Malignant cerebral edema produces diffuse signs and symptoms reflecting its more global effects on brain functioning, as opposed to the focal signs and symptoms caused by direct destruction of tissue by tumor. Subtle early changes in the patient's status are vague and usually are observed only by someone who knows the patient well. Seizure is the most common acute onset sign. Headache, another common early symptom, is due to distortion and traction of pain-sensitive structures by the edema. (pp. 736–737)

10.  **The answer is b.** Prophylactic measures to prevent new fluid from forming include elastic support sleeves or stockings; sodium restriction; and avoidance of infection, excessive use of the limb, local heat, and trauma to the limb. Preventive nursing measures are categorized as primary nursing interventions. Tertiary care is associated with the long-term care of the patient with lymphedema and includes arm elevation, continued hand and arm care measures and exercises, massage therapy, elastic wrap or sleeve to the extremity, pain control, and assessment of the patient for general functioning and ability to perform activities of daily living. (p. 739)

# Chapter 28    Sexual and Reproductive Dysfunction

## SCOPE OF THE PROBLEM

- Difficulties in the ability to be sexually intimate or to bear children have remained major problems that affect all aspects of the patient's and family's lives, sometimes influencing choices for therapy.
- Sexual or reproductive dysfunctions may be temporary or permanent.
- Various factors may affect the cancer patient's sexuality and reproductive capacity, including the biological process of cancer, the effects of treatment, the alterations caused by cancer and treatment, and the psychological issues surrounding the patient and family.

## PHYSIOLOGICAL ALTERATIONS

- See Figures 28-1 and 28-2, text page 744, along with accompanying text, for a review of normal testicular and ovarian function, and Figures 28-3 and 28-4, text page 745, for a review of ovarian failure and germinal aplasia.
- Ovarian failure and germinal aplasia can occur as a result of disease, therapy, nutritional status, psychological factors, or any combination of these
- In the male, damage to the Leydig cells results in decreased testosterone production; LH and FSH will be elevated. Continued damage results in temporary, but more often permanent, sterility.

## CLINICAL MANIFESTATIONS: EFFECT OF CANCER THERAPY ON GONADAL FUNCTION

### Surgery

- Some surgical procedures for cancer cause sexual dysfunction through the removal of sexual organs, through damage to nerves that enervate sexual organs, or through alteration in normal function.
- Organ dysfunction, either through loss of or alteration in normal function, is most common in cancers of the colon, rectum, bladder and associated urinary structures, and male and female genital tracts.

#### Cancer of the colon and rectum

- Surgery for cancer of the colon or rectum may cause sexual dysfunction in both men and women.
- Cancer of the rectum and anus may require anterior or abdominoperineal resection (APR).
  - For the patient who requires an APR, sexual dysfunction may be related to the placement of a colostomy, to removal of or interference with sexual organ function, or some combination of the two.
  - For the woman with an APR, the ovaries or uterus may be removed, thus causing dysfunction from primary inability to bear children or from alterations in normal hormonal patterns. In addition, women may have part of the vagina removed, or healing of the perineal wound may result in vaginal scarring that causes painful or incomplete vaginal intercourse.
  - For the man who has an APR, sexual dysfunction is more severe, with a suggestion that permanent sexual dysfunction may be as high as 80%.
- For all patients the removal of rectal tissue appears to be the most common denominator to organic sexual dysfunction. If the rectum remains intact, there rarely is an associated sexual dysfunction without direct tumor invasion.

## Cancers of the genitourinary tract

### Bladder cancer

- The treatment of bladder cancer may alter sexual function in men and women.
- Radical cystectomy results in sexual dysfunction for both men and women because of organ removal and/or enervation. In men, radical cystectomy consists of removal of the bladder, prostate, seminal vesicles, pelvic lymph nodes, and occasionally the urethra.
- For the woman who has radical cystectomy, the surgery usually includes removal of the bladder and urethra, the uterus, ovaries, fallopian tubes, and the anterior portion of the vagina.
- For both sexes, urinary diversion is a necessity with radical cystectomy; it may result in alterations in self-esteem and body image and may lead to a decrease or cessation of all sexual activities.

### Penile cancer/cancer of the male urethra

- Cancer of the penis and male urethra are rare.
- Treatment includes total or partial penectomy, radiation therapy, or topical chemotherapy, with radiation therapy or chemotherapy used for small, early lesions.
- Partial penectomy does not result in loss of erectile, ejaculative, or orgasmic abilities.

### Testicular cancer

- The treatment of testicular cancer includes an orchiectomy and usually retroperitoneal lymph node dissection and/or removal of a pelvic mass, usually followed by chemotherapy or radiation therapy.
- Unilateral orchiectomy will not result in infertility or sexual dysfunction, as long as the contralateral testis is normal.
- Retroperitoneal lymph node dissection (RPLND), done for staging or as treatment, may result in temporary or permanent loss of ejaculation, whereas potency and the ability to have an orgasm remain.

### Prostate cancer

- Therapy for prostate cancer consists of various combinations of surgery, chemotherapy, radiation therapy, and hormonal manipulation, all of which have a potential to alter sexual function. Surgical treatment of prostate cancer includes prostatectomy or bilateral orchiectomy. Transurethral resection of the prostate generally does not cause impotence or erectile dysfunction; however, retrograde ejaculation occurs in approximately 90% of all patients.
- Transabdominal resection of the prostate results in retrograde ejaculation in 75%–80% of patients and may cause erectile dysfunction.
- The perineal approach, or radical prostatectomy, may result in permanent damage to erectile function with concomitant loss of emission and ejaculation.
- Bilateral orchiectomy causes sexual dysfunction through gradual diminution of libido, impotence, gynecomastia, penile atrophy, and body image changes.
- Various methods, including the use of penile prostheses, suction or vacuum devices, intracorporeal injections of papaverine hydrochloride or prostaglandin $E_1$, or medications such as yohimbine hydrochloride, have been used to restore erectile potential.

### Gynecologic malignancies

#### Vulvar cancer

- Treatment will not alter fertility but may affect sexuality.
- In general, good cosmetic results occur with treatment of early disease except for the simple vulvectomy, which removes the labia and subcutaneous tissue, with retention of the clitoris.
- Evaluation of lymph nodes prior to radical surgery may allow for more limited surgeries with less compromise to sexuality.

#### Vaginal cancer

- Vaginal cancer results in some abnormality and/or need for reconstruction of the vagina.
- A shortened vagina can cause considerable sexual dysfunction.
- Total vaginectomy precludes vaginal intercourse; however, there are multiple techniques for vaginal reconstruction.

#### Cervical cancer and endometrial cancer

- Treatment for cervical intraepithelial neoplasia and carcinoma in situ includes conization, laser therapy, cryosurgery, loop electrosurgical excision (LEEP), or simple hysterectomy. All but the last usually have no effect on fertility, nor should they cause any physiological sexual dysfunction. Simple hysterectomy precludes further childbearing but should not affect sexual functioning.
- Delayed bowel and bladder function may necessitate discharge from the hospital with a urinary catheter.

#### Ovarian cancer

- Initial treatment is surgery, consisting of a radical hysterectomy with bilateral salpingo-oophorectomy and omentectomy. Fertility is lost, and the associated menopausal symptoms occur.
- Treatment usually continues with combination chemotherapy, thus further compounding sexual and reproductive dysfunctions, including alterations in libido, frequency of intercourse, and desire for close physical contact.

### Pelvic exenteration

- An anterior pelvic exenteration preserves the rectum, whereas a posterior exenteration preserves the bladder.
- A total pelvic exenteration involves removing the vagina, uterus, ovaries, fallopian tubes, bladder, and rectum (in the man, the prostate, seminal vesicles, and vas deferens are removed).
- In the woman, reproductive and sexual dysfunction are profound.

### Breast cancer

- The most likely assault to body image and sexual identity with resultant sexual dysfunction is surgical removal of all or part of the breast.
- If breast-preserving surgery is not an option, breast reconstruction can be considered. The ability to have breast reconstruction has been shown to bolster sexual self-esteem and decrease reactions to body image alterations.
- What appears to be of significance is the opportunity or perceived opportunity to select the surgical technique employed.

### Head and neck cancer

- Surgical treatment for cancers of the head and neck region are responsible for varying degrees of alteration in body image, leading to changes in sexuality and intimacy.

## Radiation Therapy

- Radiation therapy can cause sexual and reproductive dysfunction through primary organ failure, through alterations in organ function, and through the temporary or permanent effects of therapy.
- Permanent effects most commonly are related to total dose, location, length of treatment, age, and prior fertility status.
- In the woman, fertility depends on follicular maturation and ovum release.
- In the man, although the Leydig cell and mature sperm are relatively radioresistant, immature sperm and spermatogonia are extremely radiosensitive.
- In women, temporary or permanent sterility is related to the dose of radiation, the volume of tissues radiated, the time period the ovaries are exposed to radiation, and the woman's age.
- For women, movement of the ovaries out of the radiation field with appropriate shielding, has helped maintain fertility even when relatively high doses of radiation have been given.
- Women treated with radiation therapy report decreases in sexual enjoyment, libido, and the ability to attain orgasm, as well as decreased frequency of intercourse and sexual dreams; vaginal stenosis or shortening; vaginal irritation; increased risk of infection, and decreased lubrication and sensation.
- In men, temporary or permanent azoospermia also is a function of age, dose, tissue volume, and exposure time.
- The return of normal spermatogenesis is related to total testicular dose.
- The majority of men treated by external beam for prostate cancer have temporary or permanent impotence. Impotence is thought to be caused by fibrosis of pelvic vasculature or radiation damage of pelvic nerves.
- The inability to gain and maintain an erection may begin as early as two weeks into treatment and may last several weeks after treatment.
- In addition to difficulty in gaining or maintaining erection, men who receive radiation to the pelvis commonly report a decreased libido, inability to ejaculate, inability to lubricate, inability to achieve orgasm, and decreased sexual pleasure.
- General side effects and accompanying psychological effects frequently can alter sexual function.

## Chemotherapy

- Chemotherapy-induced reproductive and sexual dysfunction is related to the type of drug, dose, length of treatment, age and sex of the individual receiving treatment, and length of time after therapy.
- Adult men are more likely to experience long-term side effects regardless of age, whereas women are more apt to have permanent cessation of menses as they near the age of 40.
- Combinations of these drugs appear to prolong infertility (see Table 28-1, text page 751).

### Men

- Infertility occurs in men primarily through depletion of the germinal epithelium that lines the seminiferous tubules.
- Single-agent and combination chemotherapy have been reported to cause germinal aplasia, with alkylating agents the most extensively studied.
- Hormonal manipulation and treatment with estrogens are well known as a cause of sexual dysfunction.

## Women

- Women experience sexual and reproductive dysfunction from chemotherapy as a result of hormonal alterations or direct effects that cause ovarian fibrosis and follicle destruction.
- Age appears to play a more significant role in infertility in women than in men, with women younger than 35 able to tolerate much higher doses of chemotherapy without resultant infertility.
- Any combination of drugs that contains an alkylating agent is apt to cause infertility, and as women near menopause, permanent cessation of menses is more likely.
- When hormonal manipulation includes androgens, not only sexual and reproductive function but also body image and feelings of sexual identity are affected.
- In addition, the use of hormonal therapy, such as tamoxifen and aminoglutethimide, may be associated with menopausal symptoms and decreased desire.

## Children

- Primary effects include delayed sexual maturation and alterations in reproductive potential.
- Prepubescent boys seem to be minimally affected by chemotherapy.
- Young men treated during puberty are more likely to have gonadal dysfunction.
- The majority of girls appear to have normal ovarian function.

## Other issues

- Drugs used to manage chemotherapy side effects can alter sexual function. Table 28-2 on text page 753 lists cancer-associated drugs that affect sexual and reproductive function.

## Biologic Response Modifiers

- Most changes in sexuality are related to known BRM side effects, including fatigue, mucous membrane dryness, flu-like symptoms, and body image changes.
- Decreased libido, amenorrhea, pelvic pain, uterine bleeding, and erectile dysfunction have been reported with alfa-interferon.

## Bone Marrow Transplantation

- Late effects of BMT include chronic fatigue, body image alterations, gonadal dysfunction, and infertility.
- In survivors of BMT, major concerns included infertility, inability to perform sexually, and alterations in sexual intimacy, pleasure, and the ability to achieve orgasm and/or an erection.

# THERAPEUTIC APPROACHES AND NURSING CARE

## Sexual Counseling

- Potential side effects and possible methods for management should be discussed with the patient (and partner if available) at diagnosis, throughout treatment, and during follow-up visits.
- Nurses should include sexuality in their assessment of all patients. See Table 28-3, text page 754, for the ALARM model of evaluation. The PLISSIT model is another method of intervention (see Table 28-4, text page 754).
- Once sexual functioning has been assessed, interventions are necessary to maintain optimal sexual functioning and to promote adaptation to the sexual and reproductive side effects of disease and treatment.

## Nursing Assessment and Management

- Asking about sexual practices early in the nurse's clinical assessment will legitimize and normalize the subject and give patients permission to discuss sexual issues.
- Knowing when to make referrals and recognizing appropriate community resources is essential.

## Fertility Considerations and Procreative Alternatives

- Information about procreative alternatives, the potential for infertility, and issues related to genetic inheritance, mutagenicity, and timing of pregnancy should be thoroughly discussed with potential parents prior to attempting conception.

### Mutagenicity

- *Mutagenicity* is the ability to cause an abnormality in the genetic content of cells, resulting in cell death, alteration(s) in growth and replication, or no noticeable alteration in cell function.
- Possible germ cell mutations may not be evident for generations of offspring.

### Teratogenicity

- *Teratogenicity* is the ability of a toxic compound to produce alterations in an exposed fetus. Both chemotherapy and radiotherapy are known to have teratogenetic effects on the fetus, causing spontaneous abortion, fetal malformation, or fetal death, especially during the first trimester. Low-dose radiation has also been implicated in fetal malignancy.
- Fetal damage probably does not occur at doses < 10 cGy and is only rarely reported at doses < 50 cGy.
- In general, the alkylating agents and antimetabolites have been most often associated with fetal malformations. Table 28-5 (text page 756) lists the teratogenetic effects of chemotherapy.

## Reproductive Counseling

- It is extremely important that methods to prevent pregnancy are discussed and appropriate drugs or devices provided. It has also been suggested that following cancer therapy an individual should wait a minimum of two years before attempting conception. This suggestion is made both to prevent pregnancy during the time recurrence is most likely and to allow for the recovery of spermatogenesis or ovarian function if it has been temporarily altered by therapy.

## Sperm Banking

- Sperm banking has been used to preserve procreation abilities in men undergoing cancer therapy. Unfortunately, since sperm banking needs to be completed prior to initiation of therapy, anyone with rapidly progressing disease frequently cannot delay the start of therapy to complete the cryopreservation process.

## In Vitro Fertilization/Embryo Transfer

- In vitro fertilization may be used for male infertility due to low sperm counts or female infertility due to severe endometriosis or immunologic infertility.
- Initial results of a single oocyte-retrieval procedure have resulted in a pregnancy rate of 10%–16%.
- After four to six attempts, the rate of successful pregnancies may approach 50%–60%.

## PREGNANCY AND CANCER

- The most commonly associated cancers seen during the reproductive years are lymphoma, leukemia, malignant melanoma, and cancers of the breast, cervix, ovary, and colorectum.

- In general, most cancers do not adversely affect a pregnancy, nor does the pregnancy adversely affect the cancer outcome.
- Therapeutic abortion has not been shown to be of benefit in altering disease progression and need not be considered unless continued pregnancy will compromise treatment and thus prognosis.
- Treatment options should be evaluated as though the patient were not pregnant, and therapy instituted when appropriate.

## Medical Management of Commonly Associated Cancers

### Breast cancer

- Breast cancer is the cancer most commonly associated with pregnancy.
- Treatment of breast cancer should be the same as in the nonpregnant woman.
- Therapy can be tailored to time of gestation, physician recommendations, and patient wishes.
- In general, modified mastectomy with lymph node sampling is the standard treatment for early disease. Depending on gestational age, adjuvant chemotherapy can often be delayed until after delivery.
- For the woman desiring breast-conserving surgery, radiation therapy and chemotherapy will be delayed until delivery.
- For advanced disease, surgery and chemotherapy should be undertaken without delay. Therapeutic abortion may be suggested during the first trimester to prevent chemotherapy exposure to the fetus.

### Cancer of the Cervix

- The second most common cancer during pregnancy is cancer of the cervix.
- For carcinoma in situ the pregnancy may be allowed to continue.
- If frank invasion is found, treatment consistent with standard practice for nonpregnant women should not be delayed. During the first two trimesters, surgery or radiation therapy without therapeutic abortion usually is undertaken.
- During the third trimester, fetal viability usually can be awaited and the baby can be delivered by cesarean section, after which the appropriate cancer therapy is given.

### Ovarian cancer

- Ovarian masses are common during pregnancy. Only 2%–5% of these are malignant.
- If malignancy is diagnosed, treatment should proceed as in the nonpregnant woman. Stage IA can be managed by unilateral oophorectomy and biopsy of the other ovary. The pregnancy may be allowed to continue. For all other stages, standard therapy of radical hysterectomy, omentectomy, node biopsy, and peritoneal washings should be carried out.
- If the woman is near term, a cesarean section, followed by the appropriate therapy, may be performed.

### Malignant melanoma

- Melanoma that occurs during pregnancy more often is found on the trunk, a site associated with a poor prognosis.
- Treatment consists of wide excision with skin graft if necessary.
- For individuals with advanced disease, therapeutic abortion followed by palliative chemotherapy is advised. For the individual with brain metastasis, surgery or radiation therapy with appropriate fetal shielding may be undertaken.

## Lymphomas

- Both non-Hodgkin's lymphoma (NHL) and Hodgkin's disease (HD) occur with pregnancy, although the incidence is rare.
- HD confined to the neck or axilla usually can be treated with radiation therapy used with fetal shielding. Because more extensive disease requires combination chemotherapy, a therapeutic abortion is suggested during the first half of pregnancy.
- During the last half of pregnancy, therapy will be defined by the stage of the pregnancy.
- Although NHL is known to metastasize to the placenta and fetus and thus requires careful observations at delivery, NHL has not developed in these infants.

## Leukemia

- Leukemia treatment should be instituted immediately unless the fetus is viable or near viability. If the fetus is viable, delivery should not be delayed.
- Therapeutic abortion is suggested in the first trimester to avoid fetal exposure to chemotherapy.

## Effects of Treatment and Malignancy on the Fetus

### Surgery

- Maternal surgery can be safely accomplished with minimal risk to the fetus. Pelvic surgery is more easily accomplished during the second trimester.

### Radiation

- Radiation doses of > 250 cGy during pregnancy have been associated with fetal damage.
- Radiation to the pelvis should be avoided.

### Chemotherapy

- Chemotherapy during the first trimester has been associated with fetal wastage, malformations, and low birth weights.
- Pharmacokinetics of chemotherapeutic agents may be altered by the normal physiological changes of pregnancy. Monitoring for unexpected toxicities or altered response patterns is of extreme importance.

### Maternal-fetal spread

- Only a few cancers spread from the mother to the fetus, with melanoma, NHL, and leukemia the most common.

# PRACTICE QUESTIONS

1. Sexuality in the cancer patient may be affected by several factors, including each of the following *except*:
   a. psychosexual changes associated with mutagenicity.
   b. physiologic problems of fertility and sterility.
   c. psychologic issues such as loss of self-esteem and fears of abandonment.
   d. changes in body appearance resulting from therapy.

2. For patients who undergo surgery for gastrointestinal cancer, possible organic sexual dysfunction is most closely associated with:
   a. placement of a colostomy.
   b. removal of rectal tissue.
   c. changes in body image.
   d. responses by family and friends.

3. Treatments for prostate cancer have a potential to alter sexual function, even though prostate cancer occurs mostly in older men. Permanent damage to erectile function with loss of emission and ejaculation is most likely to occur with:
   a. radical prostatectomy.
   b. transurethral resection.
   c. bilateral orchiectomy.
   d. transabdominal resection.

4. Which of the following statements about the relationship between gynecologic malignancies and sexual dysfunction is correct?
   a. Pelvic exenteration results in relatively few problems with sexual dysfunction.
   b. The procedures commonly used to treat carcinoma in situ are not likely to affect fertility or childbearing.
   c. Menopausal symptoms are closely associated with radical hysterectomy.
   d. The majority of gynecologic cancers result in some abnormality of the vagina.

5. A woman wishing to minimize the effects of breast surgery on her sexuality would be most likely to elect:
   a. lumpectomy.
   b. modified mastectomy.
   c. radical mastectomy.
   d. any of the above might be selected by an individual woman; it is the opportunity to have input into treatment selection that is significant.

6. Which of the following side effects is least likely to occur as a result of radiation therapy?
   a. alterations in organ function, e.g., decreased vaginal lubrication
   b. enhanced hormonal activity, e.g., overstimulation of the hypothalamus or pituitary
   c. general or psychologic side effects of therapy that can alter sexual function, e.g., diarrhea, loss of sexual desire
   d. primary organ failure, e.g., ovarian failure

7. A patient is about to receive radiation for prostate cancer. He is concerned about sexual dysfunction as a result. As part of your patient education plan, you tell him that radiation therapy can cause sexual and reproductive dysfunction through:
   a. primary organ failure.
   b. alterations in organ function.
   c. temporary or permanent effects of the therapy itself.
   d. all of the above.

8. Which of the following has been implicated in sexual dysfunction in both men and women receiving chemotherapy?
   a. depletion of the germinal epithelium
   b. treatment with estrogens
   c. combination chemotherapy with MOPP
   d. treatment with androgens

9. Those at increased risk for long-term side effects from chemotherapy-induced reproductive dysfunction include:
   a. women age 40 and older.
   b. premenstrual girls.
   c. prepubescent boys.
   d. all of the above.

10. It has been suggested that after cancer therapy an individual should wait a minimum of 2 years before attempting conception. One reason for this is to allow for the recovery of spermatogenesis or ovarian function. Another important reason is that:
   a. residues from chemotherapy typically remain in the body for at least 18 months.
   b. the psychologic effects of cancer therapy may be felt for a prolonged period of time.
   c. germinal epithelium may have been damaged by chemotherapy and/or radiation therapy.
   d. recurrence is most likely within the first 2 years after cancer therapy.

11. Which of the following statements about pregnancy and cancer is false?
   a. Most cancers do not adversely affect a pregnancy.
   b. In general, pregnancy does not adversely affect the outcome of a cancer.
   c. Therapeutic abortion has been shown to be of benefit in altering disease progression.
   d. Treatment options should be evaluated as though the patient were not pregnant, and therapy should be instituted when appropriate.

12. The standard treatment for early breast cancer diagnosed in a pregnant woman consists of:
   a. immediate surgery and chemotherapy.
   b. modified mastectomy with lymph node sampling.
   c. lumpectomy with lymph node sampling if the woman is in the first trimester of pregnancy.
   d. mammogram followed by biopsy and adjuvant chemotherapy.

13. Invasion of a cervical carcinoma in situ into underlying tissue is found in a woman during the third trimester of her pregnancy. Which of the following treatments is most likely to be followed?
   a. Fetal viability is awaited and appropriate therapy is given after delivery of the baby by cesarean section.
   b. Surgery or radiation therapy, without therapeutic abortion, is undertaken immediately.
   c. A radical hysterectomy and pelvic node dissection is performed and combined with radiation therapy.
   d. Therapeutic abortion is performed immediately and followed by standard treatment for advanced disease.

14. Evaluation of the placenta for evidence of metastasis to the fetus is most likely to be carried out under which of the following situations?
    a. when the mother has received combination chemotherapy during the third trimester of pregnancy
    b. when the mother has received low does of radiation during the first trimester of pregnancy
    c. when the mother has breast cancer or invasive cervical cancer
    d. when the mother has a melanoma or lymphoma

15. Which of the following is most likely to involve risk to the fetus whose mother is being treated for cancer?
    a. pelvic surgery on the mother during the second trimester of pregnancy
    b. low doses of radiation associated with diagnostic X rays
    c. chemotherapy during the first trimester of pregnancy
    d. the use of anesthetic agents during surgery on the mother during the second trimester of pregnancy

16. In a support group you are conducting for expectant mothers with breast cancer, the question is raised: "How likely is cancer to spread from the mother to the fetus?" You explain that only a few cancers spread from the mother to the fetus. Among the following cancers mentioned by the group, the cancer least likely to spread from the mother to the fetus is:
    a. melanoma.
    b. NHL.
    c. leukemia.
    d. breast cancer.

## ANSWER EXPLANATIONS

1. **The answer is a.** Among the factors that affect the cancer patient's sexuality are those related to the biologic/physiologic process of cancer, the effects of treatment, the alterations caused by cancer and treatment, and the psychologic issues surrounding the patient and family. Physiologic problems of infertility and sterility, changes in body appearance, and the inability to have intercourse are enhanced by psychologic and psychosexual issues of alteration in body image, fears of abandonment, loss of self-esteem, alterations in sexual identity, and concerns about self. Mutagenicity and psychosexual changes are not closely related. (p. 743)

2. **The answer is b.** Choices **a**, **c**, and **d**, while all associated with sexual dysfunction resulting from gastrointestinal surgery, primarily are psychosexual and not organic issues. For all patients the removal of rectal tissue appears to be the most common denominator to organic sexual dysfunction. If the rectum remains intact, there rarely is an associated sexual dysfunction without direct tumor invasion. (p. 746)

3. **The answer is a.** Permanent damage to erectile function with loss of emission and ejaculation may occur with perineal resection, or radical prostatectomy. Retrograde ejaculation is common with transurethral and transabdominal resection; erectile dysfunction with transabdominal resection. Bilateral orchiectomy causes sexual dysfunction through gradual diminution of libido, impotence, gynecomastia, and penile atrophy. (p. 747)

4. **The answer is d.** Sexual identity, as well as sexual functioning, is often affected permanently by surgery of the vulva, vagina, uterus and uterine cervix, ovary and fallopian tube, or pelvic exenteration. Although vaginal cancer is less common than most other gynecologic malignancies, surgery for the majority of gynecologic cancers (except for carcinoma in situ) results in some abnormality

and/or reconstruction of the vagina. In women, dysfunction related to pelvic exenteration (removal of all pelvic organs) with resulting ostomies is profound and is associated with changes in body image, sexual identity, and self-esteem. Simple hysterectomy, used to treat noninvasive cervical cancer, affects fertility and childbearing. Menopausal symptoms are most closely related to removal of the ovaries and fallopian tubes, which is not part of a radical hysterectomy. (p. 748)

5.  **The answer is d.** Although it has been previously reported that the use of breast-preserving surgery (lumpectomy) has been shown to cause significantly less alteration in body image, sexual desire, and frequency of intercourse, recent studies showed no difference between women receiving lumpectomy and radiotherapy, and women undergoing mastectomy. What appears to be of significance is the opportunity or perceived opportunity to select the surgical technique employed. Thus, choices should be offered whenever possible. (p. 749)

6.  **The answer is b.** Radiation therapy can cause sexual and reproductive dysfunction through primary organ failure (e.g., ovarian failure and testicular aplasia), through alterations in organ function (e.g., decreased lubrication and impotence), and through the temporary and permanent effects of therapy associated with reproduction (e.g., diarrhea and fatigue). In addition, radiation therapy can cause decreases in sexual enjoyment, ability to obtain orgasm, libido, and frequency of intercourse and sexual dreams, as well as vaginal stenosis in women. (p. 750)

7.  **The answer is d.** Radiation therapy can cause sexual and reproductive dysfunction through primary organ failure, through alterations in organ function, and through the temporary or permanent effects of therapy related to total dose, location, length of treatment, age, and prior fertility status. (pp. 749–50)

8.  **The answer is c.** Chemotherapy-induced reproductive and sexual dysfunction is related to the type of drug, dose, length of treatment, age, and sex of the individual receiving treatment and to the length of time after treatment, as well as to the use of single versus multiple agents and drugs given to combat side effects of chemotherapy. Combination chemotherapy with MOPP (mechlorethamine, vincristine, procarbazine, and prednisone) has been shown to produce sexual dysfunction and to decrease fertility in both men and women. Androgen therapy affects sexual function in women; estrogen therapy affects sexual function in men. Chemotherapy may deplete the germinal epithelium that lines the seminiferous tubules in men. (pp. 751–752)

9.  **The answer is a.** Adult men are more likely to experience long-term side effects regardless of age, whereas women are more apt to have permanent cessation of menses as they near the age of 40. (pp. 751 and 753)

10. **The answer is d.** Those who do not believe that another pregnancy is contraindicated suggest a waiting period of 2 to 5 years after completion of all therapy inasmuch as recurrence is most likely during this time period. Further pregnancies after a diagnosis of breast cancer have been considered controversial. Some authors suggest that all women refrain from any pregnancies, whereas others suggest that a pregnancy may actually protect against recurrence. Choice **b** is true but should not seriously affect an attempt at conception; choice **c** duplicates the initial reason. (p. 757)

11. **The answer is c.** Therapeutic abortion has not been shown to be of benefit in altering disease progression and should not be considered unless pregnancy will compromise treatment and thus prognosis. Therapeutic abortion is most likely to be called for when the cancer is diagnosed at an advanced stage during the first trimester of pregnancy and the effects of combination chemotherapy are likely to damage the fetus. (p. 758)

12. **The answer is b.** Treatment of the pregnant women with early breast cancer should be as in the non-pregnant woman, with therapy tailored to time, gestation, physician recommendations, and patient desires. In general, modified mastectomy with lymph node sampling is the standard treatment for early disease. Adjuvant chemotherapy can be delayed until after delivery. For the woman who

desires breast-conserving surgery, lumpectomy with lymph node sampling may be done but radiation therapy should be delayed until after delivery. For advanced disease, surgery and chemotherapy should be undertaken without delay. Therapeutic abortion may be suggested during the first term to prevent chemotherapy exposure to the fetus. (p. 758)

13. **The answer is a.** During the first two trimesters, surgery or radiation therapy, without therapeutic abortion, is usually undertaken. Early stage disease may be treated with radical hysterectomy and pelvic node dissection, whereas in advanced disease radiation therapy is the most common treatment. During the third trimester, fetal viability usually can be awaited and the baby delivered by cesarean section, after which appropriate cancer therapy can be given. (pp. 758–759)

14. **The answer is d.** Certain malignancies, notably melanoma, non-Hodgkin's lymphoma (NHL), and leukemia, are known to spread from the mother to the fetus. If the mother has any of these cancers, the placenta should be carefully evaluated at delivery and the baby monitored for development of the disease. (p. 760)

15. **The answer is c.** Chemotherapy during the first trimester has been associated with fetal wastage, malformations, and low birth weight, although the incidence of fetal malformations is low and may be minimized or avoided with careful selection of agents. Maternal surgery can be safely accomplished with minimal risk to the fetus. Pelvic surgery is more easily accomplished during the second trimester. There is little risk to the fetus from short exposure to anesthetic agents after the first trimester, provided ventilation is adequate and hypotension is prevented. Low doses of radiation associated with diagnostic X-ray studies are not harmful if adequate fetal shielding is provided. (p. 760)

16. **The answer is d.** Only a few cancers spread from the mother to the fetus, with melanoma, NHL, and leukemia the most common. (p. 760)

# Chapter 29    Integumentary and Mucous Membrane Alterations

---

## ALTERATIONS TO THE INTEGUMENT

- Cells in a renewal system with rapid turnover and having little or no differentiation (e.g., skin cells, mucous membranes, hematopoietic stem cells) are radiosensitive.
- Cells that do not divide regularly or at all and are highly differentiated (e.g., muscle cells, nerve cells) are radioresistant.
- Damage from radiation is apparent early, within weeks to months of first exposure, in radiosensitive cells and is classified as an acute effect of radiation.
- In contrast, radioresistant cells may not manifest damage for months to years after exposure to radiation. These effects are classified as late effects of radiation.
- Acute effects are usually temporary. Late radiation effects are usually permanent and often become more severe as time goes on.
- Higher doses given over shorter periods of time to larger volumes of tissue will result in more severe acute reactions.
  - Acute damage results from the depletion of actively proliferating parenchymal or stromal cells and is characterized by vascular dilation, local edema, and inflammation.
- The severity of late effects is more dependent upon the total dose delivered and the volume of tissue irradiated.
- See Table 29-1, text page 772, for acute radiation skin effects.
- The acute skin reactions associated with radiation therapy include erythema, pruritus, hyperpigmentation, and dry or moist desquamation.
- Several factors determine the degree, onset, and duration of radiation-induced skin reactions.
  - *Dose-time-volume factors:* Higher doses given over shorter periods of time to larger volumes will result in more severe acute skin reactions.
  - *Equipment:* Electrons will produce greater skin reactions than photons.
  - *Bolus material:* Placing tissue-equivalent material on the skin reduces the skin-sparing effect of radiation therapy, allowing for maximum dose at the level of the skin.
  - *Tangential fields:* This approach is used to deliver a more homogeneous dose to the treatment area, but it simultaneously increases the skin dose.
  - *Concomitant chemotherapy:* The use of radiosensitizing chemotherapeutic agents results in increased severity of skin reactions.
  - *Anatomic location:* When treatment is targeted at areas of skin apposition, increased reaction secondary to warmth, moisture, and lack of aeration can be expected.
    - Treatment delivered over a bony prominence or surgical site may result in increased skin reactions due to alterations in vasculature and circulation.
  - *Patient-related considerations:* Normal age-related changes and nutritional status must also be considered.
- See Table 29-2, text page 775, for late radiation skin effects.
- The late skin reactions associated with radiation therapy include photosensitivity, pigmentation changes, atrophy, fibrosis, telangiectasia, and rarely, ulceration and necrosis.

## Nursing considerations

- Skin assessment should be performed prior to initiation of treatment, at least weekly during treatment, one to two weeks following completion of treatment, and at each follow-up appointment thereafter.
- A commonly used system for grading acute radiation toxicity is one devised by the Radiation Therapy Oncology Group (RTOG).
- Tissue fibrosis, ulceration, and necrosis are relatively infrequent late radiation skin effects and tend to be chronic in nature.
- Scar tissue integration therapy "breaks up" or loosens and redistributes scar tissue to increase mobility, decrease pain, and enhance lymphatic drainage.
- Surgical wound closure is often unsuccessful for the following reasons: (1) irradiated tissue is fibrotic and unyielding, making it prone to dehiscence; (2) healthy tissue often cannot be reached surgically because the ulcers are so deep; and (3) radiation injury extends beyond the ulcer to surrounding tissues.
- Myocutaneous flaps are the preferred method of surgical closure of radiation ulcers.
- See Table 29-4, text page 777, for skin care guidelines during and after radiation therapy.
- See Table 29-5, text page 778, for management of severe acute radiation skin reactions.

# Chemotherapy Effects

## Hyperpigmentation

- Hyperpigmentation occurs in individuals also experiencing busulfan-induced pulmonary fibrosis, with cyclophosphamide, with carmustine or nitrogen mustard, following 5-fluorouracil (5-FU) therapy, bleomycin, and etoposide.

## Hypersensitivity

- Cutaneous hypersensitivity reactions (HSRs) tend not to be dose-related. Cutaneous manifestations of immediate HSRs (type I reactions) generally present as urticaria angioedema or anaphylaxis. Drugs involved include L-asparaginase, paclitaxel, docetaxel, cisplatin, carboplatin, nitrogen mustard, teniposide, and etoposide.
- Other drugs producing hypersensitivity reactions include procarbazine, cytarabine, levamisole, alfa-interferon, interleukin, anthracycline antibiotics, melphalan, methotrexate, aminoglutethimide, and dactinomycin.

## Acral erythema

- *Palmerplantar erythrodysesthesia syndrome* may represent a direct toxic effect on the epidermis and dermal vasculature or an accumulation of the chemotherapeutic agent in eccrine structures and sweat, causing erythema of the palms and soles.

## Pruritus

### Etiology

- When pruritus is due primarily to systemic disease, toxic circulating substances such as peptides, histamine, bradykinin, and serotonin are thought to be the agents responsible for the itching.

### Management

- Nursing care focuses on three areas: skin care, environmental control, and administration of therapeutics.

- Adequate hydration promotes healthy skin. Drinking 3000 ml of fluid per day and eating a diet rich in iron, zinc, and protein promotes skin integrity.
- The patient is encouraged to employ alternate cutaneous stimulation methods to relieve the urge to scratch.
- Medications may be recommended based on the etiology of the pruritus.

## Photosensitivity

- Photosensitivity is caused by a variety of topical or oral medications.
- Following radiation therapy, the skin's ability to protect itself from UV rays is decreased as a result of destruction of melanocytes in the irradiated epidermis and the slower rate of melanin production in new epidermal cells in the radiation field.
- Patients are still vulnerable to UV light on cloudy days.
- Sunscreens with an SPF higher than 15 are generally recommended for use in a tropical climate or for protection following chemotherapy or radiation therapy.
- The greater the SPF, the greater the chance of skin irritation.

# HAIR

## Radiation Effects

- In order of decreasing radiosensitivity are scalp, beard, eyebrow, eyelash, axillary, pubic, and fine hair of the body.
- Hair thinning usually begins to occur after two to three weeks of treatment at a dose of 25–30 Gy and continues for an additional two to three weeks.
- If hair regrowth occurs, it usually begins eight to nine weeks following completion of treatment.
- Regrowth is unlikely if alopecia persists for greater than six months. The likelihood of hair regrowth also diminishes with age and higher doses of radiation.

## Chemotherapy Effects

### Alopecia

- Cancer chemotherapeutic agents affect actively growing (anagen) hairs.
- Chemotherapy-induced alopecia occurs rapidly and usually starts two to three weeks following a dose of chemotherapy.
- After discontinuation of the epilating drugs, regrowth is visible in four to six weeks, but complete regrowth may take one to two years.
- The severity and duration of chemotherapy-induced hair loss are related to several drug factors including the type of drug or combination of drugs, dose of drug, method of administration and pharmacokinetics, as well as patient-related factors.

## Nursing Care

- It is essential that the nurse give the patient and family an adequate appraisal of the potential for treatment-related alopecia. The timing, extent, and duration of hair loss are addressed at the onset of therapy.

## Hirsutism

- Androgens are efficacious in the treatment of women with breast cancer. Troublesome side effects include (male pattern baldness) and hirsutism.

## NAILS

- Radiation to the nail can result in decreased growth rates and the development of ridges when the nail attempts to grow.
- Pigmentation occurs most commonly with doxorubicin and cyclophosphamide but has been reported with melphalan, 5-FU, daunomycin, and bleomycin.
- Beau's lines (transverse white lines or grooves in the nail) indicate a reduction or cessation of nail growth in response to cytotoxic therapy.

## GLANDS

- Sebaceous glands are radiosensitive.
- Impairment or destruction of sebaceous glands is in large part responsible for the acute and late skin effects associated with irradiated skin such as pruritus and inelasticity.

## ALTERATIONS OF THE GASTROINTESTINAL MUCOUS MEMBRANES

- *Mucositis* describes the inflammatory response of mucosal epithelial cells to the cytotoxic effects of chemotherapy as well as localized radiation therapy.

### Stomatitis

- Virtually all patients who receive radiation therapy to the head and neck region will experience oral mucositis, especially when the total dose exceeds 50 Gy.
- Acute reactions include mucosal inflammation and ulceration, infection, and mucosal bleeding. Chronic complications occur as a result of changes in healthy tissue and include xerostomia, taste alterations, trismus, and soft-tissue and bone necrosis.
- In BMT patients, acute and chronic oral graft-versus-host disease (GVHD) is also observed.

#### Chemotherapy-induced stomatitis

##### Risk factors

- Diagnosis and aggressiveness of the chemotherapy regimen are predictors of oral complications. Breast cancer patients can have as low as a 12% risk and non-Hodgkin's lymphoma patients a 33% risk, compared with a 70% risk in leukemia patients.
- The frequency of oral problems is two to three times higher in patients with hematologic malignancies than with solid tumors.
- Those agents most associated with stomatitis are the antimetabolites and antitumor antibiotics, in particular bleomycin, doxorubicin, daunorubicin, 5-fluorouracil, and methotrexate.
- Mucositis is observed more often with 5-FU when combined with other mucositis-producing drugs and when 5-FU is given concurrently with leucovorin.

##### Direct stomatotoxicity

- Direct stomatotoxicity sequelae are a thinned atrophic mucosa and initiation of an inflammatory response (stomatitis).
- Most often affected are the nonkeratinized mucosal areas including the buccal and labial mucosa, tongue, soft palate, and floor of the mouth. Rarely is the gingiva, or hard palate, involved.
- Oral pain is the major clinical problem associated with stomatitis.

### Xerostomia

- Patients complain of dry mouth and accumulation of thick, ropy saliva that can interfere with nutrition, taste, and speech.
- Xerostomia is transient.

### Taste alterations

- Commonly induced changes include lowered threshold for bitter taste, increase threshold for sweet taste, and complaints of a metallic taste.

### Indirect stomatotoxicity

- Reduced myeloproliferation is manifested by neutropenia and thrombocytopenia; infection and hemorrhage secondary to myelosuppression can then occur.
- The lips, tongue, and gingiva are the most common sites.
- Management of bleeding with topical coagulants (thrombin-soaked gauze) and pressure is often helpful.

## Oral graft-versus-host disease

- Acute and chronic GVHD is a significant complication of patients who undergo allogeneic BMT.
- Treatment strategies include systemic immunosuppressive therapy; topical steroids, which may or may not be beneficial; and fluoride therapy for patients at risk for caries secondary to xerostomia.

## Dental evaluation and prophylactic care

- Patients should have a comprehensive oral examination by the dentist at least two to three weeks before any therapy is initiated, if possible.
- Radiation-induced oral complications can be reduced significantly with daily fluoride treatments along with good oral hygiene.

## Radiation-induced stomatitis and oral complications

- Treatment to the oral cavity may result in stomatitis, hypogeusia (loss of taste), and xerostomia. If the esophagus is included in the treatment field, patients may experience esophagitis and/or dysphagia.
- Other effects of radiation are less common and usually do not manifest for months to years after the completion of treatment. These effects include trismus, dental caries, tissue fibrosis, and tissue necrosis.
- See Table 29-12, text page 794, for radiation-induced gastrointestinal toxicities—both direct and indirect.
- As stomatitis and subsequent pain develop, patients are often unable to maintain an adequate intake of food and fluid. Early intervention and education can prevent or reduce the malnourishment that often accompanies stomatitis.
- Radiation-induced stomatitis is self-limiting and usually resolves two to three weeks after the completion of treatment if infection and further trauma are avoided. If severe, a break in treatment may be necessary.

### Taste changes (hypogeusia)

- Taste changes increase with the cumulative dose. Complete taste loss may occur.
- A positive correlation has been found between taste changes and weight loss in patients receiving radiation therapy.

### Xerostomia

- Salivary glands are highly radiosensitive, with a drastic decrease in secretion evident after just 10 Gy that is usually permanent after 40 Gy.
- Nutrition is often a problem for patients with xerostomia.
- Oral care before meals will help to freshen the mouth and stimulate appetite. Increasing fluid intake during meals and snacks will help to lubricate.
- Irritants such as tobacco, alcohol, carbonated beverages, and caffeine should be avoided. Commercial mouthwashes should be avoided.
- Vegetable or corn oil swished in the mouth may be a cost-effective alternative for artificial lubrication.
- Use of proteolytic enzymes—papain and amylase—is known to effectively dissolve and break up thick saliva in some patients.
  - Papain is found naturally in papayas.
  - Pineapple contains amylase.
- Sialagogues stimulate the secretion of endogenous saliva and include gustatory stimulants such as sugar-free lemon candy and masticatory stimulants such as sugar-free gum.
- Pilocarpine to increase saliva should be used with caution for those with cardiovascular disease because of the potential side effects of bradycardia, hypertension, and GI upset.

### Radiation-induced soft-tissue and bone necrosis

- Soft-tissue necrosis is a result of chemical, mechanical, or microbial insult. It is very painful, slow to heal, and enlarges rapidly unless treated.
- Early irrigation with saline and baking soda rinses is usually employed.
- Osteoradionecrosis is uncommon and can be a direct or indirect effect of radiation injury.
- Treatment begins with gentle debridement using saline irrigation.
- Antibiotic packs and systemic antibiotic therapy are used when infection is present.

### Radiation-induced trismus

- Trismus is the result of fibrosis of the muscles of mastication and/or fibrotic changes in the capsule of the temporomandibular joint.
- Repetition of jaw exercises should be used.
- Surgical intervention to release fibrotic tissue is used only as a last resort.

## Nursing care

### Assessment

- Critical to assessment is the availability of an oral assessment tool that can describe and quantify the physical and functional condition of the oral cavity.
- Review Table 29-13: Oral Assessment Guide (OAG), text page 798.
- A grading system depicting degree of severity of mucosal damage includes the following:
  - Grade 1—erythema of oral mucosa
  - Grade 2—isolated small ulcerations (white patches)
  - Grade 3—confluent ulcerations (white patches) covering more than 25% of oral mucosa
  - Grade 4—hemorrhagic ulceration

### Management

- Mouth rinses enhance removal of loosened debris and should be nonirritating and nondehydrating.

- Normal saline may be the least damaging; sodium bicarbonate is effective as a cleansing agent, but some patients complain of an unpleasant taste; hydrogen peroxide should be diluted to prevent damage to mucosa.
- See Table 29-15, text page 800, on the prevention and management of perioral complications of cancer treatment.
- Treatment of stomatitis remains palliative and symptom-oriented.

## Infections of the Oral Cavity

- Immunosuppression due to the treatment of cancer or the cancer itself further increases a patient's susceptibility to oral infection.
- Identification of the responsible pathogen requires culture.
- Oral *Candida* infections are traditionally treated with topical antifungal agents such as nystatin oral rinses, or clotrimazole troches.
- Alternatives for oropharyngeal candidiasis refractory to topical treatment are the systemic oral antifungal agents: ketoconazole or fluconazole.
- A course of low-dose intravenous amphotericin B is indicated for nonresponsive infection and in severe esophageal and disseminated candidal infections.
- Herpes simplex virus (HSV) is the most common viral pathogen affecting the oral cavity.
- Reactivation of latent HSV is the cause of the majority of HSV infections.
- Acyclovir prophylaxis may be used to prevent infection in selected high-risk patient populations.
- The vast majority of bacterial infections may affect three sites in the mouth: the gingiva, the mucosa, or the teeth.
- Parenteral antibiotic therapy based on causative organism is the treatment of choice.

## Esophagitis

- The most common early symptoms of esophagitis include dysphagia, odynophagia, and epigastric pain.

### Radiation-induced esophagitis

- Radiation used to treat esophageal cancer; Hodgkin's disease; head and neck, breast, and lung cancer often requires that the esophagus receive a radiation dose high enough to induce esophagitis, a common and expected transient side effect.
- Although resolution of the acute esophageal effects of radiation usually begins two to three weeks following treatment completion, late effects may be seen one to five years later. Late complications include epithelial thickening, microvascular changes, and fibrosis of muscle and connective tissue. Ulceration is seen less frequently.

### Nursing considerations

- Risk factors for developing esophagitis include alcohol consumption, tobacco use, ulcer disease, and esophageal exposure to radiation.
- All management is directed at symptom relief and supportive care.
- This is best accomplished through dietary manipulation, topical anesthesia, and systemic analgesia when needed.
- Esophageal candidiasis is most commonly treated using ketoconazole, fluconazole, or nystatin oral suspension.

### Chemotherapy-induced esophagitis

- Any patient who develops oral mucositis following chemotherapy is at risk for spread to the esophageal mucosal tissue.

- *Candida* is the most likely cause and can be fatal if disseminated systemically.
- Flexible endoscopy with brushings is more accurate than radiographic examination of the esophagus to identify the correct cause.

## Enteritis

### Radiation-induced enteritis

- A lack of acute enteritis does not preclude the development of chronic radiation enteritis; however, there is a positive correlation between the occurrence of severe acute enteritis and the development of chronic radiation enteritis.
- Several factors influence the degree, onset, and duration of radiation-induced acute and chronic enteritis: dose per fraction; treatment techniques/plan; bowel displacement techniques; previous abdominal surgery and/or radiation therapy; concomitant chemotherapy; and patient-related considerations, including compromised nutritional status, preexisting bowel disorders, diabetes, and hypertension.
- Dietary changes, specifically a low-fat, low-fiber diet, are usually initiated at the first sign of radiation enteritis and are often the only treatment necessary.
- Conservative treatment with mild antidiarrheals may be helpful initially.
- Diphenoxylate or loperamide may also be prescribed. Anticholinergics, antispasmodics, and/or bile salt sequestrating agents may also be prescribed when appropriate.
- Management of severe diarrhea may include the use of opiates such as opium tincture, paregoric elixir, and codeine to decrease peristalsis.
- Chronic radiation enteritis most frequently occurs six months to five years following completion of treatment.
- Progressive endarteritis is thought to be responsible for chronic changes in the alimentary tract.
- Conservative treatment includes decompression with a nasogastric tube and support with parenteral fluids. This is followed by maintenance on a soft-liquid diet.
- Repeated episodes of partial bowel obstruction often occur, necessitating surgical intervention. Intractable diarrhea and abdominal pain are also indications for surgery.
- There is often an increased risk of surgical complications including poor vascularity and impaired wound healing in irradiated tissue.

### Chemotherapy-induced enteritis

- Epithelial cells in the small intestine (villi and microvilli) are more vulnerable to destruction than cells in the sigmoid colon.
- Epithelial damage occurs histologically in three stages:
  1. initial injury
  2. progressive injury
  3. regeneration
- Chronic diarrhea lasts longer than two weeks.
- Because many cancer patients require antibiotic therapy at some point in their course of therapy, they are also at risk for antibiotic-associated colitis. The cause is overgrowth of *C difficile* in the colon.
- Until now, the mainstay of nonspecific therapy has been the opiates and opiate derivatives. Of these, diphenoxylate and loperamide are the most widely prescribed.
- Specific drug therapy (antibiotics) for treatment of acute infectious diarrhea is recommended in select cases based on the causative organism.

## Intestinal graft-versus-host disease

- After allogeneic BMT, diarrhea is a prominent manifestation of intestinal involvement with GVHD.
- Octreotide has been shown to be a useful agent in acute GVHD management.
- Viral infections, herpes simplex, and varicella zoster are common after BMT, although acute GVHD is the most common cause of diarrhea. Treatment choice is acyclovir.

# ALTERATIONS OF THE GENITOURINARY MUCOUS MEMBRANES

## Radiation-Induced Cystitis and Urethritis

- Radiation therapy employed to treat cancers of the genitourinary system often results in a temporary irritation of the bladder and/or urethra.
- Treatment is directed at reducing irritation. Patients should be instructed to increase fluid intake.

## Radiation-Induced Vaginitis

- The effects of radiation on the vaginal mucosa include erythema, inflammation, atrophy, fibrosis, hypopigmentation, telangiectasia, inelasticity, and ulceration.
- Fibrosis and vaginal stenosis may develop as a result of adhesions and can manifest as early as during the immediate postirradiation period.
- Women who are able to continue having intercourse during treatment have considerably less adhesion formation.
- Less commonly seen—but nonetheless the most serious complication of high-dose radiation—is tissue necrosis.
- Conservative management is usually attempted for necrosis. This includes estrogen cream, antibiotic therapy, debridement, and antiseptic douches.
- Fistula formation and hemorrhage often require surgical management; however, outcomes are often poor.
- Treatment for radiation vaginitis usually begins two weeks after the completion of radiation by vaginal dilatation and use of vaginal estrogen preparations. Dilation can be accomplished through sexual intercourse and/or use of a vaginal dilator designed to minimize fibrosis and stenosis.
- Vaginal dilatation should take place at least three times per week.
- Review of proper technique is often necessary.

## Chemotherapy-Induced Vaginitis

- Symptoms may occur three to five days after chemotherapy is given and resolve seven to ten days later.
- Signs and symptoms to report include vaginal discharge, itching, odor, pain, soreness, bleeding, or dyspareunia.
- Laboratory tests and cultures are valuable to determine causative organisms.

# MALIGNANT WOUNDS

## Description

- Malignant wounds are characterized by excessive purulent drainage, odor, and infection. They develop from local extension of tumor embolization into the epithelium and its supporting structures.
- Malignant wounds at a distant site due to metastasis often result in misdiagnosis until a lesion has become large and fungating.
- Hyperthermia used alone or in conjunction with radiation therapy and cytotoxic drugs has shown impressive response.

## Nursing Considerations

- These wounds have a very poor prognosis for healing. Malignant wounds do not undergo normal healing because of the inability of epithelial cells to migrate over active tumors and their altered vascularity.
- To maintain an optimal environment with control of infection, odor, and drainage, certain interventions are required: debridement, infection control, hemostasis, wound care, and odor control.

### Debridement

- Chemical debridement may be appropriate in the presence of a moderate amount of necrotic tissue or eschar.
- Gentle mechanical debridement is usually preferred.
- Wet to dry dressings are contraindicated.
- If eschar is dense, it may act as a splint to prevent wound contraction. This may require surgical removal.

### Infection control

- Organisms found in wound fluid are not necessarily invading. A positive wound culture of $>10^5$ bacteria is indicative of infection.
- Topical antibiotics are often more successful due to the diminished vasculature and presence of necrotic tissue that may impede systemic therapy.

### Hemostasis

- Bleeding is most often a result of trauma and can usually be prevented by proper wound care. Trauma can be greatly reduced by keeping wounds moist and using nonadherent dressings.
- If a wound and its dressing do become dry, soaking the dressing in normal saline before removal will help to prevent trauma.
- Hemolytic agents may be necessary to arrest small-vessel bleeds.

### Cleansing

- Antiseptic agents are not considered appropriate for most patients.
- If used, agents should be rinsed thoroughly from the wound.

### Wound dressing

- Petroleum-impregnated dressings should be avoided because they inhibit aeration and increase anaerobic bacterial growth.
- Creative alternatives to tape can include Montgomery straps, oversized sports bras, tube dressings, and flexible netting.

### Odor management

- The odor of these wounds is a result of bacterial invasion and the presence of debris and necrotic tissue.
- Frequent cleansing using a handheld shower (two to three times a day) will help to eliminate bacteria and excessive drainage.
- If the cause of odor cannot be eliminated, various deodorizing sprays and solutions and charcoal-containing dressings are available.
- Although unconventional, odor control using yogurt or buttermilk, either applied topically or taken orally, has been found to be useful.

## PRACTICE QUESTIONS

1. Mrs. Kelly is about to receive radiation therapy for the first time. She asks, "I have such sensitive skin. I'm worried about what effect radiation could have on my skin. What can I expect?" You tell Mrs. Kelly that acute radiation effects:
    a. result from the depletion of actively proliferating parenchymal or stromal cells.
    b. are characterized by dilation, local edema, and inflammation.
    c. are usually temporary.
    d. all of the above.

2. Which of the following is *not* true regarding radiation-induced skin reactions?
    a. Higher doses given over shorter periods of time to larger volumes will result in more severe acute skin reactions.
    b. Electrons produce greater skin reactions than photons.
    c. Placing tissue-equivalent material on the skin creates a skin-sparing effect during radiation therapy, minimizing dose at the level of the skin.
    d. When treatment is targeted at areas of skin apposition, increased reaction secondary to warmth and moisture can be expected.

3. Rachel is a new surgical nurse assisting in a center that frequently performs oncologic surgeries. She has noticed that surgical wound closure seems to be much more unsuccessful in cancer surgeries. She points this out to you and asks, "Why do you think that happens?" You explain that:
    a. irradiated tissue is fibrotic and prone to dehiscence.
    b. healthy tissue often cannot be reached surgically because the ulcers are so deep.
    c. radiation injury extends beyond the ulcer to surrounding tissues.
    d. all of the above.

4. Mrs. Kelly is experiencing hyperpigmentation. You explain to her that this may be a reaction to:
    a. L-asparaginase.
    b. bleomycin.
    c. paclitaxel.
    d. cisplatin.

5. The degree of hair loss varies depending on the area of the body exposed to radiation, the dose, and the radiosensitivity of the exposed structures. Which of the following describes the correct order of *decreasing* radiosensitivity?
    a. scalp, beard, eyebrows, eyelashes, axillary, pubic, and fine body hair
    b. fine body hair, eyebrows, eyelashes, pubic hair, scalp hair, beard
    c. beard, eyebrows, scalp, pubic hair, fine body hair
    d. All body hair is equally sensitive to radiation.

6. Following radiation therapy to the chest, your patient plans a trip to Bermuda. You instruct her to use a sunscreen with an SPF of 15 or more because radiation has undoubtedly affected her skin via:
    a. skin-sparing effect during radiation therapy.
    b. slower rate of melanin production in new epidermal cells in the radiation field.
    c. faster rate of melanin production in new epidermal cells in the radiation field.
    d. destruction of lymphocytes in the irradiated epidermis.

7. Albert is about to undergo chemotherapy that is known to cause significant hair loss. Which of the following will *not* be part of your patient education plan for Albert?

    a. Chemotherapy-induced alopecia occurs slowly and may not occur for several months after the treatment.

    b. Once chemotherapy is complete, regrowth is visible in four to six weeks.

    c. Complete regrowth of hair may take one to two years.

    d. In situations involving very high doses of alkylating agents, hair may not regrow.

8. Following four courses of chemotherapy, Albert shows you that his fingernails are having a strange reaction. They have developed transverse white lines or grooves. You explain to Albert that this symptom:

    a. is a response to doxorubicin because pigmentation has been deposited at the base of the nail.

    b. indicates a reduction or cessation of nail growth in response to cytotoxic therapy.

    c. reflects a cytotoxic reaction to cyclophosphamide.

    d. is a partial separation of the nail plate called onycholysis and is a reaction to 5-FU therapy.

9. Which of the following factors are considered risk factors for stomatitis with cancer treatment?

    a. dehydration

    b. preexisting dental problems

    c. diagnosis of leukemia

    d. all of the above

10. Mucositis is observed more often when:

    a. 5-FU is combined with other mucositis-producing drugs such as methotrexate and doxorubicin.

    b. when 5-FU is given alone.

    c. when bleomycin is used to abruptly replace 5-FU.

    d. none of the above.

11. Your patient is receiving chemotherapy and begins to complain of a dry mouth and thick, ropy saliva. The condition is beginning to interfere with his appetite and speech. "What's going on," he says, "and what can we do about it?" Which of the following will not be part of your patient education plan regarding this reaction?

    a. This reaction is permanent, and while not life-threatening, it can eventually lead to oral caries as well as candidal infections.

    b. Xerostomia is a dysfunction of the salivary gland that occurs following chemotherapy.

    c. Xerostomia is a decrease in the quality and quantity of saliva.

    d. Saliva substitutes, frequent rinses with ice water, and sugarless gum may provide relief.

12. Which is *not* part of your treatment plan for the patient experiencing xerostomia?

    a. Oral care before meals will help to freshen the mouth and stimulate appetite.

    b. Increasing fluid intake during meals and snacks will help to lubricate food and ease swallowing.

    c. Lemon glycerin is an excellent substitute for the more irritating commercial mouthwashes.

    d. Vegetable or corn oil swished in the mouth may be a cost-effective alternative for artificial lubrication.

13. What can be used to dissolve and break up thick saliva?

    a. Sugar-free lemon candy and sugar-free gum.

    b. Papain (found in papaya) and amylase (found in pineapple).

    c. Sialagogues.

    d. Pilocarpine.

14. Elise develops GVHD after undergoing allogeneic BMT. Which of the following will probably *not* be part of Elise's treatment plan?
    a. systemic immunosuppressive therapy
    b. topical steroids
    c. NSAIDs
    d. fluoride therapy

15. After radiation, Tricia begins to have trouble opening her mouth very wide. She complains of tonic muscle spasms and pain. Which of the following will *not* be part of your response to Tricia's adverse reaction?
    a. explaining to Tricia that this reaction may be the result of fibrosis of the muscles of chewing
    b. preparing Tricia as soon as possible for essential surgical intervention
    c. teaching Tricia jaw exercises
    d. explaining to Tricia that this reaction may be the result of fibrotic changes in the capsule of the temporomandibular joint

16. Tricia complains of small, isolated white patches here and there in her mouth. You determine that Tricia's mucosal damage can be classified as:
    a. grade 1.
    b. grade 2.
    c. grade 3.
    d. grade 4.

17. Tricia asks you which mouthwash would be best for her to use under these circumstances. You suggest:
    a. sodium bicarbonate.
    b. hydrogen peroxide.
    c. Listerine.
    d. saline.

18. Tricia also develops a disseminated candidal infection that spreads from her mouth to part of her esophagus. Treatment would probably include:
    a. amphotericin B.
    b. heparin.
    c. ketoconazole.
    d. fluconazole.

19. Ruth, an immunocompromised patient, has just completed a course of radiotherapy to the chest and finds that she is suffering dysphagia, odynophagia, and epigastric pain. You suspect that she may have developed:
    a. esophagitis.
    b. stomatitis.
    c. enteritis.
    d. odontogenic infection.

20. Which of the following are considered effective measures to minimize oral stomatitis?
    a. oral cryotherapy during chemotherapy treatment
    b. sucralfate oral suspension
    c. frequent oral hygiene
    d. all of the above

21. What is the best treatment approach for radiation esophagitis?
    a. symptom relief and supportive care
    b. dietary manipulation
    c. topical anesthesia and systemic analgesia when needed
    d. all of the above

22. Radiation-induced enteritis can cause significant diarrhea. Which of the following intervention would *not* be appropriate management of this problem?
    a. a liquid diet high in milk and milk products
    b. Sandostatin® given subcutatneously
    c. anticholinergics
    d. paragoric elixir

23. Mr. Brown has had a bone marrow transplant and suffers from chronic diarrhea. A likely cause for his diarrhea is most likely which of the following?
    a. viral infection
    b. GVHD
    c. herpes simplex
    d. varicella zoster

# ANSWER EXPLANATIONS

1. **The answer is d.** Acute radiation effects result from the depletion of actively proliferating parenchymal or stromal cells and is characterized by vascular dilation, local edema, and inflammation. They are usually temporary and occur after higher doses are given over shorter periods of time to larger volumes of tissue. (p. 772)

2. **The answer is c.** Factors that determine the degree, onset, and duration of radiation-induced skin reactions include the following, among others: Higher doses given over shorter periods of time to larger volumes will result in more severe acute skin reactions; electrons produce greater skin reactions than photons; placing tissue-equivalent material on the skin reduces the skin-sparing effect of radiation therapy, allowing for maximum dose at the level of the skin. Finally, when treatment is targeted at areas of skin apposition, increased reaction secondary to warmth and moisture can be expected. (pp. 772–73)

3. **The answer is d.** Surgical wound closure is often unsuccessful for the following reasons: irradiated tissue is fibrotic and unyielding, making it prone to dehiscence; healthy tissue often cannot be reached surgically because the ulcers are so deep; and radiation injury extends beyond the ulcer to surrounding tissues. (p. 776)

4. **The answer is b.** Hyperpigmentation occurs with bleomycin. Other drugs inducing this reaction include cyclophosphamide, busulfan, carmustine, nitrogen mustard, 5-FU, and etoposide. The other drugs listed as choices in this question have in common the HSRs (type I reactions). (p. 780)

5. **The answer is a.** In order of decreasing radiosensitivity are scalp, beard, eyebrow, eyelash, axillary, pubic, and fine hair of the body. (p. 783)

6. **The answer is b.** Following radiation therapy, the skin's ability to protect itself from UV rays is decreased as a result of destruction of melanocytes in the irradiated epidermis and the slower rate of melanin production in new epidermal cells in the radiation field. (p. 783)

7.  **The answer is a.** Chemotherapy-induced alopecia occurs rapidly and usually starts two to three weeks following a dose of chemotherapy. After discontinuation of the epilating drugs, regrowth is visible in four to six weeks, but complete regrowth may take one to two years. In situations involving very high doses of alkylating agents, hair may not regrow. (p. 786)

8.  **The answer is b.** Beau's lines indicate a reduction or cessation of nail growth in response to cytotoxic therapy. (p. 788)

9.  **The answer is d.** All three choices are risk factors contributing to stomatitis in the cancer patient. (p. 789)

10. **The answer is a.** Mucositis is observed more often with 5-FU when combined with other mucositis-producing drugs such as methotrexate and doxorubicin and when 5-FU is given concurrently with leucovorin to augment its cytotoxicity. (p. 790)

11. **The answer is a.** Xerostomia is a transient dysfunction of the salivary gland that occurs following chemotherapy. It is a decrease in the quality and quantity of saliva. (p. 791)

12. **The answer is c.** Oral care before meals will help to freshen the mouth and stimulate appetite. Increasing fluid intake during meals and snacks will help to lubricate food and ease swallowing. Vegetable or corn oil swished in the mouth may be a cost-effective alternative for artificial lubrication. Lemon glycerin is contraindicated as a mouthwash because it dries and irritates the mucosa and can decalcify the teeth. (p. 796)

13. **The answer is b.** Specific agents for dissolving and breaking up thick saliva include papain (found in papaya) and amylase (found in pineapple). Sialagogues stimulate the secretion of endogenous saliva and include gustatory stimulants such as sugar-free lemon candy and masticatory stimulants such as sugar-free gum. Pilocarpine to increase saliva should be used with caution for those with CV disease. (pp. 796–797)

14. **The answer is c.** Treatment strategies for GVHD include systemic immunosuppressive therapy; topical steroids, which may or may not be beneficial; and fluoride therapy for patients at risk for caries secondary to xerostomia. (p. 792)

15. **The answer is b.** Trismus is the result of fibrosis of the muscles of mastication and/or fibrotic changes in the capsule of the temporomandibular joint. Repetition of jaw exercises should be used prophylactically in patients at high risk and should be initiated in others immediately after a problem develops. Surgical intervention to release fibrotic tissue is used only as a last resort. (p. 797)

16. **The answer is b.** Grade 1 damage is erythema of oral mucosa; grade 2 is isolated small ulcerations (white patches); grade 3 consists of confluent ulcerations covering more than 25% of oral mucosa; and grade 4 involved hemorrhagic ulceration. (p. 798)

17. **The answer is d.** Normal saline is the least damaging mouth rinse; commercial rinses (like Listerine) are too harsh; sodium bicarbonate is effective but unpleasant; hydrogen peroxide breaks down new tissues and should be avoided when fresh granulation surfaces are visible in the mouth. (p. 798)

18. **The answer is a.** A course of low-dose IV amphotericin B is indicated for nonresponsive infection and in severe esophageal and disseminated candidal infection. (p. 804)

19. **The answer is a.** The most common early symptoms of esophagitis include dysphagia, odonophagia, and epigastric pain. Esophageal pain that worsens and becomes continuous and substernal indicates progressing esophagitis. (p. 805)

20. **The answer is d.** Management of stomatitis in the cancer patient includes all of these choices. (pp. 798–803)

21.  **The answer is d.** All management is directed at symptom relief and supportive care. This is best accomplished through dietary manipulation, topical anesthesia, and systemic analgesia when needed. (p. 807)

22.  **The answer is a.** Management of severe diarrhea in patients with radiation-induced enteritis include all of these choices *except* a liquid diet high in milk products. (pp. 809–810)

23.  **The answer is b.** After allogeneic BMT, diarrhea is a prominent manifestation of intestinal involvement with GVHD. (p. 814)

# Chapter 30 — Late Effects of Cancer Treatment

## SCOPE OF THE PROBLEM

- More than 8 million Americans with a history of cancer are alive today; 5 million of these cases were diagnosed five or more years ago. At least half these individuals can be considered biologically cured.
- Late effects result from physiological changes related to particular treatments or to the interactions among the treatment, the individual, and the disease.
- Unlike the acute side effects of chemotherapy and radiation, however, late effects are believed to progress over time and by different mechanisms.
- Late effects can appear months to years after treatment and can be mild to severe to life-threatening. Their impact depends on the age and developmental state of the patient.

## CENTRAL NERVOUS SYSTEM

- The late effects of CNS treatment, including neuropsychologic, neuroanatomic, and neurophysiologic changes, have been observed most commonly in children with acute lymphoblastic leukemia (ALL) and brain tumors and in adult small-cell carcinoma of the lung (SCCL) patients, all of whom received CNS treatment for the primary tumor or as prophylaxis against meningeal disease.

### Neuropsychological Effects

- The most frequently described neuropsychological late effects of CNS treatment include significant decrements in general intellectual potential and academic achievement scores, as well as specific deficits in visual-motor integration, attention, memory, and visual-motor skills.
- Neuropsychological late effects do not become apparent until 24–36 months following treatment.
- The type of CNS treatment that has been most closely associated with neuropsychological deficits is cranial radiation in combination with intrathecal (IT) chemotherapy.
- Age at the time of CNS treatment is an important risk factor for neurological sequelae. Children who receive at least 2400 cGy of cranial radiation before the age of three, four, or five years are at greatest risk for neuropsychological late effects.

### Neuroanatomic Effects

- Brain atrophy and decreased subcortical white matter are the most frequently reported abnormalities.
- The aging, as well as the developing, brain may be more vulnerable to the deleterious effects of cancer treatment involving the CNS.

### Mechanisms of Pathogenesis

- The pathogenesis of delayed injury to normal tissue after treatment of the CNS is not well understood.
- The myelin-producing glial cells in the CNS are proliferative during early childhood and therefore radiosensitive. Damage to or a reproductive loss of glial cells from radiation can disrupt the myelin membrane.
- A synergistic relationship between radiation and methotrexate may account for progressive demyelination.

- Damage to the endothelial cells of the microvasculature is believed to play an important role in the pathogenesis of delayed injury following CNS treatment.

### Vision and Hearing

- Enucleation, which may be necessary in the treatment of ocular tumors such as retinoblastoma, is the most disabling visual deficit. Cataracts have been associated with cranial irradiation.
- Hearing loss in the high-tone range is most closely associated with cisplatin.

### ENDOCRINE SYSTEM

- Table 30-1, text page 827, summarizes the major endocrine secquelae, related risk factors, and recommendations for evaluation and treatment.

### Thyroid

- Direct damage to the thyroid gland causes primary hypothyroidism with a decreased production of thyroxine ($T_4$) and triiodothyronine ($T_3$).
- When the hypothalamic pituitary axis is in the field of radiation to the nasopharynx of the CNS, secondary hypothyroidism can occur.

### Growth

- Growth hormone deficiency with short stature is one of the most common long-term endocrine consequences of radiation to the CNS in children.
- Pituitary dysfunction requires radiation doses of at least 4000 cGy, but damage to the hypothalamus occurs with lower doses.
- Chemotherapy in combination with cranial radiation may increase the risk for growth failure.

### Secondary Sexual Development and Reproduction

- Alkylating agents can cause permanent damage to the gonads.
- Primary ovarian failure, with amenorrhea, decreased estradiol, and elevated gonadotropins has been reported in women who received these agents for Hodgkin's disease, breast cancer, and ovarian germ cell tumors.
- Damage to the germinal epithelium of the testis with decreased or absent spermatogonia can occur in males treated with alkylating agents.
- The incidence of gonadal damage increases with age.
- Radiation to the cranium or nasopharynx can damage the hypothalamic pituitary axis, causing secondary gonadal failure.

### IMMUNE SYSTEM

- Immunosuppression has long been recognized as one of the most serious acute toxic effects of chemotherapy and radiation.
- Persistent immunologic impairments following radiation and chemotherapy can occur; however, there is no evidence that patients with persistent immunologic abnormalities are at greater risk for infections.
- An inversion of the helper-to-suppressor ratio can persist for as long as ten years following local radiation for breast cancer, nodal radiation for Hodgkin's disease, and total-body irradiation prior to bone marrow transplantation.
- The immunosuppressive effects of specific chemotherapeutic agents are not well-known.

## CARDIOVASCULAR SYSTEM

- One of the most serious late effects of anthracyclines is cardiac toxicity, which typically presents as cardiomyopathy, with clinical signs of congestive heart failure.
- Cumulative doses of 550 mg/m have been associated with cardiac toxicity; similar abnormalities can occur after lower doses in adults and children.
- Table 30-2, text page 830, summarizes biological late effects on selected organ systems.

## PULMONARY SYSTEM

- Pneumonitis and pulmonary fibrosis are the major biological late effects of treatment to the pulmonary system.
    - These problems can be caused by chemotherapy, radiation therapy, and recurrent respiratory infections in immunosuppressed patients.
    - Pulmonary fibrosis is the most common.

## GASTROINTESTINAL SYSTEM

- Late effects of radiation on the esophagus result primarily from damage to the esophageal wall.
- The major significant late effect of gastric irradiation is ulceration due to destruction of mucosal cells of the gastric mucosa.
- Late effects in the liver are more common and include hepatic fibrosis, cirrhosis, and portal hypertension.
- Late radiation injury to the small and large intestine can result in fecal frequency, bleeding, pain, fistula formation, and obstruction, especially in the small intestine.
- The administration of blood products as part of the supportive care of myelosuppressed patients can cause chronic hepatitis.

## RENAL SYSTEM

- Nephritis and cystitis are the major long-term renal toxicities that result from cancer treatment. Damage to the nephrons and bladder has been documented in patients treated with cyclophosphamide, ifosfamide, and cisplatin.
- Children with unilateral nephrectomy who receive ifosfamide may develop Fanconi's syndrome.
- Radiation doses of 2000 cGy or less may minimize the risk of renal toxicity.

## MUSCULOSKELETAL SYSTEM

- The treatment most frequently associated with late effects in the musculoskeletal system is radiation.
- Uneven irradiation to the vertebrae, soft tissue, and muscles for the treatment of intra-abdominal tumors frequently results in scoliosis or kyphosis, or both.
- Spinal shortening, another radiation-related effect, is caused by damage to the growth centers in the vertebral bodies.
- The late effects on long bones include functional limitations, shortening of the extremity, osteonecrosis, increased susceptibility to fractures, and poor healing.
- Altered growth of facial bones following maxillofacial or orbital irradiation or surgery causes facial asymmetry.
- Men who receive chemotherapeutic agents that impair gonadal function may lose bone mineral density.
- Late radiation damage to muscle can occur, especially following treatment of soft tissue sarcomas of the extremities.

## SECOND MALIGNANT NEOPLASMS

- Adults and children who have received chemotherapy or radiation therapy, or both, for a primary malignancy are at increased risk for the development of a second malignant neoplasm.
- In patients with Hodgkin's disease there is a 77-fold increased risk of the development of leukemia within four years of initial treatment.
- Malignant transformation of normal cells is due to nonlethal damage to the DNA that is not repaired.
- Alkylating agents and ionizing radiation are the treatments most closely linked to a second malignant neoplasm.
- In addition to the type and dose of treatment received, the risk of the development of a secondary cancer depends on several predisposing factors.
  - Some tumors have a common underlying etiologic factor (e.g., smoking).
  - Genetic susceptibility is a second factor.

### Second Malignancies Following Chemotherapy

- Acute nonlymphocytic leukemia (ANL) following treatment with alkylating agents is the most common chemotherapy-related second malignant neoplasm.
- The treatment regimen with the greatest leukemogenic potential is MOPP, presumably because of the mechlorethamine and procarbazine.
- In patients with multiple myeloma the risk or the development of ANL is unusually high.

### Second Malignancies Following Radiation

- Sarcomas of the bone and soft tissue are the most common second malignant neoplasm after radiation therapy.
- ANL following radiation therapy is uncommon but has been reported in childhood cancer and non-Hodgkin's lymphoma.

## EARLY DETECTION AND PREVENTION

- The SOMA scales (Subjective, Objective, Management, and Analytical evaluation of injury) are intended to address the need for sensitive and uniform criteria for monitoring late reactions.
- Strategies for preventing late effects are also emerging.

# PRACTICE QUESTIONS

1.  Which of the following statements about the late effects of cancer treatment is *incorrect*?
    a.  Late effects are believed to progress over time.
    b.  Late effects are believed to involve different mechanisms from those of the acute side effects of chemotherapy and radiation.
    c.  Late effects are severe but clinically subtle.
    d.  Late effects are the consequence of biologic cure.

2.  Late effects involving the central nervous system (CNS) are most likely to occur in which of the following individuals?
    a.  a child treated for Hodgkin's disease
    b.  a child treated for bone sarcoma
    c.  an adult treated for small-cell carcinoma of the lung
    d.  an adult treated for primary hypothyroidism

3.  The most frequently described neuropsychologic late effects of CNS treatment for cancer include a deterioration in general intellectual performance. If we can assume that neuropsychologic changes in the brain are related to neuroanatomic abnormalities that result from cranial radiation, then one plausible explanation for the deterioration of intellectual performance is:
    a.  a decrease in subcortical white matter.
    b.  destruction of the hypothalamus.
    c.  the formation of myelin membranes on nerve axons.
    d.  the overstimulation of thyroid tissue.

4.  Which of the following treatments is most closely associated with progressive demyelination, which may be important in the early stage of delayed injury to the brain?
    a.  methotrexate alone
    b.  radiation alone
    c.  methotrexate combined with radiation
    d.  methotrexate combined with both radiation and surgery

5.  The late effects of cancer treatment on the endocrine system result from damage to the hypothalamus pituitary axis and/or to:
    a.  target organs; e.g., the thyroid.
    b.  the cortical areas of the brain.
    c.  the chemical structure of key hormones; e.g., insulin.
    d.  epithelial tissue; e.g., blood vessel linings.

6.  Growth impairment as a late effect of treatment for cancer occurs as the result of:
    a.  overproduction of thyroxine by the thyroid gland.
    b.  deficient growth hormone release by the hypothalamus.
    c.  primary hypothyroidism.
    d.  a disruption in pituitary control of several target organs.

7.  Damage to ovaries and testes resulting in gonadal failure is most likely to be a late effect associated with which of the following malignancies?
    a.  brain cancer
    b.  bone sarcomas
    c.  acute nonlymphocytic leukemia
    d.  Hodgkin's disease

8. Which of the following statements best summarizes the late effects of cancer treatment on the immune system?
   a. There is no evidence that patients with persistent immunologic abnormalities are at increased risk for infections.
   b. Immunologic late effects have been studied most thoroughly in patients treated for hypothyroidism, liver cancer, and splenectomy.
   c. Radiation and chemotherapy are more destructive of suppressor T-cells than of helper T-cells.
   d. There is no evidence that persistent immunologic impairment follows radiation and chemotherapy.

9. An individual is admitted with congestive heart failure. Medical records indicate a history of acute leukemia, which was treated 10 years earlier with anthracyclines. The most likely late effect of this treatment is:
   a. angina.
   b. pulmonary fibrosis.
   c. pericarditis.
   d. cardiomyopathy.

10. Scoliosis and kyphosis are most likely to develop as late effects of the treatment of intra-abdominal tumors with:
    a. combination MOPP therapy.
    b. radiation to one side of the body.
    c. pelvic irradiation combined with alkylating agents.
    d. prolonged used of corticosteroids.

11. The risk of developing a second malignant neoplasm after treatment for a primary malignancy depends on several factors, including all of the following *except*:
    a. the type and dose of treatment received; e.g., radiation and alkylating agents.
    b. a common underlying etiologic factor; e.g., smoking.
    c. genetic susceptibility; e.g., genetic retinoblastoma.
    d. the timing of withdrawal of chemotherapeutic agents; e.g., MOPP latency.

12. The most common second malignancy neoplasms following radiation therapy are:
    a. breast carcinomas and gynecologic tumors.
    b. cancers of the gastrointestinal tract.
    c. sarcomas of the bone and soft tissue.
    d. tumors of the bladder and lung.

13. The most frequently reported neuroanatomic late effects include:
    a. atrophy.
    b. calcification.
    c. increased subcortical white matter.
    d. leukoencephalopathy.

14. Several years ago, a patient was given concomitant radiation therapy and chemotherapy for cancer of the bladder. Recently, she developed cystitis. If this condition is a late effect of her cancer treatment, which agent is least likely to have been the responsible agent involved?
    a. cyclophosphamide
    b. ifosfamide
    c. methotrexate
    d. cisplatin

15.  What is the most common second malignant neoplasm after radiation therapy?
     a.  leukemia
     b.  sarcoma of the bone or soft tissue
     c.  CNS neoplasm
     d.  carcinoma of the breast

---

## ANSWER EXPLANATIONS

1.  **The answer is c.** The late effects of biologic cure result from physiologic changes related to particular treatments or to the interactions among the treatment, the individual, and the disease. Unlike the acute side effects of chemotherapy and radiation, however, late effects are believed to progress over time and by different mechanisms. They can appear months to years after treatment, can be mild to severe to life-threatening, and can be clinically obvious, clinically subtle, or subclinical. Their impact appears to depend on the age and development stage of the patient. (p. 824)

2.  **The answer is c.** The late effects of CNS treatment, including neuropsychologic, neuroanatomic, and neurophysiologic changes, have been observed most commonly in children with acute lymphoblastic leukemia (ALL) and brain tumors and in adult small-cell carcinoma of the lung (SCCL) patients, all of whom received CNS treatment for the primary tumor or as prophylaxis against meningeal disease. (p. 824)

3.  **The answer is c.** Brain atrophy and decreased subcortical white matter are the most frequent abnormalities that have been observed in long-term survivors who received whole-brain radiation. Because both abnormalities affect brain function, it is reasonable to see a connection between these neuroanatomic late effects and a deterioration in general intellectual performance. Other treatment-related changes in the brain, including demyelination of nerves, calcifications, and thickening of capillary walls, no doubt also are associated with intellectual deterioration. (p. 825)

4.  **The answer is c.** Progressive demyelination (disruption of the myelin membrane that insulates nerve axons) may be due to a synergistic relationship between radiation and methotrexate. The myelin-producing glial cells in the CNS are proliferative during early childhood and therefore radiosensitive. Damage to or a reproductive loss of glial cells from radiation can disrupt the myelin membrane. Methotrexate appears to contribute to this effect. (p. 825)

5.  **The answer is a.** The target organs most commonly affected are the thyroid, ovaries, and testes. Late effects can include alterations in metabolism, growth, secondary sexual characteristics, and reproduction. (pp. 826–827)

6.  **The answer is b.** High doses of radiation to the hypothalamic pituitary axis can damage the hypothalamus and disrupt the production of growth hormone. Growth hormone deficiency with short stature is one of the most common long-term endocrine consequences of radiation to the CNS in children. (p. 828)

7.  **The answer is d.** Those at highest risk for late effects involving the gonads, including gonadal failure, are women treated for Hodgkin's disease, breast cancer, and ovarian germ cell tumors and men treated for Hodgkin's disease, pelvic and testicular tumors, and testicular leukemia. Damage occurs both with radiation and alkylating agents. (p. 828)

8.  **The answer is a.** Although persistent immunologic impairment appears to follow radiation and chemotherapy, there is not evidence that patients with persistent immunologic abnormalities are at increased risk for infections. The exception is patients who have undergone splenectomy, who are at greater risk of bacterial infection because of the protective role of the spleen against encapsulated organisms. Immunologic late effects have been studied most thoroughly in patients treated for

leukemia (ALL), Hodgkin's disease, and breast cancer. Helper T cells, and not suppressor T cells, are particularly radiosensitive. (p. 829)

9. **The answer is d.** One of the most serious side effects of anthracyclines is cardiac toxicity, which typically presents as cardiomyopathy, with clinical signs of congestive heart failure. Recent evidence, however, indicates that structural damage can occur in the absence of clinical signs and that cardiac failure may occur many years following completion of therapy. (p. 829)

10. **The answer is b.** Uneven radiation to vertebrae, soft tissue, and muscles for the treatment of intra-abdominal tumors frequently results in scoliosis or kyphosis, or both. Although recent therapies have been modified to minimize this problem, it may still occur in some children and tends to become most apparent during periods of rapid growth such as the adolescent growth spurt. (p. 833)

11. **The answer is d.** Adults and children who have received chemotherapy or radiation therapy, or both, for a primary malignancy are at increased risk for the development of a second malignant neoplasm. Alkylating agents and ionizing radiation are the treatments most closely linked to a second malignant neoplasm. In addition to the type and dose of treatment received, the risk of the development of a secondary cancer depends on several predisposing factors, including choices **b** and **c**. (p. 834)

12. **The answer is c.** Sarcomas of the bone and soft tissue are the most common second malignant neoplasms after radiation therapy, with the incidence peaking at 15 to 20 years following radiation. In a large study of survivors of childhood cancer, risk of bone cancer was highest among children treated for retinoblastoma and Ewing's sarcoma but also increased significantly in patients treated for rhabdomyosarcoma, Wilms' tumor, and Hodgkin's disease. In addition to sarcomas and leukemia, a variety of solid tumors have been linked to treatment with radiation, including carcinomas of the breast and tumors of the bladder, rectum, and uterus. (p. 835)

13. **The answer is a.** The most frequently reported neuroanatomic late effects include atrophy and decreased subcortical white matter. (p. 825)

14. **The answer is c.** Nephritis and cystitis are the major long-term renal toxicities that result from cancer treatment. Damage to the nephrons and bladder has been documented in patients treated with cyclophosphamide, ifosfamide, and cisplatin. (p. 833)

15. **The answer is b.** Sarcomas of the bone and soft tissue are the most common second malignant neoplasm after radiation therapy. (p. 835)

# Chapter 31    AIDS-Related Malignancies

## INTRODUCTION

- The devastation wreaked by HIV on the immune system, particularly the cell-mediated arm, results in the diagnosis of a malignancy at some point during the illness in approximately 30%–70% of those with acquired immunodeficiency syndrome (AIDS).
- The four most common malignancies in AIDS are Kaposi's sarcoma (KS) non-Hodgkin's lymphoma (NHL), primary central nervous system (CNS) lymphoma, and invasive squamous cell cancer (SCC) of the cervix.
- These diseases are referred to as *opportunistic* because they occur in patients with preexisting immunodeficiency. This immunodeficiency can be the result of HIV infection (which destroys the immune system), therapeutic immunosuppression (e.g., chemotherapeutic agents used in organ transplantation), or primary immunodeficiency (e.g., as the result of a genetic defect).

## KAPOSI'S SARCOMA

### Epidemiology

- Predominantly a disease that occurs in men, this malignancy is characterized as an indolent, slow-growing cutaneous nodule or plaquelike lesion. In 88% of those diagnosed, lesions will be confined to the lower extremities, distal to the knee, without invasive or disseminated disease.
- Classic KS is rarely fatal.
- In contrast, African KS (endemic) is a malignant disease that affects persons of all ages, including children, and is found almost exclusively in black Africans.
- Transplant recipients experience an increased incidence of KS.
- Within the HIV-infected population it seems that those patients who acquire HIV through sexual transmission are more likely to develop KS than those whose source is injection drug use.
- Clinical presentation ranges from localized skin lesions to disseminated disease that involves multiple body organs.
- The cause of death in patients with AIDS-related KS is usually from concomitant opportunistic infections or the pathological effects of HIV itself.

### Etiology

- A sexually transmitted agent may in fact be responsible for the development of KS and may be more readily expressed in the presence of HIV.
- KS seems to be a disease found predominantly in homosexual and bisexual men with AIDS.

### Detection

- Detection of KS is typically by self-observation of cutaneous or mucocutaneous lesions.
- Biopsy specimens of suspicious lesions are examined.
- All types of KS (endemic, classic, transplantation-induced, and epidemic) are microscopically similar.

## Clinical Manifestations

- The clinical presentation of AIDS-related KS resembles that of KS in transplant recipients.
- In AIDS-related KS, there is no characteristic site of initial involvement as there is in the classic form of the disease.
- The lesions range in pigmentation from brown, brown-red, purple, dark red, to violet; in rare cases, they may appear to be deep blue-purple, resembling ecchymosis. They may be raised, bullous nodules or flat, plaquelike lesions.
- This tumor can involve not only the skin but also the mucocutaneous surface of the buccal mucosa, the hard and soft palate, and the gums, as well as the sclera of the eyes.
- As HIV infection progresses, the immune system becomes increasingly suppressed; with it the occurrence and severity of KS also increase.
- When the gastrointestinal tract is involved, the patient may have a protein-losing enteropathy.

## Staging

- See Tables 31-2 and 31-3, text page 850, for suggested staging systems.

## Assessment

- Suspicious lesions must be biopsied before a diagnosis can be established.
- Suspected KS involvement of other organs requires more invasive diagnostic procedures; e.g., bronchoscopic examination, endoscopic examination.
- Patients with AIDS-related KS also may show laboratory abnormalities that probably are more related to HIV infection than to KS.

## Treatment

### Medical

- In AIDS-related KS, treatment of the malignancy provides only temporary remission or stabilization and does not improve survival rate.
- As with other malignancies, three treatment options exist: surgery, radiation therapy, and chemotherapy, either local or systemic. Other than enabling the provider to establish a diagnosis, surgery has almost no role.
- Radiation therapy is highly effective and plays a role in local control of lesions and in cosmetic effect.
- Chemotherapeutic agents are useful in the treatment of AIDS-related KS when a systemic effect is necessary and the benefits of treatment outweigh the risks to the patient.
- Guidelines for treatment of AIDS-related KS are outlined in Table 31-4, text page 852.
- Interferon also has shown efficacy in the treatment of AIDS-related KS.

### Nursing

- A determination of the patient's risk group and whether KS is the patient's first diagnosis or one in a long line of indicator diseases will help the nurse establish a plan of care.
- Although great strides have been made to reduce phobia concerning AIDS and homosexual men, it is important to remember that the patient may be explaining his sexual preference to his family for the first time and informing them that he has a fatal disease. Emotional support is crucial.
- What appears to differ in the AIDS population is the severity of the complications. For this reason, nurses should be aggressive in the assessment of potential complications, alert the physician promptly, and implement appropriate nursing interventions.
- Patients with KS, on receiving the first dose of vinca alkaloids, may experience severe jaw pain that may cause irreversible nerve damage.

## NON-HODGKIN'S LYMPHOMA

### Epidemiology

- NHL in a person who also is seropositive for HIV antibody or has positive culture results is considered to affirm a diagnosis of AIDS.

### Etiology

- The DNA-containing herpes virus known as EBV has been suggested as an important etiologic agent in AIDS-NHL.
- However, the role of EBV in the development of NHL remains unclear.

### Pathophysiology

- AIDS-associated NHLs are predominantly B-cell malignancies, typically intermediate to high grade. However, there have been a few isolated reports of lymphomas that are T cell in origin in men who show HIV seropositivity.
- AIDS-NHL also has been associated with a previous history of persistent generalized lymphadenopathy.

### Clinical Manifestations

- In the general population the earliest sign of NHL unrelated to AIDS is usually a painless, enlarged, discrete lymph node located in the neck. Most patients have no symptoms; however, 20% may experience fever, night sweats, and weight loss.
- In contrast, patients with HIV-related NHL have very advanced disease, which frequently involves extranodal sites.
- Extranodal sites most commonly involved include the CNS, bone marrow, bowel, and the anorectum.

### Assessment

- The diagnosis and classification of lymphoma can be made only by means of a biopsy specimen.
- To fully assess HIV-related NHL, the patient's status must be staged and graded.
  - Staging—that is, determining the extent of disease involvement—is accomplished by means of the Ann Arbor staging classification system.
  - The staging workup includes a careful history, which notes the presence or absence of "B" symptoms, and a complete physical examination with special attention to Waldeyer's ring, the liver, and the spleen.
  - It is unusual for patients with HIV-related NHL to present at a stage lower than stage III.
- A chest film and computed tomography (CT) scans of the chest, abdomen, and pelvis are not indicated for patients with NHL in the general population, but because of the extensive extranodal involvement characteristic of HIV-related NHL, they are extremely important.
- A bilateral bone marrow biopsy and aspiration, as well as a lumbar puncture, should be performed.

### Treatment

#### Medical

- Treatment options can be determined on the basis of method (surgery, radiation therapy, and chemotherapy), as well as by grade of tumor. Low-grade tumors are uncommon.
- Intermediate-grade tumors may account for as much as 50% of HIV-related NHL.
- The remaining HIV-related NHL occurs as high-grade, advanced stage disease.
- The treatment of choice for advanced intermediate/high-grade lymphoma is combination chemotherapy with CNS prophylaxis. The most active and effective single agent used in the treatment of NHL is cyclophosphamide.

- Radiation therapy may be useful for patients with limited bulky disease, for those who are unable to tolerate chemotherapy either because of poor health or low blood counts, for local control, or in some instances, for CNS prophylaxis. Surgery plays no role.

### Nursing

- Patients with large, bulky, high-grade disease are at high risk for tumor lysis syndrome.
- If left uncorrected, this condition may result in renal failure and death. The treatment of choice is prevention.
- Dialysis may be necessary if the patient's electrolyte levels continue to rise and renal function deteriorates.
- Although tumor lysis occurs in most patients 48–72 hours after the initiation of chemotherapy, some patients with HIV-related NHL may have this phenomenon sooner, usually within 24 hours.
- Some patients with HIV-related NHL have some form of tumor lysis before they receive treatment. The complications of this group are the same as those experienced by all patients with NHL: neutropenia-related sepsis, thrombocytopenia, and untreated tumor lysis syndrome.

## PRIMARY CENTRAL NERVOUS SYSTEM LYMPHOMA
### Epidemiology

- Primary CNS lymphoma is rare. Most of those diagnosed are immunocompromised.
- The cell of origin is the same as that causing NHL elsewhere in the body.

### Clinical Manifestations

- The most frequently observed symptoms of HIV-associated CNS lymphomas include confusion, lethargy, memory loss, alterations in personality and behavior, hemiparesis or aphasia, seizures, cranial nerve palsy, and headache.
- These clinical manifestations are typical of spontaneous primary CNS lymphoma. They also are typical symptoms caused by other mass lesions in the CNS.
- The most common explanation for a mass lesion in the CNS is toxoplasmosis.
- Because of the morbidity associated with brain biopsy, primary CNS lymphoma is usually a diagnosis of exclusion.
- If the lesion fails to respond to treatment for toxoplasmosis, the diagnosis of primary CNS lymphoma will then be considered.
- In most patients the radiographic findings from the CT and magnetic rsonance imaging (MRI) examinations will reveal single or multiple discrete lesions.

### Treatment
#### Medical

- Most patients with CNS lymphoma die of the concomitant opportunistic infections frequently experienced in AIDS.

### Complications

- The most frequent complication in the treatment of AIDS-associated CNS lymphoma is the patient's mental deterioration to the point of becoming moribund and comatose.

## INVASIVE SQUAMOUS CELL CANCER OF THE CERVIX

- Patients who are immune suppressed as a result of HIV are at risk of developing anogenital malignancies, in particular, invasive squamous cell cancer of the cervix.
- HIV-infected women are more likely to have advanced disease at presentation, to experience recurrence, to have evidence of HPV infection, and to have perianal involvement.

### Etiology

- HPV plays a role in the development of invasive SCC cervix in women who are HIV-positive.

### Pathophysiology

- In the general population, SCC cervix is a preventable disease; it is always preceded by dysplasia and squamous intraepithelial lesions (SIL).
- However, this process occurs more rapidly in the HIV population.

### Clinical Manifestations

- Any differences between the clinical manifestations in a noninfected woman and the woman who is seropositive have not been defined.

### Treatment

- Traditional therapy used in the HIV-infected population produced significantly shorter mean time intervals until disease recurrence and death.

#### Nursing

- Women with HIV will require more time and energy to achieve the same goals as men.

## OTHER MALIGNANCIES AND HIV

- Hodgkin's disease, squamous cell cancers of the rectum, nasopharyngeal cancers, malignant melanomas, and multiple myelomas have all been reported in patients infected with HIV.
- Response to therapy is typically poor in the person with HIV infection.

## PRACTICE QUESTIONS

1. Diseases such as Kaposi's sarcoma that are common in AIDS are referred to as *opportunistic*. This is because they:
   a. affect any or all organs and tissues in the body.
   b. normally occur in a benign state in most individuals.
   c. occur in patients with preexisting immunodeficiency.
   d. affect only HIV-infected individuals who have other diseases.

2. In contrast to patients with non-AIDS NHL, those with HIV-related NHL are most likely to:
   a. have a history of lymphadenopathy that has been present for several months.
   b. present with a painless, enlarged, discrete lymph node located in the neck.
   c. have no symptoms.
   d. have very advanced disease involving extranodal sites.

3. Which of the following would typically *not* be part of the assessment of HIV-related non-Hodgkin's lymphoma (NHL)?
   a. CT and MRI examination of the head and neck
   b. a physical examination with special attention to Waldeyer's ring, the liver, and the spleen
   c. a bilateral bone marrow biopsy and aspiration
   d. laboratory tests that screen for hypercalcemia and other conditions not directly related to NHL

4. Treatment of advanced intermediate/high-grade NHL is most likely to involve:
   a. invasive surgery.
   b. high doses of topical radiation.
   c. combination chemotherapy.
   d. cyclophosphamide combined with radiation.

5. NHL patients with big, bulky, high-grade disease are at high risk for tumor lysis syndrome. One important aspect of the nursing care for such patients is:
   a. looking for signs of motor incoordination and cognitive deficits.
   b. monitoring urine output for signs of renal failure.
   c. discontinuing vinca alkaloid treatment if signs of severe jaw pain occur.
   d. providing oral or intravenous agents that keep blood and urine acidic.

6. The most frequently observed symptoms of HIV-associated CNS lymphomas include:
   a. nerve inflammation and fever resulting from cryptococcosis or toxoplasmosis.
   b. increased metabolism and pulse due to decreased serum protein/albumin levels.
   c. "B" symptoms, including fever, chills, weight loss, and diarrhea.
   d. confusion, lethargy, memory loss, and alterations in personality or behavior.

7. Which of the following patient groups are at increased risk for classic Kaposi's sarcoma?
   a. young black Americans
   b. women with genital or breast cancer
   c. transplant recipients
   d. a and c

8.  Which of the following individuals is/are probably at greatest risk for developing Kaposi's sarcoma?
    a.  a woman who is bisexual, sexually active, and HIV-positive
    b.  an intravenous drug user with AIDS
    c.  a bisexual man with AIDS
    d.  a and c

9.  Charlie has AIDS. He is currently being assessed for possible Kaposi's sarcoma. The clinical presentation of AIDS-related KS:
    a.  generally begins as a cutaneous nodule or plaquelike lesion confined to the lower extremities.
    b.  resembles that of KS in transplant recipients.
    c.  tends to produce metastatic rather than multicentric lesions that blanch to the touch.
    d.  a and b.

10. Charlie's diagnosis is confirmed. He asks you what he can expect from treatment. You explain that in AIDS-related KS:
    a.  treatment of the malignancy provides only temporary remission or stabilization and does not improve survival rate.
    b.  radiation therapy is highly effective in local control of lesions.
    c.  radiation helps with cosmetic effect.
    d.  all of the above.

11. You are asked by an HIV specialties clinic to assist in assessment of HIV-positive patients suspected of having invasive squamous cell cancer of the cervix. These patients need to be screened for possible eligibility for participation in a study. You realize that qualified candidates will probably:
    a.  have advanced disease at presentation.
    b.  have perianal involvement.
    c.  have evidence of HPV infection.
    d.  all of the above.

## ANSWER EXPLANATIONS

1.  **The answer is c.** AIDS-related diseases such as Kaposi's sarcoma, non-Hodgkin's lymphoma (NHL), and primary CNS lymphoma are referred to as *opportunistic* because they occur in patients with preexisting immunodeficiency. This immunodeficiency can be the result of HIV infection (which destroys the immune system), therapeutic immunosuppression (e.g., chemotherapeutic agents used in organ transplantation), or primary immunodeficiency (e.g., as the result of a genetic defect). Normally these malignancies occur at a low incidence and in a more benign form. An AIDS-related opportunistic disease that is not a malignancy is *Pneumocystis carinii* pneumonia. (p. 846)

2.  **The answer is d.** Choices **a-c** are more likely to refer to patients with non-AIDS NHL. In contrast, patients with HIV-related NHL have very advanced disease, which frequently involves extranodal sites, including the CNS, bone marrow, bowel, and anorectum. These extranodal sites may be the only site of the disease; that is, peripheral lymphadenopathy may be absent. Patients may also exhibit signs and symptoms of HIV infection, AIDS-related complex, or AIDS, which makes diagnosis difficult. (p. 854)

3.  **The answer is a.** The patient's status must first be staged and graded before the diagnosis and classification of lymphoma can be made by examination of a biopsy specimen. Staging is accomplished by means of the Ann Arbor staging classification system and includes a careful history, which notes

the presence or absence of "B" symptoms; a complete physical examination with special attention to Waldeyer's ring, the liver, and the spleen; laboratory tests that assess the overall wellness of the patient and screen for conditions not directly related to lymphoma; a chest film and CT scans of the chest, abdomen, and pelvis; and a bilateral bone marrow biopsy and spiration and a lumbar puncture. If AIDS has not been previously diagnosed, then an HIV antibody test is indicated. (p. 855)

4. **The answer is c.** Whereas intermediate-grade tumors can be treated with either chemotherapy or radiation therapy, depending on the stage at presentation, advanced intermediate/high-grade lymphoma is treated with combination chemotherapy. Cyclophosphamide, the most active and effective agent, commonly is used in combination with other agents. Initial responses are usually dramatic but are not long-lived; relapse typically occurs in 4 to 6 weeks following discontinuation of chemotherapy. In addition, treatment-related neutropenia is severe and sometimes precipitates an opportunistic infection. Regardless of outcome, patients still have HIV infection and AIDS. (p. 855)

5. **The answer is b.** Tumor lysis syndrome generally occurs when the patient is initially treated. Tumor cells spill their contents into the general circulation, causing a metabolic disturbance. Renal failure and death may occur. The treatment of choice is prevention, including hydration, sodium bicarbonate, and intravenous or oral allopurinol to prevent hyperuricemia nephropathy. The patient's urine output is monitored hourly, and the physician is alerted to any sign of urinary insufficiency. Serum chemistry levels are monitored hourly, and the physician is alerted to any sign of urinary insufficiency. Serum chemistry levels are monitored every 6 hours in high-risk patients. Dialysis is administered if electrolyte levels continue to rise and renal function deteriorates. All patients with HIV-related NHL should be observed for a full 72 hours for any sign of tumor lysis syndrome. Signs and symptoms include a decreased urine output and increased lethargy. (p. 856)

6. **The answer is d.** The cell of origin for primary CNS lymphoma is the same as that causing NHL elsewhere in the body. The transformed cell, which multiplies in an area that does not allow expansion (i.e., the brain), is the cause of most presenting symptoms, including confusion, lethargy, memory loss, and alterations in personality or behavior. Seizures may also develop. Symptoms are very similar to those caused by other mass lesions in the CNS, for which toxoplasmosis is the usual explanation. (p. 857)

7. **The answer is c.** Classic Kaposi's sarcoma occurs with increased frequency in men (especially those of Mediterranean or Jewish ancestry) in the fifth to eighth decades of life, and in transplant recipients. (p. 846)

8. **The answer is c.** KS seems to be a disease found predominantly in homosexual and bisexual men with AIDS. (p. 848)

9. **The answer is b.** The clinical presentation of AIDS-related KS resembles that of KS in transplant recipients. There is no characteristic site of initial involvement as there is in the classic form of the disease. Lesions can be found on almost any skin surface. They tend to be multicentric rather than metastatic and do not blanch to the touch. (p. 849)

10. **The answer is d.** In AIDS-related KS, treatment of the malignancy provides only temporary remission or stabilization and does not improve survival rate. Radiation therapy is highly effective and plays a role in local control of lesions and in cosmetic effect. (p. 851)

11. **The answer is d.** HIV-infected women are more likely to have advanced disease at presentation, experience recurrence, have evidence of HPV infection, and have perianal involvement. (p. 859)

# Chapter 32    Bone and Soft-Tissue Sarcoma

---

## EPIDEMIOLOGY

- Incidence is slightly higher for men. The estimated number of deaths that occurred in 1995 from bone cancer is 1280.
- The estimated death toll from soft-tissue tumors was 3600.

## ETIOLOGY

- Prevention and detection of bone and soft-tissue sarcoma remain difficult because few risk factors have been identified.
  - Prior cancer therapy in the form of high-dose irradiation; exposure to chemicals such as vinyl chloride gas, arsenic, and dioxin or Agent Orange; and exposure to alkylating agents have been associated with the formation of soft-tissue sarcomas.
  - Immunosuppressed patients and persons with autoimmunodeficiency syndrome (AIDS) have a higher risk for soft-tissue sarcomas.
  - Evidence of a familial tendency in bone cancer has been demonstrated by reports of siblings with osteosarcoma, Ewing's sarcoma, and chondrosarcoma.
  - Paget's disease predisposes individuals primarily to osteosarcoma but occasionally to fibrosarcoma, chondrosarcoma, and giant cell tumor.

## PREVENTION, SCREENING, AND EARLY DETECTION

- Because of the relative low incidence of malignant bone and soft-tissue tumors, there are no screening tests available for these tumors.

## PATHOPHYSIOLOGY

- Primary malignant bone and soft-tissue tumors are derived from the cells that have a common ancestry: the mesoderm or ectoderm.
- Nearly every bone and soft tissue in the skeleton may be affected; however, individual tumors have a predilection for certain locations.
- Soft-tissue sarcomas often arise in the extremities.

## CLINICAL MANIFESTATIONS

- Bone and soft tissue sarcomas can manifest with one or more of the following presentations:
  - painful area on the musculoskeletal system
  - pain at rest
  - soft tissue or bony mass that may not be painful

## ASSESSMENT
### Patient and Family History

- The evaluation of pain assumes a major focus in the interview.
- It is important to rule out a traumatic injury to the area.
- Bone tumor pain often has a gradual onset.

- Pain can be radicular.
- Soft tissue sarcomas present as painless masses unless they are impinging on nerves, blood vessels, or viscera.
- A psychosocial assessment should be incorporated into the initial interview.

## Physical Examination

- Inspection may reveal a visible mass or swelling.
- Malignant bone tumors are not always visible or palpable. Evaluation for adenopathy and hepatomegaly also is performed. Limitations in motion of proximal joints are noted.
- An assessment of neurovascular function of the affected limb is done.

## Diagnostic Studies

- In general, radiographic changes can be appreciated only when the tumor is far advanced.
  - The geographic pattern indicates that the tumor has a slow rate of growth.
  - The moth-eaten pattern indicates a moderately aggressive tumor.
  - The permeative pattern indicates an aggressive tumor with a strong capacity for infiltration.
- A bone scan helps to detect or exclude the presence of additional lesions in the skeleton. Arteriography is not diagnostic but aids in the planning of surgical, radiation, and perfusion chemotherapy treatments by outlining tumor margins and mapping arterial blood supply to the tumor. CT provides an evaluation of the true bony extent of the disease. Fluoroscopy is used in the operating room to document the location in the bony lesion from which the biopsy specimen is taken.
- The biopsy should include the most representative section of the lesion as determined by the imaging.
- Open, or incisional, biopsy is the most common type of biopsy used for bone and soft tissue lesions.
- Closed, or needle, biopsy is utilized on the basis that it is technically simple, involves minimal patient risk, is cost- and time-effective, may be repeated without any ill effects, and makes it possible to extract material from different depths of the tumor.
- Although positive results of biopsy nearly always are accurate, biopsy yields a 20% false-negative rate.

## Prognostic Indicators

- The prognosis for individuals with bone and soft-tissue sarcoma is worse if the grade of the tumor is high, the location deep, and the tumor large.

## CLASSIFICATION AND STAGING

- Stage I includes low-grade lesions with low incidence of metastases.
- State II includes high-grade lesions with high incidence of metastases.
- The site is noted to be "A," which indicates an intracompartmental lesion, or "B," which indicates an extracompartmental lesion.
- State III includes any site or grade lesion with metastases.

## THERAPEUTIC APPROACHES AND NURSING CARE

- The goals of treatment of primary malignant bone and soft tissue cancer include eradication of the tumor, avoidance of amputation when possible, and preservation of maximum function.

## Surgery

- In the past 20 years, research has indicated that no procedure short of ablation would control or eradicate aggressive forms of osteosarcoma, fibrosarcoma, and chondrosarcoma.

- The traditional contraindications for limb salvage are as follows: (1) inability to attain adequate surgical margin, (2) neurovascular bundle involved by tumor, and (3) age-group, because of resultant limb length discrepancy.
- Limb salvage is indicated for lesions that tend to metastasize late such as surface osteosarcoma and chondrosarcomas that have not invaded soft tissue.

## Radical resection with reconstruction

- The patient needs to be aware that implant failure may occur and further surgery, including amputation, may be necessary.
- When more extensive surgery is done, the actual function cannot be predicted as readily as when an amputation is planned.
- The nurse conducts a baseline assessment of neurovascular function distal to the surgical site.
- Blood loss and anemia can result from extensive tumor resection and reconstruction.
- Position restrictions are determined by the surgeon.
- Wound necrosis can occur if large flaps are used to close the wound, especially if the surgical site was previously irradiated.
- Patients are advised in lifelong prevention of implant infection.
- Functional independence and a gradual adaptation to the changes in body image are the goals of rehabilitation.
- The three most common methods of reconstruction after sarcoma resection are arthrodesis, arthroplasty with metallic or allograft implant, and intercalary allograft reconstruction.
  - *Arthrodesis*, or fusion, results in a stiff joint, which is a handicap for the individual. This form of reconstruction, however, is sturdy and permits activities such as running and jumping.

## Allografts

- There is no donor site morbidity or size limitation.
- Bone allograft recipients do not require immunosuppressive agents, which are often given to organ recipients.
- *Osteoconduction* describes growth of capillaries and osteoprogenitor cells of the host into the allograft.
- Complications of this procedure include infection, allograft fracture, and nonunion.

## Metastatic sarcoma

- Sarcomas frequently metastasize to the lung before involving other sites. Individuals in whom lung metastases develop are good candidates for resection, provided the primary tumor is controlled, there is no indication of other visceral metastatic disease, and the pulmonary nodules are resectable.

## Amputation

- It is reasonable to assume that the person facing an amputation has fears regarding death, disability, and deformity.
- To reduce anxiety it sometimes is helpful for the person undergoing surgery to meet preoperatively those individuals who will be involved in his or her postoperative care.
- The nurse consults social service personnel to inform the patient and family about financial resources and rehabilitation programs available in the state.
- It is important for the nurse to help establish realistic expectations regarding the patient's postamputation function.
- Ideally, the goal for the individual is independent function with the use of prostheses.

### Phantom limb phenomenon

- All individuals who have had an amputation can expect to feel some phantom limb sensation.
- The physical component relates to the surgical interruption of neural reflex pathways, with resultant transmission of abnormal patterns of nerve impulses.
- Relief may be obtained simply by applying heat to the stump or by pressure, such as with elastic bandages. Distraction and diversion techniques may decrease the person's awareness of the pain. Tranquilizers, local anesthesia, or muscle relaxants are occasionally effective in managing the pain. Psychotherapy and behavioral therapy also may be useful.

### Amputation of the lower extremity

- General strengthening measures and mobility training should be initiated preoperatively by a physical therapist.
- Exercises to maintain muscle tone and prevent edema, joint contractures, and muscle atrophy are initiated on the first postoperative day.
- The goals of postoperative care are to use modern prostheses, to achieve the highest level of function possible, and to minimize the negative psychosocial consequences of amputation.
- With the conventional delayed fitting, drains frequently are inserted during surgery to remove blood and serous drainage.
- The stump usually is elevated for 24 hours after surgery to prevent edema and promote venous return.
- Stump care involves frequent wrapping with elastic bandages or stump shrinkers to facilitate stump shrinking.
- With immediate prosthetic fitting, hemorrhage is less likely because of the compression effects of the cast.
- Care must be taken to prevent the cast from slipping off the stump.
- Nursing management includes case care.
- After the swelling is diminished, fitting for a permanent prosthesis is undertaken at 12 weeks after surgery.
- The patient needs to perform daily stump hygiene with the use of a mild soap and water.
- When the wound has healed, the individual can prevent edema by putting on the prosthesis immediately after arising and keeping it on all day.
- The individual is taught the importance of never attempting to make mechanical adjustments to the prosthesis.

### Amputation of the upper extremity

- Upper limb prostheses are far less satisfactory in both appearance and function than those created for lower extremities.
- The most functional terminal (hand) device is a hook.
- Adequate cosmetic appearance can be obtained at the expense of function.
- Motion is severely limited because sources of power are unavailable.
- Rejection of the upper extremity prosthetic devices occurs more often than with prostheses of the lower extremity because of a combination of poor function, low cosmetic value, and lack of motivation.
- It is important to discuss with the individual the negative social stigma attached to the hook, as well as its functional capabilities.

## Radiotherapy

- Most bone tumors are relatively unresponsive to radiation. Consequently, radiation is reserved for palliation and may be used in conjunction with chemotherapy for inoperable tumors or in conjunction with surgery to reduce the tumor load of partially resectable tumors.
- In contrast, radiotherapy plays an integral role in the management of Ewing's sarcoma and soft-tissue sarcomas.

## Chemotherapy and Immunotherapy

- Currently chemotherapy is given preoperatively as well as postoperatively.
- The duration of treatment ranges from 6 to 12 months.
- The systemic effects of chemotherapy such as neutropenia and thrombocytopenia may create wound complications.

## CLASSIFICATION OF CERTAIN SARCOMAS

### Osteosarcoma

- Osteosarcoma is the most common osseous malignant bone tumor.
    - Central osteosarcoma includes the classic high-grade tumor.
    - Surface osteosarcoma includes these two tumor types. Periosteal osteosarcoma, a variant of osteosarcoma, occurs as a hard mass on the bone surface.
    - Parosteal or juxtacortical osteosarcomas occur also on bony surfaces.
- The tumor may be described as osteoblastic, chondroblastic, or fibroblastic, depending on which component is dominant.
- Metastatic spread occurs primarily to the lungs by the hematogenous route.
- Half of the individuals with osteosarcoma have an elevated serum alkaline phosphatase level.
- The five-year survival rate for individuals treated with surgery alone or irradiation and surgery has been approximately 10%.
- The improved results of chemotherapy have sparked interest in limb salvage resections.
- No patients survived the development of pulmonary metastases unless they had surgical resection of gross disease.

### Chondrosarcoma

- Chondrosarcoma accounts for approximately 14% of malignant bone tumors.
    - There are both primary and secondary chondrosarcomas. The former include central chondrosarcomas that arise in the medullary cavity. The latter includes those chondrosarcomas that arise from benign tumors.
- The most frequent sites of chondrosarcoma include the pelvic bone, long bones, scapula, and ribs.
- When advanced chondrosarcoma does become aggressive, it tends to metastasize via venous channels to the lungs and heart.
- At present, chondrosarcoma remains nearly totally refractory to chemotherapeutic efforts inasmuch as chondrosarcomas usually have a poor blood supply.
- Radiotherapy, usually neutrons, has limited effectiveness and is reserved for palliation of advanced or inoperable chondrosarcomas.
- The overall survival rate of individuals treated with wide resection or amputation has been reported to be 67% at five years and 50% at ten years.

### Fibrosarcoma

- Paget's disease may be a predisposing factor in the development of fibrosarcoma.

- Fibrosarcoma is a malignant fibroblastic tumor that fails to develop tumor osteoid or bone in its local invasive growth site or in its metastatic foci.
- The femur and the tibia, the most common sites of occurrence, account for 50% of all fibrosarcomas.
- When the diagnosis of fibrosarcoma has been established, surgery is indicated.
- The five- and ten-year survival rates after radical surgery have been reported at 28% and 21.8%, respectively.

## Ewing's Sarcoma

- On microscopic examination, Ewing's sarcoma is characterized by the presence of uniform cells with indistinct borders.
- No one site seems to predominate in the development of Ewing's sarcoma.
- Many individuals have fever, anemia, high erythrocyte sedimentation rates, and sometimes leukocytosis at presentation.
- Radiographs of Ewing's sarcoma show bone destruction that involves the shaft.
- Surgery or radiation alone will prevent neither the appearance of tumor foci elsewhere in the skeleton nor pulmonary metastasis.
- The tumor is extremely radiosensitive and capable of being cured locally with 50–60 Gy by means of shrinking fields.
- Limb salvage and amputation are both options to be considered. The goal is to eradicate the tumor and maintain function.

## Soft-Tissue Sarcomas

- Soft-tissue sarcomas invade surrounding tissue along the anatomic planes.
- Lymph node involvement is a poor prognostic sign.
- A tumor that is superficial and smaller than 5 cm is felt to have a better prognosis.
- The five-year survival percentages of soft-tissue sarcomas range from 30% to 95% based on subtype and grade.
- It is not uncommon for the surgeon to surgically remove a mass and, after routine pathological examination, learn it is a malignant sarcoma.
- In the optimal situation, imaging is performed prior to biopsy of the tumor. If the tumor is small and superficial, a primary myectomy may be recommended.
- The advantage of postoperative radiation is that it allows for thorough histological grading and diagnosis.
- Preoperative radiation has the advantage of a small treatment area with fewer complications.
- Patients with soft tissue sarcomas often achieve improved local control but frequently develop distant metastases.

## METASTATIC BONE TUMORS

- The three mechanisms by which a tumor spreads from the primary site to bone are direct extension to adjacent bones, arterial embolization, and direct venous spread through the pelvic and vertebral veins known as *Batson's plexus*.
- The patient commonly presents with skeletal pain that worsens with rest. The patient commonly has a prior cancer history and is greater than 40 years of age.
- Diagnostic testing includes a biopsy if the individual has no known primary tumor.
- Chemotherapy for the primary site may result in pain reduction, decrease in the size of bony lesions, and stabilization of the number of lesions.
- Radiation is most commonly given by the external beam route to the involved sites.

- The ongoing concern of those providing care to patients with metastatic bone tumors is prevention of fracture.

## SYMPTOM MANAGEMENT AND SUPPORTIVE CARE
### Pain

- Pain is often the presenting symptom of a bone sarcoma and, at times, a soft-tissue sarcoma.

### Limitations of Mobility

- The tumor may limit motion of a joint and/or the ability to use the limb.

## CONTINUITY OF CARE: NURSING CHALLENGES

- One of the ongoing issues in the care of orthopedic oncology patients is negotiating for out-of-system care from the insurance plan.
- Hospitalizations are becoming shorter. Discharge planning starts before admission and is a daily consideration.
- One of the most difficult aspects of self-care is that these previously independent individuals have short- and long-term periods in which they need family or professional assistance in the home.

# PRACTICE QUESTIONS

1.  Incidence of bone cancer is most common in people with:
    a.  a family tendency in bone cancer.
    b.  prior high-dose radiation cancer therapy.
    c.  preexisting bone conditions.
    d.  all of the above.

2.  Bone tumors originate in the blood vessels of the bone, in the bone marrow, or in collagen-producing cells. An example of a bone tumor that originates in the bone marrow is:
    a.  Ewing's sarcoma.
    b.  osteogenic sarcoma.
    c.  chondrosarcoma.
    d.  angiosarcoma.

3.  Mr. Riley is being assessed after presenting with bone pain in his leg. One characteristic of the pain associated with the presence of a bone tumor is that it:
    a.  has a sudden, unexplainable onset.
    b.  is exacerbated with activity.
    c.  is worse upon awakening.
    d.  has a gradual onset.

4.  In the presence of a known bone tumor, symptoms such as hemoptysis, cough, fever, weight loss, and malaise may indicate:
    a.  pulmonary metastases.
    b.  pernicious anemia.
    c.  radiotherapy toxicity.
    d.  infection.

5.  All of the following are goals in the treatment of primary malignant bone cancer *except*:
    a.  preservation of maximum function.
    b.  early detection and intervention in children felt to be at high risk.
    c.  eradication of tumor.
    d.  avoidance of amputation.

6.  All of the following are considered to be indications for limb-salvage surgery *except*:
    a.  a locally aggressive chondrosarcoma.
    b.  the absence of soft-tissue invasion.
    c.  a tumor that typically metastasizes late.
    d.  a child younger than 10 years of age.

7.  The most common site of metastasis for tumors of the bone is the:
    a.  GI tract.
    b.  central nervous system.
    c.  liver.
    d.  lungs.

8. After amputation, Mr. Riley reports pain in the missing leg. The nurse should be aware that this phantom limb pain:
   a. generally resolves in several months.
   b. is likely to worsen with aging.
   c. indicates a patient's inability to cope with loss.
   d. usually occurs immediately following surgery.

9. Most bone tumors are relatively unresponsive to radiation therapy. An exception is:
   a. chondrosarcoma.
   b. Ewing's sarcoma.
   c. fibrosarcoma.
   d. angiosarcoma.

10. The rationale for the use of preoperative chemotherapy in patients with osteogenic sarcoma includes all but which of the following aspects?
    a. It treats micrometastases.
    b. It decreases the size of the primary tumor, possibly facilitating limb-salvage surgery.
    c. It enhances the effect of postoperative radiation.
    d. It evaluates the effectiveness of the chemotherapy.

11. The most common sites of occurrence for chondrosarcoma are the:
    a. femur, tibia, patella, and metatarsal.
    b. vertebrae and scapula.
    c. ribs, scapula, long bones, and pelvic bones.
    d. mandible and maxilla.

12. The most effective modality currently being used to treat chondrosarcoma is:
    a. surgery.
    b. chemotherapy.
    c. radiotherapy.
    d. hormone therapy.

13. Treatment of metastases to the bone may include surgery, chemotherapy, and/or radiotherapy. When radiation therapy is used, the primary goal often is to:
    a. eliminate the need for surgical intervention.
    b. palliate pain.
    c. decrease the likelihood of further metastases.
    d. treat the primary cancer.

## ANSWER EXPLANATIONS

1. **The answer is d.** All three factors play some role in the development of bone cancer: familial tendency; prior cancer therapy in the form of high-dose irradiation; and some preexisting bone conditions such as Paget's disease. (p. 864)

2. **The answer is a.** Ewing's sarcoma is an example of a bone tumor that originates in the bone marrow reticulum. Other examples in this category are reticulosarcoma and lymphosarcoma. (p. 865)

3. **The answer is d.** The most common presenting symptom in bone cancer is pain (sometimes described as "dull" or "aching") which has had a gradual onset and may have been present for several months before evaluation is sought. Abrupt onset of pain is possible, although not common, and would most likely indicate a pathologic fracture. (p. 865)

4. **The answer is a.** Metastatic spread in bone cancer occurs primarily to the lungs by the hematogenous route. Symptoms of pulmonary metastases include weight loss, malaise, hemoptysis, cough, chest pain, and fever. (pp. 865 and 867)

5. **The answer is b.** Avoidance of amputation, preservation of maximum function, and eradication of tumor are all goals in the treatment of primary malignant bone cancer. Although there is evidence of a familial tendency in some of the bone cancers, early intervention in these cases is not common practice. (p. 868)

6. **The answer is d.** Three scenarios in which limb salvage is not a treatment option are (1) if the surgeon is unable to attain adequate surgical margin, (2) if the neurovascular bundle is involved, and (3) if the patient is younger than 10 years old. In the latter case limb salvage is contraindicated because of the resultant limb length discrepancy, although recent advances in expandable prostheses are making it possible for more children afflicted with bone cancer to retain their limbs during surgery. (p. 869)

7. **The answer is d.** Although some bone tumors metastasize to the lymph nodes (e.g., Ewing's sarcoma), few, if any, seem to metastasize to the CNS or liver. Most of the more common bone tumors metastasize to the lungs. Whether or not these metastases develop, and when, depends on the stage and aggressiveness of the disease process. (pp. 867 and 873)

8. **The answer is a.** Although phantom limb sensations (i.e., itching, pressure, tingling) are often experienced shortly after surgery, phantom limb pain (i.e., cramping, throbbing, burning) usually does not occur until one to four weeks after surgery. For most individuals, phantom limb pain resolves in a few months; 5%–10% of those who have limbs amputated have a worsening of pain over the years. This worsening may be a sign of a neuroma or of locally recurrent cancer in the stump. (p. 874)

9. **The answer is b.** Radiotherapy is mainly used palliatively and in conjunction with chemotherapy for inoperable tumors in the treatment of bone cancer. It plays an integral role, however, in the management of Ewing's sarcoma, which is one of the only bone tumors that is radiosensitive. (p. 879)

10. **The answer is c.** Currently chemotherapy is given preoperatively. The rationale for preoperative chemotherapy is to treat micrometastasis, decrease the size of the primary tumor (thereby increasing the likelihood of limb-salvage surgery) and assess the effectiveness of the chemotherapeutic agents for 2 to 3 months. The route of the chemotherapy is either intravenous or intra-arterial. (p. 879)

11. **The answer is c.** Chondrosarcoma is a tumor arising from either the interior medullary cavity of the cartilage (central chondrosarcoma) or from the bone through malignant changes in benign cartilage tumors (peripheral chondrosarcoma). The most frequent sites for this cancer are the pelvic bones, long bones, scapula, and ribs. Less common sites include the bones of the hands and feet. (p. 881)

12. **The answer is a.** Chondrosarcoma is primarily treated surgically. This form of bone cancer is almost totally refractory to chemotherapy because of its poor blood supply. Likewise, radiation therapy has limited effectiveness and is usually reserved for palliation. In terms of surgery, limb-salvage surgery as well as amputation are both options. (p. 881)

13. **The answer is b.** Radiation to the involved sites is used primarily to relieve pain, improve bone strength, and improve neurological deficits. (p. 884)

# Chapter 33    Bladder and Kidney Cancer

## BLADDER CANCER
### Epidemiology
- The four major variables related to bladder cancer incidence are race, gender, age, and geographic location.
- The age-adjusted bladder cancer rate in white men is twice the rate for black men. In whites the bladder cancer ratio of men to women is 3:1. Average age at diagnosis is 65 years.

### Etiology
- There is well-documented evidence of genetic changes in bladder cancer.
- There are four etiologic hypotheses related to bladder cancer: cigarette smoking, occupational exposure to industrial chemicals, ingestion of other physical agents, and exposure to *S haemotobium*.

### Pathophysiology
#### Cellular characteristics
- Major variables in the systems of classification are patterns of growth (in situ versus papillary versus solid), the presence or absence of invasion (the stage), and the degree of differentiation (the grade).
- Papillary tumors have a propensity for recurrence. Carcinoma in situ is usually multifocal and is associated with high recurrence rate and multicentricity.

#### Progression of disease
- Many of these tumors arise on the floor of the bladder and may involve one or both of the ureteral orifices.
- Metastasis takes place via direct extension out of the muscle of the bladder into the perivesicle fat.

### Clinical Manifestations
- Gross hematuria is the most common presenting symptom of bladder cancer.
- The bleeding is rarely profuse, often microscopic, and usually intermittent.
- Another symptom is irritability of the bladder.
- Symptoms associated with large tumor growth or metastasis also may be present.

### Assessment
#### Physical examination
- An invasive mass in the trigonal area occasionally may be revealed by rectal examination.

#### Diagnostic studies
Cytology
- Exfoliative urinary cytology is a relatively simple diagnostic tool.

### Flow cytometry

- Flow cytometry has been useful in providing prognostic information beyond grading and staging.

### Excretory urogram (intravenous pyelogram)

- Although it is not a conclusive diagnostic tool, excretory urography can help evaluate a suspected bladder tumor by possibly showing the tumor itself or by showing evidence of ureteral obstruction.

### Cystoscopy

- Cystoscopic examination can serve several purposes: tumor visualization, an opportunity for biopsy, and an opportunity for bimanual examination of the bladder.

### Tumor markers

- Tumors that elaborate A, B, or H antigens are often associated, stage for stage, with a better prognosis than tumors that do not express antigens.

### Ultrasound, computerized tomography, magnetic resonance imaging

- Both abdominal and transurethral ultrasound have been used to define the local extension and the degree of involvement of the bladder wall.

## Classification and Staging

- Grading of bladder tumors is commonly done to predict the speed of recurrence and the progression to invasion and metastases.
- The grades for cancer of the bladder are usually referred to as grade I, II, III, or IV, with IV designating the least well-differentiated.

## Treatment

### Carcinoma in situ

- Transurethral resection (TUR) and fulguration are the most common and conservative forms of management.
- Radiotherapy has no proven value in the treatment of carcinoma in situ.

### Superficial, low-grade tumors

- Standard treatment of these tumors is transurethral surgery with resection and fulguration, laser therapy, or cystectomy.
- Because the chance of recurrence is so great, intravesical chemotherapy is often given following surgery.

### Intravesical treatment

- The most widely used drug for this purpose in the United States has been thiotepa.
- Mitomycin C also has been used in the treatment of superficial disease.
- BCG is a biologic response modifier that is believed to exert its antitumor effect by stimulating various immune responses in the host.
  - Treatment with BCG has delayed progression and decreased the risk of death from bladder cancer.

- A typical BCG regimen begins one to two weeks after biopsy or transurethral resection of tumor and is repeated once a week for six treatments.

### Laser therapy

- The advantages of laser therapy are that it may be less likely than fulguration to promote tumor dissemination within the bladder, it can be performed under local anesthesia, it reduces the chance of bladder perforation, and an indwelling catheter is not necessary following the procedure.
- However, photodynamic therapy can be associated with quite severe side effects, including inflammation of the bladder mucosa.

## Invasive tumors

- High-stage tumors are generally described as stages T2 to T4 or B1 to D1.

### Radical cystectomy

- The procedure includes excision of the bladder with the pericystic fat, the attached peritoneum, and the entire prostate and seminal vesicles.
- In women, radical cystectomy includes removal of the bladder and entire urethra, the uterus, ovaries, fallopian tubes, and the anterior wall of the vagina.
- Complications of this surgical procedure include ureterocutaneous fistula, wound dehiscence, partial small bowel obstruction, wound infection, loss of sexual function, and small bowel fistula.

### Cystectomy with urinary diversion

- To help patients overcome the problem of impotence after pelvic surgery, Walsh developed a surgical approach in which nerves crucial to the mechanisms of penile erection are spared.

#### Ileal conduit

- The Bricker ileal conduit has been a popular method of diverting urinary flow in the absence of bladder function.
- Other portions of the bowel also have been used to divert the urine. Portions of the sigmoid colon are used infrequently as conduits in urinary diversions associated with bladder cancer.

#### Ureterosigmoidostomy

- Ureterosigmoidostomy involves implanting the ureters into the sigmoid colon utilizing an antirefluxing anastomosis.
- This surgical procedure is rare today.

### Continent urinary diversion

- Continent diversions offer the patient opportunity for control of voiding and urinary reflux by the creation of low-pressure reservoirs and the use of one-way valves.

#### Kock pouch

- Urinary diversion through a continent ileal reservoir provides an intra-abdominal pouch for storage of urine and two nipple valves that maintain continence and prevent ureteral reflux.
- To prevent mucus obstruction postoperatively, the Medena tube should be irrigated every four hours or more with 30–60 ml of normal saline.

### Indiana reservoir

- A continent diversion is constructed from the cecum, the ascending colon, the ileocecal valve, and the terminal ileum.

### Postsurgical sexuality

- The etiology of physiological sexual dysfunction in men is similar to that associated with treatment for prostatic cancer.
- Erectile impotence that results after radical cystectomy (or radical prostatectomy) may be helped by the insertion of a penile prosthesis.
- In women, removal of the ovaries and uterus will result in sexuality changes similar to those following hysterectomy and oophorectomy for gynecologic malignancies.
- If more than the anterior third of the vaginal wall is removed, the diameter of the introitus and the vaginal barrel can be severely compromised and intercourse may be restricted.

### Definitive radiotherapy

- External beam radiotherapy of approximately 60 Gy delivered in fractions to the pelvis in five to eight weeks is an alternative to radical cystectomy.
- The problem is that the disease often recurs after years of local control.
- Side effects of fractionated treatment are dysuria, diarrhea, and/or urinary frequency in 50%–70% of patients.

## Advanced bladder cancer

- Advanced bladder cancer may be present at diagnosis, or a result of recurrence.
- A very small fraction of patients with advanced bladder cancer can be cured.
- The focus of care for most patients with advanced bladder cancer is palliation of symptoms from a bladder tumor that often is very large.

## Nursing Care of Individuals with Bladder Cancer

### Preoperative nursing care

- Most urinary diversions have similar preoperative nursing considerations.
- Bowel preparation begins with a low-residue diet two days before surgery. The day before surgery, antibiotics, cathartics, and a clear diet are administered.
- Printed materials with explicit directions and illustrations are especially helpful preoperatively.
- The selection of a stoma site is an important preoperative consideration; the type of urinary diversion to be performed will dictate to some extent the stoma site selected.
- The abdomen is examined and the individual observed while standing, sitting, and reclining. This is done to find an area at least 3 inches in diameter that is free of wrinkles and slightly convex. The site chosen should be visible to the individual and away from bony prominences, old scars or creases, and belt lines.
- Any method of marking the site that will remain visible after the surgical scrub is acceptable.

### General postoperative care

- As with all patients who have undergone major abdominal surgery, early ambulation, use of elastic stockings, and incentive spirometry may be used to prevent pulmonary emboli or respiratory complications.
- Continent urinary reservoirs and bladder substitutes produce much mucus. They should be irrigated regularly in the early postoperative period to prevent mucus accumulation.

- The urinary diversion should produce urine from the time of surgery.

## Nursing care following urinary diversion with an ileal conduit

### Stoma characteristics

- The stoma may bleed when rubbed because of the capillaries in the area. A small amount of bleeding from the stoma is not serious, but it must be determined that the blood is from the stoma and not from the urine.
- Normal color of the stoma is deep pink to dark red. A dusky appearance ranging from purple to black may develop if circulation is seriously impaired.

### Mucus production

- Mucus will be present in all diversions using segments of the bowel for a conduit for continent pouch.

### Pouching a urinary stoma

- The fairly continuous flow of urine from a conduit requires the individual to wear an appliance at all times.
- The skin around the stoma should be clean and thoroughly dry before positioning the appliance over the stoma.
- The pouch should initially be positioned to the patient's side so that it can be attached to bed-side drainage without placing stress on the seal.
- Many of the urinary pouches today are manufactured with an antireflux valve.
- Although not always possible, an effective urinary pouch should adhere at least three days.

### Patient teaching for continuing care of a conduit

- A visit from a person who has been rehabilitated with a similar diversion may be arranged to give reassurance.
- Names and telephone numbers of resource people to call if emergencies arise are a source of reassurance to the individual.

### Follow-up nursing care

- The stoma may continue to decrease in size for several months or more. The size of the appliance opening should reflect this change.
- Alkaline encrustations around the stoma can lead to stoma stenosis as a result of skin contact with alkaline urine.
- Nurses have traditionally recommended that patients increase the intake of cranberry juice to help maintain a more acidic urine.
- Ureteral angulation, stenosis, obstruction, or lithiasis leads to hydronephrosis, or irreparable renal damage.

## Nursing care of the individual with a continent ileal reservoir for urinary diversion

- Three weeks after surgery, the individual will be readmitted to the hospital. A radiographic picture of the pouch will be taken to confirm that there is no extravasation or reflux of urine from the pouch, and then the Medena tube and ureteral stents will be removed. The patient is taught to intubate/catheterize the pouch using a #20 French or #22 French coudé red-rubber catheter every two hours during the day and every three hours at night during the first week after the Medena tube is removed. This is increased gradually (by 1 hour each week) until the pouch is being intubated and drained approximately three or four times in 24 hours.

### Nursing care for a Kock pouch to the urethra

- The patient who has chosen the continent urinary Kock reservoir is cared for postoperatively in much the same way as the patient who has had a continent reservoir procedure. The difference is that the patient has a #24 French Foley catheter inserted through the urethra into the reservoir for three weeks.
- Three weeks postoperative the patient will be readmitted for Kock pouch training.
- It takes a very motivated person three to six weeks to obtain total control during the day. It may take longer to obtain good control at night.

### Follow-up care

- Radiological studies are used to confirm the integrity of the pouch, to test the competence of the nipple valves, and to ensure complete emptying of the reservoir.

### Nursing care of the individual receiving intravesical bacillus Calmette-Guerin

- Following instillation, the patient should be encouraged to retain the drug in his or her bladder for two hours (if possible). During the first hour the patient should lie first on his or her stomach for 15 minutes, then supine for 15 minutes, then on each side for 15 minutes each. A sitting position can be resumed during the second hour.

## CANCER OF THE KIDNEY

### Epidemiology

- There are two major types of kidney cancer.
  - *Renal cell cancer* is the most common form.
  - The second major type is *cancer of the renal pelvis*.
- There is a 2:1 male predominance in kidney cancer, especially in renal cell cancer.
- One of the most important demographic risk factors for both renal cell cancer and cancer of the renal pelvis is age. Both are rare in people under 35 years of age, and thereafter the incidence increases with age.

### Etiology

#### Cigarette smoking

- The only risk factor that has been linked persistently to kidney cancer by both cohort studies and epidemiological case-controlled studies is cigarette smoking.

#### Occupation

- Exposures to asbestos and lead have each demonstrated a slightly increased risk for renal cell cancer than might otherwise be expected.

#### Analgesic use

- Heavy use of analgesics, specifically aspirin, phenacetin, or acetaminophen-containing products, has been shown to increase the risk of cancer of the renal pelvis.

### Other factors

- A strong association between renal cell cancer and obesity in women was first identified in 1974.

### Genetic factors

- Rare family constellations have been described in which multiple family members develop renal cell cancer, and predisposition to the disease is inherited in an autosomal dominant fashion.

## Pathophysiology

### Cellular characteristics

- Although the histology is diverse from tumor to tumor, renal cell carcinoma can be separated into two broad groups: clear cell tumors and granular cell tumors.
- The two major cell types in tumors of the renal pelvis are transitional cell cancer (most common) and squamous cell cancer.

### Progression of disease

- Renal cell cancers tend to grow toward the medullary portion of the kidney, whereas tumors of the renal pelvis often grow at the ureteropelvic junction and invade the underlying submucosa and muscular coats.
- Cancer of the renal pelvis and renal cell carcinoma spread through the venous and lymphatic routes.
- Renal cell carcinoma also spreads by direct extension to the renal vein and sometimes farther into the vena cava.
- Although the majority of upper urinary tract transitional cell cancers are localized at diagnosis, the most common metastatic sites are regional lymph nodes, bone, and lung.

## Paraneoplasia and Renal Cell Carcinoma

- Renal cell carcinoma may be associated with certain ectopic hormone production such as parathyroid hormone, erythropoietin, renin gonadotropins, and adrenocorticotropic hormones.

## Clinical Manifestations

### Renal cell carcinoma

- In 40% of individuals diagnosed with renal cell carcinoma, the initial symptom is gross hematuria.
- Pain is also a common presenting symptom, as is a palpable abdominal mass.

### Cancer of the renal pelvis

- Tumors of the renal pelvis originally present with hematuria, flank pain, or a palpable mass.

## Assessment

### Renal cell carcinoma

- Tests used in diagnosis and staging include kidney, ureter, and bladder (KUB) radiographs; nephrotomograms; excretory urogram; retrograde urogram; renal ultrasound (US); renal CT; and renal angiography.
- Excretory urogram and renal tomography are considered by most to be the screening tests of choice for suspected renal mass lesions, although they are only 70%–75% accurate in differentiating benign cysts from malignant lesions.

- Renal US has the apparent advantage of being easy to do, noninvasive, and relatively inexpensive, and requiring a minimal physical expenditure on the patient's part.

### Cancer of the renal pelvis

- Excretory urogram, retrograde urogram, and urinary cytology are the most useful techniques for establishing a diagnosis of cancer of the renal pelvis.

## Classification and Staging
### Renal cell carcinoma

- The size of the primary tumor is not strongly correlated with survival and may not be a significant factor in staging.

### Cancer of the renal pelvis

- Staging of renal pelvic cancers is based on an accurate assessment of the degree of tumor infiltration and parallels that staging system developed for bladder cancer.

## Treatment of Renal Cell Carcinoma
### Surgery

- A radical nephrectomy is the standard, often curative, treatment for renal cell cancer. This routinely includes removal of the kidney, Gerota's fascia, the ipsilateral adrenal, the proximal one-half of the ureter, and lymph nodes in the renal hilar area. Regional lymphadenectomy remains controversial.

### Bilateral tumors or tumors in a solitary kidney

- In bilateral tumors where there is a larger tumor in one kidney than in the other, partial nephrectomy is performed on the kidney with the smaller tumor, and several weeks later radical nephrectomy is carried out on the kidney with the larger tumor.
  - In cases where there is a tumor in a solitary kidney with no evidence of metastasis, partial nephrectomy or radical nephrectomy with subsequent chronic hemodialysis or renal transplantation are treatment alternatives.

### Radiotherapy and chemotherapy

- Renal cell carcinomas and their metastases are usually radioresistant.
- Adjuvant chemotherapy has not demonstrated any improvement in survival rates over what may be accomplished without chemotherapy.

## Treatment of Advanced Renal Cell Carcinoma

- About 30% of individuals with renal cell carcinoma present with metastases at the time of diagnosis. Another 50% will develop metastases after radical nephrectomy.

### Radiotherapy

- Radiation therapy is an important modality in the palliation of patients with metastatic renal cell cancer.

### Surgery

- Adjunctive or palliative nephrectomies have been described as approaches for individuals with metastatic renal cell carcinoma.

- Palliative nephrectomy may be justifiable for individuals who have severe disabling symptoms such as local pain, bleeding, or endocrinopathy but who otherwise have a reasonable life expectancy of greater than six months.

## Chemotherapy

- Chemotherapy has had no great impact on metastatic renal cell carcinoma.

## Biologic response modifiers

- Alfa-interferon and IL-2 act by stimulating host immunologic responses against cancer. Side effects include flu-like syndrome, fatigue, abnormal liver function, and anorexia.

## Treatment of Cancer of the Renal Pelvis

- Treatment of renal pelvic cancers should be based on tumor grade, stage and position. The standard treatment has been nephroureterectomy. To avoid recurrence in this segment, a radical nephrectomy, including the kidney, all perinephric tissue, regional lymph nodes, the ureter, and a small cuff of the bladder, is performed.

## Results and Prognosis

- For patients with tumor confined to the kidney the five-year survival is approximately 92%–95%; for T3 tumors it is approximately 18%; for metastatic disease (T4, or any T with M1) the five-year survival is low, ranging from 0% to 20%. Overall five-year survival is 40%.

## Nursing Care of Individuals with Cancer of the Kidney

- In general, the principal treatment of primary renal carcinoma is surgical excision. Radical nephrectomy is performed on all resectable lesions in stage I to III disease.

### Preoperative nursing care

- A renal infarction may be done two to three days prior to surgery in an attempt to decrease surgical hemorrhage by decreasing tumor vascularity.

### Postoperative nursing care

Pain relief

- As a result of the position on the operating table, the individual undergoing nephrectomy experiences not only incision pain but also muscular aches and pains.
- The use of moist heat, massage, and pillows to support the back while the patient is on his or her side also can provide relief. The individual should be turned from side to side at least every two hours, more often if desired.

Prevention of atelectasis and pneumonia

- The patient needs to be taught how to splint the incision while coughing.

Monitoring renal function

- The urine will be slightly blood-tinged for the first few hours after surgery. Urine output should be greater than 30 ml/hour. If the individual does not have a urinary catheter and has not voided within eight to ten hours after surgery, catheterization must be done to determine renal status.

### Paralytic ileus

- The individual is usually allowed nothing to eat or drink by mouth for the first 24–48 hours after surgery.
- A nasogastric tube and/or rectal tube is used to relieve abdominal distention.

### Hemorrhage

- Although not a frequent complication, postnephrectomy hemorrhage is a danger because the kidney is a highly vascular organ.

### Wound care

- Wound care after nephrectomy is fairly routine.

### Potential for pneumothorax

- The nurse must maintain the chest tube under water drainage and keep it free of kinks. Patients are encouraged to breathe deeply and cough to promote lung expansion.

# PRACTICE QUESTIONS

1. Up to 50% of bladder cancers in men are thought to be related to:
   a. cigarette smoking.
   b. alcohol abuse.
   c. occupational exposure.
   d. intrauterine exposure to exogenous estrogens.

2. In determining the progression of bladder cancer, the most important feature is the:
   a. degree of hematuria present.
   b. presence of bladder neck obstruction.
   c. depth of penetration into the bladder wall.
   d. presence of pain in the suprapubic region.

3. One of the treatments of choice for superficial low-grade bladder cancers is:
   a. radical cystectomy.
   b. radiation implants.
   c. laser therapy.
   d. instillation of single-agent chemotherapy.

4. In women, radical cystectomy includes removal of the:
   a. bladder, urethra, uterus, ovaries, fallopian tubes, and the anterior wall of the vagina.
   b. bladder, urethra, and anterior wall of the vagina only.
   c. bladder and urethra only.
   d. bladder only.

5. Mr. Makela has an ileal conduit placed following cystectomy for advanced bladder cancer. Which of the following would be considered normal?
   a. a delay of urinary output for 4–5 hours after surgery
   b. protrusion of the stoma 3 inches above the skin surface
   c. a stoma dark red in color and slightly edematous
   d. a small amount of leakage from the appliance

6. If the urine passing from a stoma is cloudy, it may be that:
   a. the patient is dehydrated.
   b. the stoma was formed from intestinal tissue.
   c. a leak in the stoma pouch has occurred, allowing air and bacteria to enter a sterile area.
   d. antispasmodics are indicated.

7. Ms. Nichols has just received intravesical bacillus Calmette-Guerin. The nurse should instruct her to:
   a. regard fever and cough as normal during treatment.
   b. disinfect the toilet with bleach twice daily for six days.
   c. retain the drug in her bladder for two hours.
   d. all of the above.

8. The only consistent risk factor for kidney cancer is:
   a. cigarette smoking.
   b. coffee.
   c. heredity.
   d. asbestos.

9.  In addition to cigarette smoking and occupational exposure, heavy use of which category of drugs has been shown to increase the risk of cancer of the renal pelvis?
    a.  antipsychotics
    b.  non-narcotic analgesics
    c.  narcotics
    d.  hypnotics

10. Standard treatment for renal cell cancer is most likely to take the form of:
    a.  radiotherapy.
    b.  radical nephrectomy including removal of lymph nodes in the hilar region.
    c.  chemotherapy.
    d.  regional lymphadenectomy.

11. When chemotherapy is used to treat advanced renal cell cancer, it is being used:
    a.  in combination with immunotherapy.
    b.  to achieve a response of short duration.
    c.  palliatively, to control symptoms such as pain.
    d.  to shrink tumor burden and allow for effective surgical resection.

12. In determining the survival rate for persons with cancer of the renal pelvis, the most important factor seems to be:
    a.  the stage of the tumor.
    b.  whether or not radiotherapy was used in treatment.
    c.  whether or not the tumor is hormone sensitive.
    d.  the age and physical condition of the patient at diagnosis.

## ANSWER EXPLANATIONS

1.  **The answer is a.** Recent studies have shown little or no correlation between bladder cancer and alcohol consumption. Similarly, no correlation is felt to exist between bladder cancer and intrauterine estrogen exposure. There are some occupations—among them janitors and cleaners, mechanics, miners, and printers—that place one at higher risk for developing bladder cancer, but by far the strongest correlation is between bladder cancer and cigarette smoking. Since 1956 it has been known that smokers are twice as likely as nonsmokers to develop bladder cancer, with smoking accounting for as much as 50% of all bladder cancer in American men. (p. 890)

2.  **The answer is c.** Although gross hematuria, bladder neck obstruction, and pain in the suprapubic region can all be clinical manifestations of bladder cancer, the most important indicator of disease progression is the depth of tumor penetration into the bladder wall. (p. 891)

3.  **The answer is c.** Superficial tumors of the bladder are those that remain in the epithelium and lamina propria. Standard treatment is with transurethral resection (TUR), but because the chance of recurrence is great, adjuvant treatment with combination chemotherapy, hormones, and/or laser beams is not uncommon. Partial cystectomy is indicated for some individuals; radical cystectomy is usually indicated only in high-stage, high-grade tumors. (p. 893)

4.  **The answer is a.** In women, a radical cystectomy includes the removal of the bladder, urethra, uterus, ovaries, fallopian tubes, and anterior wall of the vagina. In men, the term is synonymous with prostatectomy and includes excision of the bladder with pericystic sac, the attached perineum, the prostate, and seminal vesicles. (p. 894)

5. **The answer is c.** A urinary diversion should produce urine from the time of surgery, and flow should be more or less continuous. The stoma should protrude 1/2–3/4 inches above the skin to allow the urine to drain into the aperture of an appliance. Leakage from the appliance is abnormal and could lead to skin breakdown. The stoma itself should be deep pink to dark red in color. (p. 899)

6. **The answer is b.** The intestine normally produces mucus, and mucus will almost always be present in diversions using segments of the bowel, causing the urine to appear cloudy. Excessive mucus may clog the urinary appliance outlet, and if this occurs, and appliance with a larger outlet may be used. (p. 900)

7. **The answer is c.** If possible, following instillation, the patient is encouraged to retain the drug for two hours in the bladder. A cough can indicate a BCG infection. For home administration, the toilet is disinfected with bleach after every voiding for the first six hours. (p. 903)

8. **The answer is a.** The only risk factor that has been linked persistently to kidney cancer by both cohort studies and epidemiological studies is cigarette smoking. The links to occupational exposures (lead, asbestos) and genetics are less frequent. (pp. 905–906)

9. **The answer is b.** Heavy use of the non-narcotic analgesics aspirin and/or acetaminophen has been shown to increase the risk of cancer of the renal pelvis. Similarly, an association has been made between analgesics and renal cell cancer, but this association has not as yet been substantiated. (p. 905)

10. **The answer is b.** The treatment of choice for renal cell cancer is radical nephrectomy, which includes removal of the lymph nodes in the renal hilar area. Regional lymphadenectomy is a controversial procedure, with some experts arguing that the procedure does not improve survival and others feeling that regional lymphadenectomy in combination with radical nephrectomy is potentially curative in some individuals. Renal cell carcinomas and their metastases are usually radioresistant, making radiotherapy an unlikely choice, and adjuvant chemotherapy has not demonstrated much effectiveness against the disease. (p. 908)

11. **The answer is b.** Approximately 50% of individuals who develop metastases after radical nephrectomy have an extremely poor prognosis. These individuals, considered to have advanced renal cell carcinoma, may be treated with chemotherapy, which has demonstrated some success in achieving tumor responses, but the response is usually short-lived and the toxicity may be significant. (p. 910)

12. **The answer is a.** The overall prognosis for cancer of the renal pelvis is poor, with 5-year survival rates of only approximately 40%. This figure becomes 60% with low-grade, low-stage cancers and drops to 0%–33% for higher grades. (p. 911)

# Chapter 34    Breast Cancer

## INTRODUCTION

- Breast cancer is the most common cancer in women and the leading cause of death for women 40–44 years of age.
- Over 70% of all breast cancer occurs in women who are 50 years of age or older.
- In general, breast cancer incidence varies across the country but is about 1 in every 8 women.
- While the incidence of breast cancer has increased over the past 30 years, the mortality rate has recently demonstrated a slight decrease, reflecting better cure rates for earlier staged lesions.
- This decrease is more evident among white women than black women (Figure 34-1, text page 918).
- Whether or not the individual with breast cancer survives, the disease is determined by numerous factors, but the outcome primarily depends upon the intrinsic growth rate of the tumor, which varies dramatically; the age of the woman at diagnosis; and numerous biological parameters.

## ETIOLOGY

### Hormonal Factors

- Women are 100 times more likely to develop breast cancer than men.
- Early menarche (before age 12), nulliparity or parity after age 30 and late menopause (after age 55) are linked to the type and duration of exposure to endogenous hormones that may have an impact on the development of breast cancer.
- Hormones play a significant role in the development of breast cancer. They may act as initiators or promoters in that they alter cell proliferation, differentiation, and atrophy.
- Premenopausal women tend to exhibit decreased adrenal androgen levels. Increased testosterone production and estradiol levels appear in both pre- and postmenopausal women.
- Pregnancy (full term) has been reported to exert a deterrent effect on the development of breast cancer.
- In general, nulliparous women who began using oral contraceptives before age 20 and continued uninterrupted use for more than six years, have a minimal increased risk of developing breast cancer.
- Another increase in risk has been associated with the use of oral contraceptives during the perimenopausal years.
- Current evidence suggests either no effect on breast cancer risk from hormone replacement therapy (HRT) or an elevation in risk of less than twofold with very long-term use or relatively high doses.
- Giving breast cancer survivors estrogen therapy is a controversial issue, since the current standard of practice generally precludes prescribing these hormonal agents.

### Family History

- Family history of breast cancer is a contributing factor to the potential risk of developing the disease.
- Most women (approximately 70%) who develop breast cancer have no known risk factors. Familial and hereditary breast cancer account for a very small proportion of the diagnosed cases (20% and 9% respectively).
- Many of the genes responsible for inherited familial cancers seem to be tumor suppressor genes that are actively involved in suppressing malignant growth during the cell cycle. When these genes

undergo mutation(s), the normal function is altered, causing abnormal proliferation resulting in neoplastic and malignant cell growth.

- Inheritance of the *BRCA1* susceptibility gene is associated with a strong likelihood that the effect of the mutation will result in the disease for families with multiple breast and ovarian cancers (90%) as well as those with breast cancers diagnosed before the age of 45 (70%).
- *BRCA2* has been identified on the long arm of chromosome 13 (13q12-13). This mutation seems to be associated with male breast cancer and early-onset female breast cancer.

## Diet

- Diets high in fats have been implicated in countries that have shown a sudden increase in incidence rates, as well as high-risk countries.
- The relationship of a high-fat diet and breast cancer may be linked to the amount and ratios of hormones produced by the endocrine system. The proliferation of breast tissue may be altered by changes in estrogen, pituitary, and thyroid function, which are sensitive to dietary changes.

## Obesity

- Obesity confers a slight increased risk overall, but demonstrates more of a risk for those women who are postmenopausal than any other age group.

## Alcohol

- The most compelling evidence suggests that the relationship between alcohol and breast cancer risk is greatest for women who consume more than two drinks per day.

## Radiation

- Survivors of atomic bombs exhibited an increase in breast cancer as well as other cancers.
- A risk of breast cancer has been associated with radiation therapy.
  - The risk increases with dosage, especially if a woman is exposed in the period of young adulthood.

## Nonproliferative Disease

- Approximately 70% of biopsies reflect cellular changes that impart no risk or a very small risk to the patient and are often referred to as fibrocystic change.

## Proliferative Disease

- The presence of proliferation on a pathology slide indicates a presence of increased cell growth.
- Proliferative disease without atypia falls into the slightly increased risk category.
- The moderate risk category includes atypical ductal hyperplasia and atypical lobular hyperplasia.

## Carcinoma in Situ

- A carcinoma in situ that remains in the breast is capable of transforming to an invasive cancer but does not necessarily do so.
- Ductal carcinoma in situ (DCIS) and lobular carcinoma in situ (LCIS) are characterized by an eight- to tenfold increased risk of developing invasive cancer.

## PREVENTION OF BREAST CANCER

- Of the more than 184,000 women diagnosed yearly, only 50% will be diagnosed with stage I disease, and approximately 30% of all women with breast cancer will subsequently die of their disease.

- Newer, even more sophisticated methods of detecting breast cancer or preventing breast cancer are needed.

## Chemoprevention

- Chemoprevention for breast cancer using tamoxifen, vitamin A, 4-HPR is currently under research.
- Because of the influence of hormones in breast cancer, tamoxifen—an antiestrogen—may prevent breast cancer.
  - Tamoxifen has also been found to increase disease-free survival in node-negative, ER-positive disease, as well as node-positive disease.
  - Women taking tamoxifen for primary breast cancer have experienced a reduction in the expected incidence of contralateral breast cancer. This strengthens the possibility of a chemoprotective effect.
  - As an antagonist, tamoxifen competes with estradiol for the receptor sites in the nucleus. This mechanism causes an estrogen blockade and impedes growth of malignant cells.
  - The common toxicities of tamoxifen are hot flashes, vaginal discharge, and irregular menses.

## Prophylactic Mastectomy

- A *prophylactic mastectomy*—the removal of the majority of breast tissue including total breast, tail of Spence, and nipple areola complex—may be warranted in certain high-risk women; however, controversy exists over how much risk is enough to justify performing this procedure.
- Breast cancer has been known to occur in the chest wall or axillary region. It is therefore important for a woman to realize some risk of developing breast cancer exists after a prophylactic mastectomy.

## SCREENING

- Early detection reduces the mortality of breast cancer and provides a 90% survival rate for five years.

## BSE

- Lack of proficiency is one of the most consistent barriers to BSE practice. This can be alleviated through an education process that provides verbal and written information as well as demonstration and return demonstration.
- BSE training should have three basic components: (1) a visual exam using a mirror; (2) a palpation exam in the shower and in the supine position on the bed; and (3) proper technique emphasized during the instructional and return demonstration session.
- The monthly exam should be done one to two days after menses stops in premenopausal women or on an appointed day of the month for postmenopausal women.
- For the visual exam the woman stands before a mirror with arms relaxed, looking for any changes in breast symmetry, size, and shape, including changes in the skin or nipple/areolar complex.
  - The woman should turn to the side to inspect the lateral aspect of each breast as well. The visual inspection is repeated with arms overhead and with arms pressing on the hips.
  - The visual exam is concluded with the woman leaning forward to inspect the breasts while they are suspended.
- BSE is best performed lying on the bed.
  - Raising the arm, use the flat pads of the first three fingers to examine the breast with small circular motions. The area below the collarbone and beside the breastbone should also be included. Use the same motion to examine the armpit.
  - The woman may wish to examine herself in the shower to provide a complete and thorough monthly examination of the breasts.

## Mammography

- Asymptomatic women should begin screening mammography by the age of 40 and continue with screening mammography and clinical exams every one to two years as recommended by their physician.
- There has been recent controversy regarding the usefulness of regular screening for women aged 40–49.
- Mammograms are generally not recommended for women under age 35 because younger breasts tend to be dense, which causes the mammogram to appear white and contain very little contrast.
- Screening mammography has been proven to be beneficial in the reduction of mortality as well as technical improvements in the detection of malignancies.
- Barriers to the performance of mammography include cost, fear of the effects of radiation, lack of education regarding the benefits and recommendation guidelines for screening.
- Education is an important component in addressing these issues and encouraging screening.

## Ultrasound

- Ultrasound is not considered an adequate screening tool because of its limited sensitivity compared to mammography.
- Pregnant women, lactating mothers, or women who naturally have very dense breasts may need ultrasound as an additional or alternative screening tool.

## MULTIDISCIPLINARY BREAST CENTERS

- Ideally, the comprehensive breast center should have a full complement of disciplines available to provide an expert opinion regarding assessment of diagnostic and histopathological data.
- Breast centers will be expected to provide risk assessment for families as well as genetic counseling and testing.
- Confidentiality, informed consent, and insurance issues should be carefully addressed by the staff.
- The oncology clinical nurse specialist is often viewed as the coordinator of the comprehensive breast center. It is imperative that this professional possesses specialized knowledge in all aspects of breast cancer and its treatment as well as a compassionate, yet controlled, approach to the evaluation of a suspected breast cancer.
- The nurse is also instrumental in providing BSE instruction to all patients. The nurse also will be called on to answer questions regarding diagnostic tests, therapy regimens, clinical trials, postoperative events, and potential complications of treatment.

## PATHOPHYSIOLOGY

### Cellular Characteristics

- The majority of primary breast cancers are adenocarcinomas located in the upper outer quadrant of the breast.
- Adenocarcinoma can occur at any age, but highly malignant varieties with rapidly dividing cells affect more women in their early 50s.
- Invasive lobular carcinoma occurs in the same age range as ductal carcinoma, accounts for 5%–10% of all breast cancers, and is frequently bilateral.
- Tubular carcinoma is fairly uncommon and represents a well-differentiated adenocarcinoma of the breast.
- Medullary carcinomas account for 5%–7% of malignant breast tumors, occurring most commonly in younger women (< 50 years of age).
- Mucinous or colloid carcinoma is uncommon, occurring in women 60–70 years of age.
- Inflammatory breast cancer occurs infrequently and accounts for less than 4% of breast cancers.

## Patterns of Metastasis

- Even among women with the same histological type, clinical stage, and treatment, some will be cured, while others have emergence of metastatic disease within six months of therapy. There is no known reason for this disparity among individuals.
- Breast cancer metastasizes widely, primarily to the bone, lungs, nodes, liver, and brain. The first site of metastasis is usually local or regional involving the chest wall or axillary supraclavicular lymph nodes or bone. Women with ER(−) disease are more likely to have recurrences in visceral organs whereas women with ER(+) disease have recurrences in skin and bone.

## CLINICAL MANIFESTATIONS

### Diagnostic Studies

- Clinical manifestations that are more suspicious of malignant disease are nipple retraction or elevation.
- Skin dimpling or retraction also may be present and is possibly due to invasion of the suspensory ligaments and fixation to the chest wall. Heat and erythema of the breast skin are also signs of inflammatory breast carcinoma. Skin edema is characteristic of malignant disease.
- Ulceration of the skin with secondary infection may be present. The presence of isolated skin nodules indicates invasion of blood vessels and lymphatics.

#### Mammograms

##### Screening mammograms

- The goal of screening mammography is to detect a malignancy before it becomes clinically apparent.
- Clinical detection through the use of BSE generally occurs when a tumor is approximately the size of a walnut.
- A screening mammography allows the radiologist to detect characteristic benign and malignant masses.
- Speculated malignant lesions may present as masses, architectural distortion, asymmetric densities, or ill-defined microcalcifications. Additionally, subtle abnormalities may be noted by the radiologist that require further studies to determine whether pathology exists.

##### Diagnostic mammograms

- A diagnostic mammogram is performed when the patient reports specific symptoms, when suspicious clinical findings exist, or when an abnormality has been found on a screening mammogram.
- Diagnostic mammography provides the radiologist with additional detail, which may preclude the need for an open biopsy.

##### Digital mammography and computer assisted diagnosis (CAD)

- CAD utilizes a software program to target potentially suspicious lesions for the radiologist to review and interpret.
- The computer identification involves an algorithm from a preset database generated from probability tables.
- The specificity of the image is enhanced by real-time evaluation on a screen, allowing for manipulation of contrast, which enhances detection and permits more rapid interventional procedures.

### Sonogram

- A sonogram, or ultrasound, is used to determine whether a lesion is solid or cystic. It can also be used to guide interventional procedures such as cyst aspiration, abscess drainage, FNA, needle core biopsies, or presurgical localization.
  - Ultrasounds are appropriate in young women whose breasts have the dense fibroglandular tissue. Ultrasounds are also useful in pregnant women, who need to be spared radiation or in recently lactating women whose breasts are extremely dense.

### MRI

- MRI has become a highly accurate, though costly tool, now that specificity is enhanced by contrast infusion.
- MRI is limited in the detection of calcifications, which excludes its use for many nonpalpable lesions.

### PET

- PET may be superior to MRI in identifying viable tumor versus scar tissue, benign and malignant axillary nodes, and tumors >1 cm.
- The major limitations of PET are the high cost of the scanners and limited availability, as well as the short half-life of the radiopharmaceuticals.

### Fine-needle aspiration

- Fine-needle aspiration (FNA) is employed when an abnormality is known to be solid or to determine whether the lump is a cyst. FNA may also be used to confirm a clinically apparent positive diagnosis.
- A lesion that does not demonstrate a malignant histology may still remain clinically suspicious to the physician. In cases such as these, a biopsy will often be recommended.

### Stereotactic needle-guided biopsy

- The stereotactic needle-guided biopsy (SNB) is mainly used to target and identify mammographically detected nonpalpable lesions in the breast.
- SNB is less suitable for very small lesions or areas of calcification, superficial lesions, or those on the extreme medial or lateral area of the breast.
- The stereotactic biopsy permits diagnosis of benign disease without the trauma or scarring of an open biopsy.

### Wire localization biopsy

- The aim of this biopsy procedure is to assist the surgeon in locating the nonpalpable lesion for the purpose of excisional biopsy and to minimize the volume of tissue removed to avoid unnecessary deformity.

### Open biopsy

- The excisional biopsy is the most invasive diagnostic procedure. There are several reasons for recommending an excisional biopsy: (1) sonogram findings show the lesion to be solid and indeterminant; (2) the cytology and/or histology results are insufficient; (3) the clinical or mammographic findings are suspicious; or (4) the patient with a probable low-risk lesion requests a biopsy to allay her anxiety.

- The objective of this biopsy is to remove the lump or area identified, along with a small amount of surrounding normal tissue.

## Prognostic Indicators

- The identification of various prognostic indicators is valuable because they help in identifying various subsets of women who might benefit most from adjuvant systemic therapies, as well as establishing prognosis with increasing accuracy.
- Valuable parameters for determining the prognosis for patients with breast cancer include the status of the axillary lymph nodes, size of the tumor, the invasive nature of the neoplasm, multicentricity, nuclear grade, estrongen-progesterone receptor levels, and histological type.

### Axillary lymph node status

- Clinical assessment of the axillary nodes carries a 30% false-positive and false-negative rate. Pathological staging of the lymph nodes is mandatory.
- Prognosis worsens as the number of positive lymph nodes increases.

### Tumor size

- There is a clear relationship between increase in systemic risk of recurrence and increasing tumor size.

### Hormone receptor status

- The major benefit to hormone receptor status concerns its value in predicting which patients will respond to hormone manipulation.

### Cell proliferative indices and DNA ploidy

- Flow cytometry is used to measure DNA content and proliferative activity (S-phase fraction) of a tumor.
- Patients whose tumors have an abnormal amount of DNA are aneuploid. Those with normal DNA are diploid.
- A high S-phase calculation consistently predicts a poorer outcome compared to those patients with lower S-phase calculation.
- Tumors with positive estrogen receptor protein tend to demonstrate a low proliferative activity and tend to be more diploid than aneuploid. Comparatively, tumors that are estrogen receptor negative tend to have a more aggressive metastatic potential.

### Histological differentiation

- The more differentiated the tumor cells, the better the prognosis. Tumors are generally classified as well-differentiated, (grade I), moderately well-differentiated, (grade II), or poorly differentiated (grade III), according to their degree of anaplasia.

### Epidermal growth factor receptor

- Estrogen plays a significant role in the pathogenesis and initial proliferation of breast cancer.
- Estrogen may exert inhibitory action on epidermal growth factor receptor (EGFR) production through binding to the estrogen receptor. In the absence of this inhibition, the EGFR may actually increase proliferation of breast cancer cells.

### Her-2/*neu* oncogene

- Overexpression or amplification of this oncogene occurs in about 20% of human breast cancers and correlates positively with a poor prognosis in node-positive disease.
- Overexpression of Her-2/*neu* occurs more frequently in more advanced tumors that are more poorly differentiated.

### Cathepsin D

- High cathepsin D levels increase the probability of recurrence and poor survival in aneuploid node-negative breast cancer.

## CLASSIFICATION AND STAGING

- Once a breast cancer has been diagnosed, a complete evaluation of the disease is initiated to establish stage of disease and the most appropriate approach to treatment.
- The patient is clinically staged on the basis of the characteristics of the primary tumor, the physical examination of the axillary nodes, and the presence of distant metastases.
- Stage I—tumor 0–2 cm in size; negative lymph nodes and no evidence of metastasis
- Stage II—describes a small tumor with positive lymph nodes or a larger tumor with negative lymph nodes
- Stage III—more advanced locoregional disease with suspected but undetectable metastases
- Stage IV—distant metastases present

## THERAPEUTIC APPROACHES AND NURSING CARE

### Local-Regional Disease

- The current hypothesis governing the design of treatment alternatives for the woman with breast cancer contends that invasive breast cancer is potentially a systemic disease involving complex host-tumor interactions and that variations in local regional therapy are unlikely to affect survival outcomes.
- Patients who die from breast cancer have distant occult metastases at the time of local therapy or metastases from inadequately treated local or regional disease.
- These findings confirm the now standard approach to breast preservation, employing adjuvant radiation therapy.
- Modified radical mastectomy is indicated for larger, multicentric disease or where cosmesis is otherwise not achievable. Modified radical mastectomy may also be employed as definitive treatment following local recurrence in patients who fail conservative surgery and radiation.
- With an equivalent survival rate and preservation of the breast, conservative surgery plus radiation is now considered preferable to mastectomy for the majority of women.
- Local recurrences following mastectomy usually occur within three years of surgery.
- Radiation doses to the breast are delivered using supervoltage equipment and tangential fields to minimize lung and heart exposure. The whole-breast dose ranges from 45–50 Gy delivered in about 6 weeks.
- Some immediate side effects of radiation therapy are transient breast edema, erythema, and dry or wet desquamation. Later effects include telangiectasia, which is seen less often, and arm edema, which usually results from radiating the axilla for multiple positive nodes.

## Adjuvant Systemic Therapy

### Early stage I and II breast cancer

- Overall optimal use of adjuvant therapy can significantly improve long-term survival in women with stage I and II breast cancer and has the potential to save more lives from this disease than from any other malignancy.
- In women under 50 years of age, adjuvant chemotherapy alone reduces the annual odds of recurrence by 27%.

#### Stage I (node-negative) breast cancer

- Currently, there are important prognostic indicators that help to determine a woman's risk of recurrence, such as ploidy, proliferative indices, and tumor grade, but no one parameter is predictive of recurrence.
- Women with the lowest risk of recurrence are those with tumors less than 2 cm, a grade I malignancy, positive estrogen/progesterone receptors, and a low proliferative rate.
- Node-negative and node-positive patients may benefit from preoperative chemotherapy.

#### Stage II (node-positive) breast cancer

- Women with tumor involving the lymph nodes are recognized as having a greater likelihood for distant recurrence and death.
- The efficacy of chemotherapy in postmenopausal women has been sufficiently demonstrated.

### Locally advanced breast cancer (stage III)

- Locally advanced breast cancer is associated with high risk of developing distant metastases.
- If the tumor is fixed to the chest wall, inflammatory carcinoma is present, significant ulceration exists, or the axillary nodes are fixed to one another or other structures, the situation is generally considered to be inoperable due to the almost certain risk of recurrence.
- Results are superior when chemotherapy and radiation are included in the treatment plan.
- Significant tumor shrinkage may permit resection in previously unresectable disease, allowing for less extensive surgical procedures.
- High-dose chemotherapy with peripheral blood stem cell autologous bone marrow transplant and hematopoietic growth factor support is currently an option for treatment for women with high-risk advanced disease.

#### Adjuvant tamoxifen therapy

- The benefit with adjuvant tamoxifen is similar for node-negative and node-positive patients, but it is most evident in women over 50 years of age.
- The optimal duration of tamoxifen therapy is not known.
- Severe hot flashes, vaginal discharge and irregular menses are associated with tamoxifen therapy. Ocular toxicity has been reported in women taking conventional doses of tamoxifen, but in general, ocular toxicity is not a clinically significant danger of tamoxifen therapy.

## Nursing Considerations in the Care of the Woman with Localized Breast Cancer

- To be a supportive advocate for the woman and her family, the nurse must be knowledgeable concerning the options for therapy, the goals of therapy, measures to minimize complications of treatment, and the various resources that may need to be mobilized throughout the treatment period and beyond.

- How well a woman adjusts psychologically and socially to the diagnosis and treatment will depend upon her previous coping strategies and emotional stability. In addition, social support has consistently been found to influence a woman's adjustment through treatment.

## Surgical considerations

- The current options for surgical management of stage I and II breast cancer include breast-preserving surgery and radiation or modified radical mastectomy.
- Prior to surgery, it is important to emphasize that the breast will appear different from the other breast depending on the size of the breasts and amount of tissue removed.
- Complications following breast-preserving surgery include arm edema, seroma formation and wound infection, shoulder dysfunction, upper extremity weakness, fatigue, and limitations in mobility.
  - Postoperative complications following mastectomy include wound infection, flap necrosis, and seroma formation.
- Lymphedema following mastectomy may be transient or permanent and may occur in the early postoperative period or much later.
- Nursing care of the postmastectomy patient centers on wound care, with special attention to maintaining functioning wound drains.
- Postmastectomy exercises to maintain shoulder and arm mobility may begin as early as 24 hours after surgery. The woman is instructed to maintain the affected arm in the adducted position but to perform limited exercises involving the wrist and elbow. Flexing fingers and touching the hand to the shoulder are encouraged. Squeezing a ball is discouraged, as it increases blood flow and, if done too vigorously, leads to swelling in the early postoperative period.
- Prior to discharge, the patient should have clear instructions regarding wound care.
- Instructions regarding breast self-exam and follow-up are best given during the first outpatient visit after surgery.
- As a group, however, younger women have consistently been found to experience more episodes of depression, anger, resentment, sexual problems, and fears of recurrence compared to older women.

## Chemotherapy

- Many premenopausal women who receive chemotherapy will experience ovarian failure and early menopause, especially if a larger cumulative dose of an alkylating agent is included in the treatment regimen.
  - Premenopausal women who receive chemotherapy should be clearly informed of their risk for temporary or permanent ovarian failure.
- Other menopausal symptoms that commonly occur in women receiving chemo/hormonal therapy include hot flashes, night sweats, and irregular menses.
- Weight gain is a troublesome side effect of therapy and is commonly felt by patients to occur because of water retention. In fact, it is due to increased caloric intake.
  - Women need to receive nutritional counseling regarding the avoidance of weight gain at the outset of therapy.
- Fatigue is a common subjective complaint associated with adjuvant therapy, and symptoms such as total body tiredness, forgetfulness, and wanting to rest increase over time throughout therapy.
- Adriamycin and cytoxan (AC) are commonly used in curable breast cancer, which means many women experience total alopecia within 2 to 3 weeks of beginning therapy.
- Women on methotrexate-5-fluorouracil therapy do not lose significant amounts of hair and rarely require a wig. Women receiving CMF experience gradual thinning over the six to eight months of therapy and may require a wig only towards the end of treatment. Hair begins to grow back within a month of ending therapy at a rate of 1/4 inch per month with some variation.

### Radiation

- Skin reactions occur in all patients and generally present as itching, dryness, scaling, redness, and tenderness. The breast may feel sore and warm to touch. Patients are instructed not to use soap to wash the area and to pat dry.

## BREAST RECONSTRUCTION

- Implants are considered to be safe and effective treatment despite recent media comments to the contrary.
- Because of the adverse publicity of silicone gel implants, many women and physicians are choosing saline-filled implants, which reduce the risk of silicone contamination if rupture should occur. These implants, however, do not have the same suppleness and natural feel of silicone gel implants.
- The ideal candidate for immediate breast reconstruction is one who has early-stage disease. However, the absolute limiting factor of this surgery is a medical condition that may compromise the patient's safety during or postsurgery.
- The goals of reconstructive surgery are to achieve "acceptable" symmetry and softness, correct any deformity caused by prior treatment, and construct an adequate nipple areolar complex.

### Silicone Implants

- An ideal candidate for a silicone implant is a woman who is small-breasted with a minimum of ptosis on the contralateral breast.
- The complications that may arise are progressive contracture, hematoma, infection, and flap necrosis.

### Saline Tissue Expanders

- Saline expanders are used when an inadequate supply of skin is available at the mastectomy site or when a large and/or ptotic breast is required.
- The expander is placed behind the chest wall muscles using the lines of the mastectomy incision.
- After allowing sufficient time for wound healing, a series of injections is performed as an office procedure.
- The expansion continues until the device is overinflated by approximately 50%.
- The overfilled expander is left in place for several months to allow for accommodation of the stretched tissue.
- The expander is then removed and a permanent prosthesis of lesser fluid volume is placed.

### Latissimus Dorsi Flap

- The latissimus dorsi flap is used when inadequate skin is available at the mastectomy site and/or if additional tissue is needed to fill the supraclavicular hollow and create an anterior axillary fold following a radical mastectomy.

### TRAM Flap

- During this procedure a low transverse ellipse incision is made and abdominal muscle and fat are tunneled under the abdominal skin to the mastectomy site.
- Possible complications are hernia at the donor site, which can be remedied by the placement of synthetic mesh, and flap necrosis, which may be largely avoided by careful selection of candidates.

### Free Flap

- This procedure entails removing a portion of the skin and fat from the buttocks or lower abdomen and grafting it to the mastectomy site with microvascular anastomoses.
- The main complication is failure to maintain sufficient perfusion in the postop period.

## Gluteus Maximus Free Flap

- If a TRAM flap is unavailable or inadequate in size, a portion of the buttock skin and muscle can be an alternative donor source.

## Nipple-Areolar Construction

- Tattooing is the primary method for creating the darker pigment of the areola. Another option is a skin graft from the inner thigh. However, grafts are uncomfortable and can fade, requiring tattooing.
- Complications that may occur are failure to maintain suitable projection of the nipple, graft failure, and fading of the pigmented areas.

## METASTATIC BREAST CANCER

- African-American and Hispanic women were more likely to present with advanced disease and more likely to have ER-negative tumors and a high S-phase fraction compared with whites. These under-served minorities require intensive community screening programs aimed at education and assurance of access to care.

## Routes of Metastasis

- The most common mode of metastasis is via the lymphatics, whereby the cells may be transported to local and more distant regional nodes.
- Breast cancer most commonly metastasizes to bone, specifically the spine, ribs, and proximal long bones. Patients will commonly complain of localized, deep-seated, unrelenting pain. Pathological fracture of the proximal femur may occur spontaneously despite efforts to protect the weakened bone. Likewise, persistent back pain may herald a compression fracture and possible neurological impairment.
- Loss of appetite and abnormal liver function tests are early symptoms of liver involvement. Late symptoms include pain, abdominal distention, nausea, emesis, periodic fever, jaundice, and generalized weakness. Pulmonary involvement may begin as a subtle, nonproductive cough or shortness of breath.
- Renal involvement generally presents as oliguria and/or uremia in a woman with deteriorating mental status. Brain metastasis usually occurs in the supratentorial region, multiple sites, or as carcinomatous meningitis presenting as cranial nerve palsies, altered mentation, seizures, and/or focal paresis. Local cancer spread to the chest wall usually presents as a painless subcutaneous nodule along the mastectomy scar and adjacent chest wall areas.
- The management of patients with metastatic breast cancer is aimed at judicious use of local and systemic measures that control and/or palliate symptoms and improve quality of life.
- It may be difficult for a woman with metastatic disease to understand why her doctor is not recommending more aggressive treatment.
- The answer is based on the desire not to make the woman more ill than her disease is making her and the knowledge that these therapies, including chemotherapy, have only a small effect on the median survival of women with metastatic disease.

## Defining Extent of Disease

### Chemotherapy

- Women who have a disease-free interval of less than two years, have hormone receptor negative disease, are refractory to hormone therapy, or have aggressive disease in the liver or pulmonary system are candidates for chemotherapy.

- The rate of complete response (percentage of individuals in whom all evidence of disease disappears) consistently has been only 10%–20% of cases.
- Although radiological evidence of bone healing may take as long as six months, subjective improvement occurs within a shorter time.

## Endocrine Therapy

- Women who have estrogen receptor positive breast cancer demonstrate a consistently superior survival after recurrence compared with women who are estrogen receptor negative.
- It is thought that if the source of estrogens is removed by surgical ablation or medication manipulation, or if the hormone's access to the estrogen-receptor protein is blocked by antiestrogens, the chain of action is broken and the tumor regresses.
- Receptor-negative disease is usually associated with a short disease-free interval and more aggressive disease. Receptor-positive tumors are generally associated with a long disease-free interval between initial treatment and recurrence.

### Antiestrogen therapy

- Tamoxifen is a synthetic antiestrogen and is the most widely used hormonal therapy.
- Women who respond initially to tamoxifen and subsequently become resistant are likely to respond to ovarian ablation.

### Estrogens

- At the initiation of therapy, nausea and occasional vomiting may occur for a few days.

### Androgens

- Androgens are most effective in women who are five or more years postmenopause.

### Progestins

- This drug is generally tolerated as well as tamoxifen and is comparable in efficacy, but it is usually used only after women have failed on tamoxifen.
- The most important side effect is weight gain, which occurs in up to 50% of patients.
- Other side effects include hot flashes, vaginal bleeding, hypercalcemia, tumor flare, and thrombophlebitis.

### Aromatase inhibitors

- An important option for treatment of women with advanced, estrogen-receptor positive breast cancer is through the reduction of circulating estradiol levels by inhibiting aromatization of adrenal androgens to estrogens.

## MALE BREAST CANCER

- The anatomic structures of the male breast are the same as those of the female breast. It is the hormonal stimulation present in the female breast and absent in the male breast that accounts for the development and physiological differences between the male and female breast.
- Various factors contributing to the development of male breast cancer include undescended testes, orchiectomy, orchitis, late puberty, infertility, obesity, hypercholesteremia, and estrogen use.
- Breast cancer occurs most frequently in men aged 50–70 years with the peak incidence occurring at 60 years of age.
- The majority of male breast cancers are known to be estrogen-receptor positive.

- They typically arise from ductal elements and present as infiltrating ductal carcinoma, which is commonly fixed to underlying fascia and skin. Nipple retraction and a bloody discharge may be present.
- The lungs and bony skeleton are the most common metastatic sites.
- Adjuvant radiotherapy, hormonal manipulation, and chemotherapy are the main methods of treatment.

## SYMPTOM MANAGEMENT AND SUPPORTIVE CARE

### Bone Metastasis

- Many individuals with breast cancer will, throughout the course of their illness, experience pain due to bony destruction by tumor.
- Pain at night and pain not relieved by rest are especially suspicious.
- A more sensitive method than radiography for detecting metastatic disease, a bone scan should be obtained in all individuals with symptoms suggesting skeletal involvement.
- CA 15-3, a human breast tumor-associated antigen is a sensitive marker in breast cancer metastases and may be used as a screening test for bone metastases.
- In addition to being painful, destructive lesions involving the femur or the humerus are highly susceptible to fracture.
- Treatment is aimed at relieving pain, preventing development of pathological fractures, enhancing mobility and function, and thereby improving survival.
- In individuals with widespread bone involvement, radiation is given to areas that are painful and disabling.
- The customary ways of repositioning patients in bed are contraindicated for the individual with disease in the clavicle.
- A pull sheet should be used to reposition the person with known disease in the hip, ribs, or vertebrae. At least two people are needed to reposition the patient properly so that correct body alignment is ensured.
- In the presence of significant osteoclastic activity and bone resorption due to dissolution of bone matrix, destruction of the microarchitecture of the bone leads to increased risk of fracture and hypercalcemia.
- Biphosphonates (etidronate, clodronate, pamidronate) result in stabilization of bone mineral which inhibits bone mineral dissolution.

### Epidural Spinal Cord Compression

- Spinal cord compression constitutes an emergency because of the potential for developing paraplegia.
- If the individual is found to have compression with an isolated extradural mass, radiotherapy combined with corticosteroids may produce optimal results and return of ambulation. The person is usually fitted with a brace or maintained on bed rest throughout the course of radiotherapy.
- The mean survival of patients with breast cancer who develop epidural spinal cord compression is 4–13 months posttreatment.

### Brain Metastasis and Leptomeningeal Carcinomatosis

- Brain metastasis occurs in about 30% of individuals diagnosed with breast cancer and is often associated with devastating physical and emotional problems. The most frequent signs and symptoms of intracranial metastasis are headaches, seizures, visual defects, motor weakness, and mental changes. Symptoms generally subside with total brain irradiation and chronic steroids.
- Most chemotherapeutic agents do not achieve a therapeutic concentration in the brain or cerebral spinal fluid (CSF).

## Chronic Lymphedema

- Lymphedema is most common in women who have had axillary dissection followed by radiation in excess of 46 Gy.
- Lymphedema occurs because of an increased resistance to venous flow and a disturbance in oncotic pressure that develops in the affected arm.
- Anything that increases blood flow to the affected arm contributes to the incidence and degree of lymphedema.
- For the individual who has massive edema without evidence of infection, a program of intermittent compression with an extremity pump may be necessary.

## PREGNANCY AND BREAST CANCER

### Pregnancy and the Woman with Curable Breast Cancer

- The most important considerations in the potential effect of pregnancy in a woman with a history of breast cancer are whether or not the hormonal changes from pregnancy might stimulate growth of occult disease, the risk for genetic alterations in offspring, the woman's overall risk for recurrent breast cancer, and the risk of a second primary breast cancer.

### Pregnancy and Breast Cancer as a Simultaneous Event

- The prognosis of women diagnosed with breast cancer during pregnancy has generally been poor, not necessarily because of excessive estrogen stimulation but because pregnancy-associated breast cancer is more often diagnosed at a more advanced stage.
- The treatment of breast cancer in this population of women is determined by the extent of the disease present and the term of pregnancy or lactation.
- Radiation therapy is not recommended because of potential hazards to the fetus. Chemotherapy, if indicated, should not be administered during the first trimester, but can be more safely used in the second and third.
- A more advanced disease stage needs effective, urgent palliation and may indicate the need for termination of an early pregnancy to promptly begin treatment for the breast cancer.

## CONTINUITY OF CARE

### Support Systems

- Women with breast cancer may find a need for different support systems as they maneuver through the different phases of their diagnosis, treatment, and survival.
- Support groups are recognized as valuable sources of hope, encouragement, and education for the individual with breast cancer as well as other chronic diseases.
- Another recent advance in information and support exists through on-line Web pages.

## PRACTICE QUESTIONS

1.  Jeanne is 34 years old and has just been diagnosed with ER(+) stage I breast cancer with a 1.5 cm tumor. She is being treated with cytoxan, methotrexate, and 5-fluorouracil. Understandably, she is distressed over many aspects of the treatment, and you are trying to help her adjust. During her first week of therapy, she describes vividly how one of her aunts, who also had breast cancer, lost all of her hair during chemotherapy. She wants to know if this will happen to her as well. You tell her that:
    a.  she will not lose significant amounts of hair.
    b.  she may experience gradual thinning.
    c.  she may lose all of her hair in 2 to 3 weeks.
    d.  her hair will not start growing back for 6 months following the end of therapy.

2.  When telling Jeanne about cytoxan, methotextrate, and 5-fluorouracil you are careful to give her instructions regarding which of the following potential side effects?
    a.  severe thrombocytopenia and bleeding
    b.  symptoms of bladder infection as early signs of hemorrhagic cystitis
    c.  transient peripheral neuropathies
    d.  all of the above

3.  Which of the following statements regarding the incidence of breast cancer is/are true?
    a.  70% of breast cancer occurs in women who are 50 years of age or older.
    b.  The incidence of breast cancer has increased, but the mortality rate—especially among African-Americans and Hispanics—has decreased.
    c.  The incidence of breast cancer is approximately 1 in every 4 women.
    d.  The incidence of breast cancer has increased to epidemic proportions among premenopausal women.

4.  When your patient begins radiation treatments after her lumpectomy, she notices redness and tenderness over her breast. Her breast also itches, and the skin is scaly and dry. She comes to you when her breast has become very tender and expresses concern. You tell her that:
    a.  some patients have these reactions to the radiation treatments. If the symptoms persist, she will need to take a few days off from radiation.
    b.  she should rub the skin with baby oil just prior to her radiation treatments.
    c.  all patients have reactions to the radiation treatments. It's nothing to worry about.
    d.  her radiation dosage is obviously too high and she needs to see the radiation oncologist.

5.  Which of the following statements best describes the significance of the *BRCA1* gene?
    a.  It is an inherited gene that identifies women who are assured of having breast cancer during their premenopausal years.
    b.  It is an inherited gene mutation that identifies families at significant risk for breast cancer and ovarian cancer.
    c.  It is an inherited gene mutation that identifies women likely to have breast cancer in their postmenopausal years.
    d.  It is an inherited gene that is present in over 90% of women with breast cancer.

6.  You are holding a seminar to educate a group of women about breast cancer. Which of the following should you *not* list as a known risk factor?
    a.  early menarche
    b.  early menopause
    c.  gender
    d.  prolonged, uninterrupted contraceptive use

7. In your seminar, when you explain the proper technique for BSE, you should *not* include which of the following instructions?
   a. For the visual inspection, note symmetry, size and shape of the breasts.
   b. Examine yourself in front of the mirror with your arms relaxed at your sides.
   c. Examine yourself in front of the mirror with your hands pressed on your hips.
   d. Examine yourself in front of the mirror with your arms folded behind your back.

8. Which of the following statements regarding the *BRCA2* gene is/are true?
   a. This gene mutation is associated with postmenopausal breast cancer.
   b. This gene is related with breast cancer in men.
   c. This gene is associated with early-onset female breast cancer.
   d. b and c.

9. The best explanation as to why mammograms are *not* recommended for women under 35 is which of the following?
   a. There is little risk of breast cancer for women under 35.
   b. Younger women have firmer breasts, which are harder to examine becaue of the high fat content.
   c. Younger women have denser breasts, which are harder to image.
   d. There is increased risk of radiation damage in women under 35.

10. Mrs. Johns is pregnant and discovers a mass in the upper, outer quadrant of her left breast. Following her physical exam, the physician is most likely to order which of the following test(s)?
    a. ultrasound
    b. fine-needle aspiration
    c. mammogram (diagnostic)
    d. a or b

11. Anita has heard about prophylactic mastectomy and has been considering it for herself; however, she would like to better understand the procedure. Which of the following would you *not* tell her?
    a. In this procedure, the entire breast, tail of Spence, and nipple areola complex are removed.
    b. This procedure prevents development of breast cancer.
    c. Breast reconstruction is possible after such a procedure, using implants or a variety of surgical methods.
    d. Prophylactic mastectomy is an extreme measure, not usually considered unless a woman is at extremely high risk for breast cancer.

12. The majority of breast cancers are adenocarcinomas in the _____ quadrant.
    a. upper, outer
    b. upper, inner
    c. lower, outer
    d. lower, inner

13. All of the following are common metastatic sites for breast cancer *except* the:
    a. brain
    b. liver
    c. bone
    d. gastrointestinal tract

14. What kind of edge do you expect a benign mass to have on a mammogram?
    a. spiculated
    b. defined
    c. distorted
    d. microcalcified

15. Marcia, a patient of yours, will be commencing chemotherapy in two weeks. She asks you to explain to her the risks and side effects of chemotherapy. You tell her all of the following *except*:
    a. Chemotherapy can cause ovarian failure.
    b. Irregular menses are a common side effect.
    c. Sexual dysfunction is normal.
    d. Hot flashes and night sweats are to be expected.

16. Because of the staging of her cancer, the size of the tumor, and a number of other factors, Marcia is going to be able to undergo immediate breast reconstruction after her surgery. Her surgeon has explained that the procedure most likely to be used in her case is the TRAM flap. You explain to Marcia that this will involve removing tissue from her _____ and tunneling it to the mastectomy site.
    a. abdominal muscle
    b. latissimus dorsi muscle
    c. lower abdomen
    d. buttocks

17. Which of the following would *not* be considered to be a primary prognostic indicator in breast cancer?
    a. number of positive axillary lymph nodes
    b. size of the primary tumor
    c. Her-2/*neu* oncogene
    d. estrogen receptor positivity

18. Determining hormone receptor status is important in breast cancer because:
    a. it helps determine the menopausal status of the woman.
    b. it helps determine the cause of the cancer.
    c. it helps predict which patients will respond to hormone manipulation.
    d. it helps predict prognosis.

19. Carry asks you to explain the relationship between tumor size, node involvement, and prognosis to her. Which of the following statements is most accurate?
    a. Smaller tumors with positive node involvement have the best prognosis.
    b. Larger tumors with negative node involvement have the best prognosis.
    c. Smaller tumors with negative node involvement have the worst prognosis.
    d. Larger tumors with positive node involvement have the worst prognosis.

20. Carry is scheduled to undergo a biopsy procedure to assist in locating a nonpalpable lesion in her unaffected breast for excisional biopsy. Which of the following procedures would you expect to have to explain to her?
    a. Fine-needle aspiration
    b. Stereotactic needle-guided biopsy
    c. Wire localization
    d. Open biopsy

21. Carry is placed on tamoxifen to help control her advanced disease. She is confused by this because she is only 43 and has not yet gone through menopause. You reassure her and tell her all of the following about tamoxifen *except*:
    a. tamoxifen is also effective in premenopausal women.
    b. tamoxifen might cause irregular menses.
    c. tamoxifen may cause ovarian failure.
    d. hot flashes and vaginal discharge are common side effects of tamoxifen.

22. One of your patients, Matt, is shocked to discover that he has breast cancer. He did not think that men could develop the disease. When he asks you what risk factors men usually have, you tell Matt all of the following are risk factors *except*:
    a. undescended testes.
    b. infertility.
    c. homosexual behavior.
    d. obesity.

23. When you tell Matt that his breast cancer is estrogen receptor positive, he is confused by what you mean. Which of the following would you *not* tell Matt to clarify what the implications of ER(+) breast cancer are?
    a. ER(+) breast cancers tend to have a long disease-free interval.
    b. ER(+) breast cancers tend to be less aggressive than ER(–) breast cancers.
    c. Most men have ER(–) breast cancers.
    d. Men with ER(+) tumors are likely to undergo hormone therapy.

24. Mrs. Harris, age 41, has a 2.5 cm tumor and no positive lymph nodes. She is having a lumpectomy and radiation therapy. Her oncologist is recommending adjuvant chemotherapy. What is the best explanation for this additional treatment?
    a. In women under 50 years of age, adjuvant chemotherapy reduces risk of recurrence by approximately 27%.
    b. Lumpectomy is insufficient to prevent metastatic spread.
    c. Because of the size of the tumor, chemotherapy is essential.
    d. Adjuvant chemotherapy is not necessary in this case.

25. Mrs. Ellis has stage II breast cancer and is receiving adjuvant adriamycin and cytoxan. She has no symptoms of bone involvement but asks that a bone scan and a Ca 15-3 tumor marker be done. The most appropriate response would be which of the following?
    a. A bone scan would not be useful since Mrs. Ellis has no symptoms.
    b. Ca 15-3 is used to monitor metastatic disease, not as an early detection test.
    c. Both tests should have been done prior to surgery.
    d. a and b.

## ANSWER EXPLANATIONS

1. **The answer is b.** Cytoxan and methotrexate, the drugs which are commonly used in curable breast cancer, generally cause gradual thinning of hair. (p. 956)

2. **The answer is b.** Side effects associated with CMF include myelosuppression, hair loss, and hemorrhagic cystitis. (p. 957)

3. **The answer is a.** 70% of breast cancer occurs in women who are 50 years of age or older. (p. 917)

4.  **The answer is a.** All patients have some skin reactions to radiation treatments. The fact that the skin is reddened is normal; however, the fact that it is painful means she needs a break. (p. 956)

5.  **The answer is b.** Inheritance of the *BRCA1* susceptibility gene is associated with a strong likelihood that the effect of the mutation will result in the disease for families with multiple breast and ovarian cancers (90%) as well as those with breast cancers diagnosed before the age of 45 (70%). (p. 921)

6.  **The answer is b.** Early menopause is not a known risk factor for breast cancer. Early menarche; late menopause; early and prolonged, uninterrupted contraceptive use; and gender are all known risk factors. (p. 919)

7.  **The answer is d.** In a proper BSE, the woman should stand in front of the mirror, noting the size, shape, and symmetry of her breasts. She should examine herself with her arms relaxed at her side, with her hands pressed on her hips, and with her arms overhead, but not with her arms folded behind her. (p. 927)

8.  **The answer is d.** *BRCA2* has been identified on the long arm of chromosome 13 (13q12-13). This mutation seems to be associated with male breast cancer and early-onset female breast cancer. (p. 921)

9.  **The answer is c.** Younger women have denser breast tissue, which is harder to image properly. Mammograms tend to appear white and contain very little contrast. (p. 927)

10. **The answer is d.** Sonography is the imaging modality of choice in a young woman, a pregnant woman, or a lactating woman who has not discovered any lumps or other signs of cancer. FNA would also be appropriate. (pp. 936–937)

11. **The answer is b.** It is not true that a prophylactic mastectomy will prevent the development of breast cancer. Breast cancer can still develop in the chest wall or axillary region. (p. 925)

12. **The answer is a.** The majority of breast cancers are adenocarcinomas in the upper, outer quadrant of the breast. (p. 931)

13. **The answer is d.** Breast cancer primarily metastasizes to the bone, liver, lungs, nodes, and brain—not the gastrointestinal system. (p. 932)

14. **The answer is b.** Benign masses have defined edges on mammograms, whereas malignancies usually have a spiculated, distorted or calcified appearance. (pp. 934–935)

15. **The answer is c.** Sexual dysfunction is not a normal side effect of chemotherapy. Although it is not uncommon in conjunction with breast cancer and surgery, and it is more prevalent among younger women, sexual dysfunction can be handled, usually through therapy or a support group. The rest of these—ovarian failure, hot flashes, night sweats and irregular menses—are common side effects of chemotherapy. (p. 955)

16. **The answer is a.** The TRAM flap procedure is sometimes known as the "tummy tuck" because the muscle and fat are tunneled from the abdominal muscle to the mastectomy site. (p. 958)

17. **The answer is c.** Her-2/*neu* is not a primary independent prognostic indicator. The others are. (p. 940)

18. **The answer is c.** It helps predict who will respond to hormone manipulation. (p. 941)

19. **The answer is d.** The larger the tumor and the more positive nodes involved, the worse the prognosis is. (p. 940)

20. **The answer is c.** Wire localization is a procedure to assist in locating nonpalpable lesions for excisional biopsy. (p. 938)

21. **The answer is c.** Tamoxifen might cause irregular menses, hot flashes and vaginal discharge, and it has proven to be effective in premenopausal women; however, tamoxifen does not cause ovarian failure. (p. 924)

22. **The answer is c.** Homosexual behavior is not a risk factor for breast cancer in men. Undescended testes, orchiectomy, orchitis, late puberty, infertility, obesity and estrogen use are risk factors. (p. 967)

23. **The answer is c.** ER(+) breast cancer is associated with longer disease-free intervals and less aggressive disease. It is often treated with hormone therapy. Most men have ER(+) breast cancer. (pp. 964–967)

24. **The answer is a.** In women under 50 years of age, adjuvant chemotherapy reduces risk of recurrence by approximately 27%. (p. 948)

25. **The answer is d.** Since Mrs. Ellis displays no symptoms of bone involvement, a bone scan would not be appropriate. Ca 15-3 is used to monitor metastatic disease, not as an early detection test. (pp. 967–968)

# Chapter 35    Central Nervous System Cancers

## EPIDEMIOLOGY

- Primary CNS cancers represent 2% of all reported malignancies.
- The incidence is slightly higher in men than in women with the exception of meningiomas, which occur more often in women. CNS cancers are the second most common cancer diagnosed in children, second only to leukemia.
- The most prevalent CNS malignancy is the metastatic brain tumor, which is increasing in frequency.
- The most common primary brain tumor is the malignant glioma, accounting for more than half of all primary CNS cancers.

## ETIOLOGY

### Genetic Factors

- Approximately 5% of CNS tumors are associated with a specific genetic disorder. For example, neurofibromatosis type 1 is associated with astrocytomas. Neurofibromatosis type 2 is associated with an increased incidence of cranial and spinal nerve root tumors.

### Chemical and Environmental Factors

- Agricultural workers exposed to multiple chemicals in pesticides herbicides and ferlilizers have a higher incidence of gliomas.

### Viral Factors

- Individuals with AIDS-related primary central nervous system lymphoma (PCNSL) have been found to have a high rate of infection with the Epstein-Barr virus (EBV), and evidence of EBV has been isolated from the tumor tissue. Individuals with AIDS have an increased risk for developing PCNSL and possibly gliomas.

### Radiation

- Therapeutic irradiation of the head has been linked to the subsequent appearance of CNS tumors.
- An increased incidence of both primary and metastatic tumors, including PCNSL, has been found following immunosuppressive therapy.

## PREVENTION, SCREENING, EARLY DETECTION PROGRAMS

- No prevention, screening, or early detection programs exist for CNS cancers. However, individuals with specific hereditary syndromes that may predispose them to CNS tumors may be informed of their genetic risks.

## PATHOPHYSIOLOGY

### Anatomy and Physiology

- Anatomy and physiology of the brain and spinal cord are outlined on pages 982–988.

- Six types of glial cells are in the nervous system: astrocytes, oligodendrocytes, ependymal cells, Schwann cells, microglia, and satellite cells. These cells can undergo anaplasia and are the major source of primary tumors of the CNS.

## Physiology of intracranial pressure

- Intracranial pressure (ICP) is the pressure exerted within the skull and meninges by brain tissue, CSF, and cerebral blood volume. If any one component increases in volume, a concomitant decrease in the volume of one or both of the remaining components must occur to maintain normal ICP.
- The mechanism by which this secondary decrease in volume occurs is called *compensation.*
  - The individual with the slow-growing tumor may not exhibit clinical signs and symptoms until the compensatory mechanisms have been exhausted.
- Another important concept relating to ICP is *autoregulation.* Autoregulation maintains a normal ICP despite fluctuations in arterial pressure and venous drainage.
- Any condition that obstructs or compromises the venous outflow may also increase cerebral blood volume because more blood is backed up in the intracranial cavity.

# Gliomas

- Gliomas are the most common primary brain tumor in adults and include the astrocytomas, oligodendrogliomas, ependymomas, and mixed gliomas.

## Astrocytomas

- The majority of gliomas are astrocytomas.
- Astrocytomas generally arise in the cerebral hemispheres.
- Grade is based on the tumor's microscopic appearance and indicates its similarity to normal cells, its tendency to spread, and its growth rate.
  - Low-grade astrocytomas are most common in individuals between 20 and 40 years of age, anaplastic astrocytomas in individuals who are between 30 and 50, and GBM, the most malignant glioma, in those who are 50 or older.
  - Low-grade astrocytomas show an increased cellularity and have mild nuclear pleomorphism compared with normal brain tissue.
  - The high-grade gliomas are anaplastic astrocytoma and GBM. The histological features of the anaplastic astrocytoma are similar to the low-grade astrocytomas but are more abundant and exaggerated.
    - The GBM has these characteristics plus necrosis.
    - Anaplastic astrocytomas account for less than one-third of the gliomas, whereas the GBM is the most common adult primary brain tumor and represents more than 50% of the gliomas.
    - Individuals with anaplastic astrocytoma have a significantly better prognosis than those with glioblastomas.

## Oligodendrogliomas

- Oligodendrogliomas arise from the oligodendrocyte cell responsible for the development and maintenance of the myelin sheath. About 50% of these tumors contain oligodendrocytes, astrocytes, and ependymal cells and are referred to as *mixed gliomas.*
- Approximately 50% of oligodendrogliomas have calcifications within the tumor and adjacent brain tissue, and up to 20% are cystic.

- Like astrocytomas, oligodendrogliomas vary in malignancy. Pure oligodendrogliomas are relatively low-grade and well-differentiated.
- They tend to be slow-growing and are often present for many years before diagnosis.
- Two features separate the oligodendrogliomas from the astrocytomas: the antecedent history, averaging seven to eight years, tends to be longer, and seizures are more common, occurring in 70%–90% of patients by the time of diagnosis.
- The standard treatments for oligodendrogliomas have been surgery—when a good neurological outcome is possible—and RT.
- The PCV (procarbazine, CCNU, vincristine) regimen is particularly effective.

## Ependymomas

- Ependymomas represent less than 5% of all adult primary brain tumors and 9% of the gliomas. They occur in all age-groups but are most often seen in young adults and children. Ependymomas arise from these ependymal cells, which form the lining of the ventricles and the central canal of the spinal cord.
- Ependymomas may be differentiated as low-grade or anaplastic and high-grade.
- High-grade and infratentorial tumors are more likely to spread through the CSF pathways.
- Standard treatment of ependymomas is surgery and RT.
- Low-grade tumors are treated with local RT unless there is evidence of disseminated disease, which requires full craniospinal radiation.
- Malignant ependymomas are generally treated with craniospinal radiation.
- Chemotherapy is used primarily for recurrent ependymomas.

## Meningiomas

- Meningiomas, the most common benign brain tumors, account for up to 20% of all adult intracranial tumors.
- Meningiomas occur twice as often in women as in men and tend to occur late in life, with a peak incidence in the sixth decade for men and the seventh decade for women. The incidence of meningiomas is also higher in individuals with breast cancer.
- Malignant meningiomas account for 12% of all meningiomas and occur more often in men.
- Meningiomas produce symptoms by compression of surrounding brain tissue rather than by infiltration. Individuals may present with seizures, headache, increased ICP, focal neurological deficits such as altered mentation and hemiparesis, and cranial neuropathies.
- The primary treatment modality for meningiomas is surgery, with the extent of surgical resection the primary factor influencing the recurrence rate.
- Chemotherapy for malignant meningiomas has been generally unsuccessful.

## Vestibular Schwannomas (Acoustic Neuromas)

- Vestibular schwannomas, traditionally called *acoustic neuromas*, are benign tumors arising from the Schwann cells at the vestibular portion of the eighth cranial nerve.
- These are very slow-growing tumors whose symptoms are related to compression and stretching of cranial nerves, causing interference with their function.
- Surgery and radiosurgery are the primary treatment modalities for most individuals with vestibular schwannomas.

## Primary Central Nervous System Lymphomas

- PCNSL is an aggressive non-Hodgkin's lymphoma that arises within and is confined to the CNS.

- PCNSL has been a rare tumor; however, it is increasing in both immunocompetent and immunosuppressed individuals.
- PCNSL is almost always disseminated within the CNS.
- Ninety-five percent of patients diagnosed with PCNSL have a brain lesion, and 50% of these lesions are multifocal.
- The eyes are a direct extension of the nervous system and are involved in up to 20% of patients at diagnosis. Lymphoma may begin in the eye only. Eventually more than one-half of these patients will go on to develop brain lymphoma.
- Most PCNSLs involve the frontal lobes. Common symptoms include the following: lethargy, confusion; apathy, flat affect; headache, nausea, vomiting; hemiparesis or hemiplegia; visual disturbances; seizures (rarely).

## Metastatic Brain Tumors

- The incidence of metastatic brain tumors is increasing as patients are living longer with the cancer.
- Brain metastases occur at three sites: the brain parenchyma itself, the skull and dura, and the leptomeninges. Parenchymal brain metastases occur in more than 60% of these cases.
- The lung is the most common site of origin. If the primary tumor is not pulmonary, it may have metastasized to the lungs before reaching the brain.
- Other cancers that commonly metastasize to the brain include breast cancer, melanoma, colon cancer, and renal cancer.
- Melanoma has the highest propensity of all systemic cancers to metastasize to the brain.
- Most brain metastases occur in the cerebral hemispheres. Symptoms include signs of increased ICP (headache, nausea, vomiting), change in level of consciousness, diminished cognitive function, personality changes, hemiparesis, language problems, and seizures.
- With early diagnosis and management, brain metastases often respond to therapy. Most patients benefit from palliative treatment; an increasing number of patients experience a prolonged remission or, rarely, are cured of their cerebral disease.
- For many years WBRT has been the standard treatment for both single and multiple brain metastases.
- Tumors that metastasize to the bone, particularly metastatic tumors of the breast, prostate, and lung, may infiltrate the skull or dura by direct extension.
  - Treatment may be RT or surgical resection.
- Leptomeningeal metastasis, or meningeal carcinomatosis, is a diffuse or multifocal seeding of cancer cells throughout the meninges and CSF. The seeding pattern of growth covers the surface of the brain and spinal cord.
- The most common cancers leading to meningeal carcinomatosis are leukemia, lymphoma, melanoma, and breast, lung, and gastrointestinal (GI) cancers.
  - Treatment includes RT to symptomatic areas only, because radiation to the entire neuroaxis leads to bone marrow depression. This is followed by chemotherapy administered directly into the CSF.

## Spinal Cord Tumors

- Primary spinal cord tumors occur less frequently than primary brain tumors, accounting for only 15% of all primary CNS tumors. They occur most often in individuals between 20 and 60 years of age, and with the exception of meningiomas, which occur more often in women, spinal cord tumors are found with equal frequency in men and women.
- Spinal tumors are classified by their cell of origin and their anatomic location.
- The classification and frequency of spinal cord tumors are found in Table 35-3, text page 995.
- The neurological symptoms seen with extradural tumors result from compression rather than invasion of the spinal cord.

- Spinal cord compression (SCC) occurs either by direct extension of the tumor into the epidural space, by vertebral collapse and displacement of bone into the epidural space, or by direct extension through the intervertebral foramina.
- The thoracic spine is the most frequent location of epidural SCC, followed by the lumbosacral and cervical spine.
- Epidural SCC is a relatively common neurological complication of cancer.
- Schwannomas are the most common extramedullary tumor, followed by meningiomas. They account for most of these tumors, and both types occur most commonly in the thoracic spine.

## Pattern of Spread

- While these tumors may spread to other parts of the CNS, metastases outside the brain and spinal cord are rare.
- Most metastatic brain tumors develop from hematogenous spread of tumor cells, usually through the arterial circulation.

## CLINICAL MANIFESTATIONS
## Brain Tumors

- Clinical manifestations can be divided into three major categories: generalized effects of increased ICP, focal effects, and effects caused by displacement of brain structures.

### Generalized effects of increased ICP

- Brain tumors increase ICP by their size, cerebral edema, or obstruction of CSF pathways.
- After the brain's normal compensatory mechanisms have been exhausted, the increased ICP results in a decreased cerebral blood flow.
- The signs and symptoms of increased ICP include change in the level of consciousness or cognition, headache, pupillary changes and papilledema, motor and sensory deficits, vomiting, and changes in vital signs. Increased ICP may cause additional effects by displacing brain tissue.
- Sleeping more is the most commonly reported early sign of the tumor.
- The headache is usually bilateral in the frontal, temporal, or retro-orbital areas.
- Vomiting as a sign of increased ICP occurs more commonly in children and in individuals with infratentorial tumors.
- Changes in vital signs occur late in the course of increased ICP.

### Focal effects

- Frontal lobe tumors are associated with inability to concentrate, inattentiveness, impaired memory, personality changes, and emotional lability. Damage to Broca's area results in an inability to express oneself in words (expressive aphasia).
- Parietal lobe tumors affect sensory and perceptual functions more than motor function. Symptoms include impaired sensation, paresthesias, inability to recognize an object's shape or size by feeling it, and inability to calculate number.
- Tumors of the temporal lobe can cause impairment of recent memory, aggressive behavior, and psychomotor seizures.
- Involvement of the dominant side can lead to an inability to recall names (dysnomia), impaired perception of verbal commands, and Wernicke's or receptive aphasia.
- Occipital lobe tumors produce visual symptoms.
- Tumors located in or near the thalamus can lead to hydrocephalus, mild sensory disturbances or paresthesias and neuropathic pain, emotional lability, and sleep pattern disturbances. Hypothalamic tumors typically lead to endocrine dysfunction.

- Tumors in the cerebellum present as a wide-based ataxic gait, dysarthric speech, clumsiness, early morning headache, and vomiting.
- Brain stem tumors can produce dire consequences, since the centers that control respiration and heart rate are located here.
- Seizures, another common clinical manifestation in both primary and metastatic brain tumors, are seen primarily with supratentorial tumors.

### Displacement of brain structure

- A growing tumor mass and the associated edema cause pressure to increase within the cranial compartment. Initially the brain's compensatory mechanisms attempt to accommodate the pressure.
- Once these mechanisms are exhausted, the increased pressure can cause *herniation*.
- There are two major classifications of herniation: *supratentorial* and *infratentorial*.
  - Supratentorial tumors, located above the tentorium cerebelli, can lead to cingulate, uncal, or central transtentorial herniation.
    - Uncal herniation, usually occurring with expanding temporal lobe tumors, forces the medial portion of the temporal lobe (the uncus) into the tentorial notch.
    - *Kernohan's notch* causes a hemiparesis that is ipsilateral to the side of the lesion (and to the third cranial nerve palsy). This is a false localizing sign that may lead to confusion in determining the location of the lesion.
    - Central or transtentorial herniation results from the downward displacement of the cerebral hemispheres forcing brain contents through the tentorial notch.
    - Both central and uncal herniations cause changes in the respiratory pattern.
    - The classic vital sign changes of Cushing's triad are seen during the terminal phase of herniation.
  - Infratentorial herniation cause displacement of the cerebellum either upward through the opening in the tentorium or downward through the foramen magnum. (See Figure 35-15, text page 1000.)
  - In upward transtentorial herniation, the cerebellum compresses the midbrain. The individual may lose consciousness immediately.
    - Downward cerebellar tonsillar herniation is more common and results in the downward protrusion of the cerebellar tonsils through the foramen magnum.
    - In both types of infratentorial herniation, respiratory arrest, cardiac arrest, or both will occur if untreated.

## Spinal Cord Tumors

- The clinical manifestations associated with spinal cord tumors result from compression and, much less frequently, invasion of the spinal cord.
- A slow-growing tumor better allows the cord to accommodate the mass. Tumors can be present for years without causing significant neurological deficits. On the other hand, the spinal cord cannot accommodate a sudden mass or rapidly growing lesion.
- Pain is the most common presenting symptom of a spinal cord tumor.
- Often the pain is initially dismissed as arthritis, back strain, or disk disease.
- The pain may be localized or radicular. Localized pain and tenderness are common over the involved area. Radicular pain may be described as bandlike and follows the distribution of the spinal nerve roots (dermatomes).
- Weakness is the most readily identified objective finding and may follow the appearance of sensory symptoms.
- Specific sensory deficits will depend on where the tumor is on a cross section of the spinal cord.
  - A lateral lesion will affect pain and temperature.
  - A posterior lesion will affect awareness of vibration and proprioception.

- Anterior tumors lead to weakness and an ataxic gait. Compression affects function below the lesion.
- The effects may be symmetrical and bilateral, asymmetrical, and even unilateral.

## ASSESSMENT

- In most instances the first, earliest, and most sensitive indicator of dysfunction will be a change in the level of consciousness.
- Mental status and cognitive ability as well as motor and sensory function are also evaluated.
- Assessment of cerebellar function focuses on the ability to coordinate movement and to maintain normal muscle tone and equilibrium.
- Testing of cranial nerve function can be the most intimidating portion of the neurological assessment. The 12 pairs of cranial nerves, their function, method of testing, and desired response are listed in Table 35-4 on text page 1006.

### Diagnostic Studies

- CT is the usual preliminary study in an individual with signs and symptoms suggesting a brain tumor.
- Noncontrast CT is necessary to determine the presence of calcium or hemorrhage. Contrast is then administered to delineate the margins and extent of blood-brain barrier disruption.
- MRI is the more definitive and preferred imaging study for the individual with a CNS tumor.
- MRI can detect CT-occult tumors. An MRI may be positive when the CT is negative; this may sometimes be seen with low-grade tumors and PCNSL lesions.
- Cerebral angiography may be used to confirm that the lesion in question is a vascular malformation or an aneurysm rather than a neoplasm.
- If a lumbar puncture is indicated, it should be performed after neuroimaging studies such as MRI and CT scan, especially in an individual with a suspected tumor, because of the risk of herniation.
  - PET may also be used in individuals with brain tumors, specifically malignant gliomas.
  - Individuals having PET scans using the glucose analogue FDG should not receive dextrose intravenous solutions and should not eat for several hours prior to the test because glucose metabolism is being measured.
- SPECT is used for the imaging of functional neuroanatomy.
  - This technique has also been shown to be effective in distinguishing the presence of infiltrating tumor from solid tumor.
  - SPECT has also proved effective in differentiating lymphoma from toxoplasmosis in AIDS patients, which may lead to earlier diagnosis and treatment.
  - SPECT is used only to complement the information obtained by CT scanning or MRI, as is PET, and is not used in the initial diagnosis of brain tumors.
- CT myelography has been the standard method for identifying the location and level of spinal cord and nerve root compromise resulting from spinal tumors.
- MRI is replacing myelography as the diagnostic procedure of choice for the evaluation of both intramedullary and extramedullary spinal cord tumors.

### Prognostic Indicators

- Generally, the prognosis for a malignant brain glioma, the most common adult CNS tumor, is dismal. However, young age, lower histological grade, and high performance status are favorable prognostic indicators for astrocytomas.
- The extent of surgical resection is another important prognostic factor. There is an increase in survival for those individuals who have a complete surgical resection compared with those who have a partial resection.
- The prognosis is far better for intradural spinal cord tumors than for extradural.

- Rapid onset and quick progression are worse prognostic factors for recovery.
- Brain metastases are generally associated with a poor prognosis.

## CLASSIFICATION AND STAGING

- The World Health Organization (WHO) classification of CNS tumors first characterizes a tumor histologically by its cell of origin and then designates a grade based on its similarity to normal cells.
  - Grading assesses the degree of malignancy or aggressiveness of the tumor cells by comparing the cellular anaplasia, differentiation, and mitotic activity with normal counterparts. Tumor classification has clinical implications, dictates the choice of therapy, and predicts prognosis.
- The WHO classification of CNS tumors is found in Table 35-5, text page 1013.
- The TNM staging system classifies solid tumors by the anatomic extent of disease and evaluates the extent of the primary *tumor*, regional *lymph nodes*, and *metastases*.
- The TNM classification of brain tumors is found in Table 35-6, text page 1014.
- The highest or most malignant grade of cell found during microscopic examination determines the tumor grade, even if most of the tumor is a lower grade. Low-grade tumors can also transform and become more anaplastic over time.
- The distinction between benign and malignant tumors can be misleading when discussing classification of CNS tumors. The term *benign* suggests that a cure is possible, whereas *malignant* implies a poor prognosis. Histological features alone do not determine malignancy in the CNS.

## THERAPEUTIC APPROACHES AND NURSING CARE

### Brain Tumors

#### Surgery

- Surgery remains the initial treatment for the majority of individuals with brain tumors.
- When evaluating an individual for surgery, many factors must be considered: size and location of the tumor, relationship of the tumor to functional brain regions, presence of widespread or multiple sites of disease, and the individual's age and neurological status.
- A biopsy removes sufficient tissue to establish a histological diagnosis.
  - A stereotactic biopsy is the most precise means of obtaining a tissue sample and is the most widely used method today.
  - There are indications for a brain biopsy alone in some individuals: when the diagnosis is uncertain, the individual is unable to undergo craniotomy, the lesion involves deep brain structures, multiple lesions are present, there is a question of radiation necrosis versus tumor recurrence, or suspected tumor progression must be histologically verified.
  - Stereotactic procedures can also be used to remove tumors.
- The aim of brain tumor surgery is to remove the tumor completely and ultimately provide a cure.
- Reduction of tumor bulk or partial resection during a craniotomy decompresses the brain and becomes the next goal.
- Functional mapping of the brain, a type of intraoperative monitoring, can facilitate a more complete tumor resection, with decreased morbidity in some patients.
- A stereotactic surgical procedure may be used to place radioactive sources within the tumor. Chemotherapy wafers may be implanted surgically within a tumor to slowly and continuously release chemotherapy directly into the brain. Ommaya reservoirs may be placed to deliver chemotherapy directly into the CSF.
- Nursing interventions for patients undergoing neurosurgical procedures begin preoperatively.
- Neurological assessment is conducted on an ongoing basis.
- Postoperative cerebral edema results from the surgical manipulation of the surrounding brain tissue, changes in regional blood flow, or brain injury caused by excessive retraction.

- The effects of osmotic diuretic therapy on ICP are best evaluated by the use of an intracranial pressure monitor.
  - The signs and symptoms of cerebral edema may be similar to those of intracranial bleeding: decreased level of consciousness, progressive focal neurological deficit, increased ICP, seizures, and possible herniation.
- Venous thromboembolism is a particular concern in neurosurgery patients because of the length of surgery, immobility of some postoperative patients, and tumor-related hypercoagulable states.

### Radiation therapy

- Radiation therapy plays a central role in the treatment of malignant gliomas: low-grade gliomas; inoperable, partially resected, or recurrent benign brain tumors; and metastatic brain tumors.
- In tumors that cannot be completely excised or that recur despite aggressive resection, RT is an important adjuvant therapy.
- Malignant gliomas are radioresistant.
- In hyperfractionation two or more treatments are administered daily using fraction sizes that are smaller than conventional dose fractions to increase the total dose given over the same period of time.
- Brachytherapy involves the temporary implantation of radioactive sources directly into the brain tumor.
  - The major complication of both brachytherapy and radiosurgery is the development of symptomatic radiation necrosis requiring prolonged administration of steroids and reoperation.
  - Radiosurgery can be used for lesions that may be unsuitable for brachytherapy because of their location.
- Stereotactic radiotherapy (SRT) uses the planning technology of stereotactic radiosurgery but delivers the treatment using standard fractionation doses.
  - This approach is being used for some benign tumors and gliomas.
- Three-dimensional conformal radiation therapy (3D-CRT) not only decreases the risk of normal tissue injury but may also allow higher than traditional doses to be safely administered to patients with malignant gliomas.
- Hyperthermia has an additive effect when combined with RT.
- Particle therapy refers to the use of subatomic particles rather than photons as a form of radiation.
- In BNCT a boron compound is administered systemically and is only a focal therapy at present.
- Side effects of RT can be classified as acute reactions, early delayed reactions, and late delayed reactions.
  - The acute reactions occur during the course of treatment and are temporary.
  - The early delayed reactions generally develop one to three months after completion of therapy. These, too, are of a temporary nature.
  - Late effects of RT usually occur 6–24 months after completion of treatment. These effects are irreversible and often progressive.

### Chemotherapy

- Many factors affect the responsiveness of brain tumors to chemotherapy. These include tumor histology, tumor blood flow, the presence of inherent and acquired mechanisms of drug resistance, and the concentrations of the chemotherapeutic agents delivered to the tumor.
- Although the blood-brain barrier (BBB) can be a potential obstacle to the delivery of chemotherapy to these tumors, the most malignant brain tumors are often associated with marked disruption of this barrier.
- No other chemotherapeutic agent or combination of agents has been shown to be more effective than carmustine (BCNU) for those with GBM. Its delayed and cumulative bone marrow depression is the dose-limiting toxicity.

- Recently the oligodendrogliomas have been found to be chemosensitive. The PCV combination is now the treatment of choice for oligodendrogliomas and mixed gliomas.
- PCNSL and germ cell tumors are highly sensitive to chemotherapy. The germ cell tumors respond to a number of regimens containing cisplatin.
- Unfortunately, the addition of adjuvant chemotherapy has added little improvement to the survival of individuals with malignant brain tumors, particularly those with GBM.
- Bolus infusions of water-soluble agents with short plasma half-lives might treat the contrast-enhancing tumor ring but may never reach therapeutic concentrations within the center of the tumor.
- The instillation of chemotherapy directly into the CSF (Ommaya reservoir) is an important method of administering chemotherapy for individuals with leptomeningeal metastases, leukemic or lymphomatous meningitis, PCNSL, and primary CNS tumors such as medulloblastomas where the subarachnoid space is involved.

## Spinal Cord Tumors

### Surgery

- Surgery is the primary treatment modality for most intradural tumors. Intradural, extramedullary tumors such as schwannomas and meningiomas can often be completely resected with microsurgical techniques.
- Surgery is the initial treatment for intramedullary tumors (ependymomas and astrocytomas) with the exception of the malignant astrocytomas.
- In extradural tumors, surgery is generally indicated only in cases where the cause of spinal cord compression is unknown, there is spinal instability or bone collapse into the spinal canal, a recurrence cannot be retreated with additional RT, the tumor is known to be radioresistant, or the individual is rapidly deteriorating neurologically.
- Laminectomy generally only decompresses the spinal cord.
- In a vertebral body resection, most or all of the tumor can be removed, and the resected vertebra is replaced.
- Complications related to surgical intervention include standard surgical risks as well as neurological deficits, CSF leak, and wound dehiscence. The most significant complication to treat is a new neurological deficit in which the neurological function often may not return.

### Radiation therapy

- RT is generally not recommended for completely resected intradural spinal cord tumors.
- For those individuals with a high-grade astrocytoma, RT is often the only therapy available, and even so, the prognosis is poor.
- RT and steroids are the most widely used therapy for extradural tumors.
- Spinal RT does not cause acute clinical symptoms. The major complication of spinal cord radiation—radiation myelopathy—results from demyelination and white matter necrosis or intramedullary microvascular injury.
- The more severe late-delayed radiation myelopathy generally occurs 12–28 months following RT. The clinical manifestations are irreversible.

### Chemotherapy

- Chemotherapy does not play a large role in the treatment of spinal cord tumors.

## SYMPTOM MANAGEMENT AND SUPPORTIVE CARE

- Table 35-8, text page 1028, describes common nursing diagnoses, suggests causes of the problems, and offers some of the associated nursing interventions for the care of these individuals.
- Cerebral edema can often be managed with corticosteroids such as dexamethasone.
- Steroids help to reestablish the BBB, thus decreasing edema.
- In situations where ICP is acutely elevated, corticosteroids alone are insufficient and osmotic diuretics, also referred to as hyperosmolar agents, are required. A hyperosmolar drug, usually mannitol, is given.
- Other methods to help control increased ICP include fluid restriction, hyperventilation, sedation, and control of temperature.
- The head of the bed should be elevated to promote venous drainage.
- Unfortunately, many nursing interventions, although necessary, can further aggravate increased ICP. These include turning and positioning, range-of-motion exercises, suctioning, and pulmonary hygiene.
- Spacing the activities and care can decrease sustained elevations of increased ICP.
- Individuals with spinal cord tumors also receive corticosteroids, especially when SCC has developed.
  - Dexamethasone is the most commonly used steroid.
- While the addition of steroids provides pain relief for many individuals, others require additional analgesics.
- Neurological symptoms of SCC other than pain usually evolve quickly. If prompt treatment is not initiated, weakness leading to paralysis will occur.
- Glucocorticoid side effect can be serious: GI bleeding, bowel perforation, hyperglycemia, hallucinations, psychosis, myopathy, opportunistic infections, osteoporosis, and acute adrenal insufficiency resulting from steroid withdrawal.
- Many individuals on prolonged steroids also receive PCP prophylaxis with either trimethoprim and sulfamethoxadine or pentamadine. PCP prophylaxis generally continues for one month after the steroids have been discontinued.
- Drugs such as phenytoin, phenobarbitol, and perhaps carbamazepine increase the metabolic clearance of steroids and may decrease their therapeutic effect.
- Common anticonvulsants cause drowsiness and cognitive dysfunction.
- Anxiety and depression are often thought to be natural responses to the illness and are sometimes overlooked.

## CONTINUITY OF CARE: NURSING CHALLENGES

- Rehabilitation is important for the individual with a primary spinal cord tumor because many of these individuals have extended periods of time between recurrences.

## PRACTICE QUESTIONS

1. Which of the following has *not* been found to be associated wtih an increased incidence of primary brain tumors?
   a. inhaled steroids
   b. AIDS
   c. genetic disorders
   d. radiation to the head and neck area

2. In balancing intracranial pressure, _____ is the mechanism that specifically maintains a normal ICP despite fluctuations in arterial pressure and venous drainage.
   a. autoregulation
   b. compensation
   c. CSF displacement
   d. cerebral blood flow

3. Which of the following statements regarding metastatic brain tumors is not accurate?
   a. Metastatic brain tumors are the most comon type of brain tumor.
   b. The incidence of metastatic brain tumors is decreasing due to advances in cancer care.
   c. Tumors in the lung are the most likely of all solid tumors to metastasize in the brain.
   d. Radiation therpy is the primary mode of treatment and is palliative.

4. The glioblastoma multiforme (GBM):
   a. is most common in individuals who are between 30 and 50 years of age.
   b. has less necrosis than anaplastic astrocytoma.
   c. is the most common adult primary brain tumor.
   d. a and c.

5. The oligodendroglioma differs from the astrocytoma in that it:
   a. varies in malignancy.
   b. has a longer antecedent (prodromal) history.
   c. is more frequently associated with seizures.
   d. b and c.

6. Primary central nervous system lymphomas generally present as a single lesion. Which of the following are also true concerning PCNSL?
   a. PCNSL may be multifocal 50% of the time.
   b. PCNSL is an aggressive non-Hodgkin's lymphoma confined to the CNS.
   c. PCNSL is increasing in incidence in immunosuppressed individuals.
   d. all of the above.

7. Which of the following is considered to be a classic sign of ICP?
   a. headache at the base of the brain
   b. change in level of consciousness
   c. agitation
   d. forgetfulness

8. Spinal cord compression occurs by which of the following mechanisms?
   a. direct extension of the tumor into the epidural space
   b. vertebral collapse
   c. displacement of bone into the epidural space
   d. all of the above

9. Mrs. Johnson has complained of back pain for 6 months and now presents with weakness. Which of the following helps to explain her symptoms?
   a. Pain is rarely a symptom of spinal cord tumors.
   b. Weakness is a classic symptom of spinal cord tumors.
   c. Back pain and weakness are likely caused by her chronic steroid use.
   d. a and b.

10. After completing a course of treatment for leukemia, Shauna develops leptomeningeal metastasis. The primary treatment she is likely to receive for this is:
    a. RT to symptomatic areas only.
    b. radiation to the entire neuroaxis.
    c. chemotherapy administered directly into the CSF.
    d. concurrent, fractionated chemotherapy and radiation.

11. Mr. Allen is scheduled for a steriotactic procedure. Your teaching plan would include which of the following?
    a. The purpose of the procedure is to establish a diagnosis.
    b. Stereotactic procedures may be used to remove tumors.
    c. A stereotactic procedure is used to place radioactive sources.
    d. all of the above.

12. You will soon begin work in a clinic that specializes in the detection and treatment of spinal cord tumors. You are aware that the most common presenting symptom of a spinal cord tumor is:
    a. weakness.
    b. cold, numbness, and tingling.
    c. pain.
    d. uncoordinated ataxic gait.

13. In most instances of CNS tumors, the first, earliest, and most sensitive indicator of dysfunction will be a change in:
    a. level of consciousness.
    b. cognitive ability.
    c. motor and sensory function.
    d. all of the above.

14. Assessment of cerebellar function focuses on the ability to:
    a. coordinate movement.
    b. maintain normal muscle tone.
    c. maintain equilibrium.
    d. all of the above.

15. A patient with a brain tumor is suspected of having possible hemorrhage. The test most likely needed to determine this is:
    a. noncontrast CT.
    b. CT with contrast.
    c. MRI.
    d. cerebral angiography.

16. Out of the following possible indicators, the prognosis is far better for:
    b. intradural spinal cord tumors.
    a. extradural spinal cord tumors.
    c. rapid onset.
    d. quick progression.

17. A patient of yours is about to undergo a brain biopsy alone. You realize that this may be because:
    a. the diagnosis is uncertain despite good-quality MRI studies.
    b. the individual is unable to undergo craniotomy because of risks.
    c. there is a question of radiation necrosis versus tumor recurrence.
    d. any of the above.

18. After tumor resection, a patient suffers postoperative cerebral edema. This is most likely to result from:
    a. surgical manipulation of the surrounding brain tissue.
    b. changes in regional blood flow.
    c. brain injury caused by excessive retraction.
    d. any of the above.

19. _____ uses the planning technology of stereotactic radiosurgery but delivers the treatment using standard fractionation doses.
    a. Stereotactaic radiotherapy (SRT)
    b. Brachytherapy
    c. 3D-CRT
    d. none of the above

20. Three-dimensional conformal radiation therapy (3D-CRT):
    a. is more precise than traditional RT, but runs a slightly greater risk of normal tissue injury.
    b. enables treatment to be delivered using standard fractionation doses.
    c. may allow higher than traditional doses to be safely administered to patients with malignant gliomas.
    d. a and b.

21. Of the following chemotherapeutic agents, the most effective choice for those patients with GBM is:
    a. cisplatin.
    b. carmustine.
    c. procarbazine.
    d. etoposide.

**Questions 22 through 25 address the case of Jeffrey, who is diagnosed with an extradural CNS tumor.**

22. Jeffrey has an extradural CNS tumor that requires surgery. A possible explanation for this surgery is the fact that:
    a. the cause of spinal cord compression is unknown.
    b. there is bone collapse into Jeffrey's spinal canal.
    c. Jeffrey is rapidly deteriorating neurologically.
    d. any of the above.

23. After surgery, Jeffrey demonstrates several complications. The most significant complication to treat is:
    a. CSF leak.
    b. wound dehiscence.
    c. a new neurological deficit.
    d. none of the above.

24. Jeffrey's ICP is acutely elevated. In acute situations like his, the drug of choice is:
    a. mannitol.
    b. a corticosteroid.
    c. vincristine.
    d. vinblastine.

25. Other nonpharmacological methods you might suggest to help control Jeffrey's increased ICP include:
    a. elevating the head of the bed.
    b. range-of-motion exercises.
    c. suctioning.
    d. pulmonary hygiene.

## ANSWER EXPLANATIONS

1. **The answer is a.** Increased incidence of primary brain tumors is associated with all these choices *except* inhaled steroids. (pp. 981–982)

2. **The answer is a.** In balancing intracranial pressure, autoregulation is the mechanism that specifically maintains a normal ICP despite fluctuations in arterial pressure and venous drainage. (p. 989)

3. **The answer is b.** Gliomas are the most common primary tumor in adults. (p. 994)

4. **The answer is c.** The glioblastoma multiforme (GBM) is the most common adult primary brain tumor. It is most common in individuals who are 50 or older. It shares all the characteristics of anaplastic astrocytoma plus necrosis. (p. 991)

5. **The answer is d.** The oligodendroglioma differs from the astrocytoma in that it has a longer antecedent (prodromal) history and is more frequently associated with seizures. But, like astrocytomas, oligodendrogliomas vary in malignancy. (p. 991)

6. **The answer is d.** Chemotherapy is used primarily for recurrent ependymomas. Standard treatment of ependymomas in general is surgery and RT. Low-grade tumors are treated with local RT unless there is evidence of disseminated disease, which requires full craniospinal radiation. Malignant ependymomas are generally treated with cransiospinal radiation as well. (p. 993)

7. **The answer is b.** Change in the level of consciousness is a classic sign of ICP. (p. 997)

8. **The answer is c.** In brain metastases, the most common site of origin is the lung. Other cancers that commonly metastasize to the brain include breast cancer, melanoma, colon cancer, and renal cancer. Melanoma has the highest propensity of all systemic cancers to metastasize to the brain, but it accounts for only 1% of all cancers diagnosed. (p. 995)

9. **The answer is b.** Weakness is the most readily identified objective finding for spinal cord tumor. Choice **a** cannot be correct because pain is the most common presenting symptom of a spinal cord tumor. There is no evidence to support choice **c**. (p. 1001)

10. **The answer is a.** Treatment for leptomeningeal metastasis includes RT to symptomatic areas only because radiation to the entire neuroaxis leads to bone marrow depression. This is followed by chemotherapy administered directly into the CSF. (p. 994)

11. **The answer is d.** Stereostactic procedures are used to accomplish all of the choices given: to establish diagnosis, to remove tumors, and to place radioactive sources. (p. 1014)

12. **The answer is c.** Pain is the most common presenting symptom of a spinal cord tumor. Weakness is the most readily identified objective finding and may follow the appearance of sensory symptoms. Specific sensory deficits will depend on where the tumor is on a cross section of the spine. A lateral tumor will affect pain and temperature, causing cold, numbness, and tingling. Anterior tumors lead to weakness and an uncoordinated ataxic gait. (p. 1001)

13. **The answer is a.** In most instances the first, earliest, and most sensitive indicator of dysfunction will be a change in the level of consciousness. Mental status and cognitive ability, as well as motor and sensory function and cranial nerve function are also assessed. (p. 1004)

14. **The answer is d.** Assessment of cerebellar function focuses on the ability to coordinate movement and to maintain normal muscle tone and equilibrium. (p. 1004)

15. **The answer is a.** Noncontrast CT is necessary to determine the presence of calcium or hemorrhage. Contrast is then administered to delineate the margins and extent of blood-brain barrier disruption. MRI is the more definitive and preferred imaging study for the individual with a CNS tumor. Cerebral angiography may be used to confirm that the lesion in question is a vascular malformation or an aneurysm rather than a neoplasm. (p. 1007)

16. **The answer is b.** The prognosis is far better for intradural spinal cord tumors than for extradural. Rapid onset and quick progression are worse prognostic factors for recovery. (p. 1010)

17. **The answer is d.** The following are indications for a brain biopsy alone in some individuals: when the diagnosis is uncertain despite good-quality MRI studies, the individual is unable to undergo craniotomy because of risks, the lesion involves deep brain structures, multiple lesions are present, there is a question of radiation necrosis versus tumor recurrence, or suspected tumor progression must be histologically verified. (p. 1014)

18. **The answer is d.** Postoperative cerebral edema results from the surgical manipulation of the surrounding brain tissue, changes in regional blood flow, or brain injury caused by excessive retraction. (p. 1016)

19. **The answer is a.** Stereotactaic radiotherapy (SRT) uses the planning technology of stereotactic radiosurgery but delivers the treatment using standard fractionation doses. (p. 1020)

20. **The answer is c.** Three-dimensional conformal radiation therapy (3D-CRT) is a new method of high-precision RT. It not only decreases the risk of normal tissue injury but may also allow higher than traditional doses to be safely administered to patients with malignant gliomas. (p. 1020)

21. **The answer is b.** No other chemotherapeutic agent or combination of agents has been shown to be more effective than carmustine for those with GBM. (p. 1022)

22. **The answer is d.** In extradural tumors, surgery is generally indicated only in cases in which the cause of spinal cord compression is unknown, there is spinal instability or bone collapse into the spinal canal, a recurrence cannot be retreated with additional RT, the tumor is known to be radioresistant, or the individual is rapidly deteriorating neurologically. (p. 1026)

23. **The answer is c.** Complications related to surgical intervention, besides standard surgical risks, include neurological deficits, CSF leak, and wound dehiscence. The most significant complication to treat is a new neurological deficit in which the neurological function often may not return. (p. 1026)

24.  **The answer is a.** In situations in which ICP is acutely elevated, corticosteroids alone are insufficient and osmotic diuretics (hyperosmolar agents) are required—usually mannitol. (p. 1027)

25.  **The answer is a.** Other methods to control increased ICP include fluid restriction, hyperventilation, sedation, and control of temperature. The head of the bed should be elevated to promote venous drainage. Turning and positioning, range-of-motion exercises, suctioning, and pulmonary hygiene can aggravate increased ICP. (p. 1027)

# Chapter 36    Colon and Rectal Cancer

## EPIDEMIOLOGY

- Cancer of the colon and rectum is the third most commonly diagnosed malignancy in the United States.
- Colon and rectal cancer is also the third leading cause of death from a malignancy for both men and women.
- Overall, incidence and mortality rates have reflected a downward trend over the past decade.
- The five-year survival rate for all stages of colorectal disease between 1986 and 1991 was 62%.

## ETIOLOGY

### Age

- The number of individuals diagnosed with colorectal carcinoma begins to increase steadily after the age of 40.
- The risk of colorectal cancer then rises sharply at the age of 50 to 55 and doubles each decade thereafter up to the age of 75.

### Genetics

- Individuals who have a first-degree relative with colorectal cancer have double the risk for developing adenomatous polyps.
- An inheritable autosomal dominant trait is found in families with a high incidence of colon cancer.
- Cancers of the colon with a genetic component generally fall into two categories: *adenomatosis polyposis coli* syndrome and *hereditary nonpolyposis colorectal cancer* (HNPCC) syndrome.
- Another inherited autosomal dominant trait found in families with a higher incidence of colon cancer is familial adenocarcinomatosis.

### Diet

- A diet high in fat content is considered to be a risk factor and promoter of colon carcinogenesis.
- Diets high in fat increase the production of, and change the composition of, bile salts. These altered bile salts are converted into potential carcinogens by intestinal flora.
- Dietary fiber has been found to decrease the effects of fatty acids.
- The protective mechanism of dietary fiber increases fecal bulk, which changes the bacterial composition of the feces and accelerates the transit time in the intestinal tract.

### Alcohol

- Alcohol has been considered a risk factor in the development of colorectal cancer.
- Beer consumption places males at statistically significant higher risk for developing rectal carcinoma.

### Environment

- Solvents, abrasives, and fuel oils are substances that may increase the risk for developing this malignancy. Automotive pattern and model workers have twice the mortality rate.

## Inflammatory Bowel Conditions

- Ulcerative colitis places an individual at risk for cancer of the colon five to ten times higher than that of the general population.
- Crohn's disease is also considered to be a risk factor.

## Radiation

- Radiation therapy to the pelvis for treatment of other primary malignancies correlates with an increased risk for developing carcinoma of the colon and rectum years after the initial treatment.

## Ureterosigmoidostomy

- Ureterosigmoidostomy increased incidence of colon carcinoma 15 to 30 years after the initial surgery.

## PREVENTION, SCREENING, EARLY DETECTION

- Chemoprevention minimizes the effects of potential carcinogens.
- Antioxidants block oxidative damage to cellular DNA.
- The chemopreventive action of nonsteroidal antiinflammatory drugs (NSAIDs) is related to a reduction in endogenous prostaglandin.
- Incidence of colon cancer can be decreased with regular use of aspirin.
- Calcium, taken orally, has been shown to decrease the risk of developing colon cancer.
- The use of exogenous estrogen appears to exert a protective mechanism and decreases the risk of colon cancer in women.
- Individuals who have adenomatous polyps removed should then have a follow-up colonoscopy three years later to detect missed adenomas or subsequent adenomas. Colonoscopy may then be performed approximately every five years.
- Genes play a major role in individuals and families who are prone to developing colorectal carcinoma. The K-ras mutation occurs in 30%–50% of colorectal carcinomas.
- The *adenomatous polyposis coli* (APC) gene, the *deleted in colorectal carcinoma* (DCC) antioncogene, and the *hereditary nonpolyposis colorectal cancer* (HNPCC) gene can be used as indicators to identify a colorectal malignancy.
- Three tests are recommended by the American Cancer Society and the National Cancer Institute in the screening for colorectal cancer.
  - The first screening test is the digital rectal examination annually after the age of 40.
  - The second screening method recommended is the Hemoccult test.
  - The third recommended screening tool is flexible sigmoidoscopy every three to five years for men and women beginning at the age of 50.

## PATHOPHYSIOLOGY

### Cellular Characteristics

- The most common histological type of colorectal neoplasm is adenocarcinoma.
- The most common anatomical sites affected are the descending sigmoid colon.
- Colorectal lesions exhibit different characteristics depending on their location in the bowel.
- Right-sided tumors present as cauliflowerlike fungating masses that progress to become ulcerative and necrotic are usually well-differentiated and have a better prognosis.
  - Left-side or descending sigmoid colon lesions present as ulcerative tumors with everted edges. These tumors tend to infiltrate the bowel wall and have a poorer prognosis than right-sided tumors.
- Rectosigmoid tumors present as villous, frondlike lesions.

- Early rectal cancer symptoms include a change in the caliber of the stool and rectal bleeding. Advanced rectal cancer symptoms include tenesmus and rectal pain.

## Progression of Disease

- Adenocarcinoma of the colon and rectum develops in the bowel mucosa. The tumor will invade locally usually by direct extension protruding into the lumen of the bowel wall.
- Once the tumor has traversed the muscularis mucosa and infiltrates the submucosa, it is termed invasive.
- The major site for visceral spread is the liver.
- The median survival for individuals with distant metastasis ranges from six to nine months.

## CLINICAL MANIFESTATIONS

- The clinical manifestations of colorectal cancer relate to the anatomic location of the tumor.
- There are no signs and symptoms of early colorectal carcinoma.
- Lesions in the ascending colon may have clinical manifestations of fatigue, palpitations, and iron deficiency anemia.
- Tumors in the transverse colon can present the clinical picture of constipation alternating with diarrhea.
- The most common symptoms found in individuals with cancer of the sigmoid colon are abdominal pain and melena. Perforation becomes more of a concern with tumors in this anatomic location.
- Cancer of the rectum clinically results in bright red rectal bleeding and a change in bowel habits.
- Unfortunately, the first symptoms arising from colorectal carcinoma may be from metastatic disease.
- Jaundice, pruritis, and ascites could indicate metastatic liver involvement.
- As cancer of the colon and rectum progress, obstruction and perforation of the bowel become more likely.
- The primary symptom of intestinal obstruction is abdominal pain. Patients who present with obstruction or perforation have a poorer prognosis than those who do not. Fistula formation, general peritonitis, and abscess are the sequelae of perforation.
- Lung metastases may be revealed upon chest x-ray showing scattered densities in the lung fields.
- Anorexia and weight loss can be significant with advanced colorectal carcinoma.

## ASSESSMENT
### Patient and Family History

- Careful review of initial clinical symptoms and astute evaluation of any physiological changes can provide invaluable information.

### Physical Assessment

- A thorough abdominal assessment should progress through inspection, auscultation, percussion, and palpation.
- Inspection of the abdominal wall should include observation for any bulging, displacement, or irregularities caused by a mass.
  - Auscultation should occur in all four quadrants.
  - Suprapubic dullness should be heard over the bladder.
  - Normally liver dullness is 4 to 8 centimeters midsternally and 6 to 12 centimeters in the midclavicular area. The dullness increases if hepatomegaly is present.
  - Palpation should be done in all four quadrants.
  - While the liver is usually palpable, the spleen is normally not.

## Diagnostic Studies

- A stool sample for fecal occult blood testing needs to be obtained.
- The proctosigmoidoscopy, with the fiberoptic sigmoidoscope, provides an optimal diagnostic visualization of up to 60 centimeters of colon.
- The barium enema is commonly used in the diagnostic workup for colorectal cancer.
  - Double contrast barium enemas are considered to be diagnostically superior to the single contrast exam.
- A chest x-ray is part of the clinical evaluation for the detection of metastatic lesions in the lung.
- The plasma tumor marker carcinoembryonic antigen (CEA) is measured preoperatively and postoperatively for therapeutic effectiveness. CA 19-9 may also be monitored.
- The malignant potential of cells can be studied by evaluating their DNA content.
- Chromosomal patterns are evaluated based upon diploidy (the normal number of chromosomes) and aneuploidy (an abnormal number of chromosomes).

## Prognostic Indicators

- The prognosis is directly related to the stage of the disease at the time of diagnosis.
- At the time of diagnosis, 37% of colorectal carcinomas are localized, 37% are regional, and 19% are distant.
- Recent data from the National Cancer Institute (NCI) reflects a five-year survival rate of 92% for localized colorectal cancer, 63% for regional colorectal cancer, and 7% for distant colorectal cancer.

## CLASSIFICATION AND STAGING

- The Dukes' system, the traditional format for staging colorectal cancer, is based on classifying the depth of penetration from the tumor as well as lymph node involvement. Dukes' stages of classification are A, B, C, and D.
- The American Joint Commission on Cancer (AJCC) classification indicates the degree of penetration of the gastrointestinal mucosa by primary tumor (T), the number and site of lymph nodes involved by regional lymph nodes (N), and the presence or absence of metastases by distant metastasis (M). See Table 36-3, page 1042.

## THERAPEUTIC APPROACHES AND NURSING CARE

- Surgical intervention remains the first-line treatment for this malignancy. Surgical techniques have evolved to include laparoscopic techniques for colon resection or cryosurgery for metastatic liver disease.
- Following postoperative recovery, additional treatment regimens are implemented, including radiation therapy, chemotherapy, and immunotherapy.

## Surgery

- Adequate margins and complete excision of the tumor provide the individual with the best long-term survival.
- The location and extent of the malignancy will determine the type of surgical resection. See Figure 36-1, text pages 1044–1045.
- The ideal surgical margin surrounding the neoplasm is five centimeters.
- Regional lymphadenectomy assists in adequately staging the disease and determining who will benefit from adjuvant therapy.
- Preoperative preparation includes the cleansing of the colon and rectum. The most common infective organisms in the bowel are aerobic *E. coli* and anaerobic *Bacteroides fragiles*.
  - The commonly used mechanical bowel preparation is an isotonic lavage solution.

- Antibiotics to minimize colorectal bacteria are taken orally at specific times the day before the surgery, and intraenous antibiotics are ordered on call to the operating room the day of the surgery.
- The usual surgical intervention for tumors in the cecum and ascending colon is the right hemicolectomy.
- A transverse colectomy is the procedure of choice when the lesion involves the middle and left transverse colon.
- Carcinomas of the descending and sigmoid colon are surgically resected by left hemicolectomy.
- A method now being used for bowel resections is laparoscopic colorectal surgery.
  - Laparoscopic interventions are undertaken for ascending or sigmoid carcinomas secondary to ease of accessibility.
- For proximal and midrectal adenocarcinomas, a low anterior resection has become the technique of choice. By using this surgical technique, there is no need for a permanent colostomy because external anal sphincter control is preserved.
- Abdominoperineal resection is usually used for poorly differentiated adenocarcinoma and more advanced disease.
  - The selection for a colostomy site is done prior to surgery.
- Radiolabeled monoclonal antibodies are being given intraoperatively to identify occult disease and metastatic areas in individuals with colorectal carcinoma.
- For smaller tumors of the colon and rectum, laser therapy is being delivered to the tumor bed through a colonoscope or flexible sigmoidoscope.
- Prophylactic oophorectomy is recommended for some women diagnosed with adenocarcinoma of the colon and rectum.
- Acute complications of colorectal surgery are listed in Table 36-4, text page 1046.
- Long-term effects following an abdominoperineal resection include sexual dysfunction and impotence.
  - Sexual dysfunction may vary from partial to complete impotence.
  - The degree of dysfunction is related to surgical technique, the age of the individual, and any pre-existing medical or surgical conditions that impact on sexual function.
- The individual who undergoes surgery for colorectal carcinoma may also require a colostomy. The type of colostomy and character of the stoma is related to the anatomic site surgically removed.
  - The single barrel colostomy is formed when the proximal portion of the colon is exteriorized.
  - The double barrel colostomy has two separate stomas. The proximal stoma excretes the stool; the distal stoma secretes mucus.
  - The loop colostomy is formed by bridging the fascia under the bowel loop or looping the large bowel over a supporting bridge device.
- The character of the stool is dependent on the placement of the stoma within the intestinal tract.
- The most common site for metastatic involvement from colorectal carcinoma is the liver.
- Five-year survival rates following hepatic resection for metastatic colorectal disease are estimated at 20%–25%. Cryosurgery is also being used to treat liver metastasis from colorectal carcinoma.

## Chemotherapy

- The cornerstone of chemotherapy for cancer of the colon and rectum is 5-fluorouracil (5-FU).
  - The major side effects associated with the administration of 5-FU are hematological and gastrointestinal: anorexia, nausea, vomiting, stomatitis, and diarrhea. Leukopenia, thrombocytopenia, and anemia can occur with this chemotherapeutic agent.
- Though 5-fluorouracil is the cytotoxic agent of choice for colorectal cancer, it is most commonly administered in combination with other drugs, particularly with leucovorin (folinic acid).
  - Leucovorin enhances the cytotoxic effect of 5-FU.

- A campthotecin derivative CPT 11 (Irinotecan) is currently being evaluated for efficacy against colorectal carcinoma, particulary refractory metastatic disease.
- Advanced colorectal cancer is treated with 5-FU. Intravenous administration is preferred to oral administration.
- Leucovorin and 5-FU in combination are also used to treat metastatic disease.
- Intraportal chemotherapy administered through the portal vein or hepatic artery into the liver has also shown evidence for improved survival. One of the more traditional drugs given by intraportal infusion is floxuridine (FUDR).
- The major toxicity associated with hepatic infusion is chemical hepatitis.

## Immunotherapy

- In humans, a 30% improved survival rate for colon cancer has been demonstrated with the use of a combination of 5-FU and levamisole for one year postoperatively.
- Alpha- and gamma-interferon are also being used as immunotherapy for advanced cancer of the colon and rectum.
- Alfa-interferon combined with 5-FU yielded better response rates than when 5-FU was used alone.
  - However, central nervous system toxic effects have also been encountered with this combination.
- Gamma-interferon has been used as an adjuvant therapy in individuals with stage II, III, and IV colon cancer.
- Bacillus Calmette-Guerin (BCG) and autologous tumor cell vaccines are also being employed in the treatment of colorectal cancer.

## Radiation Therapy

- Radiation therapy has been used in preoperative, intraoperative, and postoperative treatment of colorectal cancer. Radiation therapy is used primarily, however, to treat rectal adenocarcinoma to decrease the incidence of local recurrence after surgical resection.
  - Preoperative radiation is given with the intent of decreasing the existing tumor burden.
  - Intraoperative radiation therapy can be used to treat advanced, recurrent, or inoperable rectal cancer.
  - Postoperative irradiation is used most frequently in the treatment of rectal carcinomas.
- Adenocarcinomas of the colon and rectum are radiosensitive and respond well to radiation therapy.
- The most common injury to the large bowel that occurs following radiotherapy is proctosigmoiditis, causing bleeding, tenesmus, and pain.
- Increased bowel motility, abdominal cramping, and loose, watery stools may also occur.

## SYMPTOM MANAGEMENT AND SUPPORTIVE CARE

### Hepatic Metastases

- Approximately one in four individuals with colorectal carcinoma has liver metastases at the time of initial presentation, and approximately 70% have metastatic disease to the liver by the time they die.
  - Predominant symptoms from liver metastases are right, upper quadrant abdominal pain, weight loss, anorexia, changes in bowel habits, and hepatomegaly.
- Liver metastases may be suspected if serial serum CEA levels begin to rise. Serum liver function studies may also be elevated and indicate metastases.
- Surgical resection is still believed to be the major modality. Cryotherapy may also be used with the intent of eradicating the metastatic colorectal lesion with subzero temperatures.
- Chemotherapy, radiotherapy, and immunotherapy are also used to treat liver metastases from colorectal carcinoma.
  - Palliation of symptoms is important in the management of hepatic metastases.

- Ascites can be palliatively treated with intermittent paracentesis or the insertion of an intraperitoneal Tenchoff® catheter for intermittent drainage.
- Treatment of the underlying disease to shrink the neoplasm is optimal for pain relief.
- Pharmacological approaches to pain management need to be consistently implemented to provide optimal comfort.
- Pruritis results from chemical irritation caused by excessive accumulation of bile salts in the system. Interventions to manage pruritis include increasing fluid intake, promoting capillary constriction, and applying topical anesthetic preparations.

## Bowel Obstruction

- Extrinsic compression of the bowel may occur as a result of abdominal carcinomatosis or tumor studding along the bowel. Intrinsic compression of the bowel can result from growth and progression of the tumor within the lumen of the bowel itself.
- Signs and symptoms of bowel obstructions are nausea and vomiting, abdominal distention, abdominal pain, progressive constipation, and absence of bowel sounds over the affected area.
- Initial management of a bowel obstruction associated with advanced colorectal disease is medically conservative. The placement of a nasogastric tube to decompress the gastrointestinal tract is standard.
- Total parenteral nutrition may be a consideration.

## Ureteral Obstruction

- Individuals with adenocarcinoma of the colon and rectum have ureteral obstruction in 38% of cases.
- Bilateral ureteral obstruction can occur with advanced colorectal malignancies secondary to direct tumor compression of the ureters.
- Individuals present with oliguria and an elevated serum creatinine.
- Treatment of ureteral obstruction may be accomplished.
- Urinary stents into the ureters circumvent the need for a surgical procedure.

## Pulmonary Metastases

- Colorectal carcinoma is one of the most common primary tumors with pulmonary metastases.
- It has been estimated that 85% of pulmonary metastases are asymptomatic.
- Pulmonary resection of the metastic area provides the best long-term survival for individuals. Pulmonary wedge resection is best undertaken if the lesion is isolated.
- Individuals with four or fewer metastatic pulmonary lesions have a better prognosis than do individuals with more than four.

## CONTINUITY OF CARE: NURSING CHALLENGES

- The course of colorectal carcinoma, including follow-up, can span many years.
- The average length of stay for someone who has had a surgical resection secondary to colorectal carcinoma is less than five days.
- Upon discharge the individual needs to be clear about when to call the physician for problems such as fever, chills, shortness of breath, or hemoptysis.
- Upon return for the postoperative check, an overall final pathology is shared with the individual and family if the tissue diagnosis was not available at the time of discharge.
- Provision for continuity of care is imperative.
- If the disease is advanced, palliation of symptoms is also part of the spectrum of care.

# PRACTICE QUESTIONS

1. Fat and fiber are two dietary factors that appear to be correlated with the occurrence of colorectal cancer. It is thought that they operate by affecting, in opposite ways, the:
   a. conversion of ionized bile salts into insoluble compounds.
   b. rate of uptake of calcium by the GI tract.
   c. breakdown of carcinogenic compounds by digestive enzymes.
   d. exposure of the GI tract to promoters of carcinogenesis.

2. Which of the following conditions is commonly associated with colorectal carcinoma?
   a. appendicitis or gallbladder disease
   b. hemorrhoids
   c. anal condylomata acuminata
   d. chronic ulcerative colitis

3. Which of the following tests is recommended by the American Cancer Society and the National Cancer Institute in screening for colorectal cancer?
   a. flexible sigmoidoscopy
   b. digital rectal examination
   c. Hemoccult® test
   d. all of the above

4. The prognosis for a patient with colorectal cancer is probably poorest if which of the following exists?
   a. venous and lymph node invasion
   b. high blood pressure
   c. location of the tumor above the peritoneal reflection
   d. squamous cell involvement

5. Which of the following clinical manifestations is most likely to exist in patients with a cancer of the sigmoid colon?
   a. anemia and a vague, dull, persistent pain in the upper, right quadrant
   b. abdominal pain and melena
   c. sensations of incomplete evacuation and tenesmus
   d. bright-red bleeding through the rectum

6. Physical examination and diagnostic studies of a patient with cancer of the right colon are most likely to find which of the following?
   a. a palpable mass
   b. polyps in the rectum
   c. anemia
   d. high levels of carcinoembryonic antigen (CEA)

7. Which of the following procedures is the surgeon most likely to perform when a lesion involves the middle and left transverse colon?
   a. a right hemicolectomy that includes the related lymphatic and circulatory channels
   b. a one-stage procedure involving resection of the lesion and a primary anastomosis
   c. a two-stage procedure involving a temporary colostomy or ileostomy
   d. a three-stage procedure involving a diverting colostomy, a resection of the tumor, and takedown of the colostomy

8.  For proximal and midrectal adenocarcinomas, the treatment technique of choice is:
    a.  low anterior resection, preserving external anal sphincter control.
    b.  abdominoperineal resection with a temporary colostomy.
    c.  laser therapy to the tumor bed through a colonoscope or flexible sigmoidoscope.
    d.  prophylactic oophorectomy.

9.  Although 5-fluorouracil is the cytotoxic agent of choice for colorectal cancer, it is most commonly administered in combination with:
    a.  floxuridine (FUDR).
    b.  CPR-11.
    c.  leucovorin.
    d.  none of the above.

10.  The most common injury to the large bowel that occurs following radiotherapy is:
    a.  increased bowel motility.
    b.  proctosigmoiditis.
    c.  abdominal cramping.
    d.  loose, watery stools.

11.  Predominant symptoms from liver metastases include:
    a.  rapid, unexplained weight gain.
    b.  nausea and vomiting with bile salt excretion.
    c.  liver body atrophy.
    d.  right upper quadrant abdominal pain.

12.  Colorectal carcinoma is one of the most common primary tumors with:
    a.  ovarian metastases.
    b.  renal metastases.
    c.  brain metastases.
    d.  pulmonary metastases.

# ANSWER EXPLANATIONS

1.  **The answer is d.** It is believed that dietary factors affect the exposure of the GI tract to promoters of carcinogenesis. Fats increase the production, and change the composition, of bile salts. These altered bile salts are converted into potential carcinogens. Fiber decreases the effects of fatty acids and may actually protect against the disease even in the presence of a high-fat diet. Fiber may limit the time the colon is exposed to cancer promoters by speeding intestinal transit time. (p. 1038)

2.  **The answer is d.** A number of predisposing conditions have been associated with an increased risk of colorectal cancer. These include chronic ulcerative colitis; Crohn's disease; familial polyposis; and a strong family history of predisposition to colon cancer and familial adenamatous polyposis. (p. 1038)

3.  **The answer is d.** All of these tests are recommended in screening for colorectal cancer. (pp. 1039–1040)

4.  **The answer is a.** Poor prognosis has been associated with obstructing or perforating carcinomas, occurrence in young people, location of the tumor below the peritoneal reflection, lymph node involvement, venous invasion, hepatic metastasis, and invasion of the bowel wall. (p. 1040)

5. **The answer is b.** Cancers of the sigmoid colon are most often manifested by abdominal pain and melena. The manifestations in choice **a** are those of a tumor of the right colon; manifestations in choices **c** and **d** are those of rectal cancer. (p. 1040)

6. **The answer is a.** Because the transverse colon is the most anterior and movable part of the colon, tumors here are more accessible to detection by palpation. Other possible symptoms that might have been determined by inspection, auscultation, palpation, and percussion of the abdomen include distention of the abdomen, enlarged and visible abdominal veins, occult blood in the stool, and enlarged lymph nodes or organs (especially the liver). Diagnostic examination by fiberoptic colonoscopy would confirm the presence of the tumor. Anemia is more likely to occur with cancer of the right colon. Polyps in the rectum might be present and might indicate the patient was at high risk for colorectal cancer. CEA, while useful in evaluating the efficacy of treatment, is of limited value in the detection of colon cancer. (p. 1041)

7. **The answer is b.** When a malignant lesion involves the middle and left transverse colon, the standard procedure involves resection of the lesion and a primary anastomosis. The two- and three-step procedures are riskier and less often performed. A right hemicolectomy is performed on the cecum or ascending colon. (p. 1043)

8. **The answer is a.** For proximal and midrectal adenocarcinomas, the treatment technique of choice is low anterior resection. This preserves external anal sphincter control, thus eliminating the need for a permanent colostomy. Abdominoperineal resection is usually used for poorly differentiated adenocarcinoma and more advanced disease. Laser therapy to the tumor bed through a colonoscope or flexible sigmoidoscope is used for smaller tumors of the colon and rectum, and prophylactic oophorectomy is recommended for only some women diagnosed with adenocarcinoma of the colon and rectum. (p. 1046)

9. **The answer is c.** Although 5-fluorouracil is the cytotoxic agent of choice for colorectal cancer, it is most commonly administered in combination with leucovorin. Floxuridine (FUDR) is used in intraportal chemotherapy through the portal vein or hepatic artery into the liver, in individuals with metastasis to the liver. The campthotecin derivative CPT-11 is currently being evaluated for efficacy, particularly for refractory metastatic disease previously treated with 5-FU. (p. 1047)

10. **The answer is b.** The most common injury to the large bowel that occurs following radiotherapy is proctosigmoiditis. Other commonly encountered side effects include increased bowel motility, which creates abdominal cramping and loose, watery stools. (p. 1048)

11. **The answer is d.** Predominant symptoms from liver metastases are right, upper quadrant abdominal pain, weight loss, anorexia, changes in bowel habits and hepatomegaly. Between 25% and 30% of these individuals may experience ascites and jaundice. (p. 1048)

12. **The answer is d.** While endobronchial metastases are rare, colorectal carcinoma is one of the most common primary tumors with pulmonary metastases. (p. 1049)

# Chapter 37    Endocrine Malignancies

## INTRODUCTION

- Endocrine malignancies arise from glands that secrete endocrine hormones; i.e., chemical signals released into the bloodstream to exert their effects at sites distant from their origin.
- Endocrine glands include the pituitary, the thyroid, the parathyroids, the adrenal glands, the gonads, and the islets of Langerhans.
- Individuals who inherit an autosomal dominant gene or genes that code for a MEN syndrome may experience a particular constellation of endocrine tumors, which tend to occur earlier in life than in individuals who develop sporadic endocrine tumors.

## THYROID TUMORS
### Epidemiology

- Thyroid malignancies are most commonly diagnosed in individuals aged 40–49, and women are three times as likely as men to develop a thyroid tumor. Age is an important determinant of prognosis.

### Etiology

- Ionizing radiation to the head and neck is the only clearly identified causative agent for papillary thyroid cancer, but other factors may play a role.
- Risk from radiation is inversely related to age; that is, infants and young children are more susceptible to the carcinogenic effect of radiation to the neck region than are older children.
- High rates of follicular and papillary tumors are noted in areas of endemic goiter. This supports the hypothesis that iodine insufficiency, especially in women, adolescents, and young adults, is a causative factor for thyroid malignancy.

### Pathophysiology

- Papillary and follicular tumors arise from the follicle, medullary tumors arise from parafollicular cells, and anaplastic tumors arise from differentiated papillary of follicular cells.

#### Papillary and follicular tumors

- Papillary tumors are typically multifocal and infiltrate local tissues.
- Vascular invasion and metastasis to a distant site, such as bone and lung, are more common in papillary tumors than in follicular tumors.
- Follicular thyroid cancer is more aggressive than papillary cancer.
- Follicular cancer is most often diagnosed in persons in their 50s, but those younger than 40 have the best prognosis.

#### Medullary tumors

- Medullary thyroid tumors occur equally in men and women over the age of 50.
- Fifty percent of patients have tumor spread to their cervical lymph nodes at the time of diagnosis. Regional lymph node spread is an ominous prognostic sign.
- Medullary tumors metastasize via the bloodstream and lymphatics to lung, liver, and bone.

### Anaplastic tumors

- Patients typically present with a rapidly growing firm or hard neck mass invading the structures of the neck to cause dysphagia and dysphonia.
- Anaplastic tumors have the best prognosis when the tumor is completely resectable. Unfortunately, this is often not the case.
- Metastasis is an early event, and sites may include lymph nodes, bone, and lung.

## Clinical Manifestations

- Thyroid malignancies often do not cause symptoms until the disease is advanced. Patients may seek medical attention when they notice that their necks look larger, or because their neck mass is painful and noticeably enlarging. In other instances they may be experiencing local symptoms such as recent-onset dysphagia, dysphonia, or hoarseness.

## Assessment

- Young patients with a thyroid mass tend to present with painless anterior cervical adenopathy. In older patients the first manifestation is usually regional lymph node metastasis or, rarely, distant metastasis.
- Thyroid masses are commonly found either by the patient or by a health care provider upon gentle palpation of the neck.
- Thyroid function tests are not included as part of the workup for thyroid cancer because most tumors do not alter the thyroid's functional capacity. One exception is elevated serum calcitonin levels, which are strongly suggestive of medullary hyperplasia or carcinoma.
- Ultrasound distinguishes cystic, solid, and mixed lesions.
- Fine-needle aspirate (FNA) biopsy is the procedure of choice to confirm thyroid malignancy.

## Classification and Staging

- See Table 37-1 (text page 1059) for the American Joint Committee on Cancer (AJCC) staging system.

## Therapeutic Approaches and Nursing Care

### Surgery

- While surgery is the treatment of choice for thyroid tumors, there is no consensus about how extensive surgical resection should be for well-differentiated tumors.
- Postoperative complications of thyroidectomy include vocal cord paralysis with subsequent respiratory embarrassment, thyroid storm, hemorrhage, and hypothyroidism.
- Hypothyroidism results in hypocalcemia that requires the administration of exogenous thyroid hormone to prevent the clinical effects of hypothyroidism.
- See Table 37-3 (text page 1062) for a care plan for the patient undergoing thyroid surgery.

### Radiation therapy

- Brachytherapy with oral [131]I is used to treat some cases of papillary and follicular tumors but not medullary and anaplastic tumors, which do not concentrate and retain iodine.
- Side effects of [131]I include nausea and vomiting, fatigue, headache, bone marrow suppression, salivary gland inflammation, and infrequently leukemia and radiation-induced pulmonary fibrosis.
- External-beam radiation is occasionally used to attempt local control of anaplastic tumors, but these tumors are usually radioresistant.

### Chemotherapy

- Reports of chemotherapy for refractory, metastatic, and anaplastic thyroid cancers are generally discouraging.

# PARATHYROID TUMORS

- Most people have four glands, but the normal range is two to eight.
- The chief cells produce parathyroid hormone (PTH), which is critical to maintain normal serum calcium balance.

## Epidemiology

- Parathyroid adenomas occur equally in males and females, who are usually diagnosed in their 40s and 50s.

## Etiology

- No definitive risk factors have been identified.

## Pathophysiology

- Carcinomas tend to be indolent and to recur locally after surgical resection. Metastasis of parathyroid carcinoma is most often a late event.

## Clinical Manifestations

- Hypercalcemia is the hallmark of parathyroid tumors.

## Assessment

- The diagnosis of parathyroid tumor is essentially confirmed by the signs and symptoms of parathyroid hyperplasia or tumor.
- Immunoassay typically reveals markedly increased levels of PTH.

## Therapeutic Approaches and Nursing Care

### Surgery

- Surgery is the treatment of choice for parathyroid tumors, but radical surgery may not change the course of the disease.
- Surgery for localized parathyroid adenomas and carcinomas includes unilateral neck dissection.
- After surgery, "hungry bone syndrome" signifies successful extirpation of tumor. In this syndrome calcium and phosphorus are rapidly deposited into bone, which results in symptomatic hypocalcemia.

### Chemotherapy

- Radiotherapy and chemotherapy are ineffective in treating primary and metastatic disease.

# PITUITARY TUMORS

## Epidemiology

- Pituitary adenomas occur at all ages, but 70% occur in individuals between 30 and 50 years of age.

## Etiology

- Pituitary tumors arise from epithelial cells in the anterior pituitary, but their exact pathogenesis is unknown.

## Pathophysiology

- Most pituitary tumors are localized, benign adenomas that are incapable of metastasizing.
- True pituitary carcinomas are rare.

## Clinical Manifestations

### Hormone effects

#### Prolactinomas

- In women, prolactinomas cause galactorrhea, menstrual irregularities including amenorrhea or oligomenorrhea, or infertility. In men the same tumor produces decreased libido or impotence, and in some cases, galactorrhea.

#### Growth hormone-secreting tumors

- Almost all cases of GH-secreting tumors arise in the pituitary. These tumors induce acromegaly in adults and gigantism in prepubescent children.
- As tumors enlarge, excessive GH leads to enlargement of bone, organs, and soft tissues. The result is the characteristic disfigurement of the face, arthropathies, and neuropathies.
- Other symptoms include weight gain, excessive perspiration, insulin resistance, and decreased glucose tolerance leading to diabetes.

#### Cushing's syndrome

- Most cases of Cushing's syndrome result from the sustained hypersecretion of ACTH by a pituitary adenoma. Cushing's syndrome is characterized by several signs. Almost all affected individuals have the characteristic moon face, and most have truncal obesity, hypertension, impaired glucose tolerance, and hypogonadism (menstrual irregularities, loss of libido).

### Mass effects

- Many critical structures surround the sella turcica, and if the tumor enlarges beyond the sella, mass effects occur. Extension into the optic chiasm is most common. This leads to compression of the optic nerve and bilateral visual field loss.
- Enlargement beyond the sella may also cause generalized signs of increased intracranial pressure, headache, seizures, or cerebrospinal fluid (CSF) rhinorrhea.

## Assessment

- Diagnostic procedures for all patients with suspected pituitary tumor may include evaluation of gonadal, thyroid, and adrenal functioning.
- Specific tests for stimulation and suppression of pituitary hormones are outlined in Table 37-5, text page 1068.
- Magnetic resonance imaging (MRI) and/or CT demonstrate in three dimensions the tumor size and extension preoperatively and after surgery.

## Classification and Staging

- In addition to classification by the hormone that is secreted, pituitary adenomas are classified according to their secretory ability, size, and invasiveness.
- The most common tumors are prolactinomas.
- Microadenomas are tumors that are less than 10 mm in diameter, while macroadenomas are greater than 10 mm.
- Tumors are also characterized as intrasellar and extrasellar, depending on their ability to expand outside the sella turcica, and as noninvasive or invasive, depending on whether they can infiltrate into the dural and osseous walls.

## Therapeutic Approaches and Nursing Care

- Surgery, radiation therapy, and drug therapy may be used singly or in combination.
- The optimal treatment goal is total tumor removal and rapid normalization of hormone levels, without secondary pituitary insufficiency.

### Surgery

- Surgery is the treatment of choice for almost all tumors except prolactinomas.

### Radiation therapy

- External-beam radiation is used for patients who refuse surgery or those who cannot tolerate surgery, and also in some cases of subtotal resection.
- Disadvantages include the possibility that the therapeutic effect may be too slow for patients whose tumors secrete excessive hormone and the tendency, in rare instances, for radiation to induce second CNS malignancies.

### Drug therapy

- Antineoplastic chemotherapy is not used for pituitary tumors. Other drugs are indicated as first-line therapy for microadenomas or macroadenomas before surgery or radiation in some instances, and following therapy in others.

### Nursing care

- Damage to cranial nerves, optic nerves, or the optic chiasm may lead to complete or partial visual loss or visual field defects.
- Surgical trauma may cause temporary DI followed by water intoxication, dehydration, and hypernatremia.
- If the patient develops hyponatremia, fluid restriction is instituted until DI resolves.

## ADRENAL TUMORS

- The medulla and the cortex act in concert, as the medulla rapidly responds to changes in the environment and the cortex amplifies and sustains the response.
- Adrenocortical tumors arise from the cortex, and pheochromocytomas arise from the medulla. Both types of tumors are most often benign, but both benign and malignant tumors can alter quality of life and may be life-threatening.

## ADRENOCORTICAL TUMORS

### Epidemiology

- Adrenocortical tumors are extremely rare and occur most frequently in children under 10 years of age and in adults in their 50s.

### Etiology

- There are no known risk factors for adrenal tumors.

### Pathophysiology

- Tumors of the cortex are characterized as functional or nonfunctional. Functional tumors are further characterized by the hormone(s) they produce in excess. Fifty percent of tumors hypersecrete cortisol (Cushing's syndrome), 25% secrete estradiol or testosterone, and only rare tumors secrete aldosterone. Approx-

imately 20%–25% of Cushing's syndrome results from benign or malignant adrenocortical tumors.
- Nonfunctional tumors do not produce cortical hormones and are called *incidentalomas*.

## Clinical Manifestations

- The signs and symptoms of adrenocortical tumors vary depending on the hormone or hormones secreted. Cushing's syndrome causes similar symptoms to those induced by pituitary tumors.
- Women are likely to have virilizing tumors and have symptoms reflecting hypersecretion of androgen.
- Tumors that hypersecrete estradiol are the rarest adrenal tumors and generally occur in young to middle-aged men, who experience diminished libido, testicular atrophy, and gynecomastia.
- Sex hormone-secreting tumors in children are manifested by precocious puberty.

## Assessment

- Diagnosis is confirmed by correlating physical findings with laboratory values and localization procedures.

## Classification and Staging

- Cortical tumors have been staged using the TNM system. Stage I and stage II tumors are localized.
- Stage III and IV are considered advanced disease and include positive regional lymph nodes and metastatic disease, respectively.

## Therapeutic Approaches and Nursing Care

### Surgery

- Whenever possible, surgical removal of local and metastatic disease is recommended because surgery offers the only chance for cure of malignant adrenal tumors. Cure is likely only with stage I or II tumors.

### Chemotherapy

- Chemotherapy is given in some instances.
- Mitotane, an analogue of the insecticide DDD that can cause adrenal necrosis, is the usual first-line agent. Response rates to mitotane are generally about 35%, but responses are rarely prolonged or complete, and survival does not increase.

### Symptom management and supportive care

- Because of delays in diagnosis, many patients with adrenal tumors have progressive disease that does not respond to treatment.

## PHEOCHROMOCYTOMA

## Epidemiology

- Pheochromocytomas are tumors that arise from chromaffin cells. From 85% to 95% arise from the adrenal medulla, but these tumors may also arise from other sympathetic nervous system cells.
- About 90% of pheochromocytomas in adults are benign, whereas children often have malignant tumors.

## Pathophysiology

- Both benign and malignant pheochromocytomas hypersecrete catecholamines, predominantly norepinephrine.

- This is the inverse of normal adrenal secretion.

## Clinical Manifestations

- Hypertension is the hallmark of pheochromocytoma.
- Hypertension occurs in one of three patterns: indistinguishable from essential hypertension, normal blood pressure with superimposed paroxysmal hypertension, or sustained hypertension with extreme paroxysms.
- Tumors that produce large amounts of epinephrine cause many symptoms. These may include headache, tachycardia, palpitations, sweating, tremulousness, anxiety, nausea and vomiting, and pain. Patients may experience several mental status changes, constipation, and cardiovascular complications.
- The most severe complication is pheochromocytoma crisis.

## Assessment

- The diagnosis of pheochromocytoma is often delayed because hypertension is much more likely to have other causes.
- CT, MRI, and nuclear scans may be useful to localize cortical tumors. Nuclear scan after injection of iodine meta-iodobenzylguanidine (MIBG) is used for localized or metastatic pheochromocytomas.

## Therapeutic Approaches and Nursing Care

### Surgery

- The treatment of choice for pheochromocytoma is surgery, as cure is most likely with resectable disease. Radiation therapy is indicated only for palliation of metastatic disease.
- Surgery or other invasive procedures can precipitate severe and uncontrolled hypertension, and patients require alpha-adrenergic blockade beforehand.

### Chemotherapy

- Patients may respond to drugs that are effective for other neuroendocrine neoplasms.
- Chemotherapy may induce tumor lysis.
- Treatment to induce alpha-adrenergic blockade is started at least one to two weeks before surgery or chemotherapy. Phenoxybenzamine is usually the drug of choice.

### Symptom management and supportive care

- Metyrosine is useful to decrease catecholamine synthesis in pheochromocytoma, and is given in combination with phenoxybenzamine and propranolol.

## MULTIPLE ENDOCRINE NEOPLASIA

- Multiple endocrine neoplasia (MEN) includes syndromes in which several endocrine malignancies occur. These are broadly classified as MEN type 1 and type 2.

## Multiple Endocrine Neoplasia Type 1 (MEN 1)

- The endocrine tumors that occur with MEN 1 are parathyroid, pituitary, and pancreatic islet cell.
- Parathyroid neoplasms are the most frequent, occurring in 90% of patients at the average age of 19.
- Pituitary tumors are often not discovered until autopsy.
- On the other hand, 30%–75% of patients who develop pancreatic tumors experience symptoms because their tumors secrete one of several pancreatic peptides.

## Multiple Endocrine Neoplasia Type 2 (MEN 2)

- Three separate forms, or subtypes, may arise: MEN 2A, MEN 2B, and familial medullary thyroid cancer (MTC).

### MEN 2A

- The hallmark tumor of MEN 2A is hyperplasia of thyroid C cells that progresses to MTC.

### MEN 2B

- Patients who have MEN 2B may be identified because of their physical appearance. From 85% to 95% have a marfanoid appearance and several musculoskeletal abnormalities.

## Assessment

- Ongoing screening is the major focus of management for families known to express MEN.
- Screening for MEN 2 begins in early childhood and focuses on identifying elevated serum calcitonin, which may be a marker for early MTC.

## Genetic Basis of MEN 1 and MEN 2

- Patients with familial MEN 1 or 2 develop their tumors because they have inherited a mutated gene that codes for a tumor-suppressor gene or proto-oncogene from one of their parents.

### MEN 1

- Gene linkage and marker studies indicate that the gene responsible for MEN 1 is located on the long arm of chromosome 11 q13.

### MEN 2

- The *RET* proto-oncogene, located on chromosome 10, has been clearly identified to be responsible for MEN 2.
- Genetic testing for *RET* in families with a known risk for MEN 2 (A and B) is now recommended as the diagnostic method of choice.

## Therapeutic Approaches and Nursing Care

- Preventive adrenalectomy or thyroidectomy for MEN 1 and total thyroidectomy for MEN 2 are standard therapy. In MEN 2, prophylactic thyroidectomy may be done as early as age 5. Patients whose adrenal gland or thyroid is resected will require lifelong hormone replacement.
- A major difference in the treatment of parathyroid tumors in MEN 1, and opposed to sporadic tumors, is that all of the parathyroid tissue must be located and removed.
- A small, normal-appearing parathyroid gland must be preserved to maintain calcium homeostasis. It is transplanted away from the thyroid into a muscle in the neck or forearm.

## PRACTICE QUESTIONS

1.  In endocrine malignancies, papillary and follicular tumors arise from the:
    a.  follicle.
    b.  parafollicular cells.
    c.  differentiated papillary or follicular cells.
    d.  none of the above.

2.  Eddie presents with a rapidly growing, firm neck mass. He also exhibits signs of dysphagia and dysphonia. He had been diagnosed with thyroid cancer. Of the four choices listed below, Eddie is most likely to have:
    a.  papillary tumor.
    b.  medullary tumor.
    c.  anaplastic tumor.
    d.  follicular tumor.

3.  Shortly after her 75th birthday party, Mrs. Henning is admitted for assessment for a possible thyroid mass. One early sign you might expect to find present if Mrs. Henning received a positive diagnosis would be:
    a.  painless anterior cervical adenopathy.
    b.  regional lymph node metastasis.
    c.  distant metastasis.
    d.  a and c.

4.  To confirm a thyroid malignancy, Mrs. Henning's physician would be likely to rely on:
    a.  ultrasonography.
    b.  a fine-needle aspirate biopsy.
    c.  radionuclide scanning.
    d.  a thyroid function test.

5.  Brachytherapy with $^{131}$I is used to treat some cases of:
    a.  follicular tumors.
    b.  anaplastic tumors.
    c.  papillary tumors.
    d.  a and c.

6.  Eric is treated with $^{131}$I for his tumor. The side effect he is least likely to experience is probably:
    a.  radiation-induced pulmonary fibrosis.
    b.  nausea and vomiting.
    c.  bone marrow suppression.
    d.  salivary gland inflammation.

7.  You have the opportunity to participate as a member of a team studying the occurrence and incidence of parathyroid adenomas. Appropriate subjects demographically would be most likely to include:
    a.  almost exclusively young black males.
    b.  children and the elderly.
    c.  middle-aged men and women.
    d.  postmenopausal women and sedentary teenage girls.

8. Mrs. Harris is evaluated for a possible diagnosis of parathyroid tumor. During assessment, her health care team will be assessing her for signs of:
   a. parathyroid hyperplasia.
   b. hypercalcemia.
   c. increased levels of PTH.
   d. all of the above.

9. Mrs. Harris' diagnosis is positive, and she is treated with surgery. After surgery, she exhibits signs of "hungry bone syndrome." You are aware that this signifies:
   a. successful extirpation of the tumor.
   b. that calcium and phosphorus have been rapidly deposited into bone.
   c. that Mrs. Harris is experiencing symptomatic hypocalcemia.
   d. all of the above.

10. Mr. Spenser has a pituitary tumor. He has just returned from surgery. As his nurse you need to assess him for which of the following complications of surgery?
    a. water intoxication
    b. dehydration
    c. hypernatremia
    d. all of the above

11. Harriet has an incidentalomas. This tumor is characterized by its excess secretion of the hormone:
    a. cortisol.
    b. estradiol.
    c. aldosterone.
    d. none of the above.

12. Lisa is diagnosed with a stage I adrenocortical tumor. Signs you might expect her to demonstrate include:
    a. hypersecretion of estradiol.
    b. gynecomastia.
    c. hypersecretion of androgen.
    d. a and c.

13. An appropriate treatment for a person with stage I adrenocortical tumor might be:
    a. mitotane chemotherapy.
    b. surgical removal of local and metastatic disease.
    c. ketoconazole therapy.
    d. radiotherapy combined with chemotherapy.

14. Mr. Harvey is diagnosed with pheochromocytoma. He presents with hypertension, pounding headache, and profuse perspiring. In managing his hypertension, you are aware that his is most likely:
    a. indistinguishable from essential hypertension.
    b. normal blood pressure with superimposed paroxysmal hypertension.
    c. sustained hypertension with extreme paroxysms.
    d. all of the above.

15. The treatment of choice for Mr. Harvey is most likely to be:
    a. radiation therapy.
    b. surgery alone.
    c. surgery, with alpha-adrenergic blockade one to two weeks beforehand.
    d. phenoxybenzamine alone or in combination with radiation or surgery.

16. Mr. Hill is being evaluated for possible malignancy. The chief sign he demonstrates is hyperplasia of thyroid C cells with elevated calcitonin levels. This is usually most indicative of:
    a. MEN 1.
    b. MEN 2A.
    c. MEN 2B.
    d. pancreatic islet cell tumor.

17. Bill is 17 and has scoliosis. He complains of increased joint looseness and proximal muscle weakness. On examination, you see that his lips seem enlarged and somewhat bumpy. He also seems to have delayed puberty. These signs lead you to believe Bill should be assessed for possible:
    a. MEN 1.
    b. MEN 2A.
    c. MEN 2B.
    d. pancreatic islet cell tumor.

# ANSWER EXPLANATIONS

1. **The answer is a.** Papillary and follicular tumors arise from the follicle, medullary tumors arise from parafollicular cells, and anaplastic tumors arise from differentiated papillary or follicular cells. (p. 1057)

2. **The answer is c.** Patients typically present with a rapidly growing firm or hard neck mass invading the structures of the neck to cause dysphagia and dysphonia. (p. 1057)

3. **The answer is b.** Young patients with a thyroid mass tend to present with painless anterior cervical adenopathy. In older patients, the first manifestation is usually regional lymph node metastasis or, rarely, distant metastasis. (p. 1058)

4. **The answer is b.** Fine-needle aspirate (FNA) biopsy is the procedure of choice to confirm thyroid malignancy. Thyroid function tests are not included as part of the workup for thyroid cancer because most tumors do not alter the thyroid's functional capacity. Ultrasonography and radionuclide scanning cannot accurately distinguish between benign and malignant nodules but can provide other useful information later. (p. 1058)

5. **The answer is d.** Brachytherapy with $^{131}$I is used to treat some cases of papillary and follicular tumors but not medullary and anaplastic tumors, which do not concentrate and retain iodine. (p. 1060)

6. **The answer is a.** Side effects of $^{131}$I include nausea and vomiting, fatigue, headache, bone marrow suppression, salivary gland inflammation, and infrequently leukemia and radiation-induced pulmonary fibrosis. (p. 1060)

7. **The answer is c.** Parathyroid adenomas occur equally in males and females, who are usually diagnosed in their 40s and 50s. (p. 1062)

8. **The answer is d.** The diagnosis of parathyroid tumor is essentially confirmed by the signs and symptoms of parathyroid hyperplasia or tumor. Immunoassay typically reveals markedly increased levels of PTH. (p. 1062)

9.  **The answer is d.** After surgery, "hungry bone syndrome" signifies successful extirpation of the tumor. In this syndrome, calcium and phosphorus are rapidly deposited into bone, which results in symptomatic hypocalcemia. (p. 1063)

10. **The answer is d.** Surgery can result in swelling and pressure on the pituitary stalk with diabetes insipidus followed by dehydration, water intoxication, and hypernatremia. (p. 1067)

11. **The answer is d.** Nonfunctional tumors do not produce cortical hormones and are called incidentalomas. Functional tumors are characterized by the hormones they produce in excess, such as cortisol, estradiol, or testosterone, and in rare cases, aldosterone. (p. 1072)

12. **The answer is c.** Women are likely to have virilizing tumors and have symptoms reflecting hypersecretion of androgen. Tumors that hypersecrete estradiol are the rarest adrenal tumors and generally occur in young to middle-aged men, who experience diminished libido, testicular atrophy, and gynecomastia. Sex hormone-secreting tumors in children are manifested by precocious puberty. (p. 1072)

13. **The answer is b.** Whenever possible, surgical removal of local and metastatic disease is recommended because surgery offers the only chance for cure of malignant adrenal tumors. Cure is likely only with stage I or II tumors. Chemotherapy is given in some instances, with mitotane as the usual first-line agent. Because of delays in diagnosis, many patients already have progressive disease that does not respond to treatment. Palliative treatment for these persons will reduce symptoms produced by hormone excess. Thus, drugs for Cushing's syndrome may be ketoconazole, aminoglutethimide, or metyrapone. (p. 1073)

14. **The answer is d.** Hypertension is the hallmark of pheochromocytoma. Hypertension occurs in one of three patterns: indistinguishable from essential hypertension, normal blood pressure with superimposed paroxysmal hypertension, or sustained hypertension with extreme paroxysms. (p. 1074)

15. **The answer is c.** The treatment of choice for pheochromocytoma is surgery, as cure is most likely with resectable disease. Radiation therapy is indicated only for palliation of metastatic disease. Surgery or other invasive procedures can precipitate severe and uncontrolled hypertension, and patients require alpha-adrenergic blockade beforehand. Treatment to induce alpha-adrenergic blockade is started at least one to two weeks before surgery or chemotherapy. Phenoxybenzamine is usually the drug of choice. (p. 1075)

16. **The answer is b.** The endocrine tumors that occur with MEN 1 are parathyroid, pituitary, and pancreatic islet cell. Parathyroid neoplasms are the most frequent. The hallmark tumor of MEN 2A is hyperplasia of thyroid C cells that progresses to MTC. (p. 1075)

17. **The answer is c.** Patients with MEN 2B may be identified because of their physical appearance. The large majority have a marfanoid appearance and several musculoskeletal abnormalities. (p. 1076)

# Chapter 38    Esophageal, Stomach, Liver, Gallbladder, and Pancreatic Cancers

- The gastrointestinal tract accounts for the highest incidence of malignant tumors.
- Incidence among men is compared with that among women in Table 38-1, text page 1084. Incidence in men decreases from the esophagus to the large intestine, whereas the opposite is true for women.
- The problems common to all gastrointestinal cancers stem from delay in clinical presentation.
- Gastrointestinal tumors proliferate insidiously and extend locally.
- The metastasis of gastrointestinal tumors typically occurs by local spread, blood vessel invasion, and dissemination through the lymphatic system.
- Most tumors of the gastrointestinal tract are adenocarcinomas, with the exception of the esophagus and anus, where squamous cell carcinomas predominate.
- Prognosis depends on the tumor size, degree of cellular differentiation, extent of metastases, treatment efficacy, and the individual's general health status.

## ESOPHAGEAL TUMORS
### Introduction

- Many people with esophageal cancer mistakenly attribute its signs and symptoms to more common disorders that affect older adults, for example, indigestion, heartburn and decreased appetite.
- Esophageal tumors that obstruct the lumen can cause a spillover of food, fluid, and saliva into the tracheobronchial tree, resulting in aspiration pneumonia.
- Because cancer of the esophagus grows rapidly, metastasizes early, and is diagnosed late, survival rates are poor.

### Epidemiology

- Esophageal cancer constitutes only 1% of all forms of cancer and is responsible for only 2% of total deaths from cancer.
- Only 7% of those affected will be alive five years after diagnosis.
- The incidence of esophageal cancer is much higher in African-Americans than in whites.
- Carcinoma of the esophagus develops at a younger age in African-Americans than in whites.

### Etiology

- Individuals with esophageal cancer typically have a history of heavy alcohol intake, heavy tobacco use, and poor nutrition.
- Cirrhosis, micronutrient deficiency, anemia, and poor oral hygiene may be contributing etiologic factors.
- Nitrosamines in food and vitamin deficiencies are among the factors associated with the high incidence of esophageal cancer.
- Medical conditions of chronic irritation have been cited as possible etiologic factors: these include hiatal hernia, reflux esophagitis, and diverticula.
- Chronic consumption of hot or heavily seasoned foods and liquids has been associated with this disease.

432

- Barrett's esophagus, which develops from chronic esophageal reflux, is recognized as an important risk factor for the development of adenocarcinoma of the esophagus.
- Tylosis palmaris et plantaris, a rare inherited syndrome characterized by hyperkeratosis of the palms or soles and papillomas of the esophagus, has a strong association with esophageal cancer.
- In areas with a high incidence of esophageal cancer, dietary deficiencies of selenium are correlated with esophageal cytological changes.

## Prevention, Screening, Early Detection Programs

- Counseling on nutrition, alcohol, and tobacco is an important measure for prevention. Chronic users of over-the-counter medications for gastrointestinal upsets should be encouraged to seek medical attention to evaluate potential problems.
- There are no cost-effective screening methods to permit early diagnosis.

## Pathophysiology

- Malignant lesions occur at all levels of the esophagus.
- The site of esophageal tumors is an important factor in detection and prognosis. The distribution of occurrence generally follows this pattern:
  - cervical esophagus 15%
  - upper and middle thoracic esophagus 50%
  - lower thoracic esophagus 35%

### Cellular characteristics

- Squamous cell carcinoma (85%) and adenocarcinoma (<10%) are the two major histological types of esophageal cancer.
- The esophagus is almost entirely lined with squamous epithelium; thus it follows that squamous cell carcinoma would dominate.
- An infiltrative pattern of tumor growth enriches and thickens the wall, thus leading to marked luminal narrowing. Most often the tumor has a polypoid mass projecting into the esophageal lumen.
- Because the ulcerative lesion expands in the submucosa, the lesion can be elevated to such an extent that it obstructs the lumen.

### Progression of disease

- Because there is no serosal covering to the esophagus, tumors can spread into the adjacent mediastinal tissues early in the disease.
- Squamous cell carcinomas extend beyond the lumen wall to invade adjoining structures in about 60% of cases.

### Patterns of spread

- Tumors of the esophagus metastasize principally by way of the lymphatic system.
- Hematogenous spread of tumor cells or tumor emboli is another mode of metastasis.
- Distant metastases to the lung, liver, adrenal glands, bone, brain, and kidney are common with advanced disease.

## Clinical Manifestations

- Initial symptoms include a vague sense of pressure, fullness, indigestion, and occasional substernal distress.
- Dysphagia and weight loss extending over three to six months are classic symptoms.

- A significant characteristic of esophageal cancer is the progressive nature of the dysphagia.
- Pain on swallowing occurs in about 50% of individuals with esophageal cancer.
- Weight loss of 10%–20% inevitably follows and is a dramatic symptom, equaled in frequency only by pancreatic cancer.
- A characteristic cough-swallow sequence may indicate aspiration of food or a tracheoesophageal fistula.

## Assessment

### Physical examination

- Individuals with advanced disease usually exhibit profound dysphagia and weight loss, palpable enlarged lymph nodes, and enlarged or displaced organs.

### Diagnostic studies

#### Radiological examination

- The double-contrast barium study can provide the initial assessment of the extent of the disease in the esophagus as well as any involvement of other thoracic structures.
- Computed tomography (CT) scan is an excellent modality for staging but is not appropriate to screen for esophageal cancer.

#### Endoscopy and biopsy

- Endoscopic visualization is performed to confirm the diagnosis of esophageal cancer in those individuals who have an abnormal barium swallow.
- Visualization of lesions by endoscopy has limitations and is therefore complemented by cytological examination.
- Endoscopic ultrasound enables direct visualization of the tumor and determines the depth of penetration through the wall and into surrounding structures as well as any presence of adenopathy.
- Biopsy of lymph nodes is a definitive diagnostic tool.

### Prognostic indicators

- Any invasion into the aorta and trachea is an indication of advanced disease.
- The depth of invasion, involvement of lymph nodes, and metastatic spread to other viscera are the most important variables affecting survival.

## Classification and Staging

- Unlike more accessible cancers, clinical staging of esophageal cancer is difficult to accomplish without invasive measures.
- The aggressiveness of the therapeutic approach is based on an evaluation of the individual and the extent to which the disease has progressed.
- Pathological staging is based on surgical exploration and histological examination of the resected specimen and its lymph nodes.
- The American Joint Committee for Cancer Staging and End-Results Reporting has developed a standardized classification system listed in Table 38-2, text page 1087.

## Therapeutic Approaches and Nursing Care

### Treatment planning

#### Selection of the treatment plan

- The goal of interdisciplinary planning is to select the therapies most appropriate for the extent of the tumor and for the individual.
- Surgical resection, radiotherapy, and chemotherapy are used to treat esophageal cancer.
- The most effective combination or sequence of therapies has yet to be established.
- Preoperative radiation therapy and chemotherapy have been shown to improve resectability rates but not long-term survival rates.
- The optimal candidate for curative treatment should be free of any renal, cardiac, and pulmonary diseases, be relatively well nourished, and have a tumor that is localized, responsive, and accessible to treatment (i.e., stage I or II).
- Certain findings will preclude an individual from consideration for curative treatment:
  - fixed lymph nodes (N3)
  - a fixed tumor mass (T3)
  - extension of the tumor outside the esophagus (T3, M1)
  - recurrent laryngeal nerve involvement (T3, M1)
- In cases of advanced disease, the quality of life can be improved by restoration or maintenance of a patent gastrointestinal tract.

#### Preparation for treatment

- If an aggressive treatment plan has been selected, ideally the individual will undergo pretreatment preparation to improve general health and nutrition.
- Intensive nutritional therapy (which can include total parenteral nutrition, enteral tube feedings, or high-calorie protein liquid supplements) may be given.
- The high incidence of aspiration that occurs in individuals with esophageal cancer dictates that pulmonary hygiene be a priority in pretreatment care.
- An acceptable method for controlling secretions (e.g., a nearby basin, use of oral suction equipment) should be established.

### Radiation

- Squamous cell carcinoma of the esophagus is more responsive than adenocarcinoma to radiotherapy.
- Radiation can result in rapid relief of an obstruction.
- Radiotherapy alone is not being used now because few individuals are being diagnosed in the early stages when radiation can be effective for cure.
- The most important factor in determining the appropriateness of radiation is whether the individual is potentially curable or whether palliation is the only option.
- Small localized lesions (<5 cm) with no evidence of metastases can be treated for cure with radiotherapy alone or in combination.
- About 60% of esophageal cancers are beyond potential cure at diagnosis because of distant spread.
- Radiotherapy is the treatment favored by many clinicians for stage I and II cervical esophageal lesions since surgical mortality rates are high and the larynx can be preserved with radiation.
- Esophageal fistula, stricture, hemorrhage, radiation pneumonitis, and pericarditis are possible problems.
- Side effects expected during therapy are swallowing difficulties, such as burning, pain, dryness, and skin reactions. Nursing management should be aimed at anticipating and preventing complications of the radiation therapy and concomitant therapies, maintaining adequate nutritional intake, and minimizing the discomfort of esophageal and skin irritation.

### Preoperative radiation therapy

- Preoperative radiation can reduce tumor bulk and improve surgical resectability, enable individuals with esophageal tumors to swallow, significantly improve nutritional status, and reduce operative risk.
- Increased resectability rates and decreased operative mortality rates occur when combination therapy is used.

### Postoperative radiation therapy

- Postoperative radiation therapy is administered to eradicate residual tumor cells in the area of the surgical site.

### Intracavity radiation

- Through the use of intraluminal brachytherapy, it is possible to provide a therapeutic boost to the local area involved.

## Surgery

- The goal of surgery may be cure or palliation, depending on the stage of the tumor and the overall condition of the individual.
- Curative surgery attempts to eradicate the tumor and reestablish esophageal continuity.
- Palliative surgery may aim to maintain esophageal patency.
- Surgery can be used alone or in combination with chemotherapy or radiation.
- Indications for curative surgery include a satisfactory nutritional state, a resectable tumor without evidence of invasion of adjacent structures, no distant metastases, and no serious concomitant diseases.

### Surgical approaches

- The surgical technique and approach to esophageal resection depend on the location of the tumor.
- Surgery is the best treatment for control of a local tumor and is the best treatment to provide relief of dysphagia.
- Usually a portion of the proximal stomach is removed along with the esophagus, which gives rise to the term *total* or *partial esophagogastrectomy.*
- Currently, four surgical approaches are being used: left thoracoabdominal approach, combined abdominal and right thoracotomy approach (Ivor-Lewis), transhiatal approach, and radical esophagectomy (en bloc resection). See Figures 38-2, 38-3, and 38-4, on text pages 1090–1092.
- Reconstruction following esophagectomy can be achieved by various procedures. Elevating the stomach to create an esophagogastrostomy is the most widely used reconstructive procedure.

### Special considerations: cervical esophagus

- Resection of lesions and reconstruction of the cervical esophagus require careful planning because of the difficulties imposed by location. Surgery is extensive and is recommended only if cure is the goal.

- Resection of cervical esophagus lesions involves removing all or part of the pharynx, larynx, thyroid, and proximal esophagus.
- Cervical esophageal continuity usually is reestablished by anastomosing the stomach to the pharynx, called a *gastric pull-up*.
- The postoperative period can be plagued with complications of fistula, anastomotic leak, strictures, respiratory insufficiency, pulmonary embolism, obstruction, and infection.

### Postoperative care

- Respiratory complications, fistulae, and anastomotic leaks constitute the bulk of complications following surgical resection for esophageal cancer. Severe atelectasis, pneumonia, pulmonary edema, and adult respiratory distress syndrome contribute to postoperative morbidity and mortality.
- The esophagus is a thin-walled organ drawn upward with each swallow, so an anastomosis involving the esophagus has more of a risk of developing dehiscence and anastomotic leak than any other area of the gastrointestinal tract.
- Fever or pain is usually the earliest sign of wound dehiscence or anastomotic leak.
- Contrast studies can be done four to six days after surgery to evaluate anastomotic healing.
- Virulent mouth organisms and overgrowth of pathogenic bacteria on ulcerating lesions may be a source of wound and intracavitary infections.
- Esophagocutaneous fistulae usually appear in raised, reddened, or necrotic areas along the suture line.
- The postoperative nursing care of the individual with an esophagogastrectomy includes anticipation and prevention of reflux aspiration and esophagitis.
- Feeding jejunostomy tubes may have been placed preoperatively or at the time of surgery.
- Tube feedings may be started after surgery to maintain nutrition and prevent bacterial translocation as a source of sepsis.
- Prior to surgery for colon interposition, a regimen of oral antibiotics is begun to suppress bacterial flora in the intestine.
- Foul-smelling breath is a distressing consequence of having used a segment of bowel to reconstruct the esophagus.

## Chemotherapy

- Chemotherapy in the treatment of esophageal tumors has assumed an increasingly important role.
- Combination regimens are more effective than single-agent therapy.
- Preoperative chemoradiation therapy delivers local and systemic therapy simultaneously, using combination chemotherapy, usually cisplatin and 5-FU, and fractionated radiation doses that total 3000–5000 cGy before surgery.

## Symptom Management and Supportive Care

- The objective of palliative therapy is to relieve the distressing symptoms of esophageal cancer—in particular, progressive dysphagia, which occurs in about 90% of individuals with advanced disease.
- Laser therapy is being used more frequently to alleviate esophageal obstruction or severe dysphagia.
- Palliative resection with reconstruction or surgical bypass of the esophagus will be done to relieve severe symptoms of the disease or reduce the size of the tumor.
- In some instances esophagectomy may be performed as a palliative procedure for esophageal disruption. This type of surgery is usually done as an emergency for perforation caused by palliative therapy or by the tumor itself.

- A number of synthetic esophageal funnel prosthetic tubes have been designed to create an open passage for swallowing when the esophagus is obstructed by an inoperable tumor.
- Satisfactory palliative results achieved with either type of tube are limited; however, increased food intake after tube placement occurs in about 80% of individuals.
- Other palliative treatments include hyperthermochemoradiotherapy, high-dose photoirradiation, and laser therapy.
- Gastrostomy and jejunostomy tubes are alternative palliative procedures for individuals with esophageal cancer.
- Nursing management of the individual with advanced esophageal cancer includes control of pain, nutritional support, and psychological support.

## STOMACH TUMORS

### Introduction

- Gastric cancer is epidemic in Japan, Eastern Europe, and portions of Central and South America.
- Japan has the highest incidence of gastric cancer, which is the number one cause of death nationally.
- The prognosis for individuals diagnosed with stomach cancer in the United States is extremely poor, with the five-year survival rate ranging from 5% to 15%.
- Gastric cancer is insidious in its onset and development, usually infiltrates rapidly, and can be disseminated throughout the body before overt signs are manifested. Gastric cancer mimics several other gastrointestinal maladies and diseases, such as polyps, ulcers, dyspepsia, and gastritis.
- Inappropriate use of home remedies, self-medication, and misdiagnosis are major challenges.

### Epidemiology

- Japan has the highest incidence in the world of gastric cancer for both men and women, and the disease is the country's major cause of death.
- In the United States the incidence of gastric cancer is low.
- It is predominantly a disease of men worldwide, occurring about twice as often in men as in women.

### Etiology

- Factors believed to contribute to or be associated with gastric cancer are largely environmental and genetic.
- The fact that immigrants exhibit incidence rates similar to those of their country of origin has led researchers to accept exogenous influences such as environment and diet.
- A high intake of smoked or salted meats and fish and nitrates, along with low consumption of fresh vegetables and fruits, have all correlated with increased gastric cancer risk in populations.
- High intake of grains and low intake of animal fats and proteins appear to be associated with a decreased risk.
- Those at greatest risk for the development of gastric cancer are older than 40 years of age and exhibit one or several of the following factors:
  - low socioeconomic status
  - poor nutritional habits
  - vitamin A deficiency
  - family history
  - previous gastric resection for benign disease
  - pernicious anemia
  - *Helicobacter pylori* infection
  - gastric atrophy and chronic gastritis
  - occupational risk factors (rubber and coal workers)

## Prevention, Screening, Early Detection Programs

- Screening tests usually include barium x-ray or upper endoscopy, which has 90% sensitivity and specificity. The detection of early gastric cancer in the screened populations has been substantial and has resulted in a high cure rate.

## Pathophysiology

### Cellular characteristics

- Approximately 95% of gastric cancers are adenocarcinomas.
- Most gastric cancers arise in the antrum, the distal third of the stomach.

### Progression of disease

- Because initial symptoms are vague, gastric cancer is usually locally advanced or metastatic when an individual is first symptomatic.

### Patterns of spread

- There are four characteristic routes by which gastric carcinoma spreads and metastasizes: (1) by direct extension into adjacent structures such as the pancreas, liver or esophagus; (2) local or distant nodal metastases mostly on the left side of the neck (Virchow's node); (3) bloodstream metastases; and (4) intraperitoneal dissemination, particularly to the ovary, perirectal area, and periumbilical nodules.
- The pattern of metastatic spread of gastric cancer correlates with the size and location of the tumor.
- Distant metastatic sites are the lung, adrenals, bone, liver, rectum, and peritoneal cavity.

## Clinical Manifestations

- The initial symptoms of gastric cancer are vague and nonspecific, with variable duration.
- Pain in the epigastrium, back, or retrosternal area is often cited as an early symptom that was ignored or self-treated.
- The individual may complain of a vague, uneasy sense of fullness, a feeling of heaviness, and moderate distention after meals.
- As the disease advances, progressive weight loss can result from disturbances in appetite, nausea, and vomiting.
- Weakness, fatigue, and anemia are common findings.

## Assessment

### Patient and family history

- Areas to include in a nutritional history and assessment are as follows:
  - food and fluid intake patterns
  - symptoms associated with eating
  - change in dietary habits or appetite
  - weight
  - bowel patterns and habits
  - medications
  - previous and/or concurrent illness

### Physical examination

- The physical examination includes palpation of the abdomen and lymph nodes, particularly the supraclavicular and axillary lymph nodes.
- Enlarged lymph nodes and hepatomegaly indicate the need for biopsy.
- Advanced gastric cancer can result in anemia and jaundice.

### Diagnostic studies

- Upper endoscopic gastroduodenoscopy (EGD) is now considered the study of choice to establish a diagnosis of gastric cancer. Biopsy and brushings for cytology can be performed at the same time.
- Usually, six to ten biopsy samples need to be obtained to yield an accurate diagnosis.
- Flexible endoscopic gastroscopy is more comfortable for the individual and less traumatic to the gastrointestinal tissues.
- A double-contrast upper gastrointestinal series will reveal the mucosal pattern, character of mobility, distensibility, and flexibility of the stomach wall.
- CT scanning is useful in defining tumor extension and systemic metastases.
- EUS has been used to accurately stage gastric cancers.
- Laboratory analyses include hematologic profiles, which may reveal anemia resulting from gradual blood loss in both gastric cancer and chronic gastric ulcer.

### Prognostic indicators

- Karyometric studies of DNA content have correlated high-ploidy gastric tumors with a higher incidence of lymphatic and vascular invasion.
- Strong predictors of outcome in gastric cancer have been shown to be lymph node metastases and the number of positive lymph nodes at the time of surgery.

## Classification and Staging

- The prognosis and treatment plan depend on the stage of the disease and the general well-being of the individual.
- Table 38-3 on text page 1098 lists the TNM classification for gastric carcinoma.

## Therapeutic Approaches and Nursing Care

- Localized gastric carcinomas are treated with aggressive surgery alone or in combination with chemotherapy or radiotherapy for curative intent. Approximately 50% of individuals are candidates for curative resection.
- Advanced tumors that are partially resectable, unresectable, or disseminated are treated with combination therapy including surgery and chemotherapy, with or without radiotherapy, and palliative surgery.

### Surgery

- Surgery is the only treatment modality that can potentially cure localized gastric cancer. It is also the most effective approach for palliation. Definitive or palliative gastrectomy should always be considered, even in individuals with known metastatic disease. Consideration for surgery is given to any individual with a good performance status and no major medical contraindications.
- Measures to prepare an individual for surgery include correction of fluid and electrolyte imbalances, correction of anemia from chronic blood loss, and attention to nutritional status.
- Gastric cancers should not be considered unresectable or incurable based on the size of the tumor.

## Total gastrectomy

- A total gastrectomy may be performed for a resectable lesion located in the midportion or body of the stomach. Linitus plastica is usually treated with a total gastrectomy because of the extensive involvement of the gastric wall.
- Pneumonia, infection, anastomotic leak, hemorrhage, and reflux aspiration are possible complications.
- Overall mortality rates are 10%–15% for individuals who have a total gastrectomy.

## Radical subtotal gastrectomy

- Lesions located in the middle and distal portions of the stomach are treated by radical subtotal gastrectomy. A Billroth I or Billroth II operation will be performed.
- The Billroth I involves a limited amount of resection, and as a result generally produces lower cure rates than a Billroth II. A Billroth I is usually selected if the individual is debilitated and needs restricted intraoperative time.
- A Billroth II is a wider resection, thereby decreasing the possibility of nodal or metastatic recurrence.
- Gastric emptying is altered by the Billroth I and II procedures resulting in the following: dumping syndrome, nausea, vomiting, diarrhea, steatorrhea, weight loss, vitamin deficiency, and anastomotic leak.

## Proximal subtotal gastrectomy

- A proximal subtotal gastrectomy may be performed for a resectable tumor located in the proximal portion of the stomach or cardia.
- Potential complications include pneumonia, anastomotic leak, infection, reflux aspiration, and esophagitis.

## Surgical palliation

- Resection is the most effective palliative treatment for advanced gastric cancer if the individual is a suitable candidate for the procedure. Although the survival time with palliative surgery is disappointing, it appears to be longer than without resection.
- Relief of gastrointestinal symptoms, such as vomiting, can be achieved with a palliative resection. Palliative resection may increase the effectiveness of adjuvant therapy.

## Postoperative care

- Pneumonia, infection, anastomotic leak, hemorrhage, and reflux aspiration are frequent complications following radical gastric surgery.
- Dumping syndrome is a potential sequela of subtotal gastrectomy and total gastrectomy that affects many but not all individuals.
- Vitamin $B_{12}$ deficiency will occur in an individual with a total gastrectomy.

## Radiation

- Gastric adenocarcinomas are generally radiosensitive. Radiation therapy is somewhat prohibitive because the stomach lies deep in the abdomen, and the tumor is often widely disseminated.
- Radiation therapy can be administered as adjuvant therapy along with chemotherapy and surgery and is useful for inoperable cancer or locally advanced or recurrent local disease.
- Excessive weight loss is the main dose-limiting toxicity that can delay or halt treatment.
- Radiotherapy is used to augment locoregional control of residual or unresectable gastric cancer.

- Radiotherapy may contribute to the palliation of symptoms and prolongation of survival in individuals with gastric cancer.
- Intraoperative radiotherapy (IORT), used extensively in Japan, allows direct visualization of the site to be irradiated and the opportunity to move the radiosensitive tissues away from the field during the radiation.

### Chemotherapy

- No specific chemotherapeutic regimen alone has been able to establish a clear impact on survival from gastric cancer.
- Combination drug therapy appears to be superior to single agents.
- The combination regimens used most commonly are FAM (5-FU, doxorubicin mitomycin C); FAP (5-FU, doxorubicin, platinol); FAMTX (5-FU, doxorubicin, leucovorin); and EAP (etoposide, doxorubicin, cisplatin).

### Symptom Management and Supportive Care

- Advanced gastric cancer can result in an individual's rapid deterioration.
- As gastric cancer advances, nutrition becomes a serious problem because of disruption of stomach continuity or stomach dysfunction.
- Nutritional surveillance and aggressive approaches to maintaining a high level of nutrition are nursing priorities.
- Individuals with gastric cancer commonly die of bronchopneumonia or lung abscess secondary to malnutrition or immobility.

## LIVER TUMORS

### Introduction

- Hepatocellular cancer is one of the ten most common cancers in the world. Liver cancer is the main cause of cancer death in Africa and Asia.
- Liver cancers have unusual clinical features and are commonly diagnosed at an advanced stage.
- At present, no specific treatment effectively controls this aggressive malignancy, and the outlook remains poor.

### Epidemiology

- An unusual epidemiological aspect of liver cancer is its geographic distribution.
- Liver cancer is the most common cause of death in males worldwide. In all populations, the incidence rate increases with age.
- The average age of onset is 60–70 years in the United States.

### Etiology

- Hepatocellular carcinomas are associated with environmental and hereditary factors, hepatitis B and hepatitis C viruses, and cirrhosis.
- Aflatoxins, produced by the molds *Aspergillus flavus* and *Aspergillus parasiticus*, are suspect as etiologic agents.
- The macronodular cirrhosis associated with chronic hepatitis B virus is a major risk factor for liver cancer.
- Alcoholic cirrhosis is a common risk factor for cancer in the United States.
- Ingestion of estrogens, androgens, and oral contraceptives has been reported to be associated with liver tumors.

## Prevention, Screening, Early Detection Programs

- Efforts are under way in parts of China to reduce or eliminate hepatocellular carcinoma by aggressive programs to vaccinate newborns against hepatitis B virus.
- The present recommendation in the United States to vaccinate all newborns against hepatitis B virus may prevent future cases of hepatocellular carcinoma.
- Prevention of hepatitis B and hepatitis C infection is the ideal measure.
- In the United States those with the greatest risk are hepatitis B–positive males with a family history of the disease, individuals older than 45 years, or individuals who have cirrhosis.
- Ultrasound (US) and serum alfa-fetoprotein (AFP) tests are inexpensive and relatively effective tools to screen for hepatocellular carcinoma in high-risk populations.

## Pathophysiology

- Tumors of the liver may be a primary cancer of the liver or secondary tumors that have metastasized from other sites.

### Cellular characteristics

#### Primary liver cancer

- Most primary tumors of the liver are adenocarcinomas of two cell types: about 90% are hepatocellular carcinomas arising from the liver cells; about 7% are cholangiocarcinomas arising from the bile ducts.
- Hepatocellular carcinoma originate mainly in the right lobe of the liver.
- The tumor may be multicentric in origin, or it may start with a single focus that subsequently develops satellite lesions.
- Cholangiocarcinomas tend to invade surrounding parenchyma in a disorderly, irregular manner and tend to metastasize late.
- Liver tumors are often well-differentiated lesions with clearly defined margins.
- About 50% of individuals with primary liver cancer will not develop extrahepatic spread of tumor.
- Regional lymph node metastasis is uncommon—a definite characteristic of liver cancer.

#### Secondary liver cancer

- The liver is 20 times more likely to harbor a metastatic deposit than a primary liver cancer.
- Metastases to the liver usually are from the following high-incidence sites: lung, breast, kidney, and the intestinal tract (gallbladder, extrahepatic bile ducts, pancreas, stomach, colon, rectum).
- Metastatic tumors in the liver usually indicate that the primary cancer is incurable.

### Progression of disease

- Liver failure and hemorrhage have been cited as the cause of death in about 50% of individuals with liver cancer.
- Esophageal varices and unrelenting ascites are common sequelae of either primary or secondary liver cancer.
- Overall five-year survival rate is about 5%.
- If the disease is untreated, death usually occurs within six to eight weeks following diagnosis.

### Patterns of spread

- Liver cancer tends to advance by direct extension within and around the liver.

- About 50% of individuals with liver cancer will have distant metastases to regional lymph nodes, lungs, bone, adrenal glands, and brain.
- Liver tumors typically alter the pattern of blood flow within the liver.

## Clinical Manifestations

- The tumor can grow to huge proportions before symptoms appear. In adults the most common presenting complaint is right upper quadrant abdominal pain that is not severe, but rather dull and aching.
- Profound, progressive weakness and fatigue are characteristic of liver cancer. Fullness in the epigastrium, especially after meals, and constipation or diarrhea are common manifestations. Anorexia and weight loss are indicators of advanced disease.
- Mild jaundice may be present.
- Cirrhosis is found in 30%–70% of persons with hepatocellular carcinomas.
- Ascites and signs of portal hypertension that result from portal vein compression frequently accompany advanced disease.

## Assessment

- The only definitive diagnostic tool is tissue diagnosis. Unfortunately, the risk of hemorrhage following needle biopsy is significant; therefore, noninvasive measures are relied on heavily.

### Patient and family history

- A history of cirrhosis, hepatitis B or hepatitis C virus infection, or exposure to mycotoxins or other agents that cause chronic liver failure will aid in confirming the diagnosis.

### Physical examination

- A complete physical examination usually reveals a painful, enlarged liver and such manifestations as ascites, edema, an audible arterial bruit, jaundice, and splenomegaly.

### Diagnostic studies

- A simple radiograph of the abdomen may establish hepatomegaly and displacement or deformity of adjoining structures.
- US of the abdomen, CT scan of the abdomen and lungs, and MRI are noninvasive techniques used in the diagnostic evaluation of liver cancer.
- Radionuclide scanning is an effective noninvasive technique for outlining primary and metastatic tumors of the liver.
- Selective hepatic arteriography is the best way to delineate hepatic artery anatomy and the presence of vascular invasion or encasement.
- Combining CT scan with an arteriogram (CTA) can help detect lesions less than 1 cm in diameter.

### Laboratory studies

- In the absence of cirrhosis, tumor growth can extensively involve parenchyma before liver function is impaired.
- AFP is a tumor marker that is elevated in the serum of 70%–90% of individuals with primary hepatocellular carcinoma.
- Elevated levels of CEA are not indicative of primary liver cancer but may signify metastatic involvement.

Biopsy

- Biopsy is required to establish a histological diagnosis.
- If the tumor appears to be unresectable, a percutaneous needle biopsy can be performed, usually as a fine-needle aspiration (FNAB) with US or CT scan guidance. Needle biopsy should be performed only on a cooperative individual with normal hemostatic function.
- Potential complications following liver biopsy are hemorrhage, shock, peritonitis, and pneumothorax.

## Classification and Staging

- Table 38-4 on text page 1106 lists TNM classifications for liver cancer.
- The staging system has not been universally accepted but is available for use.

## Therapeutic Approaches and Nursing Care
### Treatment planning

- For individuals with solitary, localized liver cancer, advances in surgery, radiotherapy, and chemotherapy offer hope of cure or palliation.
- The choice of treatment depends on type and extent of tumor, concomitant diseases, liver function and reserve, individual/family preference, hematologic status, nutritional status, age, and skill of the principal clinicians.

### Pretreatment therapy

- Most individuals with primary liver cancer have some degree of anemia, which must be corrected.
- Deficits in clotting mechanisms can exist, and vitamin K is administered, fluid and electrolyte imbalances are corrected, and measures to prevent trauma or bleeding are taken.
- Vitamins A, C, D, and B complex can be given to reduce the effect of jaundice. Pruritus, which frequently accompanies jaundice, is precipitated by irritation of the cutaneous sensory nerve fibers by accumulated bile salts. Meticulous skin hygiene and efforts to reduce itching are instituted.
- Most individuals with liver cancer are in poor nutritional state and benefit from a diet high in proteins and carbohydrates and moderate in fats.

### Objectives of treatment
#### *Primary liver cancer*

- Cure is the objective of the therapy if the primary liver tumor is a localized, solitary mass without evidence of regional lymph node involvement or distant metastases.
- Only about 25% of individuals with primary liver cancer are candidates for radical resection.
- Aggressive efforts toward eradicating residual cancer cells and possible micrometastases with adjuvant chemotherapy and radiotherapy usually are initiated.
- Palliation of the disabling effects of liver cancer may be the objective of treatment for advanced disease.

#### *Secondary liver tumors*

- Aggressive therapy is employed if the metastatic deposit is a solitary or well-defined mass in a single lobe of the liver.
- The aim of aggressive treatment of metastatic tumors in the liver is to control the tumor, increase survival time, and palliate debilitating symptoms such as jaundice, anemia, and pain.

## Surgery

- Surgical excision is the most definitive treatment for primary liver tumors and depends mainly on tumor size, location, and the condition of the uninvolved liver.
- Contraindications to major hepatic resection include the following: (1) severe cirrhosis; (2) distant metastases; (3) jaundice; (4) ascites; (5) poor visualization on angiographic studies; (6) poor liver function; and (7) involvement of the inferior vena cava and the portal vein bifurcation by tumor.
- Greater than three-quarters (80%–85%) of the noncirrhotic liver can be removed safely unless the tumor is in the posterior segment of the right lobe.
- Right or left hepatic lobectomy, trisegmentectomy, and lateral segmentectomy are the classic liver resections.
- Cryosurgery with liquid nitrogen has been employed for local destruction of tumors in individuals with multiple primary or metastatic tumors in both lobes of the liver.
- Liver transplantation is controversial and fraught with a high incidence of recurrent cancer in the transplanted liver.
- Hepatic artery occlusion or embolization is used to deprive the tumor of its blood supply, causing tumor necrosis.
- Percutaneous injections of liver tumors with ethanol under US guidance have been used as both palliative and curative treatment.

### Postoperative care

- Overall surgical mortality (death rate of individuals who do not survive the hospitalization period) is less than 10% with hepatic resection.
- The major complications following liver resection include the following:
  - hemorrhage
  - biliary fistula
  - subphrenic abscess
  - infection
  - pneumonia
  - atelectasis
  - transient metabolic consequences
  - portal hypertension
  - clotting defects

### Postoperative complications

#### Hemorrhage

- Hemorrhage usually will appear within the first 24 hours following surgery.
- Nursing assessments include frequent monitoring of vital signs; measurement of abdominal girth; frequent checks for bleeding from incision sites, urine, and stool; and close attention to fluid and electrolyte levels and blood profiles.

#### Biliary fistula

- Excessive drainage of bile through the subhepatic drain could indicate a biliary fistula pouring large amounts of bile into the subhepatic space.
- Fever, pain, distended abdomen, and altered vital signs may accompany a biliary fistula.

### Subphrenic abscess

- Incomplete or insufficient drainage of the surgical defect can precipitate a subphrenic abscess.
- Development of sharp, piercing right upper quadrant pain later in the postoperative course and a low-grade fever are other warning signs.

### Infection

- Individuals with cirrhosis are more prone to infection following hepatic resection than individuals without cirrhosis.
- The mortality associated with serious infection is high.

### Pneumonia and atelectasis

- Aggressive pulmonary toilet is especially important.
- Early ambulation, administration of analgesics prior to pulmonary exercise, incisional support, and avoidance of contact with persons with respiratory infections are important nursing care measures.

### Transient metabolic consequences

- Jaundice is common during the first postoperative week.
- More often, jaundice results from multiple blood transfusions and anoxia of the hepatocytes caused by vascular occlusion during surgery.

### Portal hypertension

- Portal hypertension is the result of the surgical rerouting of portal venous flow through a small remnant of liver, which leads to sequestration in the splanchnic circulation.

### Clotting defects

- The prothrombin time may be delayed during the first postoperative week.

## Chemotherapy

- Chemotherapy may be the treatment of choice for unresectable liver tumors.
- Chemotherapeutic agents can be administered by two approaches: systemic administration of single or combination drug regimens, and regional infusion into a hepatic artery or portal vein.
- Chemotherapeutic agents used with primary and secondary liver cancer include doxorubicin, floxuradine (FUDR), 5-FU, cisplatin, streptozocin, etoposide, mitomycin C, folinic acid, mitoxantrone, epirubicin, methyl CCNU, and teniposide.
- Regional therapy provides a high concentration of drug directly and continuously to the tumor, with minimal systemic exposure.
- Catheters for regional therapy administration are placed into the specifically defined vessels identified as the major source of blood supply to the tumor.
- In general, regional infusion is considered superior to systemic chemotherapy.
- Intraperitoneal administration of 5-FU has been well tolerated by individuals and produces results comparable to those with regional therapy.

## Radiation therapy

- Because of the poor tolerance of normal liver tissue, the role of radiotherapy in liver cancer therapy is limited to palliation.

- Relief of pain, improvements in strength, increased appetite, and increased liver function have been reported with doses ranging from 1900 cGy to 3100 cGy over a period of 2 to 20 days.
- Radiation therapy has been enhanced without damage to normal liver tissue by the use of $^{131}$I-Lipidiol, a radiolabeled iodinated contrast medium.
- Radiotherapy is used in conjunction with surgery or chemotherapy to palliate symptoms or to eradicate micrometastases.
- The major side effects of radiotherapy to the liver are nausea, vomiting, anorexia, and fatigue.

### Biological and hormonal therapy

- Interferons have been used in combination with chemotherapeutic agents in randomized trials showing tumor regression and longer survival than in those individuals who received no antitumor therapy.

### Symptom Management and Supportive Care

- The prognosis for the individual with liver cancer is dismal. Most individuals die within six months of diagnosis.
- Pain is one of the most difficult problems to manage.
- Ascites can become severe in advanced disease.
- Anorexia and vomiting may be late-stage manifestations in liver cancer.
- Jaundice with pruritus may present an ongoing problem.
- Hepatic coma occurs with profound liver dysfunction as the liver fails to work and toxins accumulate in the body.

### Continuity of Care: Nursing Challenges

- Anticipatory management will be necessary when an individual fails or no longer desires aggressive therapy.

## GALLBLADDER CANCER
### Introduction

- The two most common malignancies of the biliary tree are adenocarcinoma of the gallbladder and bile ducts (cholangiocarcinoma).
- Carcinoma of the gallbladder is rare.

### Epidemiology

- Although gallbladder cancer is a rare form of cancer, it is the most common cancer of the liver and biliary passages.
- Women develop gallbladder cancer three times more often than men.
- Gallbladder cancer is rare in individuals under 50 years of age, with the average age at diagnosis being 60 years.

### Etiology

- Gallstones are the most common factor.
- Gallbladder cancer is more likely to occur in individuals with a single large gallstone than with multiple smaller stones.
- Individuals with a choledochal cyst may develop carcinoma throughout the biliary tree, but most tumors arise in the gallbladder.
- Various chemical carcinogens have been suspected to cause biliary cancers.

- An increased incidence of gallbladder cancer has been reported in rubber plant workers.
- Typhoid carriers have an increased risk of gallbladder and bile duct cancers.

## Prevention, Screening, Early Detection Programs

- At present there is no effective method of screening for gallbladder cancer.
- The presenting symptoms of the disease usually occur with advanced disease, making early detection almost impossible.

## Pathophysiology

### Cellular characteristics

- The vast majority of gallbladder cancers are adenocarcinomas, which occur in 85% of individuals.

### Progression of disease

- Gallbladder cancer is a locally invasive tumor that may extend directly into the gallbladder bed in the liver, extrahepatic bile ducts, duodenum or transverse colon, portal vein, hepatic artery, or pancreas.

### Pattern of spread

- The pattern of spread predictably follows lymphatic and venous drainage of the gallbladder. Venous drainage of the gallbladder is directly into the adjacent liver. The most common pattern of spread of gallbladder cancer is through direct extension into the liver.
- These tumors can spread into and around the cystic duct and can extend into the common bile duct, causing biliary obstruction.

## Clinical Manifestations

- The signs and symptoms of gallbladder cancer are similar to those of gallstones. Right upper quadrant pain, discomfort, and dyspepsia can result from both.
- Individuals with gallbladder cancer commonly have advanced disease and present with nonspecific signs of malaise, weight loss, nausea, vomiting, and anorexia. Almost half present with jaundice.
- In advanced stages of the disease, individuals may present with a palpable mass in the right upper quadrant.

## Assessment

### Patient and family history

- The individual may have had no previous symptoms or vague, chronic complaints of right upper quadrant pain.

### Physical examination

- Jaundice with pruritus may be evident in individuals with an obstructing gallbladder cancer. An individual may have a visibly palpable gallbladder when supine. Severe weight loss may be evident.

### Diagnostic studies

- With the exception of jaundice, no specific laboratory abnormalities are present.
- Ultrasonography, CT scan, MRI, cholangiography, and angiography may all be helpful in evaluating individuals with suspected gallbladder cancer.

- Cholangiography can be useful for diagnosing gallbladder cancer in an individual with jaundice.
- Percutaneous transhepatic cholangiography (PTC) or endoscopic retrograde cholangiopancreatography (ERCP) may both be beneficial.
- Angiography may be the most useful radiological study for staging gallbladder cancer.

### Prognostic indicators

- Histological grade has significant prognostic implications.
- Individuals with metaplasia have a better prognosis. Metaplasia is more common in women.
- Papillary tumors are less likely to directly invade the liver and have a lower incidence of lymph node metastasis.
- Tumors with the best prognosis are those found incidentally at the time of cholecystectomy for symptomatic gallstone disease.

## Classification and Staging

- The American Joint Committee for Cancer Staging and End-Results Reporting has established the TNM classification listed in Table 38-5, text page 1114.

## Therapeutic Approaches and Nursing Care

- Special attention must be given to any liver problems, as cirrhosis and portal hypertension will increase the risk from surgery.
- Local invasion of the adjacent liver is a common finding that can sometimes be managed with a wedge resection of the liver.
- More extensive liver involvement may require a larger liver resection.
- Multiple metastases in both lobes of the liver, or peritoneal or distant metastases are considered contraindications to resection of the primary gallbladder tumor.

### Surgery

- Less than 25% of cancers of the gallbladder are resectable, but the most effective treatment for cancer of the gallbladder is resection of the primary tumor and areas of local invasion.
- Cholecystectomy is the primary treatment of stage I gallbladder carcinoma.
- Laparoscopic removal of the gallbladder is not recommended, since tumor implantation at the trocar sites has been found.
- When the cancer involves deeper layers of the gallbladder wall, the prognosis is grim. A radical or extended cholecystectomy has been recommended.
- Extended cholecystectomy should be considered the therapy of choice for preoperatively recognized and potentially resectable gallbladder cancer.
- For stage I tumors, the five-year survival after routine cholecystectomy is greater than 85%. For stage II, III, and IV tumors, five-year survivals are approximately 25%, 10%, and 2%.

#### Postoperative care

- The main concerns are control of hemorrhage, replacement of blood loss, prevention of infection and pneumonia, and appropriate supportive care. Postoperative complications include hemorrhage, biliary fistula, infection, transient metabolic consequences, subphrenic abscess, pneumonia, atelectasis, portal hypertension, and clotting defects.

### Palliative therapy

- Most therapies for gallbladder cancer are palliative since most individuals are unable to be resected with negative margins.
- Recurrent jaundice and cholangitis are problems that may recur during the course of the disease due to tumor obstruction of the biliary tree or biliary tubes.
- Pain should be treated aggressively to improve the individual's quality of life.
- Opiates, radiation therapy, and percutaneous celiac nerve block may be helpful.
- Operative palliation may be helpful to establish a diagnosis, remove the gallbladder to prevent acute cholecystitis, relieve or prevent pain, and treat or prevent gastric outlet obstruction.
- The addition of any internal-external percutaneous transhepatic biliary stents depends on the extent of the disease and the choice of the physician in treating jaundice.
- The majority of individuals with gallbladder cancer have unresectable disease at the time of diagnosis.
- Less than 5% of all individuals with gallbladder cancer are alive after five years.

### Radiation therapy

- Used to treat individuals with resected as well as unresectable tumors.
- There has been no proven survival advantage with external-beam radiation alone after surgery.

### Chemotherapy

- Chemotherapy agents for the treatment of gallbladder cancer have been limited due to poor tumor response.
- Mitomycin C and 5-FU have been most commonly used.

## Symptom Management and Supportive Care

- Obstructive jaundice, liver abscess, and liver failure are potential complications.
- Persistent pain, fever, chills, and recurrent jaundice may be symptoms of a liver abscess caused by obstructed bile ducts.
- With progressive liver failure, ascites and increased abdominal girth may cause problems with pain, discomfort, and dyspnea.
- Supportive measures include aggressive pain management and proper body positioning. Ascites can be controlled by fluid and sodium restriction along with diuretic therapy.
- Liver failure usually develops as the disease progresses.

## Continuity of Care: Nursing Challenges

- Most individuals present at an advanced stage and rapidly decline from gallbladder carcinoma.

## PANCREATIC CANCER

### Introduction

- Cancer of the pancreas is the fifth leading cause of death from cancer in the United States. It is ninth among all cancers in incidence in the United States.
- Less than 20% of affected individuals survive one year after diagnosis, and the overall five-year survival is only 3%.
- Pancreatic cancer onset is insidious, with signs and symptoms that occur late, are vague and misleading, and mimic other diseases.
- Recent progress in both surgical management and improved responses to combined therapy have begun to improve overall results.

## Epidemiology

- Pancreatic cancer accounts for 2% of new cancer cases.
- The incidence of pancreatic cancer increases with age, with peak incidence between ages 60 and 70.
- The incidence of pancreatic cancer is slightly higher in African-Americans.

## Etiology

- Cigarette smoking has been the strongest risk factor associated with the development of pancreatic cancer.
- A diet high in animal fat has been associated with an increased risk of pancreatic cancer. Likewise diets high in fresh fruits and vegetables appear to provide a protective effect.

## Prevention, Screening, Early Detection Programs

- Cancer of the pancreas is an insidious disease, with little known about the cause.
- Abnormalities in the expression of the tumor-suppressor gene *p53* and the oncogene *K-ras* seem to be the most common mutations recognized, with each occurring in over 70%–80% of individuals.
- Familial cases of pancreatic cancer are being studied to identify genetic alterations that are inherited through the germ line.

## Pathophysiology

- The most common pathological form of pancreatic cancer is an adenocarcinoma that originates from the cells lining the pancreatic duct. Tumors of the pancreas develop in both the endocrine and the exocrine parenchyma.
- Approximately 90% of tumors arise from the exocrine pancreas, which contains two major types of epithelium: acinar and ductal.
- Cystic neoplasms of the pancreas also arise from the exocrine pancreas.
- Cystic tumors, less common than ductal adenocarcinomas, are found throughout the entire gland, and tend to occur in women.
- Endocrine or islet cell tumors constitute the remainder of pancreatic malignant tumors.

### Cellular characteristics

- Adenocarcinomas of the pancreas usually are tannish, hard, nodular, firm masses with a large amount of fibrosis.
- Often, pancreatic lesions are associated with an extensive desmoplastic reaction that can make diagnosis on the basis of needle biopsy difficult.
- The presence of metastases is the most reliable criterion for establishing malignancy.

### Progression of disease

- Pancreatic cancer arises in the head of the pancreas in 60%–70% of cases. About 15% of tumors develop in the body of the gland, another 10% develop in the tail, and the remaining 5%–15% are diffuse.
- Extension beyond the confines of the pancreas is the rule rather than the exception with ductal carcinoma of the pancreas.
- The bile duct is invaded early in the course of the disease.
- Tumors tend to invade local structures, such as the duodenum and retroperitoneum, either directly or via the course of autonomic nerves of the celiac plexus. Some degree of perineural invasion is present in 90% of cases.

## Patterns of spread

- At the time of detection, large tumor masses may be fixed to tissues behind the pancreas or to the vertebral column. The tumor may directly invade surrounding organs, such as kidney, spleen, or diaphragm. Invasion of the celiac nerve plexus may account for unrelenting pain.
- Characteristically, tumors of the pancreas grow slowly, with late signs and symptoms of pathology.
- The liver peritoneum, and regional lymph nodes are the most commonly involved structures.

## Clinical Manifestations

- The early signs and symptoms of pancreatic cancer are vague, nonspecific, and gradual, which often contributes to a delay in diagnosis.
- Weight loss and abdominal pain are the most prominent symptoms.
- Weight loss and clinical wasting are classic symptoms of cancer of the pancreas, particularly when it is located in the head of the gland.
- Tumor involvement of the pancreas prevents secretions of the digestive pancreatic enzymes and may diminish insulin production. Malabsorption can lead to diarrhea, constipation, steatorrhea, and muscle weakness.
- New onset of diabetes is found in 15%–20% of individuals.
- Metabolic disturbances such as hyperglycemia, glycosuria, and hypoalbuminemia may occur.
- Pain is often vague and nonspecific.
- A dull, intermittent pain in the epigastric region is initially experienced by most individuals.
- The intensity of the pain is affected by activity, eating, and posture. The pain is often ameliorated when the individual sits forward or lies in the fetal position.

### Head of pancreas

- When carcinoma involves the head of the pancreas, the signs and symptoms often appear earlier than a tumor in the body or tail of the pancreas. A classic triad of symptoms is seen in individuals with cancer of the head of the pancreas: jaundice, pain, and weight loss.
- Jaundice is the symptom that invariably causes individuals to seek medical attention.
- Other symptoms, less common and nonspecific, include weakness, food intolerance, and anorexia.
- Depression and anxiety may be part of the initial presentation of pancreatic cancer, independent of pain and other somatic symptoms.

### Body of pancreas

- Tumors in the body of the pancreas produce signs and symptoms late in the disease process, making early detection virtually impossible.
- Severe epigastric pain three to four hours after a meal usually is the first and predominant symptom.
- Cancer located in the body and tail produce more pain and weight loss than lesions in the head of the pancreas.
- There is no jaundice with tumors of the body and tail of the pancreas.

### Tail of pancreas

- Cancer in the tail of the pancreas has the most silent and insidious progression of disease. Individuals may complain of left upper quadrant abdominal pain, generalized weakness, vague indigestion, anorexia, and unexplained weight loss. Metastatic disease is usually present when cancer in the tail of the pancreas is diagnosed.

## Assessment

### Patient and family history

- Careful attention to an individual's presenting symptoms and risk factors, and a heightened awareness of the possibility of pancreatic cancer by the clinician are important.

### Physical examination

- A palpable liver is the most common finding.
- A hard, well-defined, mass palpable in the left upper quadrant of the abdomen is found in individuals presenting with lesions in the body and tail of the pancreas and is uncommon in lesions in the head of the pancreas.

### Diagnostic studies

#### Radiological examination

- US can detect intrahepatic and extrahepatic bile duct obstruction, a pancreatic mass, liver metastases greater than 1 cm in diameter, and ascites.
- CT scan is the diagnostic procedure of choice for the jaundiced individual with a suspected malignancy, especially in older individuals.
- Cholangiography is indicated in the evaluation of the jaundiced individual to define the site of biliary obstruction, by either the endoscopic or the percutaneous approach. Using ERCP, both biliary and pancreatic ductal systems can be visualized.
- ERCP may be most useful in the nonjaundiced individual with vague gastrointestinal symptoms in whom an early nonobstructing cancer is suspected.
- PTC with percutaneous transhepatic biliary drainage (PTBD) is usually reserved for those individuals who fail ERCP.
- The use of biliary stents preoperatively has not been shown to improve overall operative risk.
- Preoperative angiography is performed selectively to determine vascular invasion and to delineate the important vascular anomalies that might alter the operative approach.
- EUS is a relatively new technique.
- Laparoscopy and direct visualization are best used for staging cancer of the pancreas.
- Percutaneous FNAB of pancreatic tumors is useful in selected individuals, especially when guided by CT scan or US.
- It is not indicated in individuals who are candidates for resection or surgical palliation.
- FNAB is primarily used in an individual with an unresectable mass in the body or tail of the pancreas, based on CT scan evidence.

#### Laboratory tests

- With obstructive jaundice, increased serum bilirubin, alkaline phosphatase, and often elevated levels of aminotransaminases are found. Mild coagulopathy, as evidenced by prolonged prothrombin time and anemia, may also be evident.

#### Tumor markers

- The carbohydrate antigen 19-9 (CA 19-9) is tumor-associated, not tumor-specific, and has been the most useful and important tumor marker. This test is nonspecific for pancreatic carcinoma.
- CEA levels are not elevated in early pancreatic cancer and are not specific to pancreatic cancer. CA 494, a glycogen antigen, has shown promise as a marker for pancreatic cancer.

## Classification and Staging

- The goal of staging is to determine the optimal treatment.
- The staging of pancreatic carcinoma is based on the tumor-node-metastases (TNM) system.
- Four stages in the diagnosis of pancreatic cancer are listed in Table 38-6, text page 1123.

## Treatment

- Surgery, radiotherapy, and chemotherapy are the major treatment modalities used for pancreatic cancer. Surgical resection still remains the best therapeutic option even though few individuals are cured.
- Cure is the objective if the tumor is localized and not fixed to other structures, and if there is no evidence of regional or distant metastases.
- Control or palliation is the goal of therapy if the tumor is unresectable or has metastasized to regional or distant nodes or to other organs.

### Surgery

- Surgical resection of pancreatic carcinoma still remains the best therapeutic option. Pancreatic resection provides the only opportunity for cure.
- Only about 10% of carcinomas of the head of the pancreas are resectable and potentially curable at surgery. The survival rate for tumors in the body and tail is much lower.
- The surgical approach most used when cure is the objective is a pancreaticoduodenectomy (Whipple procedure). Total pancreatectomy may be performed for tumor involvement of the entire gland. An extended or radical pancreaticoduodenectomy has also been performed as a modification of the original regional pancreatectomy.

#### Pancreaticoduodenectomy (Whipple procedure)

- The Whipple procedure is the most commonly performed operation for carcinoma of the pancreas. The classic Whipple procedure includes resection of the distal stomach, gallbladder, distal common bile duct, head of the pancreas, and duodenum.
- A modification, called a *pylorus preserving pancreaticoduodenectomy*, is preferred by some surgeons. This procedure preserves the entire stomach, including the pylorus, and a small cuff of proximal duodenum.
- Pancreatic fistula and delayed gastric emptying are the most common serious complications after a pancreaticoduodenectomy.

#### Extended pancreaticoduodenectomy

- This operation consists of a pancreaticoduodenectomy or sometimes a total pancreatectomy, along with an extensive retroperitoneal lymph node and soft-tissue resection.
- Evidence suggests that wide lymphatic resections, wider than those commonly performed with the standard Whipple procedure, may prolong survival.

#### Total pancreatectomy

- A total pancreatectomy includes an en bloc resection of the distal stomach, duodenum, gallbladder, and distal common bile duct, along with the entire pancreas, spleen, and a wide margin of peripancreatic tissue including lymph nodes.
- Individuals who have total pancreatectomy develop pancreatic endocrine and exocrine insufficiency and as a result are brittle diabetics with difficult-to-control glucose levels.

## Distal pancreatectomy

- In rare cases, when tumors of the body and tail of the pancreas are detected early enough to be considered curable, a distal pancreatectomy with a splenectomy is performed.

## Palliative procedures

- Currently, only approximately 15% of individuals with pancreatic cancer are resectable for cure at the time of presentation.
- Obstructive jaundice, duodenal obstruction, and pain are the most frequent symptoms requiring palliative intervention.
- A choice must be made between operative and nonoperative palliation.
- Individuals in poor health or those not expected to live for a prolonged time should be considered for nonoperative palliation.
- Conventional surgical palliation for an individual with a tumor in the head of the pancreas is directed toward relief of obstructive jaundice, gastric outlet obstruction, and pain.
- The surgical options for palliation of obstructive jaundice include an internal biliary bypass by means of a choledochojejunostomy or a cholecystojejunostomy.
- Nonoperative palliation of obstructed jaundice by either percutaneous or endoscopic drainage methods is also effective.
- Endoscopically placed biliary stents offer an advantage over the percutaneous technique, with fewer procedure-related complications and better individual acceptance.
- Percutaneous biliary drainage is indicated in individuals in whom endoscopic biliary drainage is unsuccessful and in individuals with recurrent jaundice following surgical bypass.
- A gastrojejunostomy can be performed to treat or prevent gastric outlet obstruction.
- Duodenal obstruction can be alleviated by placement of a percutaneous endoscopic gastrostomy (PEG) decompression tube.
- For most individuals with pancreatic cancer who are not surgical candidates, the appropriate use of oral agents can successfully manage pain. Chemical splanchnicectomy (alcohol block) is an alternative therapy available to those individuals who do not benefit from oral analgesia or cannot tolerate oral intake due to gastric outlet obstruction.
- Another modality used for control of pain due to unresectable pancreatic cancer is external-beam radiation.

## Postoperative care

- Hemorrhage in the early postoperative period can be life-threatening.
- Also, hypovolemia, hypotension, pulmonary complications, pneumonia, anastomotic leakage, and prolonged ileus and delayed gastric emptying are potential complications.
- Endocrine function, the secretion of insulin, and the production of glucagon may be altered after a pancreatic resection.
- Endocrine consultants should be contacted soon after surgery to assist with glucose management and insulin adjustment.
- Alteration of exocrine function by removal of pancreatic tissue can result in a malabsorption syndrome characterized by an inability to use ingested forms of fat and protein.
- Pancreatic enzymes are replaced with oral enzyme supplements.
- After pancreatic surgery when the individual is able to tolerate food, several small feedings consisting of foods that are low in fat and high in carbohydrates and protein are tolerated better than large meals. Restrictions include overindulgence, caffeine, and alcohol.
- The stool should be examined daily for the characteristic signs of steatorrhea.

## Chemotherapy

- Because most individuals present with unresectable cancer of the pancreas, the use of chemotherapeutic agents has been tried. The overall survival results have been dismal.
- Some chemotherapeutic agents have been used as single agents in the treatment of pancreatic cancer: 5-FU, mitomycin C, streptozocin, ifosfamide, and doxorubicin. The results have been minimally effective.
- Combination chemotherapy has shown no survival advantage over treatment with single agents.
- A more realistic objective of treatment may be the improvement in the quality of life with prolonged survival being a secondary benefit.
- A new cytotoxic agent, gemcitabine, has been evaluated in the treatment of individuals with unresectable pancreatic cancer.
- Clinical benefit response is a novel approach to assess the clinical effectiveness of gemcitabine based on marked improvement in pain control, analgesic consumption, and performance status.

## Radiation therapy

- External-beam radiation therapy has been used for both palliation and curative therapy of pancreatic cancer.
- Radiation therapy in combination with surgery has been used to improve local disease control and survival. Radiation therapy is given postoperatively as tumor may still remain in adjacent tissue and lymph nodes, or it is given preoperatively to reduce tumor size to permit subsequent resection.
- Adjuvant combined chemotherapy and radiation therapy is used after surgical resection.

## Symptom Management

- The individual who has had surgery for pancreatic cancer usually dies of locally recurrent disease. The most common harbingers of imminent demise are recurrence of pain, jaundice from obstruction or intrahepatic metastases, and the development of ascites.
- The goal of palliative therapy is to reduce the debilitating symptoms of the disease and to improve the quality of remaining life.
- Relief of pain is a primary objective, particularly in advanced disease.
- Eliminating the source of the pain is the first objective.
- The most effective approach to pain therapy in individuals with advanced disease is to prevent the pain from peaking by routinely administering the selected relief measures.
- The goal of pain management should be to permit an acceptable level of functioning and to allow the individual to die as free of pain as possible.
- Malnutrition, cachexia, muscle weakness, and fatigue all contribute to depression, causing a cycle of difficulties.
- Nutritional support may pose a difficult problem as a result of the obstructive nature of advanced pancreatic cancer.
- Oral feedings should be maintained as long as the individual can meet caloric requirements. Frequent, small feedings and supplemental mixtures may be tolerated better than larger meals.
- Bowel obstruction caused by tumor may necessitate the placement of a gastric tube for decompression.
- The administration of continuous subcutaneous opiate infusions by means of a PCA pump has the advantage of delivering analgesics to individuals with impaired gastrointestinal function and for whom oral analgesics are not appropriate.
- Malabsorption may result from steatorrhea and pancreatic exocrine insufficiency.
- Lactose intolerance treatment consists of a diet high in protein and carbohydrate and replacement of pancreatic enzymes.

- Individuals with cancer of the pancreas frequently have liver involvement, resulting in abdominal distention from malignant ascites. The treatment is difficult, but symptom control can be accomplished with the careful use of diuretics.
- Palliation of obstructive jaundice can be provided with endoscopic or percutaneous procedures. Insertion of internal biliary stents by endoscopy can relieve jaundice and its concomitant symptoms.
- Almost 90% of individuals with pancreatic cancer die within a year of diagnosis.

## Continuity of Care: Nursing Challenges

- Individuals in the terminal stage of pancreatic cancer may not wish to eat, may become extremely cachectic, and may have decreased or no urine output as hepatorenal failure ensues.

# PRACTICE QUESTIONS

1. In the United States, the highest incidence of esophageal cancer is found among:
   a. women aged 29 to 39 years.
   b. African-American men.
   c. perimenopausal women.
   d. men aged 30 to 40 years.

2. Individuals with esophageal cancer typically have a history of:
   a. occupational exposure to radiation.
   b. obesity.
   c. oral contraceptive use.
   d. heavy alcohol intake.

3. Which of the following conditions usually precludes an individual with esophageal cancer from consideration for curative treatment?
   a. extension of the tumor outside of the esophagus
   b. excessive weight loss (i.e., >25% of ideal body weight)
   c. age greater than 65 years
   d. tumor location in the cervical esophagus

4. Individuals with advanced esophageal cancer are considered at high risk for the development of:
   a. other gastrointestinal cancers.
   b. superior vena cava syndrome.
   c. aspiration pneumonia.
   d. xerostomia.

5. Complications and side effects of radiotherapy for esophageal cancer include all of the following *except*:
   a. esophageal stricture.
   b. radiation pneumonitis.
   c. skin reaction.
   d. diarrhea.

6. Within a week of surgery for esophageal cancer, contrast studies are likely to be done to check for:
   a. local edema.
   b. any signs of residual tumor.
   c. anastomotic leaks.
   d. swallowing ability.

7. Early detection of gastric cancer is unlikely because:
   a. the cancer metastasizes readily.
   b. people tend to self-medicate themselves for gastrointestinal distress.
   c. risk factors for the disease have not yet been identified.
   d. none of the diagnostic tests or procedures currently available accurately detect gastric cancer in its early stages.

8. The country with the highest incidence of gastric cancer is:
   a. Japan.
   b. China.
   c. England.
   d. the United States.

9. The use of radiotherapy in the treatment of gastric cancer is limited by the:
   a. radiosensitivity of the tumor.
   b. close proximity of the liver, kidneys, and spinal cord.
   c. severity of the side effects experienced.
   d. size of the tumor mass.

10. Liver cancer is often associated with:
    a. a long smoking history.
    b. obesity.
    c. cirrhosis.
    d. a bacterial infection.

11. One of the common sequelae of liver cancer is:
    a. esophageal varices.
    b. visual disturbances.
    c. fat intolerance.
    d. urinary retention.

12. A liver tumor may be suspected if laboratory tests reveal elevated levels of:
    a. gastrin.
    b. cholesterol.
    c. alpha-fetoprotein.
    d. amylase.

13. The individual who has recently had an ultrasound-guided percutaneous needle biopsy of the liver must be monitored closely for symptoms of:
    a. spinal cord compression.
    b. hematemesis.
    c. headache.
    d. hemorrhage.

14. Nursing care of the individual with liver cancer involves:
    a. meticulous skin care for pruritus.
    b. providing a low-protein, high-fat diet.
    c. continuous administration of anticoagulants.
    d. assistance with an abdominal binder.

15. All of the following are possible contraindications to hepatic resection for liver cancer *except*:
    a. jaundice.
    b. severe cirrhosis.
    c. chemotherapy failure.
    d. ascites.

16. The primary treatment of stage I gallbladder carcinoma is:
    a. cholecystectomy.
    b. laparoscopic removal of the gallbladder.
    c. internal-external percutaneous transhepatic biliary stent.
    d. external-beam radiotherapy.

17. Individuals with pancreatic cancer generally die within _____ year(s).
    a. one
    b. two
    c. five
    d. three

18. The three classic signs of a pancreatic tumor located in the head of the pancreas are progressive jaundice, profound weight loss, and:
    a. pain.
    b. projectile vomiting.
    c. confusion.
    d. hyperkalemia.

19. The treatment of choice of pancreatic cancer, and the treatment presently offering the only hope for cure, is:
    a. systemic chemotherapy.
    b. intra-arterial chemotherapy.
    c. surgery.
    d. radiotherapy.

20. Postoperative care of an individual who has undergone palliative surgery for pancreatic cancer includes all of the following *except*:
    a. administration of pancreatic enzyme supplements.
    b. providing a diet that is low in fat, high in protein, and includes a glass of red wine with lunch and dinner.
    c. observing for hemorrhage, hypovolemia, and hypotension.
    d. examining stools for steatorrhea.

## ANSWER EXPLANATIONS

1. **The answer is b.** In the United States, African-American men have a significantly higher incidence of esophageal cancer than white men; similarly, African-American women have a higher incidence of the disease than white women. This type of cancer also seems to develop at a younger age in African-American persons than it does in white persons. (p. 1084)

2. **The answer is d.** Esophageal cancer appears to be associated with heavy alcohol intake, heavy tobacco use, and poor nutrition; cirrhosis, vitamin deficiency, anemia, and poor oral hygiene may be contributing factors. (p. 1084)

3. **The answer is a.** The findings that usually preclude an individual from consideration for curative treatment are: (1) fixed lymph nodes; (2) fixed tumor mass; (3) extension of the tumor outside of the esophagus; and (4) recurrent laryngeal nerve involvement. A combination of surgery, radiotherapy, and/or chemotherapy appears to offer the greatest hope of cure, although the most effective combination or sequence has yet to be established. (p. 1088)

4. **The answer is c.** When an esophageal tumor gets so large that it causes saliva, food, and liquids to spill over into the lungs, affected individuals are at high risk for the development of aspiration pneumonia. Because of this potential, pulmonary hygiene and aspiration precautions should be a focus of nursing care for the person with esophageal cancer. (pp. 1084 and 1088)

5. **The answer is d.** Esophageal fistula, stricture, hemorrhage, radiation pneumonitis, and pericarditis are all possible complications of radiotherapy for esophageal cancer. Side effects to be expected are swallowing difficulties, including burning, pain, dryness, and skin reactions. (p. 1089)

6. **The answer is c.** Because the esophagus is thin-walled and draws upward with each swallow, an anastomosis involving the esophagus has more of a tendency to leak than any other area of the gastrointestinal tract. It is for this reason that contrast studies are performed 4 to 6 days after surgery to check for patency of the anastomosis. Small leaks usually close spontaneously; larger leaks often require surgical approximation. (pp. 1091 and 1093)

7. **The answer is b.** The earliest symptoms of gastric cancer, such as a sense of fullness or heaviness and moderate distention after meals, are usually vague in nature. Home remedies and self-medication are often employed successfully for a while until other symptoms appear. Because of the elusive nature of gastric disorders, this type of cancer is usually quite advanced by the time medical attention is sought out. (p. 1095)

8. **The answer is a.** Japan has the highest incidence of gastric cancer in the world, and stomach cancer is the major cause of death in that country. The incidence of gastric cancer is low in the United States. The dramatic differences in geographic distribution of the disease remain an enigma to epidemiologists. (p. 1095)

9. **The answer is b.** Gastric adenocarcinomas are generally radiosensitive; however, the close proximity to dose-limiting organs in the abdomen (i.e., the liver, kidney, and spinal cord) restricts the use of radiotherapy as a treatment modality. (p. 1100)

10. **The answer is c.** Hepatocellular carcinomas are associated with environmental and hereditary factors, hepatitis B and hepatitis C viruses, and cirrhosis. Alcoholic cirrhosis is a common risk factor for cancer in the United States. Ingestion of estrogens, androgens, and oral contraceptives has been reported to be associated with liver tumors. (p. 1102)

11. **The answer is a.** As liver cancer advances, serious complications, usually involving many body systems, arise. Portal vein obstruction may lead to necrosis, rupture, and hemorrhage. Esophageal varices and unrelenting ascites are also common sequelae of either primary or secondary liver cancer. (p. 1104)

12. **The answer is c.** Alpha-fetoprotein is a tumor marker that is elevated in the serum of 70% to 90% of individuals with primary hepatocellular carcinoma, but because levels of alpha-fetoprotein are not specific for liver cancer, histologic diagnosis is required. (p. 1105)

13. **The answer is d.** Because most liver tumors are highly vascular, the person having an ultrasound-guided percutaneous needle biopsy of the liver must be monitored closely for intra-abdominal hemorrhage. In general, this procedure is rapid, safe, and commonly used; however, there are those clinicians who strongly believe that needle biopsies should be avoided at all costs if there is any potential for curative resection, because of the potential for seeding and spreading the cancer during the procedure. (p. 1105)

14. **The answer is a.** Pruritus, which frequently accompanies jaundice, is precipitated by irritation of the cutaneous sensory nerve fibers by accumulated bile salts. Therefore, an individual with liver cancer must have meticulous skin hygiene and efforts to reduce itching should be implemented. Depending on the extent of liver dysfunction, deficits in clotting mechanisms may exist, occasionally necessitating the use of vitamin K to prevent bleeding. Most individuals with liver cancer are in a poor nutritional state and benefit greatly from a diet high in proteins and carbohydrates and low in fats. (p. 1106)

15. **The answer is c.** Possible contraindications to major hepatic resection for liver cancer include the following: (1) severe cirrhosis; (2) distant metastases in the lung, bone, or lymph nodes; (3) jaundice, which is often indicative of obstruction of the common bile duct; (4) ascites, which is usually indicative of liver failure and an inability to tolerate a surgical procedure; (5) poor visualization on angiographic studies, which may jeopardize the certainty with which the surgeon resects the tumor; (6) certain biochemical changes which indicate poor liver function and lower the probability of survival; and, (7) involvement of the inferior vena cava or portal vein which would make surgical intervention hazardous. (p. 1107)

16. **The answer is a.** Cholecystectomy is the primary treatment of stage I gallbladder carcinoma. Laparoscopic removal of the gallbladder is not recommended. The addition of stents are palliative only, and there has been no proven survival advantage to external-beam radiation. (pp. 1115–1117)

17. **The answer is a.** Of those diagnosed with cancer of the pancreas, less than 20% will survive one year after diagnosis. The cause of death will usually be cachexia, infection, or liver failure. (p. 1117)

18. **The answer is a.** A classic triad is apparent with cancer of the head of the pancreas: progressive jaundice, profound weight loss, and pain. Jaundice, which is precipitated by common bile duct obstruction, is the presenting symptom in 80% of all cases of cancer of the head of the pancreas, and is the symptom that inevitably leads individuals to seek medical attention. (p. 1120)

19. **The answer is c.** In general, palliative procedures are the mainstay of therapy for cancer of the pancreas because the disease is usually far advanced, with both local and distant metastases, by the time it is diagnosed. For a few individuals whose disease is detected early, the goal of surgery will be to obtain a cure. Current applications of chemotherapy have failed to produce significant results in the treatment of pancreatic cancer. If the cancer is unresectable, many clinicians advocate use of a combination of chemotherapy and radiotherapy, which occasionally controls local tumor growth and relieves the patient of some debilitating symptoms. (p. 1124)

20. **The answer is b.** Hemorrhage, hypovolemia, and hypotension pose the greatest threats to the individual who has just undergone surgery for cancer of the pancreas. As soon as possible after pancreatectomy, small feedings will be started with a diet that is usually bland, low in fat, and high in carbohydrates and protein. Restrictions will include caffeine, alcohol, and overindulgence. The stool should be examined daily for the characteristic signs of steatorrhea: frothy, foul-smelling stool with fat particles floating in the water. (pp. 1130–1131)

# Chapter 39    Gynecologic Cancers

## INTRODUCTION
- Gynecologic cancers account for about 14% of all cancers in women.
- The majority occur in the middle years (cervical), perimenopausal years (ovarian), and post-menopausal years (endometrial, vulvar, and vaginal).

## ENDOMETRIAL CANCER
### Epidemiology
- Cancer of the endometrium is the predominant cancer of the female genital tract.
- Although am estimated 34,000 new cases of endometrial cancer were diagnosed in the U.S. in 1996, only approximately 6000 women died of the disease that year.
  - This low mortality rate reflects the fact that 79% are diagnosed with localized disease. Survival rates for endometrial cancer by stage are 76% for stage I, 50% for stage II, 30% for stage III, and 9% for stage IV.
- Endometrial cancer is primarily a disease of postmenopausal women.
- The median age at diagnosis is 61 years, with the majority of women diagnosed between 50 and 59 years of age.

### Etiology
- Multiple risk factors include obesity (more than 20 pounds overweight), nulliparity, late menopause (after age 52), diabetes, hypertension, infertility, irregular menses, failure of ovulation, a history of breast or ovarian cancer, adenomatous hyperplasia, and prolonged use of exogenous estrogen therapy.
- Excessive endogenous estrogen metabolism or production has been implicated in the development of endometrial cancer. Several hormonal aberrations can be linked to obesity. Increased body size plays a role in androgen conversion to estrogen. Obese women with an upper body fat pattern have a 5.8-fold increase in risk over women who are nonobese or have a lower body fat pattern.
- Use of unopposed exogenous estrogen has been linked to an increased incidence of endometrial cancer.

### Prevention, Screening, Early Detection
- Two factors appear to have a protective effect against the development of endometrial cancer: oral contraceptives and cigarette smoking.
  - However, the risks of developing other health problems well outweigh any protection gained from smoking against endometrial cancer.
- There is no sensitive and specific screening test for endometrial cancer.
- Endometrial biopsy is 90% effective in detecting a cancer and can be accomplished in the outpatient setting. However, it is not without morbidity and cost and should not be applied as a screen.

### Pathophysiology and Cellular Characteristics
- Endometrial cancer develops in the epithelial layer of the uterine corpus.
- Tumors that arise in the lower uterine segment involve the cervix sooner and have a higher incidence of pelvic and para-aortic lymph node involvement.

- Tumors that have deep myometrial invasion tend to be more aggressive and have a poorer survival rate.
- Over 90% of endometrial cancers are adenocarcinomas.

## Clinical Manifestations

- Cancer usually starts in the fundus and may spread through direct extension and infiltration to the myometrium, endocervix, cervix, fallopian tubes, and ovaries.
- Metastatic spread is usually to pelvic and para-aortic lymph nodes and has been positively correlated with myometrial invasion.
- Less common sites of metastases include the vagina, peritoneal cavity, omentum, and inguinal lymph nodes. Hematogenous spread often involves the lung, liver, bone, and brain.
- Histological differentiation is one of the most sensitive indicators of metastases and prognosis. The less differentiated the tumor, the poorer the prognosis.
- The greater the degree of myometrial invasion, the poorer the prognosis.
- Fortunately, the abnormal vaginal bleeding associated with endometrial cancer causes women to seek medical attention promptly.

## Assessment

- Postmenopausal bleeding, any serosanguinous vaginal discharge, or new heavy bleeding should be evaluated.
- Premenopausal onset of irregular or heavy menstrual flow may be significant.
- A thorough pelvic examination is performed. A Pap smear will only occasionally detect an endometrial cancer. A more reliable technique is endometrial biopsy.
- If the endometrial biopsy is negative and symptoms persist, a fractional dilatation and curettage (D & C) is performed.
- Other diagnostic tests include chest radiograph, intravenous pyelogram (IVP), complete blood count (CBC), and blood chemistry profiles. Cystoscopy, barium enema, and proctoscopy are performed if bladder or rectal involvement is suspected.

## Classification and Staging

- See Table 39-2 on text page 1149 for corpus cancer staging.
- Staging helps to define primary tumor size and location as well as extent of spread beyond the uterus.
- Surgical staging and treatment can involve an extensive evaluation of the abdomino-pelvic cavity and use of the following procedures: bimanual examination under anesthesia, peritoneal cytology, inspection and palpation of all peritoneal surfaces, biopsy of suspicious areas, selective pelvic and para-aortic lymphadenectomy, total abdominal hysterectomy (TAH), bilateral salpingo-oophorectomy (BSO), and possible omentectomy and resection of tumor implants.

## Therapeutic Approaches and Nursing Care

### Primary

- Primary surgical staging prior to any radiation therapy is advantageous because many women with early-stage disease will not need additional postoperative therapy and thus can avoid the time, effort, and morbidity associated with pelvic radiation therapy.
- Selection of adjuvant radiation therapy for early endometrial cancer is determined by stage, histology, and cytopathology.
- Patients with stage I, grade 1 disease and no myometrial invasion require no further treatment after TAH, BSO. Patients with stage I, grade 2 disease and less than 50% myometrial invasion require intravaginal radiation to reduce the risk of central recurrence.

- Indications for pelvic external beam radiation therapy include disease localized to the pelvis, a high-grade tumor, or greater than 50% myometrial invasion.
- Whole-pelvis radiation, in contrast to intravaginal radiation, allows treatment of all pelvic tissue including nodes and lymphatics.
- Adjuvant hormonal therapy in endometrial cancer is considered unproven and remains controversial.

### Advanced or recurrent disease

- Endometrial cancer is one of the most difficult cancers to treat if metastasis or recurrence has occurred.
- Women with vaginal recurrences can be treated successfully with surgery or radiotherapy.
- Recurrences outside the upper vagina are not easily treated. Hormonal therapy or chemotherapy is essential to treat recurrent and advanced disease.
- Palliative radiation can be employed to control heavy vaginal bleeding in patients who present with advanced, incurable disease.

#### Hormonal therapy

- The most commonly used systemic therapy for recurrent endometrial cancer has been synthetic progestational agents. Response rates range from 30%–37%.
- Positive estrogen and progesterone receptor status correlates with a better response to progestin therapy regardless of the grade of the tumor.
- Side effects of progestational agents include fluid retention, phlebitis, and thrombosis.
- Oral preparations of megestrol acetate or intramuscular medroxyprogesterone acetate are effective agents against endometrial cancer.

#### Chemotherapy

- Cytotoxic agents have a limited role in advanced endometrial cancer.
- Only a few agents have demonstrated activity equal to or greater than progestin therapy.
- Administration of high doses (100 mg/m$^2$) of cisplatin has achieved response rates of 46% in women with no prior chemotherapy.
- Though the majority of women are diagnosed with early-stage disease, women still die from recurrent or advanced disease.
- Patient information needs are summarized in Table 39-3, text page 1152.

### Symptom Management and Continuity of Care

- For the vast majority of women with endometrial cancer, the major nursing challenges are those that relate to regular follow-up.
- For those women who present with advanced disease or who have a recurrence, the challenges of care will vary according to the type of therapy they are receiving.

## OVARIAN CANCER

### Epidemiology

- Ovarian cancer accounts for approximately 33% of all gynecologic cancers and 55% of deaths from cancer of the female genital tract. It is the most common cause of death from gynecologic cancers and the fifth leading cause of cancer death in women in the United States. Ovarian cancer is a leading cause of death in industrialized countries (except Japan) but is rare in developing nations.
- It is estimated that 1 of every 71 women will develop ovarian cancer, with most cases seen in women between 55 and 59 years of age.

- The overall five-year survival rate for women with ovarian cancer is between 30% and 35% and has not changed over the past 30 years.

## Etiology

- Multiple risk factors have been identified including environmental, hormonal, menstrual, reproductive, dietary, and hereditary indicators. Specifically, these include infertility; first pregnancy after 35; nulliparity; low number of pregnancies; hereditary ovarian cancer; breast and ovarian cancer; and the Lynch II syndrome of breast, ovarian, and colon cancer.
- Early menarche, late menopause, and hormonal therapy have also been identified as affecting the risk for ovarian cancer. However, conflicting data exist.

## Prevention, Screening, Early Detection

- Prevention of ovarian cancer may be achieved, at least temporarily, with the use of oral contraceptives; however, even the prophylactic removal of the ovaries does not provide absolute protection. In addition, avoiding the use of talc and maintaining a diet low in fat may be preventative.
- Routine pelvic examination will detect one ovarian carcinoma in 10,000 examinations of asymptomatic women. Despite this, pelvic examinations remain the most usual method for detecting early disease.
- Transvaginal ultrasound in conjunction with CA-125, a tumor-associated antigen, is gaining popularity as a screening method.
- Current screening tools for ovarian cancer have not detected disease at a stage when treatment could alter the outcome.
- An annual pelvic examination including a rectal-vaginal examination is a general recommendation.

## Pathophysiology and Cellular Characteristics

- Epithelial ovarian cancers arise from a malignant transformation of the ovarian surface epithelium. How this transformation occurs is not known.
- Ovarian cancer includes several histological types that may occur in different age groups, exhibit different methods of spread, and respond to different therapeutic regimens: epithelial, germ cell, and stromal tumors.
- Epithelial tumors constitute 80%–90% of all malignant ovarian neoplasms.
- Epithelial ovarian tumors of low malignant potential (LMP) constitute a separate clinical and pathological entity between benign and invasive disease and represent about 15% of epithelial tumors.
- Tumors of LMP usually occur in women less than 40 years of age and have a favorable prognosis regardless of stage.
- Grade seems to be of greater prognostic significance in stage I and II disease, where the more differentiated tumors respond better to treatment.

## Clinical Manifestations

- Most ovarian malignancies originate from the epithelial surface of the ovary. As the tumor grows, it invades the stromal tissue and penetrates the capsule of the ovary. The most common mechanisms of spread are by direct extension and peritoneal seeding.
  - Direct extension occurs when tumor cells on the surface of the ovary invade the adjacent structures, including fallopian tubes, uterus, bladder, and rectosigmoid and pelvic peritoneum.
  - Peritoneal seeding occurs when cells exfoliate into the peritoneal cavity, where they are carried in fluid via the posterior paracolic spaces to the subdiaphragmatic surfaces.
  - Tumor nodules or seeds may be found on the peritoneal surfaces of the liver, diaphragm, bladder, and large and small bowel.

- Ovarian lymphatics may also have a role.
- Death is usually secondary to intra-abdominal tumor dissemination. Bowel and mesentery are most commonly involved.
- Women with intra-abdominal tumor dissemination gradually deteriorate and eventually die of electrolyte imbalance, sepsis, or cardiovascular collapse.

## Assessment

- Unfortunately, there are typically no early manifestations of ovarian cancer. Localized disease limited to the ovary is asymptomatic in the majority of women.
- As the mass enlarges, the woman may experience abdominal discomfort, dyspepsia, indigestion, flatulence, eructations, loss of appetite, pelvic pressure, or urinary frequency. These vague complaints are often attributed to personal stresses and midlife changes and may precede other symptoms by months.
- Often evaluation does not occur until the woman has a palpable mass or ascites. As a result, the cancer has spread beyond the ovary in 75% of patients at the time of diagnosis.
- Routine diagnostic tests may help rule out another primary tumor as the source of the pelvic mass: barium enema, proctosigmoidoscopy, gastrointestinal series, chest radiography, and IVP. Ultrasound (US) and computed tomography (CT) scans are used.
- A laparotomy is necessary to confirm the diagnosis and to adequately determine the stage or extent of disease.

## Classification and Staging

- The staging of ovarian cancer is based on surgical evaluation and forms the basis for planning subsequent therapy.
- Table 39-4, text page 1156, summarizes the surgical staging for ovarian cancer.
- The initial surgical exploration enables the surgeon to determine the precise diagnosis and accurate stage and to perform optimal debulking. Careful evaluation of all peritoneal surfaces is required to ensure accurate staging.
- Size of residual disease is an important prognostic factor.
- Unfortunately, accurate surgical staging is not obtained in all patients presenting with early ovarian cancer.

## Therapeutic Approaches and Nursing Care

- Initial ovarian cancer therapy includes thorough evaluation, staging, and cytoreduction. A TAH-BSO, omentectomy, selected pelvic and para-aortic lymph node sampling, and maximal cytoreduction are performed when surgically feasible.
- Selection of the appropriate therapy is based on stage, grade, size and location of residual tumor, and presence of ascites or peritoneal washings that contain malignant cells.

### Stage I

- Patients with stage I, grade 1 tumors have a greater than 90% survival with surgery alone.
- There is no standard adjuvant therapy defined for other stage I ovarian cancers.
- A platinum-based chemotherapy regimen is considered beneficial for patients with stage IC, grade 3 tumors who are at high risk for recurrence.
- Approximately 20% of patients with early-stage disease still relapse and die.

### Stage II

- Following the surgical staging and cytoreduction, intraperitoneal $^{32}$P, whole-abdominal radiation, single-agent chemotherapy, or platinum-based combination chemotherapy may be employed.

- Few women are diagnosed at this stage.

### Stage III, IV

- When the patient is a surgical candidate, aggressive staging and cytoreductive surgery are advocated to reduce the tumor burden and amount of residual disease.
- If the tumor is cytoreduced and the patient has no area of residual disease greater than 1 cm in diameter, she may be treated with a platinum-based paclitaxel regimen of chemotherapy or whole-abdominal and pelvic radiation.
- Platinum-based combination chemotherapy including paclitaxel is administered for stage III with residual disease greater than 1 cm and for stage IV disease.

### Recurrent or persistent disease

- The benefits of salvage therapy are limited.

#### Second-look surgery

- A second-look operation is performed on patients who have a complete clinical response following the full course of chemotherapy as evidenced by a negative tumor marker (CA-125) and negative CT scan or US.
- This surgery is advocated for the following reasons: (1) to determine whether the patient had a complete remission and therapy can be stopped, (2) to assess the response and determine whether a change in the therapy is indicated, and (3) to perform secondary cytoreductive surgery to attempt to prolong survival.

#### Tumor-associated antigens

- If tumor-associated antigens specific for epithelial ovarian cancer could be detected in the bloodstream, they would provide a means for diagnosis at an early stage when patients could be cured.
- One monoclonal antibody can detect an antigen (CA-125) in the blood of women with ovarian cancer. However, CA-125 is not specific for ovarian cancer alone.
- Elevations of CA-125 have preceded clinical disease recurrence by 1–11 months.
- CA-19-9 is another tumor marker used in combination with CA-125.

### Chemotherapy

#### Single-agent therapy

- The mainstay of adjuvant therapy for stage III and IV epithelial ovarian cancer is chemotherapy.
- Cisplatin is now considered the single most active agent for treatment of ovarian cancer, with response rates reported as high as 55% depending on dose.
- Paclitaxel, a new drug with a 30% response rate in previously untreated patients is considered to be an important drug in the initial treatment of advanced ovarian cancer.
- See Table 39-5, text page 1159, for a list of single agents active in advanced ovarian adenocarcinoma.

#### Combination chemotherapy

- The overall response rates for combination chemotherapy vary, with clinical complete remission seen in up to 40%–50% of women. See Table 39-6 on text page 1160 for selected regimens for combination chemotherapy in advanced ovarian cancer.
- The addition of cisplatin into combination chemotherapy regimens has markedly improved response rates.

- Carboplatin, a platinum analogue, is an alternative to cisplatin.
  - Like cisplatin, carboplatin has a significant dose-response relationship and can be given to patients who are not platinum refractory yet can no longer tolerate the neurotoxicity or nephrotoxicity associated with cisplatin.
- Colony stimulating factors (CSF) may allow higher doses of myelosuppressive drugs and are currently being incorporated into treatment regimens.
- Since the majority of patients suffer disease recurrence despite response to initial chemotherapy, efforts continue to identify active new second-line agents.
- Current single-agent response rates range from 0%–6% in women who have received prior cisplatin therapy.

### Drug resistance

- The development of multidrug resistance severely limits the effectiveness of chemotherapy.
- Patients with ovarian cancer die from chemotherapy-refractory disease. Drug resistance is likely due to multiple factors.
- Debulking surgery to reduce tumor burden to aggregates of 1 cm or less improves the response to postoperative chemotherapy by reducing the potentially refractory disease.

### Intraperitoneal chemotherapy

- The current aim of intraperitoneal chemotherapy (IP) approach is to increase cytotoxic drug levels to the tumor sites.
- Patients who will benefit most from IP therapy are those with: (1) minimal residual disease following systemic therapy, (2) high-grade tumors with a surgically defined complete response, (3) high-grade stage I/II with the risk of covert disease in the upper abdomen, (4) advanced disease with all or some drugs administered IP, and (5) advanced disease with IP therapy following a limited course of intravenous therapy with or without secondary surgical debulking.
- The technique for IP administration includes placement of a semipermanent Tenckhoff dialysis catheter or implanted port system into the abdominal cavity so that a large volume of fluid can be instilled.

## Hormone therapy

- Hormone therapy for ovarian cancer has resulted in uneven responses.
- Tamoxifen has been investigated as a second-line drug in individuals who have failed combination chemotherapy.
- Further clinical trials are needed.

## Radiotherapy

- Radioactive chromic phosphate ($^{32}$P) and radioactive gold ($^{198}$Au) have been used as adjuvant therapy in women with stage I ovarian cancer.
- See Figure 39-3, text page 1152, for the method of administration of radioactive colloidal chromic phosphate into the peritoneal cavity.
- Complications of $^{32}$P can include small bowel obstruction and stenosis and are higher in women who have uneven distribution of the radioactive material in the peritoneal cavity.
- The efficacy of external beam radiotherapy in advanced disease is directly related to the volume of disease at the time radiation is administered.
- Whole-abdominal radiation (WAR) appears to be most effective in those selected individuals with little or no gross residual disease.

### Biologic therapy

- Immunotherapy, including monoclonal antibodies, adoptive cellular immunotherapy, and interferon, may soon become the fourth modality of therapy for ovarian cancer (in addition to surgery, radiation, and chemotherapy).
- These promising agents have cytotoxic mechanisms that are probably unrelated to the other treatment modalities and are most likely different enough from each other to enable sequential use.
- Recombinant alfa-interferon has shown some promise in patients with small-volume residual disease who are given the drug intraperitoneally.
- Despite aggressive multimodality therapy, the overall survival rate of ovarian cancer remains poor.

## Symptom Management and Continuity of Care

- Table 39-7, text page 1164, summarizes some common nursing management issues specific to the woman with ovarian cancer.
- The overwhelming issue in caring for women with ovarian cancer is that the majority are diagnosed in late stages when the hope for cure is grim.
- Many women will have to deal with abdominal ascites either as a presenting sign or as a sign of recurrent, progressive disease.
- These women will need to learn self-care measures such as the care of a peritoneovenous shunt, monitoring weight gain, and measuring for increase in abdominal girth.

## CERVICAL CANCER

### Epidemiology

- The number of deaths from cervical cancer has decreased in women over age 45, while mortality in women under 35 years has increased. However, cervical cancer remains a significant health problem in women aged 65 years and older.
- Though the incidence of invasive cancer has decreased by nearly 50%, the incidence of carcinoma in situ (CIS) has climbed dramatically.
- Women in their 20s are most often diagnosed with cervical dysplasia; those aged 30 to 39 with in situ cancer; and those over age 40 with invasive cancer.

### Etiology

- Personal risk factors and preventive measures associated with malignancies of the lower genital tract are listed in Table 39-10 on text page 1166.
- Higher incidence of the disease occurs in lower socioeconomic groups; smokers; blacks; Hispanics; and women who become sexually active prior to age 17, have many sexual partners, and are multiparous.
- Women with HIV infection are at higher risk for developing squamous intraepithelial lesions (SIL) of the cervix.
- Cervical carcinoma is infrequent in women who are nulliparous, and those who are lifetime celibates or lifetime monogamous.
- Some types of human papillomaviruses (HPV) are associated with genital warts, precancerous lesions, or invasive cervical carcinoma.
  - The prevalence of HPV 16 appears to increase with the severity of the lesion.
  - HPV 18 is the most common papillomavirus found in women with adenocarcinoma of the cervix, whereas HPV 16 was more commonly associated with squamous carcinomas.
- The male plays a role in the etiology of cervical cancer.
  - Women married to men whose previous spouses had cervical cancer seem to be at a higher risk of developing cervical cancer.

- The male partner's age at first coitus, smoking habits, visitation of prostitutes, and number of sexual partners also may affect relative risk.
- Several factors that may lower a woman's risk include barrier-type contraception, vasectomy, recommended daily allowances of vitamin A, beta carotene, vitamin C, limiting the number of sexual partners, and initiating sexual activity at a later age.
- Several researchers have cited the use of vitamins as chemopreventive agents.

## Pathophysiology

### Cellular characteristics

- Histologically, 80%–90% of cervical tumors are squamous and 10%–20% are adenocarcinomas.
- Adenocarcinomas, generally in younger women, impose a greater risk because the tumor can become quite bulky before it becomes clinically evident.

### Progression of disease

- Cancer of the cervix is a culmination of a progressive disease that begins as a neoplastic alteration of the squamocolumnar junction and can progress to involve the full thickness of the epithelium and invade into the stromal tissue of the cervix.
- The initial preinvasive or premalignant changes are called cervical intraepithelial neoplasia (CIN).
  - *Cervical intraepithelial neoplasia* (CIN) defines epithelial cervical abnormalities. CIN classification demonstrates the progression of the disease process rather than delineating distinctly different abnormalities.
  - The term *CIN I* is used to describe dysplasia or atypical changes in the cervical epithelium involving less than one-third the thickness of the epithelium.
  - *CIN II* describes neoplastic changes involving up to two-thirds the thickness.
  - *CIN III* or carcinoma in situ describes a lesion that has neoplastic changes involving up to full thickness of the epithelium with no areas of stromal invasion or metastases.
- See Table 39-11 on text page 1169 for the Bethesda System, which is used to report cervical/vaginal cytological diagnoses.
- Low-grade squamous intraepithelial lesions (SIL) include cellular changes associated with HPV or mild dysplasia (CIN I). High-grade SIL includes lesions formerly designated as moderate dysplasia (CIN II) and severe dysplasia or CIS (CIN III). The use of the word *grade* as it is used with the SIL terminology does not imply invasive carcinoma.

### Patterns of spread

- Each type of SIL (CIN) lesion can regress, persist, or become invasive. High-grade SIL (CIN III) is more likely to progress than the milder forms, which may regress spontaneously to normal.
- Cervical cancer develops in one of three types of lesions: exophytic, excavating (or ulcerative), or endophytic.
- Exophytic lesions are the most common and appear as cauliflowerlike, fungating cancers that are very friable and bleed easily.
- The excavating of ulcerative lesion is a necrotic lesion that replaces the cervix and upper vagina.
- The endophytic lesion is located within the endocervical canal and is without visible tumor or ulceration.
- Once invasive, cervical cancer spreads by three routes: direct extension, via lymphatics, and by hematogenous spread. Direct extension is the most common route and the lesion may spread in any direction.

## Clinical Manifestations

- Cervical cancer is usually asymptomatic in the preinvasive and early stages, although women may notice a watery vaginal discharge. In the majority of cases the disease is discovered by PAP smears during routine examinations.
- The later symptoms that often prompt the woman to seek medical attention are postcoital bleeding, intermenstrual bleeding, or heavy menstrual flow.
- A common complaint in advanced cervical malignancy is that of a serous, foul-smelling vaginal discharge.
- End-stage disease may be characterized by edema of the lower extremities due to lymphatic and venous obstruction.

## Assessment—SIL

- The Pap smear is an effective, accurate, and economical screening technique to detect cervical neoplasia.
- The American Cancer Society recommends that all women who are or have been sexually active or who are 18 years or older should have an annual Pap test and pelvic examination. After a woman has had three or more consecutive normal annual examinations, the Pap test may be performed less frequently at the discretion of her physician.
- Sexually active women should have annual Pap smears. Those who have any pelvic symptoms such as pain, vaginal discharge, or abnormal bleeding should be evaluated by their physician promptly.
- When the Pap smear report shows SIL, referral for biopsy, colposcopy, and/or treatment is indicated.

## Therapeutic Approaches and Nursing Care—SIL

- The Pap smear, colposcopy, and biopsy determine the extent and severity of the cervical lesion, differentiating between SIL and invasive carcinoma of the cervix. Treatment for SIL may include a direct cervical biopsy, electrocautery/cryosurgery, laser surgery, electrosurgery, cone biopsy, or hysterectomy.
- Cryosurgery, the most commonly used method for outpatient treatment of SIL in the United States, freezes cervical tissue.
  - Cryosurgery is a cost-effective and painless treatment with low morbidity that can be performed in the office.
- Approximately 80% to 90% of SIL can be eradicated by laser while minimizing removal of disease-free tissue.
- Treatment of SIL using the loop electrosurgical excision procedure (loop diathermy excision) (LEEP) is an increasingly popular alternative.
- Conization involves removal of a cone-shaped piece of tissue from the exocervix and endocervix. (See Figure 39-6 on text page 1172.)
- Total vaginal hysterectomy (TVH) may be employed for treatment of individuals with high-grade SIL (CIS). Total abdominal hysterectomy is appropriate for individuals with high-grade SIL (CIS) who have completed childbearing.
- Ultimately, the therapy selected is based on the extent of the disease, the patient's wishes to preserve ovarian and reproductive function, and the physician's experience.
- Interferon (IFN) has been used sparingly in the treatment of low-grade SIL.
- Figure 39-7 on text page 1173 summarizes the appropriate management of a patient with an abnormal Pap smear.

### Continuity of care: Nursing challenges

- The primary nursing responsibilities for women with SIL focus on education.
- The importance of follow-up must be stressed because there is a possibility of treatment failure or recurrence of the SIL.
- Table 39-13 on text page 1174 summarizes issues specifically related to nursing management.

## Assessment—Invasive Disease

### Diagnostic studies

- A thorough clinical examination under anesthesia includes cervical biopsies, endocervical curettage, cystoscopy, and proctosigmoidoscopy. Additional diagnostic tests may include chest radiograph, IVP, barium enema, CBC, and blood chemistries. If liver enzymes are elevated, a liver scan (or CT scan) is indicated.
- Lymphangiogram may be indicated in selected individuals.
- Additional studies that are helpful in defining the extent of disease but do not alter clinical staging include CT and MRI.
- Clinical staging is not changed on the basis of surgical findings, but treatment may be altered.

## Classification and Staging—Invasive Disease

- Cervical cancer is staged clinically, with confirmation obtained from examinations completed with the patient under anesthesia. This allows for a more accurate staging.

## Therapeutic Approaches and Nursing Care—Invasive Disease

- Treatment is based on the woman's age, general medical condition, extent of the cancer, and the presence of any complicating abnormalities. Either surgery or radiation therapy can be used equally effectively for patients with early-stage disease.

### Stage Ia

- Stage Ia1 should be treated by TAH or TVH if the patient is healthy and does not desire further childbearing. Conization can be done for those who are poor surgical risks or who wish to preserve fertility.
- Stage Ia2 disease is treated by TAH or TVH if invasion is less than 3 mm and there is no lymphovascular involvement.

### Stage Ib and IIa

- Stage Ib and Stage IIa disease can be treated with radical abdominal hysterectomy and pelvic lymphadenectomy or with definitive radiation, which may include external beam and/or intracavitary insertions.
- Surgery is preferred to radiotherapy by some gynecologic oncologists because ovarian function can be preserved.
- Patients with Bulky disease (barrel-shaped cervix) have a higher incidence of central recurrence, pelvic and para-aortic lymph node metastases, and distant dissemination. An increased dose of radiation to the central pelvis or radical hysterectomy, or both, have been advocated in patients with bulky disease.

### Stage IIb, III, and IVa

- Women with stage IIb, III and IV cervical cancer are usually treated with high doses of external pelvic radiation, with parametrial boosts, intracavitary radiation, or a pelvic exenteration.

- The number of total pelvic exenterations has decreased dramatically because the incidence of isolated pelvic recurrence has decreased.
- Surgical staging of advanced disease before initiating treatment is advocated in an attempt to gain a more precise evaluation of the extent of the disease.
- At present, chemotherapy alone has not proved useful as initial therapy for women who are at high risk for recurrence, but it continues to be investigated.

### Recurrent or persistent disease

- Approximately 35% of women with invasive cervical cancer will have recurrent or persistent disease. Therefore, thorough, regular follow-ups after treatment are mandatory and critical to early detection of recurrence.
- Almost 80% of recurrences manifest within two years after therapy. Signs and symptoms may be subtle and include unexplained weight loss, leg edema (excessive and often unilateral), pelvic or thigh and buttock pain, serosanguinous vaginal discharge, progressive ureteral obstruction, supraclavicular lymph node enlargement (usually of the left side), or cough, hemoptysis, and chest pain.
- About 75% of all recurrences are local (cervix, uterus, vagina, parametrium, and regional lymph nodes); the remaining 25% involve distant metastases to the lung, liver, bone, mediastinal, or supraclavicular lymph nodes.
- One-year survival rates are 10% to 15%.

### Surgery

- When cervical cancer recurs centrally following radiotherapy, pelvic exenteration may be considered. This includes radical hysterectomy, pelvic lymph node dissection, and removal of the bladder and rectosigmoid colon.
- Because the goal of the surgery is curative, only a small percentage of women with recurrence are candidates for pelvic exenteration.
- Extensive preoperative evaluation must be done to ensure that there is not disease outside the pelvis and that renal function is adequate.
- At laparotomy, the entire abdomen and pelvis is explored for metastases. A selective para-aortic lymphadenectomy, bilateral pelvic lymphadenectomy, and biopsies of the pelvic sidewalls are done and sent for frozen section. If any of these is positive, the disease is considered incurable.
- Immediate postoperative problems include pulmonary embolism, pulmonary edema, cardiovascular accident, hemorrhage, myocardial infarction, sepsis, and small bowel obstruction. Long-term problems include fistula formation, urinary obstruction, infection, and sepsis.

### Radiotherapy

- In previously irradiated individuals, metastatic disease may be treated to provide local control and relieve symptoms.
- For women treated initially with surgery, full-dose radiotherapy using a combination of external and intracavitary implants may afford excellent palliation or even cure.
- Intraoperative radiation therapy could be beneficial in selected cases of recurrent cervical cancer involving the pelvic wall.

### Chemotherapy

- In women who have recurrent cervical cancer, chemotherapy may be the only hope for cure. In general, there is no long-term benefit, with responses lasting four to eight months with variable lengths of survival.

- Of the single agents, cisplatin remains the drug with the greatest antineoplastic activity although carboplatin may be used as first-line treatment as well. Even so, objective response rates with cisplatin only range between 17%–30% and provide no increase in survival time for patients.
- Combination chemotherapy has not been proven more effective than single agents.
- Chemotherapy can be used as a radiation sensitizer, particularly hydroxyurea.
- Initial treatment of cervical cancer with chemotherapy is generating increased interest.
- Chemotherapy has not been shown to be useful as adjuvant therapy after definitive treatment in high-risk women.

### Biologic response modifiers

- Antitumor biological therapies have the potential to be effective agents in the treatment of cervical malignancies.

### Complications of surgery

- The major complications of radical hysterectomy include ureteral fistulas, bladder dysfunction, pulmonary embolus, lymphocysts, pelvic infection, bowel obstruction, rectovaginal fistulas, and hemorrhage.

### Complications of radiotherapy

- Morbidity resulting from properly administered radiotherapy in cervical cancer is usually manageable.
- The major complications related to radiotherapy include vaginal stenosis, fistula formation, sigmoid perforation or stricture, uterine perforation, rectal ulcer or proctitis, intestinal obstruction, fistulas, ureteral stricture, severe cystitis, pelvic hemorrhage, and pelvic abscess.
- Sexual dysfunction secondary to vaginal atrophy, stenosis, and lack of lubrication is a known effect of the radiation therapy.

### Complications of chemotherapy

- The complications of chemotherapy may manifest themselves in any organ system and depend on the agent, dose, and route used.

## Continuity of Care: Nursing Challenges

- Given the complexity of treatment modalities provided in the hospital environment, outpatient setting, and in the home, continuity of care across health care settings should be a priority for all women with gynecologic malignancies.

## VULVAR CANCER

### Epidemiology

- Vulvar carcinoma accounts for 3%–4% of all gynecologic cancers. It is a disease of elderly women, with peak incidence occurring in the seventh decade of life.
- Vulvar cancer is categorized as either VIN or invasive. Vulvar intraepithelial neoplasia (VIN) describes epithelial abnormalities of the vulva. VIN is divided into categories I, II, or III that differentiate the degree of epithelial involvement by neoplastic cells.

### Etiology

- The etiology of VIN and invasive vulvar cancer is largely unknown.

- Risk factors for vulvar cancer include HPV type 16, multiple sexual partners, venereal warts, cigarette smoking, herpes simplex type 2, and a history of breast, cervical, or endometrial malignancy. (See Table 39-16, text page 1181.)

## Pathophysiology

### Cellular characteristics

- Squamous cell cancer accounts for about 90% of vulvar malignancies. The remaining 10% include malignant melanoma, basal cell, Pagets, Bartholins gland, adenocarcinoma, and sarcoma.

### Progression of disease

- VIN is divided into three categories: VIN I, VIN II, and VIN III.
- VIN I is used to describe mild dysplasia. VIN II describes moderate dysplasia. VIN III, or carcinoma in situ (CIS), describes severe dysplasia and suggests full thickness changes of the epithelium.

### Patterns of spread

- Although primary disease can develop anywhere on the vulva, the labia are the most common sites, followed by the clitoris.
- The lesions occur three times more frequently on the labia majora than on the labia minora.
- The most common routes of metastatic spread are through direct extension and lymphatic dissemination to regional lymph nodes.

## Clinical Manifestations

- The symptoms of VIN and invasive vulvar carcinoma are variable and insidious. In VIN, 50% of women are asymptomatic whereas others may complain of vulvar pruritus or burning (vulvodynia). Up to 20% of women with vulvar cancer are asymptomatic, with lesions detected only during routine pelvic examination.
- The most common complaint is the presence of a mass or growth in the vulvar area.
- Delay in diagnosing the woman with vulvar cancer may occur because she may be too embarrassed to seek medical assistance because of the intimate area of the body that is involved.

## Assessment—VIN

- Careful inspection of the vulva remains the most productive diagnostic measure.
- A 1% toluidine blue solution can be used to stain suspicious areas but this technique has a high false-positive rate.
- Multiple vulvar biopsies should be done if lesions are noted.

## Therapeutic Approaches and Nursing Care—VIN

- Controversy exists about the treatment of choice for patients with VIN. Current treatment is a wide local excision followed by primary-closure skin flaps or skin graft to restore normal anatomy.
- For multicentric disease, a skinning vulvectomy is performed.
- An alternative to excision of the vulvar lesion is to treat it locally with cautery, laser surgery, or cryosurgery.
- Topical 5% 5-FU may be used for VIN.

### Continuity of care: Nursing challenges

- For women with VIN, education is an essential responsibility of nursing. Explaining the difference between VIN and invasive cancer is key.

## Assessment—Invasive Disease

- Vulvar cancer is diagnosed by local excisional biopsy of the lesions. Colposcopy is useful for defining areas to biopsy. Pap smear of the cervix is essential because 10% of women with vulvar neoplasia also have cervical SIL or invasive cancer.
- Metastatic evaluation includes chest radiograph, proctosigmoidoscopy, cystoscopy, barium enema, IVP, and biochemical profile. Computerized axial tomography or MRI of the pelvis may help to evaluate retroperitoneal nodal areas.

## Classification and Staging

- Survival rate for vulvar cancer can be correlated with stage and nodal involvement.
- Overall 5-year survival rate is between 70%–75% for all stages. For patients with stage I and II disease, the survival rate is 85%–90%; and for those with stage III disease, 51%–74%. Stage IV disease carries a poor prognosis of only 18%–30%.

## Therapeutic Approaches and Nursing Care—Invasive Disease

### Surgery

- The trend has been away from radical surgery that has been associated with disturbances in sexual function and body image.
- Recently, there is more emphasis on individualized treatment of the patient, taking into account age, location of disease, extent of disease, and psychosocial consequences.
  - Stage I carcinomas of the vulva are treated with modified radical vulvectomy or hemivulvectomy with ipsilateral inguinofemoral lymphadenectomy.
  - Stage II lesions may require a radical vulvectomy and bilateral inguinal femoral lymphadenectomy.
  - For stage III patients, radical vulvectomy often involves removal of a portion of the distal urethra or vagina and may require excision of a portion of the anus.
  - Patients with stage IV disease may require pelvic exenteration in addition to radical vulvectomy if the bladder or rectum is involved. If the tumor is fixed to the bone or distant metastases have occurred, treatment is usually palliative and mainly consists of radiotherapy.
- The major immediate complication after radical surgery is groin wound infection, necrosis, and breakdown.
- The major late complication of radical surgery is chronic leg edema.

### Radiation

- The role of radiation therapy in the management of carcinoma of the vulva is still evolving. Radiation therapy is being used more often in combination with surgery.
- Postoperative irradiation should consist of at least 4500–5000 cGy.
- Patients who receive external radiation to the vulva can develop severe erythema, swelling, and radiation cystitis.

### Chemotherapy

- To date, chemotherapy has not been effective in the treatment of vulvar cancer.
- Chemoradiation also appears to enhance locoregional control in recurrent or advanced disease.
- About 80% of recurrences will develop within the first two years after initial treatment, which demands initial close follow-up.
- Patients with less than three positive nodes generally have a low incidence of recurrence.
- Over half of the recurrences are local and in close proximity to the original lesion.

- A combination of radiation and chemotherapy may be used as a palliative measure in metastatic disease.

## Continuity of Care: Nursing Challenges

- Coordination of care from hospital to home is essential. The patient may face problems such as chronic leg edema, urinary difficulties, and wound infection.

## VAGINAL CANCER

### Epidemiology

- Carcinoma of the vagina, a rare malignancy, accounts for 1%–2% of gynecologic malignancies. Usually, the vagina is a secondary site of malignant dissemination from primary cancers of the cervix or other sites.
- The peak incidence of squamous carcinoma of the vagina, the most common cell type, occurs in women between 50 and 70 years of age. In contrast, the peak incidence for clear cell adenocarcinoma of the vagina occurs in women aged 18–19.
- Vaginal intraepithelial neoplasia (VAIN) is much less common than cervical (CIN) (SIL) or vaginal (VIN).
  - VAIN is divided into three categories (I, II, III) with each higher number indicative of increasing epithelial involvement. Unlike CIN (SIL), VAIN is generally multifocal in nature.

### Etiology

- Incidence of squamous cell cancer of the vagina increases with age.
- Rates are higher in the black population and for persons of low socioeconomic level.
- Other related risk factors include a history of HPV, vaginal trauma (douching with preparations other than water or vinegar), previous abdominal hysterectomies for benign disease, and absence of regular PAP smears, and prior radiation therapy.

### Pathophysiology

#### Cellular characteristics

- Squamous cell carcinoma makes up 75%–95% of the cases. Other histological types include adenocarcinoma, melanoma, sarcoma, and verrucous carcinoma.

#### Patterns of spread

- Vaginal cancers occur most commonly on the posterior wall of the upper third of the vagina. The second most common site is the anterior wall in the lower one-third of the vagina.
- The tumor spreads by direct extension into the obturator fossa, cardinal ligaments, lateral pelvic walls, and uterosacral ligament.
- The incidence of lymph node metastasis is directly proportional to the stage of the vaginal cancer.

### Clinical Manifestations

- The most frequent initial symptoms of invasive vaginal cancer are abnormal vaginal bleeding, foul-smelling discharge, and dysuria. Even in early-stage disease, urinary symptoms are more common when vaginal tumors are in close proximity to the bladder neck and compress the urethra.

### Assessment

- Clinical diagnosis of a vaginal neoplasm is made by careful visual examination and palpation of the vagina. Pap smear is helpful for squamous carcinoma, but not for adenocarcinoma.

- Colposcopy is particularly helpful for directed biopsies of abnormal vaginal areas.
- Women with invasive vaginal cancer should have a history and physical examination, chest radiograph, biochemical profile, IVP, barium enema, cystoscopy, and proctosigmoidoscopy.
- Colposcopic exam, which allows visualization and determination of location, number, and size of lesions, is essential for planning appropriate therapeutic management.

## Classification and Staging

- Vaginal cancer is staged clinically using the staging classification system shown in Table 39-19, text page 1186. The overall 5-year survival rate for all stages of squamous vaginal carcinoma is between 40%–50%. The survival rate is 80% for patients with stage I.
- The 5-year survival rate in patients with adenocarcinoma is 75%.
- Clinical stage is the most important prognostic indicator in vaginal cancer. A better prognosis is associated with early diagnosis, small tumor burden, and negative nodal involvement.
- Well-differentiated tumors respond better to treatment and overall survival is improved.

## Therapeutic Approaches and Nursing Care—VAIN

- Location of the lesion, the size of the lesion, and whether it is a single focus or multiple foci are considered in determining the treatment option.
- Local excision is appropriate for single lesions or for several lesions clustered in a single portion of the vagina.
- Surgery for diffuse multiple lesions may result in a shortened or absent vagina.
- Local application of 5-FU cream can completely eradicate preinvasive lesions.
- Laser therapy can cure between 69% and 80% of patients with vaginal intraepithelial lesions.

## Therapeutic Approaches and Nursing Care—Invasive Disease

- Radiotherapy is the treatment of choice for most invasive vaginal cancers, especially for patients with stage I and II disease.
- If the tumor is adenocarcinoma, surgery may be used in stage I. A radical hysterectomy and vaginectomy with radical lymph node dissection is performed. All other stages of adenocarcinoma can be treated with radiation therapy.
- Lesions of any cell type that fail to respond to radiation can be treated effectively with surgery.
- For women receiving radiation therapy to the vagina, and for women who have had a reconstructed vagina, sexual intercourse or the use of vaginal dilators is encouraged.

## PRACTICE QUESTIONS

1. One of the primary risk factors associated with the development of endometrial cancer is:
   a. late menopause.
   b. oral contraceptive use.
   c. radiation exposure.
   d. sex at an early age.

2. Endometrial cancer is known to spread to:
   a. local lymph nodes only.
   b. the lungs, liver, bone, and brain only.
   c. local lymph nodes as well as distant sites (e.g., lungs and bone).
   d. none of the above; it does not readily metastasize.

3. The most effective method of detecting endometrial cancer is with a(n):
   a. Pap smear.
   b. endometrial biopsy.
   c. laparotomy.
   d. blood test.

4. The primary systemic agent used in the treatment of recurrent endometrial cancer is:
   a. synthetic progestin.
   b. cyclophosphamide.
   c. alpha-interferon.
   d. tumor necrosis factor.

5. One of the factors that seems to place a woman at higher risk for the development of ovarian cancer is:
   a. occupational exposure.
   b. a great many sexual partners.
   c. DES use by the mother.
   d. a history of breast cancer.

6. The treatment of choice for women with a diagnosis of stage I (noninvasive) ovarian cancer is:
   a. intracavitary radiotherapy.
   b. combination chemotherapy.
   c. surgery alone.
   d. hormone therapy.

7. One of the early signs of ovarian cancer is:
   a. frequent urinary tract infections.
   b. thin, bloody vaginal discharge.
   c. heavy and painful menstruation.
   d. none of the above; there are usually no early signs of ovarian cancer.

8. A common site of metastasis for ovarian cancer is the:
   a. lung.
   b. bladder.
   c. brain.
   d. bone.

9. A method of detecting recurrent ovarian cancer that also may be helpful in early detection of the disease is the use of:
   a. LAK cells.
   b. open biopsies.
   c. paracentesis.
   d. tumor-associated antigen.

10. One of the factors that seems to put a woman at higher risk for developing cervical dysplasia is:
    a. DES exposure.
    b. hypertension.
    c. diabetes.
    d. human papillomavirus.

11. Incidence of cervical cancer is highest in women who are:
    a. nulliparous.
    b. lifetime celibate.
    c. lifetime monogamous.
    d. multiparous.

12. CIN III (cervical intraepithelial neoplasia stage III) is characterized by neoplastic changes involving up to full thickness of the epithelium with no areas of stromal invasion or metastases. CIN III is also known as:
    a. preclinical invasive carcinoma.
    b. carcinoma in situ.
    c. adenocarcinoma.
    d. verrucous carcinoma.

13. One of the first symptoms of cervical cancer is:
    a. pelvic pain.
    b. malaise.
    c. regional lymphedema.
    d. watery vaginal discharge.

14. The most effective method of detecting cervical neoplasia is with:
    a. x-rays.
    b. routine visual examination/inspection.
    c. biopsy.
    d. a Pap smear.

15. The American Cancer Society recommends that all women who are sexually active or who are 18 years of age or older have a Pap smear performed:
    a. every three years.
    b. every two years.
    c. annually.
    d. biannually.

16. All of the following are commonly used in the diagnosing/staging of cervical cancer *except*:
    a. PAP smear.
    b. colposcopy.
    c. biopsy.
    d. laparoscopy.

17. The treatment(s) of choice for advanced cervical cancer is:
    a. local surgery.
    b. chemotherapy and surgery.
    c. internal or external radiotherapy.
    d. chemotherapy.

18. The chemotherapeutic agent felt to have the greatest antineoplastic activity in the treatment of recurrent cervical cancer is:
    a. ifosfamide.
    b. cisplatin.
    c. cyclophosphamide.
    d. methotrexate.

19. Vulvar intraepithelial neoplasia is usually discovered by means of:
    a. intravenous pyelography (IVP).
    b. inspection.
    c. a Pap smear.
    d. a patient history.

20. Vulvar cancer is most commonly detected during:
    a. childbirth.
    b. urinary catheterization for an unrelated illness or condition.
    c. routine pelvic examination.
    d. monthly self-examination.

21. Surgical excision of a stage I vulvar tumor generally includes:
    a. radical vulvectomy only.
    b. radical vulvectomy and bilateral groin dissection.
    c. surgery is not commonly used to treat vulvar cancer.
    d. individualized surgical treatment.

22. Of the following symptoms, the one most likely to be experienced by a woman who has vaginal cancer is:
    a. pain with urination.
    b. bilateral leg pain.
    c. night sweats.
    d. changes in libido.

# ANSWER EXPLANATIONS

1. **The answer is a.** The risk factors associated with the development of endometrial cancer are obesity, nulliparity, late menopause, irregular menses, failure to ovulate, infertility, diabetes, hypertension, history of breast or ovarian cancer, adenomatous hyperplasia, and prolonged use of exogenous estrogen therapy. The more of these factors that apply, the greater the risk of developing endometrial cancer. (p. 1147)

2. **The answer is c.** Endometrial cancer metastasizes primarily to pelvic and para-aortic lymph nodes; less common sites of metastasis include the vagina, peritoneal cavity, omentum, and inguinal lymph nodes. Hematogenous spread occurs to the lungs, liver, bone, and brain. (p. 1148)

3.  **The answer is b.** The most reliable technique for detecting endometrial cancer, if it is suspected, is an endometrial biopsy. A Pap smear is not a reliable method of detecting endometrial cancer, although it too may be performed. (p. 1149)

4.  **The answer is a.** For patients with recurrent endometrial cancer, the synthetic progestational agents have shown some degree of effectiveness. Response appears to be related to tumor grade, the length of disease-free interval, the woman's age, and the presence of areas of squamous metaplasia within the tumor. (p. 1150)

5.  **The answer is d.** Hormonal factors such as nulliparity, infertility, and estrogen therapy have been connected to the development of ovarian cancer. A family history of breast cancer or colon cancer doubles the risk of ovarian cancer. (p. 1153)

6.  **The answer is c.** Patients with stage I, grade I tumors have a greater than 90% survival with surgery alone. At the present time no one adjuvant therapy is being recommended. (p. 1155)

7.  **The answer is d.** Ovarian cancer is typically asymptomatic in its early stages. As the disease progresses, women may experience vague abdominal discomfort leading to loss of appetite, flatulence, or urinary frequency, but more often than not these symptoms are no more than annoying and not taken seriously by the patient and her physician. By the time a diagnosis of ovarian cancer is made, the cancer has spread beyond the ovary in 75% of cases. (p. 1155)

8.  **The answer is b.** The most common mechanisms for the spread of ovarian cancer are direct extension and peritoneal seeding. Both of these mechanisms involve neighboring organs such as the bladder and bowel. Ovarian lymphatics may also play a role. Hematogenous spread to distant sites (e.g., lungs and bone) is the least common. (p. 1154)

9.  **The answer is d.** At least two of the tumor-associated antigens specific for ovarian cancer (CA-125 and CA-19-9) have been identified to date, and both seem to correlate relatively closely with disease status. If this method is perfected, then early detection, at a point where the disease can still be cured, becomes a possibility. (p. 1158)

10. **The answer is d.** Human papillomaviruses have been implicated in an increased risk for both precancerous cervical lesions and invasive cervical carcinoma. The virus is sexually transmitted and can cause a variety of warty infections. (p. 1165)

11. **The answer is d.** Cervical carcinoma is infrequent in women who are nulliparous and those who are lifetime celibates or monogamous. Multiparity is among the risk factors listed in Table 39-10. (p. 1166)

12. **The answer is b.** The term *carcinoma in situ* describes a lesion characterized by full thickness neoplastic change with no evidence of stromal invasion or metastases. Figure 39-4, text page 1167 is a schematic representation of the different categories of cervical neoplasia. (p. 1167)

13. **The answer is d.** The first symptom of cervical cancer may be a watery vaginal discharge that frequently goes unrecognized. The symptoms that usually prompt the woman to seek medical attention are postcoital bleeding, intermenstrual bleeding, or heavy menstrual flow. If the bleeding is chronic, she may complain of symptoms related to anemia. Pelvic pain and regional lymphedema are late symptoms that usually indicate advanced disease. (p. 1168)

14. **The answer is d.** The Pap smear is one of the most effective, accurate, and economical techniques used to detect cervical neoplasia. (p. 1170)

15. **The answer is c.** Presently, the American Cancer Society recommends that all women who are or have been sexually active or who are 18 years of age or older should have annual Pap smears. After a woman has had three negative annual Pap smears, the test may be performed less frequently at the discretion of the physician. (p. 1170)

16. **The answer is d.** The Pap smear is an effective technique for detecting cervical cancer. When the Pap report shows SIL, biopsy, colposcopy and/or treatment is indicated. (p. 1171)

17. **The answer is c.** Women with later, more advanced forms of cervical cancer are usually treated with high-doses of external pelvic radiation, with or without the addition of interstitial parametrial implants. Either radical surgery or radiation therapy is used equally effectively for the earlier stages. (p. 1177)

18. **The answer is b.** In general, chemotherapy is not the treatment of choice for women with cervical cancer, because these women often have decreased pelvic vascular perfusion, a limited bone marrow reserve, and poor renal function related to previous treatment with radiation and/or chemotherapy. However, of the single agents, the only one to show significant activity when used alone is cisplatin. (p. 1178)

19. **The answer is b.** The most important diagnostic tool available in vulvar intraepithelial neoplasia is thorough inspection, possibly followed by biopsy. A 1% toluidine blue solution can be used to stain suspicious areas, although it has a high false-positive rate. (p. 1182)

20. **The answer is c.** Vulvar cancer's peak occurrence is in the seventh decade of life. It is an indolent disease, usually without symptoms in its early stages, and may be detected during routine pelvic examination. (p. 1182)

21. **The answer is d.** Traditionally, stage I lesions were treated with radical vulvectomy and bilateral groin dissection, but this has been associated with disturbances in sexual function and body image. Recently, the trend has moved away from radical surgery to more emphasis on individualized treatment of the patient, taking into account age, location of disease, extent of disease, and psychosocial consequences. (p. 1184)

22. **The answer is a.** The most common presenting symptoms of vaginal cancer are vaginal bleeding, foul-smelling discharge, and dysuria. Urinary symptoms are present because vaginal tumors are in close proximity to the bladder neck and can compress the urethra at an early stage of the disease. (p. 1186)

# Chapter 40    Head and Neck Malignancies

## EPIDEMIOLOGY

- Head and neck cancer represents about 4% of all malignant tumors in the United States.
- The ratio of male to female incidence remains 3:1. The incidence of squamous carcinomas of all sites of the upper aerodigestive tract has risen in females. This rise can be attributed to an increased incidence of consumption of alcohol and tobacco in this group.
- In some tumors of the head and neck, pain occurs very late, causing a delay in medical treatment. On initial presentation, 80%–90% of oral cancers are 2 cm or more in diameter.

## ETIOLOGY

- Tobacco use remains the primary risk factor in the development of head and neck cancer. This includes not only cigarette use but the use of smokeless tobacco as well. The sites at greatest risk for developing cancer from tobacco used are the oral cavity, pharynx, larynx, and esophagus.
- Over 95% of the cases of head and neck cancer can be attributed to the use of tobacco and alcohol together.
- As many as 15% of patients with head and neck cancer may have a viral etiology associated with the development of their tumors. The Epstein-Barr virus (EBV) has long been associated with the development of nasopharyngeal cancers.
- Nutritional deficiencies are also seen in patients with head and neck cancer.

## PREVENTION, SCREENING, EARLY DETECTION PROGRAMS
### Primary Prevention

- Avoiding use of tobacco and alcohol is key to prevention of head and neck cancer.

#### Retinoids

- Isotretinoin has shown some activity in suppressing oral premalignancies and in preventing second primary tumors in patients with squamous cell cancer of the head and neck.

### Screening and Early Detection

- Early detection remains the key to successful control of disease.
- Diagnosis may be delayed because pain may not be present, and denial of symptoms and a fear of treatment are common.

## PATHOPHYSIOLOGY

- Approximately 95% of all head and neck carcinomas are squamous cell in origin.
- The typical mucosal lesion can appear as an ulceration, roughened or thickened area, cauliflowerlike lesion, or a combination of all of these.
- The majority of head and neck tumors invade locally, deep into underlying structures as well as along tissue planes or nerves.
- Lymphatic spread occurs both locally at the primary site and regionally through lymphatic channels when tumor implantation into the lymph nodes occurs.

486

- The presence or absence of histologically proven lymph node metastasis is an important factor in determining prognosis.
- The greatest risk of a second primary tumor occurs within the initial three-year period following treatment for primary cancer.

## CLINICAL MANIFESTATIONS

### Carcinoma of the Nasal Cavity and Paranasal Sinuses

- Eighty percent of cancers in the nasal cavity and paranasal sinus area are squamous cell in origin.
- The incidence of nasal cavity carcinoma is increased in persons with occupations in nickel plating, furniture manufacturing, and leather working.
- Symptoms may be similar to those of chronic sinusitis.
- General prognosis is more favorable if tumors are located anterior and inferior to a plane connecting the medial canthus to the angle of the mandible.

### Carcinoma of the Nasopharynx

- An enlarged node in the neck may be the first indication of nasopharyngeal carcinoma in many patients.
- Invasion of tumor through the base of the skull results in cranial nerve involvement.
- Malignant tumors of the nasopharynx are one of the few tumors in the head and neck that metastasize widely.

### Carcinoma of the Oral Cavity

- The assessment and finding of oral cavity lesions are frequently first made in the dentist's office.
- *Field cancerization* is the development of multiple primary cancers that occur either concurrently or subsequently in the same patient.
- More than 90% of oral cavity tumors are squamous cell carcinomas. Adenocarcinomas rank second in frequency. Squamous cell cancers are more often seen in men and older age groups, while adenocarcinomas predominate in younger-aged women.

### Carcinoma of the Hypopharynx

- Patients with cancer of the hypopharynx typically present with odynophagia (painful swallowing), referred otalgia (usually unilateral), and dysphagia (difficulty swallowing).

### Carcinoma of the Larynx

- Cancer of the larynx cannot be considered one disease but, rather, as cancer involving different areas within the larynx such as the glottis, supraglottis, and subglottis.

#### Subglottic carcinoma

- Subglottic tumors, like supraglottic tumors, are more likely to be poorly differentiated when compared with glottic carcinomas.

#### Glottic carcinoma

- This area includes the true vocal folds and the anterior and posterior glottic commissures. Tumors in this area tend to be well-differentiated, grow slowly, and metastasize late.
- Important diagnostic information includes the mobility of the cords, evidence of fixation of the cord, involvement of the anterior commissure, and involvement of cervical lymphatic vessels.

### Supraglottic carcinoma

- Lesions that lie superior to a horizontal plane passing through the floor of the ventricles and including the epiglottis, aryepiglottic folds, arytenoids, and ventricular bands (false cords) are classified as supraglottic tumors.
- There are few early symptoms. The patient may complain of pain and poorly defined throat and neck discomfort that occurs during swallowing. Many patients complain of referred otalgia in combination with throat pain.

## ASSESSMENT
### Physical Exam

- Bimanual examination is essential.
- Regional metastasis in the neck is the *only* presenting symptom in more than one-third of patients with head and neck cancers.

### Diagnostic Studies

- Biopsies of suspicious areas, conventional radiography, computerized tomography (CT), magnetic resonance imaging (MRI), and positron emission tomography (PET) are valuable tools.

## CLASSIFICATION AND STAGING

- Head and neck tumors are classified and staged according to the TNM classification system proposed by the American Joint Committee on Cancer and the International Union Against Cancer.
- An overview of the distinctions in the TNM method is outlined in Table 40-3, text page 1206.

## THERAPEUTIC APPROACHES AND NURSING CARE
### Surgery

- Surgery and radiation given alone and in combination therapy remain the standard treatment options for this disease.

### Carcinoma of the nasal cavity and paranasal sinuses

Anatomy

- Symptoms of ethmoid sinus involvement can include decreased vision, epiphora (excessive tearing), medial orbital swelling, and olfactory changes. Distant metastasis from the paranasal and nasal cavity area can occur, but death is usually caused by tumor extension to the brain.
- Tumor extension in the area of the sphenoid sinus can cause compression of the third, fourth, and sixth cranial nerves, resulting in diplopia. In addition, pressure on the optic nerve can result in gradual loss of vision.

Treatment

- Maxillectomy remains the treatment of choice for tumors in the maxillary sinus.
- Before surgical excision, the maxillofacial prosthodontist will take an impression of the hard and soft palate to create an obturator, which is placed following resection and before the patient leaves the operating room suite.

- An oral irrigating device with controlled pressure of the jet stream will effectively cleanse the cavity.
- There is minimal facial deformity following maxillectomy because the incision along the nose generally blends in with facial lines and fades over time. However, if an orbital exenteration is performed, the patient loses the eyeball and orbital contents.

## Cranial base surgery

- The craniofacial approach, one of the most challenging areas of head and neck surgery, is used to resect tumors involving the skull base.
- Malignant diseases of the nose and paranasal sinuses, nasopharynx, or infratemporal fossa may be resected via the craniofacial approach.

## Nursing considerations

- Following cranial base surgery the patient is on bed rest with the head of the bed elevated 20–30 degrees. A lumbar subarachnoid drain is left in place 24–48 hours postoperatively with the drainage bag suspended at the level of the orbit to maintain a low-normal cerebrospinal fluid pressure.
- The purpose of a lumbar drain is to relieve pressure at the operative site through cerebral spinal fluid decompression.

## Carcinoma of the nasopharynx

### Anatomy

- The diagnosis of nasopharyngeal carcinoma is made by careful examination of the area using a head-mirror, tongue depressor, and laryngeal mirror to visualize the area, CT scans and other radiological evaluations.

### Treatment

- Radiotherapy remains the primary treatment for nasopharyngeal carcinoma.
- Carcinoma of the nasopharynx should be considered a malignant neoplasm that is distinct from squamous cell cancer of the head and neck.
- Selected patients with recurrent or metastatic carcinoma of the nasopharynx should receive aggressive combination chemotherapy.

## Carcinoma of the oral cavity

### Anatomy

- A steady, persistent growth pattern is demonstrated by most squamous cell tumors.

### Treatment

- The most common historical complaint may be a painless lesion that has existed for some time. Pain may or may not be present at the primary site.
- Referred pain is an important sign that can indicate induration, ulceration, or pressure affecting adjacent nerves. As the lesion increases in size, the individual may experience difficulty chewing foods and swallowing.
- Surgery and radiation alone have comparable cure rates in early-stage lesions.
- While chemotherapy alone cannot cure oropharyngeal cancer, complete and partial response rates as high as 90% have been demonstrated for platinum-based combinations.

### Surgery

- An ipsilateral neck dissection is often done because there is a high frequency of metastasis to ipsilateral nodes.
- A typical resection may include removal of the base of the tongue, a portion of the posterior pharyngeal wall, and a segment of the mandible.

### Laser therapy

- The $CO_2$ laser has the advantage of being very precise, and it contributes to decreased possibility of tumor spread by sealing lymphatics as tissue is removed.

## Cancer of the hypopharynx

### Etiology

- Most lesions in the hypopharynx are squamous cell in origin. There is a tendency for submucosal spread.
- Carcinoma of the hypopharynx tends to metastasize superiorly to the base of the skull.

### Anatomy

- The pyriform sinuses are best visualized during phonation.
- Diagnostic studies include CT, which can help to define the extent of the primary tumor and may demonstrate nonpalpable metastases in the lateral or retropharyngeal cervical lymph nodes. Direct laryngoscopy and biopsy are performed to confirm a tissue diagnosis.
- If both cords are mobile, invasion by tumor has not occurred and the lesion is exterior to the larynx. If one cord is fixed, the individual may be a candidate for a partial laryngectomy in continuity with the primary site.
- The posterior pharynx is often used to reconstruct the site after resection, but involvement by tumor would obviate its use for reconstruction, and alternate tissues would need to be used.
- Pooling of saliva in or around the pyriform sinus and pharynx could indicate cervical esophageal extension or obstruction of the opening of the cervical esophagus, which would require aggressive treatment.
- Treatment planning is based on the stage of disease, as outlined in Table 40-5, text page 1212.

### Treatment

- Surgery is generally done first, followed by radiation therapy. Postoperative radiation therapy is preferred in most centers because it allows the surgeon to deal with tumor margins that have not been altered by treatment. In addition, it reduces the chance of delayed healing and other problems that typically occur when irradiated tissues are resected.
- Because most hypopharyngeal tumors are locally advanced, either partial or total pharyngectomy is required.
- $CO_2$ laser microsurgery can produce effective tumor ablation with satisfactory functional results.

### Rehabilitation needs

- Swallowing is often a problem following surgical resection for hypopharyngeal carcinoma.
- Patients who have undergone surgical resection will be at increased risk for fistula formation.

## Cancer of the larynx

- The staging of glottic laryngeal cancer is based on the assessment of the depth of tumor invasion and the extent of mucosal disease (Table 40-6, text page 1213).
- When there is no evidence of cord fixation, a conservative laryngeal resection is usually the treatment of choice. Conservative surgery for glottic cancer includes laryngofissure, partial laryngectomy, or hemilaryngectomy.

### Surgery

#### Early disease (T1 or T2)

- When tumor extends forward to the anterior commissure or posteriorly to or beyond the vocal process, the surgery that is most effective is hemilaryngectomy.
- Radiotherapy is used as an option for cure in early lesions.

#### Advanced disease (T3 to T4)

- A total laryngectomy is reserved for patients who have persistent or recurrent disease after radiotherapy or who present with advanced disease.
    - Total laryngectomy involves removal of all laryngeal structures between and including the thyroid bone, thyroid cartilage, cricoid cartilage, and two to three tracheal rings.
    - Radical neck dissection is indicated for any patient who presents with obvious metastasis to the lateral neck nodes. This is most frequently seen in patients with larger, high-grade tumors or vocal cord fixation.
- Use of an electrolarynx, esophageal speech, and esophageal prosthetic voice restoration are three options for speech on a long-term basis.
- Many patients may ultimately use all three speech methods at different times in the rehabilitation period: artificial larynx immediately after surgery; esophageal voice therapy a month or so after surgery; and, after a few months, surgical voice restoration or TE puncture.

#### Postoperative care

- In the immediate postoperative period, most patients will have a laryngectomy tube placed.
- The provision of adequate humidity will remain a lifelong concern for the laryngectomized patient.
- Hyposmia occurs to some degree in every laryngectomized patient. This is a permanent loss recognized early on by the patient.
- The ability to taste is also reduced.
- Due to the absence of thoracic fixation after laryngectomy, the patient's ability to lift heavy objects is compromised. The patient is instructed not to lift more than ten pounds for four months after surgery.

### Supraglottic cancer

#### Assessment

- The diagnosis of supraglottic cancer is usually made through indirect laryngoscopy, with direct laryngoscopy used for obtaining a biopsy specimen.

#### Treatment

- Early supraglottic cancers can be treated effectively by irradiation or by surgery with the possible addition of irradiation to control the neck disease.

- The standard supraglottic laryngectomy consists of resection of the following structures: the hyoid bone, epiglottis, pre-epiglottic space, thyrohyoid membrane, superior half of the thyroid cartilage, and the false vocal cords.
- Postoperative airway obstruction is common following supraglottic laryngectomy. For this reason, patients will have a temporary tracheostomy tube.
- Aspiration during swallowing is one of the major complications following supraglottic laryngectomy.
- The mechanisms of action in the supraglottic swallow are outlined in Table 40-9, text page 1216.
- A cine-esophogram and videofluoroscopy are usually obtained before the tracheostomy tube is removed to evaluate the patient's ability to swallow without aspirating.
- Liquids are the most difficult thing for the patient to swallow without aspirating.
- The cuff of the tracheostomy tube should be deflated because it will inhibit elevation of the laryngeal remnant against the base of the tongue. If aspiration during meals is severe, the cuff will need to be inflated to protect the airway.

## Methods of Reconstruction

- The goal of reconstructive procedures in the head and neck is to restore function while simultaneously retaining socially acceptable cosmesis.

### Myocutaneous flap

- The myocutaneous flap is especially useful when large amounts of tissue have been resected and bulk is needed to reconstruct the defect.
- The muscles most often used to reconstruct defects in the head and neck area include the pectoralis major, sternocleidomastoid, trapezius, and latissimus dorsi.

### Free flap

- The free flap is completely removed from its donor site and placed into the recipient site using microvascular anastomosis. Donor sites that have been used successfully include the groin and the radial forearm.
- Major advantages are that immediate function reconstructive replacement of removed tissue is possible, the donor site is not exposed, and bulky exposed pedicles are avoided.
- Disadvantages include prolonged operating time and the need for microsurgical expertise and two teams of operating surgeons.

### Deltopectoral flap

- The deltopectoral flap brings well-vascularized tissue to a previously irradiated surgical bed from an area that had not been treated with radiation. There is no muscle included in the deltopectoral flap.
- The disadvantages of this flap include strictures, fistulae, and the fact that several stages are necessary. Because of its thinness, the deltopectoral flap has a limited role in head and neck reconstruction.

### Nursing care of flaps and grafts

Skin grafts

- Split-thickness skin grafts are used frequently to reconstruct a primary defect or to protect a major structure such as the carotid artery.
- A commonly used donor site is the anterior thigh on the operative side.

- Pain in the donor site is due to exposure of nerve endings and bruising of the underlying muscle during resection of the graft.

## Skin flaps

- Circulation is very important. The viability of any flap depends on adequate vascularization.
- More flap deaths occur from venous blood that is unable to flow out of the flap than from not enough blood flowing into the flap. The following indicators should be assessed:
  - *Color:* Color is usually the best indicator of adequate blood supply. The flap color is usually a pale pink in Caucasians.
    - A white color indicates a dearterialized flap that has lost its blood supply, and a blue color indicates venous congestion.
    - It may be more difficult to detect subtle changes in color in African-Americans.
  - *Temperature:* The flap should feel warm to the touch.
    - A flap that is cool to the touch indicates that arterial inflow is decreased.
  - *Capillary refill:* The tissue of the flap should blanche with gentle pressure applied to the flap and return to normal color quickly.
- The criteria of temperature and capillary refill are not applicable to the assessment of intraoral flaps.
- External factors can also compromise flap viability. Care must be taken to avoid circumferential pressure on the flap from either dressings or tracheostomy ties.

# Chemotherapy

- In the presence of metastatic or recurrent head and neck cancer, the addition of chemotherapy is an appropriate standard approach to treatment. The goals of chemotherapy in this situation are palliation of symptoms.

## Primary/neoadjuvant chemotherapy

- Primary chemotherapy involves giving a specified number of chemotherapy cycles before standard, local, or regional therapy is instituted.
- Besides organ preservation, the goal of neoadjuvant chemotherapy is to decrease the size of the tumor, thereby enhancing disease control, and to increase the chance of cure (survival) with subsequent surgery and radiation.

## Adjuvant/concurrent chemotherapy

- There is strong evidence that chemotherapy allows increased larynx preservation without alteration of overall survival.
- The goal of concomitant chemoradiotherapy is to enhance the efficacy of each modality without undue toxicity.
  - Each has a different toxicity profile, so while the combination may cause additional toxicities, the toxicity of each is not potentiated.
- The radiosensitizing effects of certain chemotherapy drugs (e.g., 5-fluorouracil, cisplatin, carboplatin, and paclitaxel) are known to enhance radiation effects.
- Interrupted schedules permit the use of multiple agents but may also result in delay in treatment (radiation) due to toxicity.
- Alternating/sequential chemoradiotherapy for potentially curable disease is considered a standard approach to treatment in many settings.

### Palliative chemotherapy

- Chemotherapy may be used to effectively palliate the symptoms of advanced, nonresectable, or recurrent disease.
- High-dose therapy using agents such as methotrexate or cisplatin has not proven more effective than standard low-dose therapy, and toxicity is markedly less with standard therapy.
- Intra-arterial or regional chemotherapy is a local way of delivering high drug levels to the tumor with less systemic toxicity.

### Biologic response modifiers

- IFN and IL-2 immunotherapy may result in tumor regression in some patients with advanced malignancies.

## Radiation Therapy

- The goal of any radiation treatment is to eradicate tumor while preserving function and cosmesis.
- Standard radiation therapy consists of five daily treatments per week for five to seven consecutive weeks.
- The success of radiation therapy depends on cell death during division. The damage occurs in the DNA during cell division. Head and neck tumors are in the middle range of sensitivity to radiation. They can be controlled with radiation but will require a higher dose than other tumors such as lymphomas that are more radiosensitive.

### Implant therapy (brachytherapy)

- Implant therapy is the use of radioactive sources placed directly into the tumor.
- The sources are placed using a procedure called *after-loading*.
- Implants may be used as a curative therapy for early-stage lesions in the floor of the mouth and anterior tongue or may be used to boost a tumor that has received prior external beam therapy.
- Another common approach is to combine external beam therapy with intracavitary or interstitial implantation of radioactive sources.
- Radioactive seeds may also be implanted permanently at the time of surgery.

### Hyperthermia with radiation

- Hyperthermia is rarely used in head and neck cancer but may be combined with radiation to enhance tumor response.

### Concomitant radiation therapy and chemotherapy

- The goal of therapy is to control regional disease, thereby decreasing the high incidence of persistent disease.
- Chemotherapy can be successful at eliminating systemic micrometastases while concurrently enhancing the activity of radiotherapy in the irradiated field.
- Cisplatin, 5-FU, and bleomycin have all been used as single agents in combination with radiotherapy with concomitant radiotherapy have been promising.

### Nursing management of patients undergoing radiation therapy

- The following side effects are usually experienced by any patient who receives radiation therapy to the head and neck area: mucositis, xerostomia, loss of taste, anorexia, fatigue, and local skin reaction.

## Mucositis

- Mucositis is an inflammatory response of the oral mucosa to radiation therapy. The soft palate, tonsillar pillars, buccal mucosa, pharyngeal walls, and lateral tongue are most susceptible.

## Xerostomia

- Xerostomia is a drying of the oral mucosa that results from loss of saliva due to damage that occurs to the salivary glands subsequent to radiation therapy to the head and neck.

## Loss of taste

- This symptom occurs when the taste buds are included in the radiated field and is compounded by mucositis and xerostomia.
- Anorexia is an accompanying symptom that can interfere with an optimal nutritional status.

## Trismus

- If the posterior mandible is included in the irradiated field, the patient may experience jaw hypomobility or trismus.

## Fatigue

- Patients should be aware that this is a normal side effect that can occur at any time during the treatment course.
- Depression and poor nutritional intake can also contribute to fatigue.

## Skin reactions

- Wet and/or dry desquamation can occur in the tissues of the radiated site.

# SYMPTOM MANAGEMENT AND SUPPORTIVE CARE

## Management of the Altered Airway

- Tracheostomy is effectively used in situations where airway obstruction or compromised pulmonary function is anticipated or already exists. The massive edema that develops after oropharyngeal procedures necessitates tracheostomy at the time of surgery.

### The tracheostomy tube

- The type of tracheostomy tube used will depend on the surgical procedure and clinical objectives.

### Tracheal suction

- If the procedure is performed correctly, the patient should not experience pain.
- Only suction after a thorough respiratory assessment reveals that the patient cannot clear the airway effectively.
- Limit suctioning to 10 seconds or less at 120 mm Hg or less.
- Hyperoxygenation and hyperinflation of the lungs are advised both before and after the procedure to prevent suction-induced hypoxemia and subsequent arrhythmias.

### Inner cannula care

- Tubes that are constructed of a polyvinyl chloride or other plastic material can be cleaned with hydrogen peroxide and saline. Inner cannulas from metal tracheostomy tubes should be cleaned with saline or sterile water only.

### Tracheostomy site care

- If there are flaps or grafts or a large amount of edema in the area, breakdown can occur at pressure points of the neck flange of the tube.

### Humidity

- The most commonly used device to provide supplemental humidity in the immediate postoperative period is the tracheostomy high-humidity collar. In the home setting, the patient should have a large, nine- to ten-gallon room humidifier in the living area of the home and a small bedside humidifier during the nighttime.

### Instillation of normal saline

- The action of the saline is to lavage and irritate the trachea and bronchi: coughing is precipitated and secretions are mobilized.

### Cuffed tracheostomy tubes

- The purpose of a cuff on a tracheostomy tube is to protect the airway from aspiration of blood or secretions.
- The recommended procedure for cuff inflation is the "minimal leak technique."
- A sample teaching plan that summarizes the specifics of preparing a patient to go home with a tracheostomy can be found in Table 40-11, text pages 1225–1227.

### Laryngectomy care

- The provision of adequate humidity is a lifelong concern for the laryngectomy patient.

## Nutritional Management

### Enteral therapy

- Any obstruction in the GI tract is usually seen in the upper area of the tract, therefore requiring enteral support to be delivered below the level of the obstruction. Options available for enteral access include transnasal intubation, percutaneous endoscopic gastrostomy or jejunostomy, and surgical gastrostomy or jejunostomy.
- If enteral support is anticipated to be necessary for a prolonged period of time, a feeding gastrostomy tube may be recommended.

### Oral feeding

- The movement from a regular to soft to blenderized diet may be gradual as the patient begins to experience dysphagia.
- The psychosocial aspects of long-term enteral nutrition or even an altered method of eating should not be overlooked.

## Oral Care

- Not only can halitosis be a significant problem, but, more important, the surgical site of the oral cavity should be kept clean to prevent infection.
- Oral care via lavage or power spray is most effective.

## Swallowing Rehabilitation

- The four phases of the normal swallow include the oral preparation phase, the oral phase, the pharyngeal phase, and the esophageal phase. The sequence of events in a normal swallow is outlined in Table 40-12, text page 1229.
- The assessment of the oral and pharyngeal stages of swallow are completed by a modified barium swallow, or "cookie swallow," in which the patient ingests small amounts of liquid, paste, and semi-solid materials that have been coated with barium.

## Wound Care

- A wound that requires debridement will be treated with wet to dry dressings until all necrotic tissue is removed and evidence of tissue growth in the wound is seen.

### Wound breakdown

- Wound breakdown with subsequent exposure of the carotid artery is one of the most serious and life-threatening sequelae of either the disease process itself or of surgical therapy.
- The nursing actions during a carotid hemorrhage focus on maintenance of the airway and control of bleeding. If the patient has a tracheostomy, the cuff should be inflated to prevent aspiration.
  - Firm pressure should be applied to the neck using a towel or dressing material. If an internal carotid bleed is suspected, a vaginal pack or fluff dressing should be used to tightly pack the oral cavity and oropharynx.
  - The patient is then transported to the operating room for ligation of the carotid artery.
- Numbness or tingling of the extremities on the ipsilateral side, diplopia, blindness, progressive motor loss, and changes in the level of consciousness will alert the nurse to possible cerebral ischemia secondary to carotid artery ligation.

### Carotid hemorrhage in the terminal patient

- The goal following carotid hemorrhage in the patient who is terminal will not be ligation but providing an atmosphere that minimizes anxiety and ensures death with dignity.

## Pain Management

- The type of pain usually experienced by the patient with head and neck cancer is described as "throbbing, pounding, or pressurelike."

## Psychosocial Issues

- The psychological investment in the head and neck area is greater than that in any other part of the body. This is because social interaction and emotional expression depend greatly on the integrity of the face, especially the eyes. This is of even greater concern for the head and neck cancer patient who cannot hide the structural changes that result from treatment and must therefore deal with constant exposure to others.
- Two parameters must be considered in the adjustment process: disfigurement and dysfunction.

## CONTINUITY OF CARE: NURSING CHALLENGES

## Home Care

- The patient with head and neck cancer routinely receives either a portion of or the entire course of chemotherapy in the home.
- If the patient has a laryngectomy or tracheostomy and should require resuscitation, mouth-to-stoma rather than mouth-to-mouth resuscitation will be needed.

## Quality of Life in Head and Neck Cancer

- It may be helpful to structure a system that allows for all physicians involved in the patient's care to evaluate the patient in a clinic setting prior to treatment planning as well as at predetermined intervals following each phase of treatment.

## PRACTICE QUESTIONS

1. Mr. Roberts is a retired welder who is diagnosed with a tumor in his oral cavity. You might predict that this tumor is most likely to be:
   a. adenocarcinoma.
   b. basal cell carcinoma.
   c. squamous cell carcinoma.
   d. sarcoma.

2. Stan has a well-differentiated tumor on his true vocal folds that seems to be growing fairly slowly. Stan's tumor is most likely to be a _____ tumor.
   a. subglottic
   b. supraglottic
   c. glottic
   d. either a or c

3. Once a skin flap has been transposed, its survival is based on many things. Which of the following factors is most often the cause of flap failure?
   a. inadequate circulation
   b. trapped venous blood
   c. pressure along suture lines
   d. infection

4. Which of the following are considered accepted means of communication for the person who has undergone a laryngectomy?
   a. artificial larynx
   b. esophageal voice
   c. tracheosophageal puncture (TP)
   d. all of the above

5. Mrs. Blase has carcinoma of the oral cavity. Although her main complaint initially concerned a painless lesion that she believed she had had for some time, she has recently begun to report a referred pain in her jaw and increased difficulty chewing and swallowing. This kind of referred pain can indicate:
   a. induration.
   b. ulceration.
   c. pressure affecting adjacent nerves.
   d. any of the above.

6. Mrs. Blase's physician tells her that he intends to perform a resection. This may include removal of:
   a. the base of the tongue.
   b. a portion of the posterior pharyngeal wall.
   c. a segment of the mandible.
   d. all of the above.

7. Mr. Larson has cancer of the hypopharynx. Both vocal cords are mobile, however. This suggests that:
   a. invasion by tumor has not occurred.
   b. the lesion is not exterior to the larynx.
   c. Mr. Larson may be a candidate for a partial laryngectomy in continuity with the primary site.
   d. a and c.

8. Mr. Cassidy has difficulty swallowing and on physical exam shows signs of saliva pooling around the pyriform sinus and pharynx. What might this suggest?
   a. cervical esophageal extension
   b. lesion exterior to the larynx
   c. obstruction of the opening of the cervical esophagus
   d. either a or c

9. Mr. Fox has cancer of the larynx with no evidence of cord fixation. On further examination, the physician is able to determine that the tumor extends forward to the anterior commissure or posteriorly to or beyond the vocal process. The surgery that is most effective is:
   a. laryngofissure surgery.
   b. partial laryngectomy.
   c. hemilaryngectomy.
   d. total laryngectomy.

10. Six months after his surgery, Mr. Fox, after participating in extensive speech rehabilitation, learns to speak by diverting exhaled pulmonary air through a surgically constructed fistula tract directly into the esophagus. This method of speech is produced through:
    a. an artificial larynx made available immediately after surgery.
    b. esophageal voice therapy.
    c. surgical voice restoration or tracheoesophageal (TE) puncture.
    d. none of the above.

11. Through use of indirect laryngoscopy, Ms. Eliot is diagnosed with supraglottic cancer. She is told that she will need a supraglottic laryngectomy. This means a resection of the:
    a. hyoid bone and thyrohyoid membrane.
    b. epiglottis and pre-epiglottic space.
    c. superior half of the thyroid cartilage, as well as the false vocal cords.
    d. all of the above.

12. After surgery, part of Ms. Eliot's rehabilitation process involves restoring the swallowing function, because aspiration during swallowing is one of the major complications following supraglottic laryngectomy. Initially, _____ will be the most difficult thing for Ms. Eliot to swallow without aspirating.
    a. soft, mashed foods
    b. dry, crunchy foods
    c. liquids
    d. hard, bulky food boluses (especially meats)

13. After laryngectomy, heavy lifting is restricted because of the:
    a. lack of thoracic fixation.
    b. risk of aspiration.
    c. risk of hiatal hernia.
    d. reduction in cough effectiveness.

14. Ms. Leonard is to undergo interrupted or split-course chemoradiotherapy. As part of Ms. Leonard's patient education plan, you explain that interrupted schedules:
    a. permit the use of multiple agents.
    b. involve alternating radiation and chemotherapy.
    c. may also result in delay in treatment (radiation) due to toxicity.
    d. all of the above.

15. Michelle has been diagnosed with a tumor that includes neck node involvement. She is about to receive a fractionated schedule of radiation. Her physician tells her, "The shorter the course of treatment, the better." After the physician leaves, Michelle asks you, "How will this work?" As part of Michelle's patient education, you explain that:
    a. it may be necessary to destroy not only all of the tumor cells present at the beginning of the course of therapy, but also those that may result in cell divisions during the course.
    b. more than one fraction must be administered on each treatment day to give an increased number of treatments.
    c. combining hyperfractionation with treatment acceleration will reduce the overall duration of treatment.
    d. all of the above.

16. After treatment, Michelle complains of a dry mouth and within three weeks develops a thick, ropy saliva. The side effect Michelle is experiencing is:
    a. xerostomia.
    b. mucositis.
    c. trismus.
    d. desquamation.

17. You are asked to demonstrate proper suctioning of a tracheostomy for a group of student nurses. Points you will be sure to make during the demonstration include:
    a. "Limit suctioning to 10 seconds or less at 120 mm Hg or less."
    b. "Hyperoxygenation is advised before and after suctioning."
    c. "Hyperinflation of the lungs is advised both before and after the procedure to prevent suction-induced hypoxemia and subsequent arrhythmias."
    d. all of the above.

18. Jane has had a standard supraglottic laryngectomy and has a tracheostomy tube postoperationally. Which of the following points are important to include in your teaching plan?
    a. The tracheostomy tube may be removed intermittently but is probably permanent.
    b. The tracheostomy tube is only temporary, and as soon as she can swallow without aspirating, the tube well be removed.
    c. She will be placed on a liquid diet and gradually will learn to swallow more solid food.
    d. The cuff must be inflated at all times unless the patient experiences emesis.

19. Mr. Jessup, who has a tracheostomy, is having a carotid hemorrhage. Besides controlling the bleeding, what should you do first to prevent aspiration of the blood?
    a. Suction his throat and oral cavity.
    b. Deflate the cuff and remove the trach to clear the airway.
    c. Inflate the tracheostomy cuff.
    d. Transport him immediately to the operating room for ligation of the carotid artery.

20. After his emergency treatment, Mr. Jessup begins to experience tingling in his extremities on the ipsilateral side, as well as progressive motor loss and changes in the level of consciousness. You suspect, therefore, that he might have:
    a. Cushing's syndrome, in response to progressive tumor.
    b. intermittent pulmonary failure with cardiac episodes, secondary to carotid artery ligation.
    c. cerebral ischemia secondary to carotid artery ligation.
    d. none of the above.

## ANSWER EXPLANATIONS

1. **The answer is c.** More than 90% of oral cavity tumors are squamous cell carcinomas. Adenocarcinomas rank second in frequency. Squamous cell cancers are more often seen in men and older age groups, while adenocarcinomas predominate in younger-aged women. (p. 1204)

2. **The answer is c.** The glottic area includes the true vocal folds and the anterior and posterior glottic commissures. Tumors in this area tend to be well-differentiated, grow slowly, and metastasize late. Lesions that lie superior to a horizontal plane passing through the floor of the ventricles and including the epiglottis, aryepiglottic folds, arytenoids, and ventricular bands (false cords) are classified as supraglottic.

3. **The answer is b.** Although circulation is very important, more flap deaths occur from venous blood that is unable to flow out of the flap than from not enough blood flowing into the flap. (p. 1218)

4. **The answer is d.** Many patients may ultimately use all three speech methods at different times in the rehabilitation period: artificial larynx immediately after surgery; esophageal voice therapy a month or so after surgery; and, after a few months, surgical voice restoration or TE puncture. (pp. 1214–1215)

5. **The answer is d.** Referred pain is an important sign that can indicate induration, ulceration, or pressure affecting adjacent nerves. As the lesion increases in size, the individual may experience difficulty chewing foods and swallowing. (p. 1211)

6. **The answer is d.** A typical resection may include removal of the base of the tongue, a portion of the posterior pharyngeal wall, and a segment of the mandible. (p. 1211)

7. **The answer is a.** If both cords are mobile, invasion by tumor has not occurred and the lesion is exterior to the larynx. If one cord is fixed, the individual may be a candidate for a partial laryngectomy in continuity with the primary site. (p. 1212)

8. **The answer is d.** Pooling of saliva in or around the pyriform sinus and pharynx could indicate cervical esophageal extension or obstruction of the opening of the cervical esophagus, which would require aggressive treatment. Treatment planning is based on the stage of disease. (p. 1212)

9. **The answer is c.** When there is no evidence of cord fixation, a conservative laryngeal resection is usually the treatment of choice. Conservative surgery for glottic cancer includes laryngofissure, partial laryngectomy, or hemilaryngectomy. When the tumor extends forward to the anterior commissure or posteriorly to or beyond the vocal process, the surgery that is most effective is hemilaryngectomy. A total laryngectomy is reserved for patients who have persistent or recurrent disease after radiotherapy or who present with advanced disease. (p. 1214)

10. **The answer is c.** TE puncture enables the patient to divert exhaled pulmonary air through a surgically constructed fistula tract directly into the esophagus. (p. 1214)

11. **The answer is d.** The standard supraglottic laryngectomy consists of resection of the following structures: the hyoid bone, epiglottis, pre-epiglottic space, thyrohyoid membrane, superior half of the thyroid cartilage, and the false vocal cords. (p. 1216)

12. **The answer is c.** Liquids are the most difficult thing for the patient to swallow without aspirating. (p. 1217)

13. **The answer is a.** Due to the absence of thoracic fixation after laryngectomy, the patient's ability to lift heavy objects is compromised. (p. 1215)

14. **The answer is d.** Two basic schedules of concomitant radiotherapy are used: continuous (synchronous) and interrupted or split-course (alternating radiation and chemotherapy). Interrupted schedules permit the use of multiple agents but may also result in delay in treatment (radiation) due to toxicity. Alternating/sequential chemoradiotherapy for potentially curable disease is considered a standard approach to treatment in many settings. (p. 1220)

15. **The answer is d.** It may be necessary to destroy not only all of the tumor cells present at the beginning of the course of therapy, but also those that may result in cell divisions during the course. Therefore, the shorter the course of treatment, the less opportunity there is for cellular proliferation. To achieve this goal, many different fractionation schedules of treatment have been tried. More than one fraction must be administered on each treatment day to give an increased number of treatments and to reduce the overall duration of treatment. This is referred to as combining hyperfractionation with treatment acceleration. (p. 1221)

16. **The answer is a.** Mucositis is an inflammatory response of the oral mucosa to radiation therapy. The oral cavity appears inflamed, and white patchy areas may be seen. The patient will complain of a sore throat and mouth. Xerostomia is a drying of the oral mucosa that results from loss of saliva due to damage that occurs to the salivary glands subsequent to radiation therapy to the head and neck. It manifests itself in a thicker saliva. Trismus or jaw hypomobility may occur if the posterior mandible is included in the irradiated field. (pp. 1222–1223)

17. **The answer is d.** Some points to remember regarding suctioning a tracheostomy include limiting suctioning to 10 seconds or less at 120 mm Hg or less. Hyperoxygenation and hyperinflation of the lungs are advised both before and after the procedure to prevent suction-induced hypoxemia and subsequent arrhythmias. (p. 1224)

18. **The answer is b.** Postoperative airway obstruction is common following supraglottic laryngectomy due to edema in the surgical area. For this reason, patients will have a temporary tracheostomy tube placed at the time of surgery. The tube will be removed following successful swallowing without aspiration within 10 to 14 days after surgery. (p. 1216)

19. **The answer is c.** The nursing actions during a carotid hemorrhage focus on maintenance of the airway and control of bleeding. If the patient has a tracheostomy, the cuff should be inflated to prevent aspiration. Firm pressure should be applied to the neck using a towel or dressing material. If an internal carotid bleed is suspected, a vaginal pack or fluff dressing should be used to tightly pack the oral cavity and oropharynx. The patient is then transported to the operating room for ligation of the carotid artery. (p. 1229)

20. **The answer is c.** Numbness or tingling of the extremities on the ipsilateral side, diplopia, blindness, progressive motor loss, and changes in the level of consciousness will alert the nurse to possible cerebral ischemia secondary to carotid artery ligation. (p. 1230)

# Chapter 41    Leukemia

## INTRODUCTION

- Leukemia is the name given to a group of hematologic malignancies affecting the bone marrow and lymph tissue.
- The term *leukemia* now includes abnormalities of proliferation and maturation in lymphocyte and myeloid (nonlymphocyte) cell lines.
- The acute leukemias are marked by an abnormal proliferation of immature blood cells with a short natural history (one to five months).
- Chronic leukemias have an excessive accumulation of more mature-appearing but still ineffective cells and a slower, progressive course (two to five years).

## EPIDEMIOLOGY

- Leukemia represents 3% of the cancer incidence. Approximately one-half of the cases are acute and the remaining cases are chronic, but the number of new cases per year is greater in adults than in children.
- The most common types of leukemia in adults are acute myelogenous leukemia (AML) and chronic lymphocytic leukemia (CLL), while acute lymphocytic leukemia (ALL) accounts for 80% of all childhood leukemias.

## ETIOLOGY

- The cause of leukemia is not known. The etiologic factors most commonly considered are genetic predisposition, radiation, chemicals, drugs, and viruses.

### Genetic Factors

- There is evidence of familial clustering with a four- to sevenfold increased risk in individuals with a family member diagnosed with leukemia. In addition, 10%–20% of monozygous twins of individuals with leukemia develop the disease.
- Certain genetic disorders are associated with increased incidence of leukemia (e.g., Down's syndrome, Bloom's syndrome, etc.). Also, diseases such as ataxia telangiectasia and congenital agammaglobulinemia are also prone to terminate in acute leukemia.

### Radiation

- Populations exposed to ionizing radiation have an increased incidence of leukemia, especially AML.
- Radiation remains the most conclusively identified leukemogenic factor in human beings.

### Chemicals

- Chronic exposure to certain chemicals, such as benzene, has been associated with an increased incidence of pancytopenia and subsequent AML. In addition to those who work with benzene in unleaded gasoline, rubber cement, and cleaning solvents, other populations at risk include explosives handlers, distillers, dye users, painters, and shoemakers.

## Drugs

- Drugs that have demonstrated a relationship to the etiology of acute leukemia include certain alkylating agents, chloramphenicol, and phenylbutazone. AML is the most frequently reported second cancer following aggressive chemotherapy and is associated with treatment for Hodgkin's disease, multiple myeloma, ovarian cancer, non-Hodgkin's lymphoma, and breast cancer.

## Viruses

- The role of viruses in the etiology of human leukemia is unclear. Reverse transcriptase has been detected in human leukemic blood cells, but not in normal blood cells.
- HTLV-II has been identified in a rare form of hairy cell leukemia and is also prevalent in intravenous drug addicts.

## CLASSIFICATION

- Leukemias are classified as either chronic or acute and as either myeloid or lymphoid.
- In chronic leukemia the predominant cell is mature-appearing, although it does not function normally.
- The predominant cell in acute leukemia is undifferentiated or immature, usually a "blast" cell.
- All cell lines arise from the same totipotent stem cell. From this cell, which has the potential to differentiate into a variety of cells, the myeloid and lymphocyte series are derived.
- The type of leukemia is named according to the point at which cell maturation is arrested.
- The classification system for leukemias, developed in 1976 by the French-American-British (FAB) Cooperative Group is based on morphology and number of cells; this has been revised and updated.

## PATHOPHYSIOLOGY

- In leukemia, the bone marrow's control of cell proliferation and maturation is absent or abnormal. The results are (1) arrest of the cell in an early phase of its maturation process, causing the accumulation of immature cells; (2) an abnormal proliferation of these immature cells; and (3) crowding of other marrow elements, resulting in inhibited growth and function of these elements and eventual replacement of the marrow by leukemic cells.
- Manifestations of leukemia are related to three factors: (1) excessive proliferation of immature leukocytes within blood-forming organs; (2) infiltration of proliferating leukocytes into various organs of the body; and (3) decrease in the number of normal leukocytes, erythrocytes, and thrombocytes as a result of crowding of the bone marrow by proliferating leukemic cells.

## ASSESSMENT OF ACUTE LEUKEMIA

- Factors that influence the symptoms and physical findings are: (1) the type of leukemic cell, (2) the degree of leukemic cell burden (early-stage or advanced disease), (3) involvement of organs or systems outside of the bone marrow or peripheral circulation, and (4) the depression of normal marrow elements by the leukemic process.

## Patient History

- Acute leukemia presents with a large and rapidly growing population of leukemic cells. Usually, signs and symptoms have been present for less than three months, and perhaps for only a few days.
- The most common complaints of the patient are nonspecific—fatigue, malaise, weight loss, and fever. The presenting symptoms are the manifestations of the effects of leukemic cells on the normal marrow elements. Infections are recurrent in the common sites.
- Neurological complaints are frequent and may signal either leukemia infiltration (especially in ALL) or intracerebral hemorrhage. These include a history of headache, vomiting, visual disturbances, or seizures.

- Occupational exposure and family history of genetic abnormalities or cancer contribute to the total epidemiological picture.

## Physical Examination

- The physical findings of acute leukemia usually relate directly to the effects of pancytopenia. Vital signs may demonstrate fever, tachycardia, and tachypnea. The skin and mucous membranes generally appear pale, with readily apparent ecchymoses or petechiae.
- Generalized or localized adenopathy may be present.

## Diagnostic Studies

- Diagnosis is suggested by the peripheral smear but requires a full examination of the bone marrow. The white blood cell count may be low, normal, or high, and 90% of patients have blast cells present in the peripheral blood.
- Neutropenia is frequent, and thrombocytopenia is present in 40% of patients.
- Blood chemistry studies may reveal hyperuricemia and increased lactic dehydrogenase, as well as altered serum and urine muramidase.
- Bone marrow contents are usually hypercellular.
- Cytogenetic analysis and immunologic studies are performed at the time of diagnosis.

## ACUTE MYELOGENOUS LEUKEMIA

### Classification

- Acute myelogenous leukemia (AML), also referred to as acute nonlymphocytic leukemia (ANLL), is a disease of the pluripotent myeloid stem cell. The malignant clone arises in the myeloid, monocyte, erythroid, or megakaryocyte lines. The exact event that triggers the malignant transformation is not known.
- By the time an individual is diagnosed with AML, the bone marrow and peripheral blood contain up to $10^{12}$ leukemic cells.
- If the disease is left untreated, death occurs within a few months due to infection or uncontrolled bleeding.

### Treatment

- The goal of antileukemic treatment for AML is the eradication of the leukemic stem cell. Complete remission is defined as the restoration of normal peripheral counts and <5% blasts in the bone marrow.
- Treatment regimens are composed of several drugs and are divided into two stages: (1) induction and (2) postremission therapy.

#### Induction therapy

- The goal of induction therapy is to cause severe bone marrow hypoplasia. The cornerstone for remission induction is administration of the cell cycle-specific antimetabolite cytosine arabinoside plus an anthracycline.
- The impact of chemotherapy is assessed at one week after the completion of therapy with a bone marrow biopsy and aspiration on the 14th day.
- Only 20% of patients remain in complete remission. Relapse occurs in the remaining cases within 1–2 years. Thus, postremission therapy is essential.

### Postremission therapy

- By the addition of postremission therapy, the median duration of remission can be increased from 4–8 months to 10–15 months.
- The goal of further therapy is to prevent leukemic recurrence related to undetectable, resistant disease, also called *minimal residual disease*. Postremission therapies include consolidation, intensification, maintenance, and allogeneic or autologous bone marrow transplant:
  - Consolidation therapy consists of one or two courses of very high doses of the same drugs used for induction.
  - Intensification may be initiated right after remission induction (early intensification) or several months later (late intensification). Different drugs are used with the hope that they will be non–cross-resistant with the induction drugs.
  - Maintenance therapy is treatment with lower doses of the same or other drugs given monthly for a prolonged period of time.
- Patients who relapse after induction and postinduction chemotherapy have a 30%–60% likelihood of achieving a second remission. Patients who relapse quickly or who have resistant leukemia should be considered for clinical trials or bone marrow transplant (BMT).

## ACUTE LYMPHOCYTIC LEUKEMIA

- Acute lymphocytic leukemia (ALL) is a malignant disease of the lymphoid progenitors. The abnormal clone originates in the marrow, thymus, and lymph nodes, but the exact etiologic event is unknown.
- Although the defect does not involve the myeloid cell lines, the secondary effect of the high leukemic cell burden on the bone marrow interferes with normal hematopoietic activity.

### Classification

- The FAB classification for ALL is based on several cell properties: size ratio of nucleus to cytoplasm; number, size, and shape of nucleoli; and amount and basophilia of the cytoplasm.
- Another classification system is based on immune features. Four subtypes are identified by the presence of certain markers on the cell surface.
- Leukemic cells infiltrate into the CNS early in the disease and are sheltered from the cytotoxic effects of drugs that penetrate poorly into the cerebrospinal fluid. Over time, the leukemic cells proliferate and cause relapse. Cells can also be harbored in the testes. In addition, 80% of patients have lymphadenopathy and/or splenomegaly at the time of diagnosis.
- The prognosis for long-term survival is more favorable for individuals with ALL than AML since drugs are available that are uniquely effective against lymphocytes.
- Long-term survival and cure for individuals with ALL is possible only if a complete remission is achieved.

### Treatment

- Chemotherapeutic regimens proven effective against ALL contain drugs that are selectively toxic to lymphoblasts and relatively sparing of normal hematopoietic stem cells.
- The focus of therapy for ALL is to eradicate all leukemic cells from the marrow and lymph tissue and eliminate any residual foci of disease within the CNS. Treatment is divided into three stages: (1) induction, (2) CNS prophylaxis, and (3) postremission therapy.

#### Induction therapy

- Although it is possible to achieve complete remission in 93% of children with ALL by using a combination of vincristine, prednisone, and L-asparaginase, the same drugs—even with the addition of an anthracycline—produce remission rates of only 70%–75% in adults with ALL.

### CNS prophylaxis

- Meningeal leukemia is known to occur in up to 50% of patients with ALL in the absence of CNS prophylaxis. By comparison, in patients with AML, the incidence is less than 5%.
- CNS prophylaxis should start within a few weeks of the initiation of therapy. Treatment usually includes intracranial radiation and intrathecal methotrexate.

### Postremission therapy

- As in AML, even after complete remission, patients with ALL harbor remaining leukemic cells. Relapse occurs in two to three months if there is no continuing therapy. Prolonged chemotherapy may lead to a 40% overall cure rate, but the type and duration are not completely defined.
- The outlook for patients in whom relapse occurs during therapy is quite poor, and younger patients with an HLA-matched donor should be immediately referred for BMT.
- If relapse occurs after the completion of therapy, treatment is continued with high-dose methotrexate, tenoposide, and cytarabine or high-dose cytosine arabinoside with an anthracycline or amsacrine.
- Second remission can be achieved in up to 50% of cases.
- Because patients treated with allogeneic BMT show a trend toward longer survival if the transplant is performed during the first remission, it is important to identify patients with an unfavorable prognosis in the early stages of disease.

## MYELODYSPLASTIC SYNDROMES

- Myelodysplastic syndromes (MDS) are a group of hematologic disorders with an increased risk of transformation to AML. They are characterized by a change in the quantity and quality of bone marrow products.
- MDSs are believed to occur as the result of an altered stem cell. The cause is unknown.
- Approximately 30% of patients diagnosed with AML initially present with preleukemic syndrome. MDS may be considered to be different stages of the same disease.
- Even if the evolution to acute leukemia never occurs, life-threatening anemia, thrombocytopenia, and/or neutropenia invariably occur.
- The median age of patients diagnosed with MDS is 60. The incidence is slightly higher in males than females.
- About half of patients with MDS develop AML.
- Treatment for MDS is as aggressive as the course of the disease. Serial bone marrow and peripheral blood examinations allow the physician to monitor the pace of the disease. Supportive therapy includes replacement of RBCs or platelets and antibiotics for infection. Differentiation inducers, especially cytosine arabinoside, are thought to induce differentiation of immature myeloid cells in 25%–35% of patients with MDS.

## CHRONIC MYELOGENOUS LEUKEMIA

- Chronic myelogenous leukemia (CML), also called chronic granulocytic leukemia, is a disorder of the myeloid stem cell characterized by marked splenomegaly and in increased production of granulocytes, especially neutrophils. Approximately 90% of patients with CML have a diagnostic marker, the Philadelphia chromosome (Ph[1]).
- There is no known specific cause for CML, except exposure to ionizing radiation.
- The natural course of CML is divided into a chronic and terminal phase. The initial chronic phase is characterized by excessive proliferation and accumulation of mature granulocytes and precursors. There is an absence of lymphadenopathy, but 90% of patients have palpable splenomegaly.

- Within 30–40 months the disorder transforms into a terminal phase consisting of accelerated and blastic phases.
  - The accelerated phase includes progressive leukocytosis with increasing myeloid precursors, increasing basophils, splenomegaly, weight loss, and weakness. There is increasing resistance to therapy.
  - The blastic phase resembles AML, with 30%–40% of the bone marrow cells being blasts or promyelocytes. A crisis occurs as blast cell counts rise rapidly, often exceeding 100,000/dl.
- Median survival after the onset of the terminal phase is 3 months.

## Assessment

- CML in up to 20% of affected individuals is diagnosed in the absence of any symptomatology. Most patients, however, present with a history that reflects the gradual accumulation of a white blood cell mass that is 10–150 times normal.

### Patient history

- The initial symptoms typically are related to massive splenomegaly due to infiltration of the spleen by leukemic cells: left upper quadrant pain, early satiety, and vague abdominal fullness may be the presenting complaints.

### Physical examination

- Examination of the eyes, ears, nose, and throat may reveal leukemic infiltration. Splenomegaly and hepatomegaly are common.
- The physical examination of the patient in blast crisis is similar to that for the patient with acute leukemia.
- Rapid diagnosis and treatment to reduce the number of proliferating blasts are essential.

### Diagnostic studies

- A complete blood count in the chronic phase reveals anemia and severe leukocytosis. The differential count of the leukocytes demonstrates WBCs in every stage of maturation, with a predominance of more mature cells.
- The presence of functional but leukemic granulocytes in these individuals accounts for the low incidence of infection during the chronic phase.

## Treatment

- The only chance for cure of CML is with ablation of the Ph[1] chromosome and absence of the *bcr-abl* fusion gene. Currently this occurs after high-dose therapy followed by allogeneic BMT.

### Chronic phase

- The standard therapy during the chronic phase is single-agent oral chemotherapy.
- Busulfan, an alkylating agent, is active against primitive hematopoietic stem cells. Treatment is stopped if the WBC is less than 20,000/mm$^3$.
- Hydroxyurea is cytostatic to cycling cells. It acts on late progenitor stem cells causing rapid disease control.
- Interferon-alfa (IFN) is approved for previously untreated or pretreated patients with chronic phase, Ph positive CML. It is recommended that therapy begin within one year of diagnosis.

### Terminal phase

- CML is a chronic neoplasm with a 100% incidence of blastic transformation. This transformation is a gradual failure of response to treatment and failure of production of erythrocytes and platelets.
- However, bone marrow aspirations are required, which are costly and uncomfortable for the patient. The current trend is to continue chronic phase therapy until evidence of the blastic phase appears.
- It is difficult to predict survival, although life expectancy is less than 1 year.
- Blast crisis requires intensive chemotherapy, similar to that used in the treatment of AML.
- Although BMT remains the only chance for cure, it is an option for only 25% of patients. The best results have been obtained in patients receiving allogeneic BMT during the chronic phase, with 55%–70% being disease-free at three to five years.

## CHRONIC LYMPHOCYTIC LEUKEMIA

- A progressive accumulation of morphologically normal but functionally inert lymphocytes is found in chronic lymphocytic leukemia (CLL). As the disease progresses, the abnormal lymphocytes accumulate in the bone marrow, spleen, liver, and lymph nodes. In 95% of the cases, there is clonal expansion of neoplastic B-lymphocytes. The median age at diagnosis is 60 years; the majority of cases are male.
- The clinical course is variable, and, as with other hematologic malignancies, many attempts have been made to correlate a staging system with prognosis. The two most commonly used systems are Rai and Binet.
  - The Rai staging system has five levels based on the extent of tissue involvement and compromise of bone marrow function.
  - The Binet system identifies three groups, each with a subsequently worsening prognosis.
- In general, treatment is withheld until the patient shows evidence of hemolytic anemia, cytopenia, disfiguring or painful lymphadenopathy, symptomatic organomegaly, or marked systemic symptoms.

### Assessment

- One-fourth of individuals with CLL are diagnosed during a routine physical examination.

#### Patient history

- Early CLL may be asymptomatic. However, because CLL is a disease of immunoglobulin-secreting cells, a history of recurrent infections, especially of the skin and respiratory tract, may be elicited.
- Progressive infiltration and accumulation in nodal structures and the bone marrow gradually produce the symptoms that are typical of more advanced disease.
  - Vague complaints of malaise, anorexia, and fatigue are common, as is noticeable and bothersome lymphadenopathy. Splenomegaly may cause early satiety and abdominal discomfort.

#### Physical examination

- Splenomegaly may be the only clinical finding. Lymphadenopathy occurs in 60% of patients.

#### Diagnostic studies

- Peripheral blood examination reveals lymphocytosis with normal or immature lymphocytes.
  - The lymphocyte is greater than $20,000/mm^3$ in early disease and may be over $100,000/mm^3$ in advanced disease.

## Treatment

- In general, treatment consists only of observation until the patient is symptomatic with cytopenias or organomegaly.
- Chlorambucil and cyclophosphamide are used to treat CLL.
- Corticosteroids are used to control leukocytosis and immune-mediated cytopenias. When the patient no longer responds to steroid therapy, splenectomy may provide relief of symptoms.
- Radiation therapy may be used to treat lymphadenopathy or painful splenomegaly. Total body irradiation (TBI) and extracorporeal irradiation of blood to reduce lymphocyte counts are treatment options that may induce a temporary remission.
- For patients with advanced disease (stage III or IV) and anemia or thrombocytopenia, combination therapy is recommended. This includes cyclophosphamide, vincristine, doxorubicin, and prednisone.

## HAIRY CELL LEUKEMIA
### Etiology

- An unusual variant of the chronic leukemias is *hairy cell leukemia* (HCL), so named for the prominent cytoplasmic projections on circulating mononuclear cells.
- Distinguishing characteristics are massive splenomegaly and little or no adenopathy. The characteristic hairy cells stain positively for tartrate-resistant acid phosphatase. Two-thirds of individuals with HCL have pancytopenia.

### Treatment

- The goal of therapy in HCL has progressed from palliative to cure with the use of nucleoside analogues and interferon. Splenectomy is the treatment of choice for patients with marked pancytopenia, recurrent infections, massive splenomegaly, or rapid disease progression and may allow prolonged survival of up to 15 years.
- Recombinant alfa-interferon is considered the treatment of choice for those in whom disease progresses either before or after splenectomy.

## SUPPORTIVE THERAPY
### Education

- The teaching plan for all patients includes pertinent information about the diagnosis, strategies for self-care in the prevention and treatment of side effects, and methods to facilitate coping and adaptation to the illness.
- Include the basic physiology of the bone marrow in the teaching plan. From this base, individualized instruction related to the specific leukemia is given.

### Physical Care

- The nurse must regularly conduct a thorough physical examination in order to detect any subtle evidence of infection; the usual signs and symptoms are diminished or absent.
- The nurse caring for the patient with acute leukemia must be experienced in the use of right atrial catheters (RACs) and vascular access devices (VADs). Patients undergoing aggressive induction therapy in the hospital often have a double or triple lumen RAC placed prior to the start of therapy.
- Patients who require ongoing treatment but less frequent blood sampling and no simultaneous infusion of multiple fluids may have a VAD placed subcutaneously.

## Symptom Management

### Bone marrow depression

- The desired effect of cytotoxic therapy is bone marrow hypoplasia. The duration of pancytopenia is variable, depending on the type of therapy and the person's ability to recover.

### Neutropenia

- It takes 9–10 days for immature cells formed in the bone marrow to become mature granulocytes; any interruption in their production quickly places the patient at risk for developing an infection. Neutropenia is commonly defined as an absolute neutrophil count less than 1000/mm$^3$. Neutropenia eliminates one of the body's first lines of defense against infection.
- Most infections are due to organisms endogenous to the host or present in the environment.
- Empiric antibiotic therapy is used to treat high-risk (neutropenic and febrile) patients until an infecting organism is identified.
- Amphotericin B is used to treat life-threatening fungal infections in myelosuppressed, immunosuppressed individuals. It is indicated if fever continues for five to seven days after the start of antibiotic therapy, if there is no identified source of infection, and if continued neutropenia is expected.
- Symptom management includes interventions to prevent or treat fever, chills or rigors.
- Fever is usually the first sign of infection. Early indications of pneumonia are shortness of breath or cough. Vital signs are assessed every four hours. At the onset of fever over 100°F in the neutropenic patient, blood, urine, and sputum cultures are obtained and empiric antibiotic therapy is initiated.
- Prevention of infection focuses on restoring host defenses, decreasing invasive procedures, and decreasing colonization of organisms.
- To decrease the number of gram-negative organisms, uncooked fruits and vegetables are avoided.
- Granulocyte transfusions are a controversial therapy.
- Colony-stimulating factors have been used to treat leukemia.

### Erythrocytopenia

- Transfusions of RBCs is provided for symptomatic anemia or sudden blood loss due to bleeding.

### Thrombocytopenia

- The first evidence of bleeding may be petechiae or ecchymoses.
- Random donor platelets are given to keep the platelet count above 20,000/mm$^3$.

## Complications

### Leukostasis

- Individuals with extremely high numbers of circulating blasts are at risk of leukostatic-induced hemorrhage. This occurs most often in patients with ALL. Intracerebral hemorrhage is the most common and most lethal manifestation of this complication. Treatment consists of high doses of cytotoxic drugs.

### Disseminated intravascular coagulation

- Disseminated intravascular coagulation (DIC) is most frequently associated with acute promyelocytic leukemia. Correction depends on the succcessful treatment of the leukemia. Nursing care focuses on the prevention of injury, administration of prescribed therapy, and monitoring of the appropriate lab results.

### Retinoic acid-APL syndrome

- This syndrome appears clinically similar to the capillary leak syndrome associated with interleukin-2 therapy and is characterized by fever, respiratory distress, pulmonary infiltrates on chest x-ray, and weight gain. Nursing care is focused on early detection of fluid retention, fever, and pulmonary distress.

### Oral complications

- Gingival hypertrophy due to massive infiltration by leukemic cells is associated with acute myelomonocytic and monocytic leukemia. Stomatitis due to the toxicity of chemotherapeutic agents renders the patient at high risk for oral infection. Oral care consists of regular cleansing with a solution of one quart of water with one teaspoon each of salt and sodium bicarbonate, treatment of infection with nystatin mouth rinses, and appropriate analgesia as needed.

### Cerebellar toxicity

- Cerebellar toxicity is a CNS toxicity associated with the administration of high-dose cytosine arabinoside (HDCA). The syndrome may begin with signs of ataxia and nystagmus and progress to dysarthria and adiadochokinesis. This toxicity may be irreversible if not detected early.

## PSYCHOSOCIAL SUPPORT

- A primary objective of supportive care must be to facilitate the most effective coping mechanisms for the individual and family as well as to enable the patient to live as full and normal a life as possible.
- Assessment of the individual's needs and degree of stress will facilitate the planning of suitable intervention.
- The stage and "curability" of the disease are other factors to be considered. It is imperative that the nurse understand the implications of the planned therapy and assist the patient in making appropriate decisions.

## PRACTICE QUESTIONS

**Questions 1–4 concern Ms. Jantzen, who is diagnosed with AML.**

1.  Four years ago, Ms. Jantzen successfully completed treatment for breast cancer. Now she is diagnosed with acute myelogenous leukemia (AML). Which is most likely to have contributed to Ms. Jantzen's AML?
    a.  Alkylating agents
    b.  Anthracyclines
    c.  Vinca alkaloids
    d.  Antimetabolites

2.  Ms. Jantzen will soon begin induction therapy. As her oncology nurse, you explain that the goal of therapy will be to cause severe bone marrow hypoplasia, using:
    a.  busulfan and hydroxyurea.
    b.  cytosine arabinoside and daunorubicin.
    c.  vincristine, prednisone, L-asparaginase, and daunorubicin.
    d.  chlorambucil and cyclophosphamide.

3.  Treatment is well underway, but Ms. Jantzen begins to experience slight difficulty with articulation of words. She smiles apologetically and says, "I guess I didn't get enough sleep. My mouth is pretty dry, too." Your response is to:
    a.  do an oral examination and offer mouth care. Ms. Jantzen needs to be given HDCA therapy.
    b.  withhold her medication and do a neurological evaluation.
    c.  withhold her medication and check her renal function tests.
    d.  take the time to interview Ms. Jantzen to identify factors contributing to her sleeplessness, which is also contributing to her dry mouth.

4.  Ms. Jantzen is in complete remission after two courses of induction therapy. She is beginning postremission therapy, in which she will receive very high doses of the same drugs used for induction therapy. She asks, "What's the point of this? I'm so sick of treatment. I'm in remission, aren't I?" You explain that this type of postremission therapy is:
    a.  consolidation therapy to prevent leukemic recurrence related to minimal residual disease.
    b.  intensification therapy to treat substantial toxicities, including extended myelosuppression and cerebellar dysfunction.
    c.  maintenance therapy, which is used to help prevent a recurrence in some specific cases.
    d.  CNS prophylaxis to prevent leukemic recurrence related to minimal residual disease.

**Questions 5–7 concern Liza, a 10-year-old who may have AML or ALL.**

5.  Ten-year-old Liza is to be assessed for possible acute myelogenous leukemia (AML) and acute lymphocytic leukemia (ALL). This proves to be quite a challenge since the two have similar symptoms. This makes Liza's mother anxious; she is, naturally, eager for treatment to begin. You explain that even though they appear similar, it is essential to differentiate between the two before beginning treatment because:
    a.  the response rate and survival rate are better in AML than in ALL.
    b.  patients with AML are more susceptible to viral infections.
    c.  bone marrow transplant is the treatment of choice in AML.
    d.  CNS prophylaxis is given routinely in ALL but not in AML.

6.  It is determined that Liza has ALL. Liza begins treatment with a combination of vincristine, prednisone, and L-asparaginase. The physician begins to express strong hopes for a remission, but Liza's mother takes you aside and says, "My husband's aunt died of AML at age 40—and she was very robust and athletic! What hope does a mere ten-year-old have? Liza's not exactly robust to begin with, and she's so young." You answer that:

    a.  The physician is aware of the fact that the prognosis is grimmer when ALL affects children, but that psychosocial support for Liza can make a world of difference in survival rate.

    b.  Age and athletic ability have been shown to make no difference in demographics of remission and survival rates in ALL.

    c.  Complete remission is achieved in 93% of children with ALL, as opposed to 70%–75% in adults.

    d.  Remission rates in patients with ALL depend on etiology and stage of disease and are not reflected by age or activity levels.

7.  You are monitoring Liza to ensure that she does not develop complications associated with leukostasis. The most common and most lethal complication to watch for is:

    a.  intracerebral hemorrhage.

    b.  cerebellar toxicity.

    c.  blast crisis.

    d.  disseminated intravascular coagulation.

8.  Ms. Drake has myelodysplastic syndrome (MDS). She reports being asymptomatic "forever," and asks you why she still has to endure ongoing monitoring. The best explanation you can offer is that:

    a.  T-cell abnormalities increase the risk of opportunistic infections.

    b.  Compliance with the prescribed treatment will delay or prevent the onset of symptoms.

    c.  All patients with MDS eventually develop anemia, thrombocytopenia, and/or neutropenia.

    d.  All patients with MDS eventually develop acute leukemia.

**Questions 9–11 concern Mr. Jackson, a leukemia patient.**

9.  You are the new oncology nurse in a large hospital. On your first day you meet Mr. Jackson. His physician neglects to tell you what type of leukemia Mr. Jackson has, but she does tell you, "He still has the Philadelphia chromosome, so we don't exactly have a cure yet." From this you are able to discern that Mr. Jackson has:

    a.  acute lymphocytic leukemia.

    b.  acute myelogenous leukemia.

    c.  chronic lymphocytic leukemia.

    d.  chronic myelogenous leukemia.

10. Mr. Jackson, from the previous question, is being treated with busulfan. He complains of left upper quadrant abdominal pain, early satiety, and vague abdominal fullness. These symptoms are most likely to be related to:

    a.  toxicities of busulfan.

    b.  bowel obstruction.

    c.  splenomegaly.

    d.  hypercalcemia.

11. Mr. Jackson's busulfan therapy will be stopped if his white blood count is less than:
    a.  1000 WBC/mm$^3$.
    b.  3000 WBC/mm$^3$.
    c.  10,000 WBC/mm$^3$.
    d.  20,000 WBC/mm$^3$.

**Questions 12–14 concern Ms. Camara, who is being treated for hairy cell leukemia.**

12. Ms. Camara is being treated for hairy cell leukemia. Her disease continues to progress. You are about to sit down with her family to plan her course of treatment. She has already begun receiving supportive therapy with transfusions of red blood cells and platelets. In addition, you explain, she needs:
    a.  aggressive chemotherapy requiring hospitalization.
    b.  aggressive chemotherapy requiring hospitalization plus CNS prophylaxis.
    c.  recombinant alfa-interferon; also, a splenectomy may be considered.
    d.  chemotherapy followed by a bone marrow transplant.

13. Ms. Camara develops neutropenia. You are monitoring her regularly for signs of infection. Which of the following are you most concerned about?
    a.  Viral infection
    b.  Fungal infection
    c.  Infection from gram-positive organisms
    d.  Infection from gram-negative organisms

14. As you continue to monitor Ms. Camara, you remind yourself that the usual symptoms of infection will very likely be absent or muted in this particular patient because:
    a.  most infections are due to organisms that are part of the body's normal flora.
    b.  the WBCs drop rapidly and recovery time is slow.
    c.  neutrophils are necessary to produce an inflammatory response.
    d.  the immunoglobulins are reduced.

15. Mr. Chross has acute myelomonocytic leukemia. He complains of swelling, necrosis, and infection of the gums, and you are able to discern that he has gingival hypertrophy. "What can you do about it?" he asks. "It's really uncomfortable." You explain each of the following treatments, all of which are appropriate. But, you assure him, the most effective course of action will be:
    a.  oral care with a solution of one quart water with one teaspoon each of salt and sodium bicarbonate.
    b.  antifungal mouth rinses.
    c.  a local analgesic the physician has ordered.
    d.  initiating chemotherapy.

---

# Answer Explanations

1.  **The answer is a.** Alkylating agents have a demonstrated causative relationship to acute myelocytic leukemia. AML is the most frequently reported second cancer following aggressive chemotherapy for Hodgkin's disease, non-Hodgkin's lymphoma, multiple myeloma, ovarian cancer, and breast cancer. These cancers are treated with aggressive chemotherapy regimens containing alkylating agents. (p. 1237)

2. **The answer is b.** The cornerstone of induction therapy in AML is the cell-cycle-specific antimetabolite cytosine arabinoside, plus an anthracycline such as daunorubicin. (p. 1261)

3. **The answer is b.** The cytosine arabinoside (HDCA) Ms. Jantzen has been taking should be withheld because her dysarthria is a symptom of cerebellar toxicity from the drug. HDCA can cause cerebellar toxicities that may be irreversible. A full neurological examination should be done before each dose, even in the absence of symptoms. (p. 1255)

4. **The answer is a.** The purpose of postremission therapies is to prevent leukemic recurrence related to minimal residual disease. The three types of postremission therapies are consolidation therapy, intensification therapy, maintenance therapy, and bone marrow transplant (BMT). Consolidation therapy consists of one or two courses of very high doses of the same drugs used for induction (up to 30 times the induction doses of cytosine arabinoside for AML). Intensification regimens use different drugs in the hope that they will not be cross-resistant. Maintenance therapies use lower doses for a prolonged period of time. Maintenance therapy is not currently recommended in the treatment of AML. (p. 1243)

5. **The answer is d.** Leukemic infiltration of the CNS occurs more frequently in ALL. Meningeal leukemia occurs in up to 50% of patients who do not receive CNS prophylaxis. Choices **a**, **b**, and **c** are incorrect because the response rate and survival rate are better in ALL than in AML; patients with ALL and patients with AML are equally susceptible to viral infections; and the role for BMT in AML remains controversial. (p. 1245)

6. **The answer is c.** Although it is possible to achieve complete remission in 93% of children with ALL, the same drug treatment—even with the addition of an anthracycline—produces remission rates of only 70%–75% in adults with ALL. (p. 1245)

7. **The answer is a.** Leukostasis occurs as the leukemic blast cells accumulate and invade vessel walls, causing rupture and bleeding. Patients with extremely high numbers of circulating blasts (WBC >50,000/mm$^3$) are at increased risk for leukostasis. Intracerebral hemorrhage is the most common and most lethal manifestation of this complication. (p. 1254)

8. **The answer is c.** All patients with MDS will eventually develop life-threatening anemia, thrombocytopenia and/or neutropenia. Regular evaluation of patients with MDS is important in order to monitor the need for supportive therapy with red blood cells, platelets, or antibiotics. MDS can transform to acute leukemia; however, this does not occur in all patients with MDS. (p. 1247)

9. **The answer is d.** Approximately 90% of patients with CML have the diagnostic marker, Philadelphia chromosome Ph$^1$. As long as this marker is present, the disease is not cured. (p. 1247)

10. **The answer is c.** Symptoms of splenomegaly are the result of infiltration of the spleen by leukemic cells. (p. 1247)

11. **The answer is d.** Busulfan is taken daily in the chronic phase of CML. Blood counts begin to drop in 10–14 days after therapy is begun. To prevent prolonged or severe myelosuppression, treatment is stopped if the WBC is less than 20,000 WBC/mm$^3$. (p. 1248)

12. **The answer is c.** Splenectomy is the treatment of choice for patients with marked pancytopenia, recurrent infections, massive splenomegaly, or rapid disease progress. Recombinant alfa-interferon is considered the treatment of choice for those with hairy cell leukemia in whom disease progresses either before or after splenectomy. (p. 1250)

13. **The answer is b.** Fungal infections are difficult to treat in the neutropenic and immunocompromised patient, and recovery of the marrow is the best hope for survival. (p. 1253)

14. **The answer is c.** The patient with neutropenia is unable to mount an inflammatory response. Fever is usually the first sign of infection. Choices **a**, **b**, and **d** are all true, but they explain why the neutropenic patient is at greater risk for infection rather than why the usual signs and symptoms of infection are often absent. (p. 1253)

15. **The answer is d.** While all of these treatments will help, Mr. Chross's gingival hypertrophy is the result of infiltration of the gums by leukemic cells, so chemotherapy will treat the underlying cause. The other measures may reduce infection and add to his comfort. (p. 1254)

# Chapter 42    Lung Cancers

## INTRODUCTION

- Lung cancer is the most frequent cause of cancer death in men and women in North America. Cigarette smoking has been estimated to cause 80%–90% of all lung cancer deaths. Despite the use of multimodality treatments for lung cancer, overall cure rates remain a discouraging 14%.

## EPIDEMIOLOGY

- Today lung cancer kills more women than any other cancer in the United States; worldwide, U.S. women are second only to those in Denmark in age-adjusted death rates for lung cancer per 100,000 population.
- Although the mortality rate for men with lung cancer began to decline in the mid-1980s, lung cancer continues to cause over 2.5 times more deaths in men than prostate cancer, the second leading cancer killer among men in the United States.
- Mortality rates among African-American men are slightly higher than for white men, but are comparable among African-American and white women.
- The highest incidence of lung cancer is in the elderly.

## ETIOLOGY

### Cigarette Smoke

- The risk of lung cancer development in heavy smokers is estimated to be 10–25 times the risk of nonsmokers.
- Risk from smoking is determined by multiple factors: number of cigarettes smoked per day, duration of smoking, age at which smoking began, inhalation patterns, and tar content of cigarettes.
- Benefit from smoking cessation begins five years after quitting and increases steadily over time, although the risk for lung cancer among former smokers will remain higher than the risk for lifetime nonsmokers.
- Tar, the most carcinogenic compound in cigarettes, causes basal cell hyperplasia, then dysplasia with displacement of the normal, healthy ciliated and mucus-secreting cells.
- Tobacco smoke is a complete carcinogen, containing both initiator and promoter substances. Initiators can cause irreversible gene mutations. Repeated exposure to promoters may cause a cell to exhibit malignant behaviors, although cellular repair may occur if promoters are withdrawn.

### Passive Smoke

- Environmental tobacco smoke (ETS) contains nearly all of the carcinogens contained in mainstream smoke inhaled by smokers, but because it is not filtered, greater numbers of carcinogens are inhaled passively.
- The Environmental Protection Agency (EPA) considers ETS to be a human carcinogen. Exposure to ETS accounts for 30% of all lung cancers.

### Asbestos

- Asbestos exposure is the most common occupational etiology of lung cancer, causing 3%–4% of all cases. Asbestos and smoking are synergistic for the development of lung cancer.

## Radon

- Radon particles act as both initiators and promoters. Synergy with cigarette smoke has been reported.
- Radon is present in rock and soil and is known to seep into homes and office buildings through basements and crawl spaces. The U.S. EPA estimates that over 14,000 lung cancer deaths per year are caused by radon, mostly in smokers.

## Occupational Agents

- An increased incidence of lung cancer has been documented in individuals working with arsenic, copper, silica, lead, zinc, gold, chloromethyl ether, diesel exhaust, chromium, coal, hydrocarbons, nickel, ionizing radiation, cadmium, beryllium, fur, and vineyard environments.

## Indoor Air Pollution

- Indoor environments may be contaminated with other harmful pollutants including radon, cigarette smoke, building materials, household aerosol products, combusion devices, and the entry of outdoor air contaminants. Data regarding risk are inconclusive.

## Dietary Factors

- Although the relationship of diet to lung cancer requires further investigation, early evidence suggests an inverse relationship between lung cancer risk and consumption of vitamin A or beta-carotene, vitamin C, vitamin E, and selenium.

## PREVENTION, SCREENING, EARLY DETECTION PROGRAMS

### Primary Prevention

- Primary prevention of lung cancer depends on identifying successful strategies for smoking prevention and cessation. If smoking were totally eliminated, 85% of lung cancers would disappear.
- Today's death rate from lung cancer in women is 500% higher than that of 1935. Over 22 million women in the U.S. smoke, including 25% of those who are pregnant.
- Of the 1 million Americans who become smokers each year, most are children or adolescents. Ninety percent of smokers begin smoking before they are 20 years old, and most are girls.
- In the United States, higher smoking rates are seen in individuals of a lower socioeconomic status, particularly women, although male blue-collar workers continue to be the heaviest smokers. Education appears to be inversely related to smoking rates.
- During the 1970s, 1980s, and 1990s, significant progress was made to limit and/or ban smoking in the workplace and other public places. In 1995 President Clinton approved an FDA regulatory plan to restrict seductive advertising directed at minors and to reduce easy access to their cigarettes. Almost all states have passed legislation prohibiting the sale of tobacco to minors.

### Secondary Prevention

#### Smoking cessation

- Smoking cessation can reduce the risk for lung cancer in a smoker. Because it has been shown that smokers respond to direct, unequivocal messages from nurses and physicians to quit smoking, such messages should be given at every opportunity.
- Smoking cessation rates after behavioral interventions alone have been discouraging. Nicotine replacement using chewing gum or the transdermal patch has been shown to relieve withdrawal symptoms and has improved success rates to as high as 27.5% at one year when combined with smoking cessation counseling.

- Research has found that the brains of living smokers have significantly lower levels of the enzyme monoamine oxidase B (MAO B) than the brains of nonsmokers and former smokers. Low MAO B enhances the addictive aspects of nicotine. These data may have implications for smoking cessation strategies.

### Chemoprevention

- Chemoprevention, also called chemoprophylaxis, is treatment with agents that may prevent or reverse the promotion phase of carcinogenesis.
- The leading cause of death in early-stage lung cancer is the development of second primary tumors. The most commonly studied groups of chemoprevention agents are the retinoids and carotenoids, along with dietary intake of beta-carotene and vitamin A. Investigators are searching for cell markers that might verify the effects of these agents before a malignancy actually develops.

### Screening and Early Detection

- Screening can detect lung cancer at an earlier stage but does not improve long-term survival. Therefore, mass screening for lung cancer is not currently recommended.
- Dominant oncogenes, whose expression promotes neoplastic growth, include the *ras* and *myc* families. The *ras* oncogenes appear to function early in the process of carcinogenesis and may be a good target for early detection.

## PATHOPHYSIOLOGY
### Cellular Characteristics

- All lung cancers are thought to arise from a pluripotent stem cell originating from a primitive endodermal structure, eventually differentiating into multiple different histological subtypes.
- Bronchogenic cancers have been grouped into two broad categories: small-cell lung cancer (SCLC) and the non–small-cell lung cancers (NSCLC), which include squamous cell carcinoma, adenocarcinoma, and large-cell carcinoma.
- Many tumors are heterogenous, containing cells from more than one histological type, which makes accurate classification more difficult.

### Small-cell lung cancer

- SCLC is an epithelial tumor that invades the submucosa and is thought to arise from Kulchitsky cells, neuroendocine cells that secrete peptide hormones.
- Most SCLC tumors are centrally located, developing around a main bronchus and eventually compressing the bronchi externally. Responsible for 25% of all lung cancers, SCLC is an agressive tumor and often is metastatic at the time of diagnosis. Its doubling time is shorter than that of any other lung cancer type.
- The World Health Organization (WHO) has classified SCLC into three subtypes: oat cell, which accounts for 90% of cases; intermediate; and combined (oat cell with adenocarcinoma or squamous cell carcinoma component).
- All SCLC cells are several times larger than a mature lymphocyte, have scant cytoplasm, and show multiple atypical mitoses. Genetic abnormalities include absence of two suppressor genes, the retinoblastoma (RB) gene and the *p53* gene. Amplification of the *myc* family of proto (dominant) oncogenes has been observed.
- About 70% of SCLCs produce neuroendocrine markers. Early identification of these markers may aid in the diagnosis and management of SCLC and may have prognostic significance. Lung cancer cells can produce autocrine growth factors, such as gastrin-releasing peptide (GRP).

### Non–small-cell lung cancer

#### Squamous cell carcinoma

- Squamous cell carcinomas constitute 30% of all lung cancers and are more common in males than in females. These tumors arise from the basal cells of the bronchial epithelium and usually present as masses in large bronchi.

#### Adenocarcinoma

- Adenocarcinomas are the most common lung cancers in males, in females, and in nonsmokers, accounting for 40% of all tumors. They arise from the bronchial epithelium.
- The WHO has classified adenocarcinomas of the lung by four histological subtypes: (1) acinar, (2) papillary, (3) solid carcinoma with mucus formation, and (4) bronchoalveolar, although there is controversy regarding whether the latter should be considered a separate entity.

#### Large-cell carcinoma

- Large-cell carcinoma is the least common type of lung cancer, representing about 10%–15% of all cases. Large-cell tumors usually arise as peripheral nodules and metastasize early, often to the GI tract. The average doubling time is about three months.
- Large-cell carcinomas are classified by the WHO into two types: (1) clear cell and (2) giant cell.

## Progression of Disease

- Lung cancers spread by direct extension, lymphatic invasion, and hematogenous routes. In SCLC, metastasis to distant sites has already occurred in up to 63% of cases at the time of diagnosis. NSCLC cancers are more likely to spread by direct extension or lymphatic invasion.

## CLINICAL MANIFESTATIONS

- A summary of symptoms associated with lung cancer is presented in Table 42-1 on text page 1271.

## Local-Regional Symptoms

- Lung tumors may be present for as long as five years before symptoms are experienced. The most common symptoms of local-regional disease include cough, dyspnea, hemoptysis, wheezing, chest pain, and postobstructive pneumonia.
- Although peripheral tumors cause chest pain in as many as 50% of patients, central tumors are more likely to cause symptoms associated with airway obstruction. Apical tumors may involve the cervical and first thoracic nerves. As a lung tumor with mediastinal involvement grows, it may eventually compress the superior vena cava, causing superior vena cava syndrome (SVCS).

## Symptoms Due to Extrathoracic Involvement

- Signs and symptoms of extrathoracic metastases depend upon the site of involvement.

## Systemic Symptoms with or without Paraneoplastic Syndromes

- Systemic symptoms of lung cancer include generalized weakness and fatigue, anorexia, cachexia, weight loss, and anemia.
- Small-cell lung cancer is associated with paraneoplastic syndromes more frequently than the non–small-cell tumors. These include Cushing's syndrome, the Lambert-Eaton myasthenic syndrome (LEMS), and humoral hypercalcemia of malignancy (the most frequent paraneoplastic syndrome in NSCLC).

## ASSESSMENT

- An accurate health history should include a description of the problem(s), an assessment of past history and family history, a thorough psychosocial history, and a review of systems, examination of the pulmonary and lymphatic systems, and inspection, palpation, percussion, and auscultation.

## Diagnostic Studies

### Imaging studies

- The chest radiograph is probably the most helpful diagnostic study for lung cancer. However, lesions not seen on the chest radiograph can be detected on computed tomography (CT). The chest CT can be particularly helpful in evaluating mediastinal lymph nodes. Magnetic resonance imaging (MRI) of the chest may be superior in evaluation of the perihilar and paravertebral regions and may be employed when CT scan results are not definitive.

### Tissue diagnostic studies

#### Sputum cytology

- The diagnostic yield for sputum cytologies is up to 80% for central tumors but drops to below 20% for small peripheral tumors. Squamous cell carcinomas are the most frequent type diagnosed by sputum cytology; adenocarcinomas are least often diagnosed by this test.

#### Bronchoscopy

- In fiberoptic bronchoscopy, when central lesions can be visualized, the diagnoses can be made more than 90% of the time.

#### Fine-needle aspiration

- Percutaneous fine-needle aspiration is used when lung lesions cannot be visualized by bronchoscopy but are accessible percutaneously.

#### Mediastinoscopy

- Mediastinoscopy allows for more direct visualization and palpation of mediastinal lymph nodes.

#### Video-assisted thorascopic surgery

- VATS has been used for the staging and diagnosis of lung cancer.

#### Thoracotomy

- On rare occasion thoracotomy is necessary to make a diagnosis of lung cancer. Adequate tissue samples are almost always obtained, although morbidity and mortality are higher than with mediastinoscopy.

## Prognostic Indicators

### Small-cell lung cancer

- The most favorable prognostic factor in SCLC is limited-stage disease. Ambulatory performance status, female gender, and a normal serum lactic dehydrogenase (LDH) are also favorable prognostic factors for SCLC. The tumor marker neuron-specific enolase (NSE) is a promising prognostic indicator.
  - SCLC has the poorest survial rates of all lung cancer types.

### Non–small-cell lung cancer

- Stage of disease is the most significant prognostic factor for NSCLC with early-stage cancers responding better to treatment and demonstrating longer survival. The presence of mediastinal lymph node metastases usually indicates a very poor prognosis, although patients with ipsilateral node involvement may be curable with multimodality treatment.
- Factors associated with shortened survival include weight loss, poor performance status, male gender, elevated serum LDH, and bone or liver metastases.

## CLASSIFICATION AND STAGING

### Non–Small-Cell Lung Cancer

- The American Joint Committee on Cancer (AJCC) revised the TNM staging system for lung cancer. (See Table 42-3 on text page 1276.) Lung cancer is divided into six stages, each of which is distinct relative to treatment and five-year survival statistics.

### Small-Cell Lung Cancer

- Although the AJCC has aways recommended that SCLC be staged using the TNM system, most clinicians use the two-stage system. *Limited-stage disease* is defined as tumor confined to one hemithorax and regional lymph nodes with or without pleural effusion. It is meant to include all tumors that can be encompassed within a single radiotherapy portal. *Extensive-stage disease* refers to tumor that has spread beyond the boundaries of limited disease.

## THERAPEUTIC APPROACHES AND NURSING CARE

### Surgery

- Surgical resection is considered standard treatment for stage I and stage II NSCLC and is performed with the intent to cure the patient. The five-year survival rates following surgical resection exceed 50% for stage I and 35% for stage II tumors.
- Controversy exists regarding the appropriate treatment for stage IIIa patients. Most surgeons consider individuals with stage IIIb and stage IV lung cancer to be inoperable.
- Surgical resection may be an option for the limited number of SCLC patients who present with a small, solitary mass, no lymph node involvement, and no distant metastases. Cardiopulmonary status and cardiac studies should be done before surgery is chosen.

### Surgical procedures

#### Pneumonectomy

- Pneumonectomy is now performed only if a tumor cannot be completely excised by lobectomy. Pneumonectomy is chosen when the tumor involves the proximal bronchus, is widespread throughout the lung, or is fixed to the hilum.

#### Lobectomy

- Lobectomy is the most common surgical procedure performed for primary lung cancer confined to a single lobe of the lung.

#### Sleeve resection with bronchoplastic reconstruction

- When the tumor is confined to the bronchus or pulmonary artery and there is no evidence of metastasis, the affected area can be removed and the bronchus reattached.

### Segmental resection (Segmentectomy)

- The role of this procedure has yet to be clearly defined.

### Wedge resection

- Wedge resection, the most conservative surgical approach, is done to remove small peripheral nodules or as the procedure of choice in individuals whose physical condition will not permit more extensive surgery.

### Types of incisions

- The most common approach is the posterolateral thoracotomy, which gives the surgeon access to both the lung and the mediastinum. Others include the anterolateral thoracotomy, the median sternotomy, and the axillary incision.

## Complications

- Perioperative complications may include air leak, bleeding, atelectasis, and other well-known intraoperative complications. The most common postoperative complications are pain and atelectasis. Infection and sepsis, as well as cardiac arrhythmias and myocardial infarction, may occur postoperatively.

## Nursing care

- A plan of care or critical pathway should be developed based on the following nursing diagnoses and appropriate nursing interventions:

### Knowledge deficit

- Preoperative education with particular emphasis on the patient's participation in pulmonary toilet activities

### Alteration in comfort

- Frequent pain assessment along with intravenous or epidural infusion of narcotics for control of incisional pain; teaching the patient position changes and range-of-motion exercises; offering antiemetics

### Potential for impaired gas exchange

- Assessing vital signs and arterial blood gases, sputum production, and patency of chest tubes

### Potential for infection

- Institution of preventive nursing measures for wound management

### Alterations in bowel elimination

- Consulting a dietician concerning both diarrhea and constipation

### Potential for ineffective coping/anxiety

- Encouraging patient and family to express their feelings; offering realistic responses

## Radiation Therapy

### Non–small-cell lung cancer

- The usual dosage of external beam chest irradiation is 50–60 Gy delivered in fractions of 1.8–2.0 Gy five days a week over five to six weeks. Although surgery offers the best chance for cure for stage I and stage II disease, RT offers a potentially curative alternative in patients who refuse surgery or are not surgical candidates.
- Postoperative RT is the standard of care for selected stage IIIa patients undergoing surgical resection and for patients with unresectable stage III disease.
- New methods of fractionation of RT dosages are being tested.

### Small-cell lung cancer

- Combined-modality treatment results in lower recurrence rates and appears to confer a modest survival advantage over chemotherapy alone. The usual dosage of chest RT for SCLC is 45–50 Gy over three to four weeks.
- Prophylactic cranial irradiation (PCI) in limited-stage SCLC is an area of considerable debate.

### Palliative radiation therapy for all lung cancer types

- RT can be used as an effective palliative treatment for many of the distressing symptoms caused by metastatic lung cancer.
- One of the most common indications for palliative RT is major airway obstruction by endobronchial lesions.

### Side effects of radiation therapy for lung cancer and nursing care

- Side effects of RT are generally related to the area being irradiated. Side effects of chest RT include skin irritation; esophagitis, manifested by dysphagia; radiation pneumonitis, manifested by dry cough; dyspnea on exertion, and fever; pericarditis, with chest pain, electrocardiogram abnormalities, and a pericardial friction rub; and fatigue.

## Chemotherapy

### Non–small-cell lung cancer

- Chemotherapy is used to treat stage III and stage IV patients. Response rates of 50%–70% are seen in stage III patients when chemotherapy is added to surgery or RT, and some chemotherapeutic agents act as radiation sensitizers. Cisplatin-based chemotherapy protocols are the standard of treatment.
- Patients with distant metastases (stage IV) have traditionally been treated with either chemotherapy alone or with supportive care.
- Palliation of symptoms, quality of life, and length of survival, in addition to response rates, must be evaluated when chemotherapy is given for metastatic NSCLC.
- Promising new chemotherapeutic agents used in the treatment of NSCLC include camptothecin analogues, taxanes, vinorelbine (a vinca alkaloid), and antimetabolites.

### Small-cell lung cancer

- SCLC is initially much more sensitive to chemotherapy than NSCLC. Chemotherapy, with or without RT, has been the mainstay of treatment for many years.
- Currently, etoposide and cisplatin (EP regimen) are standard induction therapy for SCLC.

### Complications of chemotherapy and nursing care

- Complications are many and are dependent upon the drugs given. Side effects may be acute or chronic. Acute side effects include myelosuppression, nausea, vomiting, diarrhea, mucositis, constipation, anorexia, alopecia, skin changes, hemorrhagic cystitis, hypersensitivity reactions, myalgias, and arthralgias.

## Biotherapy

- In general, results of clinical trials with biological therapies have not been encouraging. The hematopoietic growth factors [both granulocyte (G) and granulocytomacrophage (GM) colony-stimulating factors (CSFs)] have been the most useful biologic response modifiers in treatment of lung cancer.

## Photodynamic Therapy

- Photodynamic therapy (PDT) has been used in an investigational setting to treat lung cancer. It is most useful in early-stage lung cancer.

## SYMPTOM MANAGEMENT AND SUPPORTIVE CARE
### Cough

- The dry, irritating cough must be distinguished from the productive cough. Although it may be appropriate to suppress a dry, persistent, and debilitating cough, this should not be attempted at the expense of removal of secretions.
- Narcotic medications are generally used for cough suppression, along with warmed and humidified inspired air; cigarette smoking is discouraged, and deep breathing and effective cough techniques are taught and reinforced.

## Hemoptysis

- Mild hemoptysis is common. If the volume of bleeding is less than 50 ml in 24 hours, the patient usually is treated conservatively on an outpatient basis. Hospitalization and careful monitoring are required for patients with profound hemoptysis. Bleeding of over 200 ml in 24 hours requires immediate attention. The patient should be positioned with the suspected bleeding lung in a dependent position.

## Dyspnea

- Dyspnea may be associated with destruction of lung tissue by tumor, pleural effusions, airway obstruction by endobronchial lesions, and increased mucus production. Teach the patient to assess patterns of occurrence, plan coping strategies, and conserve energy and minimize fatigue.
- Dyspnea in lung cancer is often associated with pleural effusions. Large volumes of fluid can be removed by thoracentesis. When pleural effusions reaccumulate, pleurodesis is the recommended therapy.

## Pain

- Chest pain occurs in half of all patients with lung cancer; bone pain is common, as is pain related to metastases to other distant sites. Narcotic analgesics commonly used include morphine, hydromorphone, and fentanyl. The key to pain management is its accurate assessment.

## Fatigue

- Disability related to fatigue and weakness has been reported to be the source of greatest suffering among persons with lung cancer. Significant correlations have been reported between pain and fatigue in individuals with lung cancer, and between fatigue and mood states.

## Gastrointestinal Disturbances: Nausea/Vomiting, Anorexia/ Cachexia, and Elimination

- Nausea and vomiting related to the disease process in the person with lung cancer have several etiologies, including GI obstruction, liver metastases, increased intracranial pressure from brain metastases, and narcotic analgesics.
- Anorexia and cancer cachexia are common manifestations of lung cancer. As many as 50% of all individuals with lung cancer lose weight prior to their diagnosis, which is generally considered to be a poor prognostic factor. Constipation may occur as a result of any combination of factors.

## Psychosocial Issues

- The goal of nursing care relative to psychosocial issues is to foster appropriate coping responses of the patient and family members. The recurrence of lung cancer can be a greater crisis than the initial diagnosis.
- The patient should be allowed to explore fears, concerns, and wishes regarding death.
- Correlates of depression have included psychiatric history and the presence of metastatic disease.

## CONTINUITY OF CARE: NURSING CHALLENGES

- Access to care can be impeded by competition for patients and territoriality among agencies.
- Communication is promoted through the use of multidisciplinary discharge planning team conferences, case management critical pathways, multidisciplinary documentation tools, and written communication to referral agencies upon discharge. It is the nurse in the ambulatory care setting who is positioned to facilitate continuity of care over a period of months or years.
- The difficulty in predicting when death will occur makes referrals to hospice difficult since Medicare reimbursement requires that a hospice patient have a life expectancy of six months or less.

# PRACTICE QUESTIONS

1. Your brother-in-law tells you that he is tired of "all the negative talk about smoking. There's more prejudice against it than there is real danger." What percentage of lung cancer deaths are caused by cigarette smoking?
   a. 45% to 50%
   b. 50% to 60%
   c. 75% to 85%
   d. 80% to 90%

2. Most epidemiologic trends in lung cancer over the last century include a(n):
   a. overall increased incidence, and a decreased mortality among nonwhites.
   b. increased incidence, but decreased mortality among women.
   c. higher mortality rate for African-American men than white men, but with comparable mortality rates among African-American and white women.
   d. mortality that is increasing three times as fast for men as for women.

3. What percentage of lung cancers is considered preventable?
   a. 45%
   b. 50%
   c. 75%
   d. 85%

4. During his physical examination, Mr. Pederson, a coal miner, asks you about his relative risk of developing lung cancer. The best response to his question would be to:
   a. tell him that his risk is due to his exposure to coal.
   b. ask him about his family history of lung cancer, and explain that multiple factors cause the disease.
   c. get his demographic information, and ask him about his exposure to tobacco smoke.
   d. ask him about his diet and his smoking history.

5. The leading cause of death in early-stage lung cancer is:
   a. lower levels of the enzyme monoamine oxidase B (MAO B).
   b. dopamine breakdown.
   c. second primary tumors.
   d. dietary intake of beta-carotene.

6. The *ras* oncogenes:
   a. have a screening usefulness of about 45%.
   b. function early in the process of carcinogenesis.
   c. are a late event.
   d. are not effective as targets for early detection.

7. Two patients have been diagnosed with bronchogenic cancer. You know that this does not mean both patients will necessarily have a similar symptomatology or course of treatment because bronchogenic cancers are grouped into two broad categories:
   a. small-cell lung cancer (SCLC) and the non–small-cell lung cancers (NSCLC).
   b. adenocarcinoma and large-cell carcinoma.
   c. heterogeneous and histological.
   d. hyperplasia and carcinoma in situ.

8. Most SCLC tumors:
   a. are not associated with necrosis.
   b. are responsible for 55% of all lung cancers.
   c. are centrally located, developing around a main bronchus, eventually compressing the bronchi externally.
   d. have a longer doubling time that that of any other lung cancer type.

9. Ms. St. Charles has small-cell lung cancer. If you were asked to predict the cell subtype one would be most likely to find, you would predict that subtype would be the:
   a. oat cell.
   b. mediary cell.
   c. adenocarcinoma.
   d. squamous cell carcinoma.

10. Adenocarcinomas:
    a. constitute 30% of all lung cancers and are more common in males than in females.
    b. arise from the basal cells of the bronchial epithelium and usually present as masses in large bronchi.
    c. are the most common lung cancer in males, in females, and in nonsmokers, accounting for 40% of all tumors.
    d. are the least common type of lung cancer, representing approximately 10%–15%.

11. Mrs. Alexander has been diagnosed with local-regional lung tumor. You are told she has a central, rather than peripheral, tumor. What kinds of symptoms will Mrs. Alexander be most likely to have?
    a. Symptoms due to extrathoracic involvement
    b. Chest pain
    c. Symptoms associated with airway obstruction
    d. Weakness, anorexia, and cachexia

12. Mrs. Wilson is about to have a sputum cytology. She asked the nurse to "explain this type of test. I already had a chest x-ray. Why isn't that enough?" The best answer would be to explain that sputum cytology:
    a. is probably the most helpful diagnostic study for lung cancer.
    b. can be particularly helpful in evaluating mediastinal lymph nodes.
    c. has a diagnostic yield of up to 80% for small peripheral tumors.
    d. has a diagnostic yield of up to 80% for central tumors.

13. Mrs. Hilliard is diagnosed with small-cell lung cancer (SCLC). The most favorable prognostic factor in Mrs. Hilliard's case is:
    a. the fact that she is a female.
    b. limited-stage disease.
    c. a normal serum lactic dehydrogenase (LDH).
    d. undeterminable, since not enough information is given.

14. The most significant prognostic factor for NSCLC is:
    a. stage of disease.
    b. the presence of mediastinal lymph node metastases.
    c. male gender.
    d. mutations of the *K-ras* oncogene.

15. The AJCC staging system for lung cancer uses:
    a. six stages, each of which is distinct relative to treatment and five-year survival statistics.
    b. the TNM letters.
    c. the simple two-stage system.
    d. two defining terms—limited-stage disease and extensive-stage disease—to stage lung cancers.

16. Mr. Keller has NSCLC that is in stage I; Ms. Harris' is a stage II. Mr. DeBalivere has stage IIIa, Mrs. Jensen has stage IV, and Ms. Jording has stage IIIb NSCLC. Who will benefit most from surgical resection?
    a. Mr. Keller and Ms. Harris
    b. Mr. DeBalivere and Ms. Jording
    c. Ms. Jording and Mrs. Jensen
    d. Mr. Keller only

17. Tomorrow morning, Steven, an oncology nursing candidate, will observe a pneumonectomy for the first time. You know he is prepared when he tells you that pneumonectomy is:
    a. never performed if a tumor cannot be completely excised by lobectomy as well.
    b. performed for primary lung cancer confined to a single lobe of the lung.
    c. chosen when the tumor involves the proximal bronchus, is widespread throughout the lung, or is fixed to the hilum.
    d. used when the tumor is confined to the bronchus or pulmonary artery and there is no evidence of metastasis.

18. Mr. Keller is diagnosed with stage I non–small-cell lung cancer and is to undergo a lobectomy of his disease. He asks you about his preparation for surgery and whether you think he will need any radiation. "If I do," he says, "will I get that before or after surgery?" Patient teaching would include all of the following *except*:
    a. describing pulmonary function tests.
    b. talking to him about the importance of preoperative chest physical therapy.
    c. telling him that he would probably need radiation postoperatively, but not pre-operatively.
    d. telling him that bronchoscopy or photoirradiation would have to be used to localize the tumor.

19. Four patients complain of the symptoms listed below. Which one will benefit most from palliative RT?
    a. Harry has esophagitis, manifested by dysphagia.
    b. Bette has radiation pneumonitis, manifested by a drug cough and dyspnea on exertion. She also has a fever.
    c. Paul has pericarditis with chest pain, ECG abnormalities, and a pericardial friction rub.
    d. Jack has major airway obstruction by endobronchial lesions.

20. Ms. St. James has distant metastasis (stage IV). The treatment that will most likely be recommended for her is:
    a. surgery alone.
    b. radiation alone.
    c. palliation of symptoms only.
    d. either chemotherapy alone or with supportive care.

21. Etoposide and cisplatin (the EP regimen):
    a. have more severe combined side effects than CAV.
    b. are standard induction therapy for SCLC.
    c. appear to not be synergistic.
    d. are not as effective as CAV.

22. Granulocyte (G) and granulocyte-macrophage (GM) colony-stimulating factors (CSFs):
    a.   increase febrile episodes.
    b.   decrease myelosuppression.
    c.   decrease mucositis.
    d.   decrease anorexia.

23. Ms. Howe has persistent productive coughing, which, she says, is exhausting. Which treatment modality should not be used?
    a.   Inspired air is warmed and humidified.
    b.   Cigarette smoking is discouraged.
    c.   Deep breathing and coughing techniques are taught and reinforced.
    d.   Narcotic medications are used for cough suppression.

24. Mr. Cunningham is brought to the ER with profound hemoptysis, associated with lung cancer. Suggest a response to his current condition.
    a.   Mr. Cunningham can be treated conservatively with oxygen supplementation as needed; under the circumstances, surgery is not possible.
    b.   Cough suppressants should be prescribed.
    c.   Reassure him about the fear of bleeding to death.
    d.   He should be positioned with the suspected bleeding lung in a dependent position.

25. Ms. Green complains of dyspnea and a sensation of smothering. You will *not* instruct her:
    a.   to assess patterns of occurrence.
    b.   in planning coping strategies.
    c.   to identify ways to conserve energy and minimize fatigue.
    d.   that she will receive chemotherapy for a malignant pleural effusion.

26. You notice that a number of patients with lung cancer experience nausea and vomiting that does not seem to be a side effect of any treatment regimen. Which is *not* as likely an appropriate etiology to suggest?
    a.   GI obstruction
    b.   Liver metastases
    c.   Flu due to lowered resistance
    d.   Increased intracranial pressure from brain metastases

27. You are working with Mr. Gunther and his family, who have just discovered not only that his lung cancer has recurred, but that it is terminal this time. Which is not likely to be true regarding Mr. Gunther's psychosocial needs?
    a.   When coping with a difficult disease like lung cancer, it is the discovery of meaning in the disease that gives one a sense of mastery.
    b.   The recurrence of lung cancer can be a greater crisis than the initial diagnosis.
    c.   Often the fear of dying is not as profound as the fear of suffering in the process.
    d.   Patients who are allowed to indulge excessively in expressing their fears, concerns, and wishes regarding death are more prone to morbid depression.

# Answer Explanations

1.  **The answer is d.** Eighty to ninety percent of lung cancer deaths are estimated to be caused by cigarette smoking. (p. 1261)

2.  **The answer is c.** Lung cancer is now the source of most male and female cancer deaths. Although the lung cancer mortality rates are higher for African-American males than for white males, mortality rates for African-American women and white women are comparable. (p. 1261)

3.  **The answer is d.** Eight-five percent of lung cancers could be prevented if people did not smoke. The relative risk of cancer increases with the number of cigarettes smoked per day and the number of years of smoking history. (p. 1264)

4.  **The answer is c.** It is misleading to suggest that coal poses the most obvious risk. By asking Mr. Pederson for demographic information, the nurse would be able to assess his exposure to air pollution and possibly his exposure to radon (certain areas have been identified as higher in radon activity than others). Since tobacco has an interactive and synergistic effect on the development of lung cancer when combined with other carcinogens, this would also be a good factor to explore. Genetics and diet have not been shown to have a significant effect on the development of lung cancer. (p. 1264)

5.  **The answer is c.** The leading cause of death in early-stage lung cancer is SPTs. Living smokers have lower levels of the enzyme monoamine oxidase B (MAO B)—but this in itself is not the leading cause of death. MAO B helps break down dopamine, a neurotransmitter involved in feelings of pleasure associated with nicotine, so it seems unlikely that dopamine would cause death. Finally, dietary intake of beta-carotene has been associated with a decreased risk of lung cancer, not a cause of death. (p. 1266)

6.  **The answer is b.** The *ras* oncogenes appear to function early in the process of carcinogenesis and may be a good target for early detection. (p. 1267)

7.  **The answer is a.** Bronchogenic cancers have been grouped into small-cell lung cancer (SCLC) and the non–small-cell lung cancers (NSCLC), which include squamous cell carcinoma, adenocarcinoma, and large-cell carcinoma. Many tumors are heterogeneous, containing cells from more than one histological type. In both types of cancer, we see both hyperplasia and carcinoma in situ. (p. 1267)

8.  **The answer is c.** Most SCLC tumors are centrally located, developing around a main bronchus as a whitish gray growth that invades surrounding structures, eventually compressing the bronchi externally. Necrosis is frequently seen, and SCLC is responsible for 25% of all lung cancers, not 55%. Its doubling time is shorter, not longer, than that of any other lung cancer type. (p. 1267)

9.  **The answer is a.** The oat cell accounts for 90% of all cases. The two other subtypes established by the WHO are the intermediate and the combined type (oat cell with adenocarcinoma or squamous cell carcinoma component). (p. 1268)

10. **The answer is c.** Adenocarcinomas are the most common lung cancer in males, in females, and in nonsmokers, accounting for 40% of all tumors. It is the squamous cell carcinomas that constitute 30% of all lung cancers and are more common in males than in females. They are also the ones that arise from the basal cells of the bronchial epithelium and usually present as masses in large bronchi. Finally, it is the large-cell carcinomas, not the adenocarcinomas, that are the least common type of lung cancer, representing approximately 10%–15%. (pp. 1269–70)

11. **The answer is c.** Central tumors are more likely to cause symptoms associated with airway obstruction, such as wheezing, stridor, dyspnea, atelectasis, and pneumonia. Chest pain is associated with peripheral tumors, which cause chest pain in as many as 50% of patients. Weakness, anorexia, and cachexia are systemic symptoms. (pp. 1270–71)

12. **The answer is d.** Sputum cytology has a diagnostic yield of up to 80% for central tumors, but less than 20% for small peripheral tumors. But it is the chest radiograph that is probably the most helpful diagnostic study for lung cancer, and it is CT that can be particularly helpful in evaluating mediastinal lymph nodes. (pp. 1273–1274)

13. **The answer is b.** The most favorable prognostic factor in SCLC is limited-stage disease. Female gender and normal serum lactic dehydrogenase are also favorable prognostic factors. (p. 1274)

14. **The answer is a.** Stage of disease is the most significant prognostic factor for NSCLC, with early-stage cancers responding better to treatment and demonstrating longer survival. The presence of mediastinal lymph node metastases usually indicates a very poor prognosis. Male gender is also associated with shortened survival. Point mutations of the *K-ras* oncogene also appear to be an important prognostic factor for NSCLC. (p. 1275)

15. **The answer is b.** The AJCC staging system for lung cancer uses the TNM letters. **T** designates primary tumor and is divided into categories relative to size, location, and invasion. **N**, with three categories, represents regional lymph node status. **M** designates the absence or presence of distant metastases. Lung cancer is also divided into six stages, each of which is distinctive relative to treatment and five-year survival statistics. Small-cell lung cancer is usually staged using a simple two-stage system. Since most SCLC patients have metastatic disease at the time of diagnosis, this system describes the extent of disease as either "limited" or "extensive." (p. 1275)

16. **The answer is a.** Surgical resection is considered standard treatment for stage I (like Mr. Keller's) and stage II (like Ms. Harris') NSCLC and is performed with the intent to cure the patient. Controversy exists regarding the appropriate treatment for stage IIIa patients, particularly those who have ipsilateral mediastinal lymph node involvement. Most surgeons consider stage IIIb and stage IV lung cancer to be inoperable. (p. 1276)

17. **The answer is c.** Pneumonectomy is performed only if a tumor cannot be completely excised by lobectomy. It is chosen when the tumor involves the proximal bronchus, is widespread throughout the lung, or is fixed to the hilum. It is sleeve resection with bronchoplastic reconstruction that is used when the tumor is confined to the bronchus or pulmonary artery, and there is no evidence of metastasis. Finally, lobectomy is the most common surgical procedure performed for primary lung cancer confined to a single lobe of the lung. (p. 1277)

18. **The answer is c.** Postoperative radiation has not been shown to affect survival rates in patients with NSCLC. (p. 1279)

19. **The answer is d.** One of the most common indications for palliative RT is a major airway obstruction by endobronchial lesions. The other patients seem to have side effects of RT that are related to the area being irradiated. (p. 1280)

20. **The answer is d.** Patients with distant metastases (stage IV) have traditionally been treated with either chemotherapy alone or with supportive care. (p. 1281)

21. **The answer is b.** Currently, etoposide and cisplatin (EP regimen) are standard induction therapy for SCLC. They appear to be synergistic, have comparable efficacy to CAV, and combined side effects are less severe than with CAV. (p. 1282)

22. **The answer is b.** Granulocyte (G) and granulocyte-macrophage (GM) colony-stimulating factors (CSFs) decrease myelosuppression, febrile episodes, and number of hospital days when given in conjunction with chemotherapy. Both mucositis and anorexia are complications of chemotherapy and have no relationship to biotherapy. (p. 1283)

23. **The answer is d.** Although it may be appropriate to suppress a dry, persistent and debilitating cough, this should not be attempted at the expense of removal of secretions. The other strategies suggested promote comfort. (p. 1284)

24. **The answer is d.** A patient with profound hemoptysis requires immediate attention and should be positioned with the suspected bleeding lung in a dependent position to prevent blood spillage into the unaffected lung. Emergency surgery may be required. (p. 1284)

25. **The answer is d.** Not all pleural effusions are malignant. Etiology should be established before palliative treatment is initiated. All other teaching strategies suggested in this question are appropriate. (p. 1284)

26. **The answer is c.** Nausea and vomiting related to the disease process in the person with lung cancer have several etiologies, including GI obstruction, liver metastases, increased intracranial pressure from brain metastases, and narcotic analgesics. (p. 1285)

27. **The answer is d.** The patient should be allowed to express his fears, concerns, and wishes regarding death; this can provide comfort and emotional healing. When coping with a difficult disease like lung cancer, it is the discovery of meaning in the disease that gives one a sense of mastery. The recurrence of lung cancer can be a greater crisis than the initial diagnosis. Often the fear of dying is not as profound as the fear of suffering in the process. (p. 1286)

# Chapter 43    Malignant Lymphomas

## INTRODUCTION

- The malignant lymphomas constitute a diverse group of neoplasms that arise from the uncontrolled proliferation of the cellular components of the lymphoreticular system.
- Based on histologic characteristics, the lymphomas are divided into two major subgroups—Hodgkin's disease (HD) and non-Hodgkin's lymphoma (NHL).
- The distinctions between HD and NHL are important because their clinical courses, prognoses, and treatments are substantially different.

## THE IMMUNE SYSTEM AND NEOPLASIA

- The incidence of lymphomas, particularly NHL, is escalating, and it has now become the fifth most common cancer in the United States. See Figure 43-1, text page 1293, for organs of the immune system.
- Lymphomas are preeminently a malignancy of the lymphocyte, and the process by which a lymphoid neoplasm is generated may be thought of as a series of cellular changes whereby a once normal lymphoid cell (or cell clone) becomes refractory to the regulation of its differentiation and proliferation.
- Once transformed, the new clone of malignant cells follows the behavior pattern of the stage at which lymphocyte alteration took place.

## MATURATION OF THE LYMPHOCYTE

- At each step along the path of differentiation, a cell loses its capacity to proceed along an alternate route.
- In the first step, the stem cell matures so that it is either the precursor of the lymphocyte series or of all the other cellular series of the blood (erythrocyte, megakaryocyte, polymorphonuclear neutrophil, or monocyte).
- The lymphocyte precursor then develops into one of a number of types of mature lymphocytes.
- See Figure 43-2, text page 1294, for major lymph node groups.
- See Figure 43-3, text page 1294, for sites of lymphocyte transformation in the lymph node.
- An early step in the differentiation of the maturing lymphocyte occurs when the cell is programmed either by the bone marrow (bursa equivalent) or by the thymus to become a B-lymphocyte or a T-lymphocyte respectively.
- Eighty percent of lymphomas manifest B-cell origin, and most patients initially present with disease involving bone marrow or lymph nodes.
- See Figure 43-4, text page 1295, for maturation sequence of the lymphocyte.
- Lymphomas derived from T-lymphocytes usually arise in bone marrow, thymus, lymph nodes, and skin.

## HODGKIN'S DISEASE
### Historical Perspective

- All lymphomas were called HD until around the turn of the century when the giant, multinucleated cells in the nodal material of HD patients were characterized by Reed and Sternberg, and their names have been associated with the pathognomonic cell of HD ever since.

- The Reed-Sternberg cell is useful in prognosis since lymphocytic malignancies that are similar in pathological appearance behave differently according to the presence or absence of this cell.

## Epidemiology

- The disease has a world-wide distribution, and its most prominent epidemiological feature pertains to the distinct age-related incidence patterns that have been observed.
- In developing countries the incidence of HD is clearly bimodal. In these areas the disease is infrequent in children under 10 years old. Incidence rises rapidly in adolescence and has its first peak among young adults ages 20–30. Subsequently, it falls until after age 45.

## Etiology

- The etiology of HD remains unclear.
- The Epstein-Barr virus (EBV) is now recognized as being associated with several forms of lymphoma.

## Cellular Abnormalities

- Patients in all stages of HD exhibit a molecular defect characterized by markedly reduced cellular immunity.
- This deficit is manifested by impaired delayed hypersensitivity skin reactions and reduced T-cell proliferation following antigenic stimulation.
- They also display increased susceptibility to infectious complications from opportunistic pathogens such as herpes zoster, cytomegalovirus, and *Pneumocystis carinii*.

## Clinical Manifestations

- A typical HD patient presents with a slow, insidious, superficial lymphadenopathy.
- Nodes of variable size are firm, rubbery, and freely movable.
- A second common presentation, mediastinal adenopathy, is often recognized during routine chest roentgenogram.
- B symptoms (constitutional symptoms of fever, malaise, night sweats, weight loss, and pruritus) appear in about 40% of affected individuals.
  - These manifestations are more common in patients with advanced disease.
- The spread of HD is via contiguous nodal groups, and the pattern is quite predictable. Symptomatology and prognosis are related to the location and number of disease sites.

## Assessment

- The diagnosis of HD can be established only by biopsy of involved tissue, usually a lymph node.
- Some causes of lymphadenopathy include upper respiratory infections, infectious mononucleosis, allergic reactions, and other nonspecific causes.
- Older persons with cancers of the head and neck also may present initially with enlarged cervical nodes.

## Histopathology

- Hodgkin's disease is distinguished from other lymphomas by the presence of the Reed-Sternberg cell.
- Unlike most cancers, this characteristic cell represents only a small fraction of the cells in a malignant lymph node.
- Four distinct subtypes of HD are: nodular sclerosis, lymphocyte-predominant, mixed cellularity, and lymphocyte-depleted.

- Nodular sclerosis (NS), with its unique age incidence (between ages 15 and 34) and its different sex incidence (females more commonly than males), has a singular histological makeup.
- See Table 43-1 on text page 1298 for Rye classification of Hodgkin's disease.
- Most patients with nodular sclerosis (NS) HD are asymptomatic at presentation and exhibit stage I or II disease.
- The *lymphocyte-predominant (LP)* is characterized by sheets of mature-appearing small lymphocytes and few Reed-Sternberg cells. Patients usually present with localized stage I or II disease, primarily in the cervical lymph nodes. Peak incidence occurs in the fourth or fifth decades.
- In *mixed cellularity (MC)* HD there is a wide age range that peaks in the 30- to 40-year-old age group, and male cases predominate. Most patients have stage III or IV disease.
- *Lymphocyte-depleted (LD)* HD is marked by a paucity of small lymphocytes and an increased number of Reed-Sternberg cells. Patients often present with bone marrow infiltration and peripheral lymphadenopathy. Usually, these patients are elderly males with advanced-stage disease and B symptoms.

## Staging

- See Figure 43-5 on text page 1299 for the Ann Arbor staging system for Hodgkin's disease.
  - Lymph node involvement in just one area is designated as stage I disease. Involvement of two or more areas confined to one side of the diaphragm constitutes stage II. In stage III, lymph node groups above and below the diaphragm are affected.
  - Stage III is subdivided further into stage $III_1$ for disease limited to the upper abdomen, and stage $III_2$ for disease involving the lower abdomen.
  - Stage IV is marked by diffuse extralymphatic progression.
  - Clinical staging (CS) rests on history, physical examination, initial diagnostic biopsy, laboratory tests, and radiographic evidence. Pathological staging (PS) adds definitive histopathologic information, obtained through biopsy of strategic sites.
- See Table 43-2 on text page 1300 for the staging evaluation for Hodgkin's disease.

## Treatment

- Radiation therapy is curative in most patients with limited disease. Several important factors have an impact on its effectiveness—skilled use of linear accelerators, careful field simulation, administration of tumoricidal doses, and comprehensive follow-up.
- See Table 43-3 on text page 1301 for the guidelines for treatment of Hodgkin's disease.
- See Figure 43-6 on text page 1301 for the standard radiation fields for Hodgkin's disease.
- Whereas radiotherapy is curative in local and regional HD, chemotherapy may be curative in both early and advanced disease.
- Because of their high response and durable remission rates, the MOPP regimen and the ABVD regimen have become the benchmarks for combination chemotherapy in HD.
- See Table 43-4 on text page 1302 for the MOPP regimen for Hodgkin's disease.
- The success of aggressive chemotherapeutic regimens is quite dependent on the dosage and timing of drug administration because even minor alterations can have a substantial impact on efficacy.
- Specific subsets of patients appear to benefit from combined chemotherapy and radiation therapy.
- When relapse occurs less than 12 months after initial remission, or when patients are refractory to initial therapy, the prognosis is grave.
- See Table 43-5 on text page 1302 for the ABVD regimen for Hodgkin's disease.

# NON-HODGKIN'S LYMPHOMAS

## Historical Perspective

- The non-Hodgkin's lymphomas are a diverse group of neoplasms derived from the different developmental and functional subdivisions of the lymphoreticular system.

## Epidemiology

- In the United States, NHL is diagnosed nearly six times as often as HD, and its death rate is 13 times greater.
- Like HD, higher mortalities are associated with higher socioeconomic status and urban residence.

## Etiology

- The heterogeneity of NHL suggests that a variety of factors including viral infections, genetic abnormalities, and immune disturbances interact in the pathogenesis.
- Environmental factors and exposure to chemicals in the workplace also are implicated in the pathogenesis of NHL.
- One form of lymphoma, gastric lymphoma of mucosa-associated lymphoid tissue (MALT), has recently been reported to be due to the same bacteria that induces gastric ulcers, *Helicobacter pylori*.

## Cellular Abnormalities

- In most cases, chromosomal translocations facilitate the identification of the genetic lesion responsible for oncogenesis.
- Cytogenetic analysis of lymphoma cells has identified other abnormalities as well.

## Clinical Manifestations

- In contrast to HD, 80% of patients with NHL present to their physicians with advanced disease (stage III or IV).
  - This is usually reflected by painless, generalized lymphadenopathy. Systemic B symptoms (fever, night sweats, and/or weight loss) are the initial complaint.
- Gastrointestinal involvement is fairly common at presentation.
- See Table 43-6 on text page 1304 for the systemic alterations in non-Hodgkin's lymphoma.

## Assessment

- Careful histological evaluation is the most important step.
- In general, the principles governing assessment of NHL are the same as those previously identified for HD.

## Histopathology

- Few areas of pathology have evoked as much controversy and confusion as the classification of NHL, and the lack of consistent standardization makes international analysis and comparison extremely difficult.
  - The major classifications in the Working Formulation and their pathological counterparts in the Rappaport and Lukes-Collins systems are compared in Table 43-7, text page 1306.

### Low-grade lymphomas

- The low-grade category includes three tumors: small lymphocytic lymphoma; follicular, predominantly small cleaved cell lymphoma; and follicular mixed (small cleaved and large-cell) lymphoma.

- The usual presenting problems for patients with low-grade lymphomas are connected with a painless, progressive, often symmetrical generalized lymphadenopathy.
  - Except for liver and bone marrow involvement, extra-nodal extension is uncommon.
- Most low-grade lymphomas have a long natural history that appears to be largely unaffected by treatment.

### Intermediate-grade lymphomas

- There are four neoplasms under the intermediate-grade category.
- The follicular, predominantly large-cell NHL has a more aggressive clinical course.
- The three diffuse subgroups of intermediate-grade lymphomas occur mainly in adults, and unlike follicular NHL, patients with diffuse neoplasms often present with disease limited to one side of the diaphragm.

### High-grade lymphomas

- High-grade lymphomas consist of three quite distinct diseases that are grouped together because of their aggressive clinical behavior and poor prognosis.
- The first of this group are immunoblastic lymphomas.
- Anemia, B symptoms, and advanced stage are common at presentation, and high incidence of cutaneous disease has been reported.
- Lymphoblastic lymphoma is a high-grade, usually T-cell malignancy. Adolescents and young adults account for the majority of cases.
- Approximately two-thirds of the patients present with a prominent anterior mediastinal mass suggestive of a thymic origin.
- Within the category of small, noncleaved cell lymphomas are two distinct subtypes, Burkitt's lymphoma (BL) and non-Burkitt's lymphoma.
- Burkitt's lymphoma (BL) occurs endemically in tropical Africa and New Guinea, where it is associated with the Epstein-Barr virus.
- Non-Burkitt's lymphoma is a relatively uncommon malignancy.
- These neoplasms respond better to chemotherapy than the indolent, low-grade lymphomas, and they have a greater potential for cure, especially if complete remissions are sustained for at least two years.

### Mycosis fungoides (cutaneous T-cell lymphoma)

- Involvement of the skin is a hallmark of cutaneous T-cell lymphoma (CTCL) that results from the clonal proliferation of T-lymphocytes. CTCL tends to be initially indolent, but it may evolve into a widely disseminated malignancy.

### Mantle cell lymphoma

- Mantle cell lymphoma, also called centrocytic or intermediate lymphoma, has a very aggressive clinical course and poor prognosis.

## Staging

- Once a histological diagnosis of NHL has been confirmed by biopsy, a careful, comprehensive staging workup is essential. Baseline studies for all patients should include complete history and physical examination with particular emphasis on all lymphoid tissue including liver, spleen, Waldeyer's ring, and lymph nodes. Also required are complete blood counts, blood chemistries including liver and kidney function tests, erythrocyte sedimentation rate, uric acid, serum immunoglobulins, and bone marrow biopsy.

- Unlike HD, where the disease sites are more predictable and orderly, the multiplicity of potential NHL locations and the variety of their clinical presentations forestall the adoption of a single radiological scheme.
- Additional studies that may be appropriate in certain circumstances include multiple biopsies of the liver, removal of the spleen for pathological study, and exploratory laparotomy for biopsy of multiple lymph node groups.
- After clinical evaluation is complete, patients are classified according to the criteria previously outlined for HD in the Ann Arbor-Cottswolds staging system.

## Treatment

- The treatment of NHL is determined by histology of the tumor, stage of the disease, and physiological performance status of the patient.
- See Table 43-8 on text page 1309 for the staging procedures for non-Hodgkin's lymphoma.

### Indolent lymphomas

- Some physicians advocate a policy of "watchful waiting" until systemic symptoms require intervention.
- An alternative approach is the use of intensive combination chemotherapy regimens to induce a complete remission.

### Aggressive lymphomas

- The recognized treatment of choice for advanced-stage aggressive NHL is combination chemotherapy.
- See Table 43-9 on text page 1311 for chemotherapeutic regimens for aggressive lymphomas.
- It is believed that CHOP is the best treatment for intermediate-grade and high-grade NHL.

### Salvage Therapy

- Refractoriness to treatment is the rule rather than the exception; thus, cure is rarely possible with recurrent aggressive NHL.
- With the advent of high-dose therapy followed by autologous bone marrow transplantation (ABMT), a substantial number of relapsed patients with aggressive lymphoma are achieving durable second complete remissions.

## COMPLICATIONS OF TREATMENT

- The most common reactions associated with mantle irradiation are loss of taste, dry mouth, redness of skin, dysphagia, loss of hair at the nape of the neck, nausea, and vomiting.
- Depending on the particular drug regimen administered, other reactions can include alopecia, myalgia, chills, fever, euphoria, fluid retention, stomatitis, gastrointestinal disturbances, hemorrhagic cystitis, and mental depression.
- The most serious side effect produced by all combination regimens is bone marrow suppression, which renders the individual susceptible to infection and hemorrhage.

## CONSEQUENCES OF SURVIVAL

- No organ system is immune to alteration.
- An extension of injury to the lungs is common in mantle irradiation, and it may develop as early as one to three months after RT is completed.

- See Table 43-10 on text page 1313 for long-term complications in patients cured of malignant lymphoma.
- Tumors on the right side of the superior mediastinum have the potential to obstruct the return of blood to the heart from the superior vena cava.
- Acute and chronic pericarditis are not uncommon, and a patient often presents with a spectrum of symptoms ranging from cough and chest pain to edema, paradoxical pulse, cardiac tamponade, and hemodynamic compromise. Coronary artery disease and cardiomyopathy are also seen following extensive mediastinal radiation.
- Because both chemotherapy and radiotherapy are immunosuppressive, bacterial as well as other unusual infections may occur.
- The two fungal infections diagnosed most often are candidiasis and aspergillosis.
- Herpes zoster may be seen at any time during the course of illness, from initial treatment to relapse.
- Chronic progressive radiation myelopathy symptoms include paresthesias, weakness, and bowel/bladder dysfunction.
- Rare as a presenting symptom but commonly seen in progressive lymphoma, compression of the spinal cord represents a complication that is dreaded because of its potential to cause paraplegia in a person who might otherwise have many productive years remaining.
- Two of the most devastating complications associated with lymphoma treatment are sterility and carcinogenesis.
- Second malignancies may develop after curative treatment for lymphoma.
  - A regimen such as ABVD might be associated with a lower rate of leukemia than MOPP.

## SUPPORTIVE CARE

- Supportive care of the lymphoma patient begins at diagnosis with an explanation of the disease, a description of the steps that will be taken for staging and treatment, and a generation in the patient of a feeling of confidence in the multidisciplinary team responsible for care.
- After the primary treatment there will be a prolonged period during which the patient must be observed for a recurrence of disease.
- The nurse must be aware that whereas the treatment team views this as a "routine" visit for a patient who has responded very well to therapy, the individual perceives every word or facial expression as a potential clue that the cancer has recurred.

## PRACTICE QUESTIONS

1. Which of the following statements about lymphomas is correct?
   a. Non-Hodgkin's lymphoma (NHL) is distinguished from Hodgkin's disease (HD) primarily on the basis of its different clinical manifestations.
   b. Lymphomas are preeminently a malignancy of the lymphocyte.
   c. There seems to be a single malignancy for all stages in the developmental sequence from primitive to mature lymphocyte.
   d. In general, B-lymphocyte malignancies are more aggressive than T-lymphocyte malignancies.

**A 52-year-old male presents with signs and symptoms of lymphoma. Subsequent assessment and diagnostic tests confirm stage IIB Hodgkin's disease. Answer questions 2–8 with this diagnosis in mind.**

2. Mortality in this individual, if it occurs as a result of HD, is most likely to result from:
   a. spinal cord compression.
   b. superior vena cava obstruction.
   c. failure of the liver or kidneys.
   d. infection or hemorrhage.

3. Which of the following was the most likely presenting symptom in this patient?
   a. edema in the upper part of the body
   b. enlarged cervical lymph nodes
   c. a palpable mass in the axillary or inguinal lymph nodes
   d. an upper respiratory infection

4. The diagnosis of either HD or NHL usually is established by:
   a. cytologic examination of the Reed-Sternberg cells.
   b. CT and MRI scans of the nodular tissue.
   c. lymph node biopsy.
   d. exploratory laparotomy.

5. Which of the following statements about the staging of this patient's cancer is correct?
   a. Stage II malignancy was determined by a positive bone marrow biopsy.
   b. Stage II determination is important because it influences what treatment option will be used.
   c. Stage II presentation is usually indicative of a more aggressive HD type.
   d. HD rarely presents as stage II.

6. Accurate staging of this patient was least likely to include which of the following procedures?
   a. a chest radiograph
   b. an exploratory laparotomy
   c. blood chemistries, including liver and kidney function tests
   d. a complete blood count

7. The prognosis for this patient is most closely related to:
   a. elevated lactic dehydrogenase level.
   b. histologic type.
   c. abdominal lymph node involvement.
   d. stage at presentation.

8. If careful laparotomy staging has been conducted, the patient is most likely to be treated with:
   a. total or subtotal nodal radiation only.
   b. chemotherapy only.
   c. total or subtotal nodal radiation combined with chemotherapy.
   d. subtotal radiation only.

9. The vast majority of patients with NHL present to their physicians with advanced disease (stages III and IV), reflected largely by:
   a. painless, generalized lymphadenopathy.
   b. fever.
   c. night sweats.
   d. weight loss.

10. Lydia has intermediate-grade NHL, and George has high-grade NHL. Which combination treatment would they both be most likely to receive?
    a. CVP
    b. CHOP
    c. C-MOPP
    d. COP-BLAM

11. Althea has received both extensive mediastinal radiation and chemotherapy. Toxic effects to monitor for include:
    a. pericarditis and hemodynamic compromise.
    b. chest pain, edema, and cardiac tamponade.
    c. coronary artery disease and cardiomyopathy.
    d. all of the above.

# ANSWER EXPLANATIONS

1. **The answer is b.** Lymphomas are preeminently a malignancy of the lymphocyte. However, there seems to be a separate malignancy for each sequential stage in the developmental sequence from primitive to mature lymphocyte. At each stage of development, the potential exists for the normal maturing lymphocyte to be transformed into a cancer cell. Once transformed, the new clone of malignant cells follows the behavioral pattern of the stage of the lymphocyte at which the transformation occurred. For example, if the function of the maturing cell at the time it is transformed is secretion of an antibody, the tumor cells will continue to secrete that normal protein in abnormal quantities. HD and NHL are distinguished on the basis of the Reed-Sternberg giant cells in NHL. The information in choice **d** is reversed. (p. 1293)

2. **The answer is d.** In this early stage, only infection or hemorrhage could be the cause of death. All the others would not occur at this stage. (pp. 1292–1293)

3. **The answer is b.** Three-fourths of lymphoma patients present with enlargement of cervical or supra-clavicular lymph nodes, but enlarged axillary or inguinal nodes may be the presenting symptoms. Such nodes are characteristically painless, firm, rubbery in consistency, freely movable, and of variable size. Weakness, fatigue, and general malaise may be a part of the presenting picture. (p. 1297)

4. **The answer is c.** The diagnosis of lymphoma can be established only by a biopsy of involved tissue, usually a lymph node. Because there are many causes of lymphadenopathy, however—including upper respiratory infection, infectious mononucleosis, allergic reactions, and, in older people, cancer of the head and neck—a careful history and physical examination must first determine if an

enlarged lymph node should be biopsied. For persistent lymphadenopathy or when etiology is not present, a biopsy is usually indicated. (p. 1297)

5.  **The answer is b.** Determination of the stage of disease in HD is important because it influences which treatment option (radiation therapy or combination therapy) will be used. Radiation is very effective for localized HD and is therefore used in early-stage disease. Chemotherapy is more effective than radiation for late-stage disease, when the number of lymph node groups involved is greater, but it also is as effective as radiation in early-stage disease. NHL, on the other hand, is almost always treated with chemotherapy because it usually presents at an advanced stage. A positive bone marrow biopsy indicates a stage IV tumor. A stage II presentation for HD is more likely to indicate a slow-growing malignancy; it is not at all uncommon. (p. 1298)

6.  **The answer is b.** All of the other choices, along with a history and physical examination, are standard procedures used in the staging of lymphoma. Other procedures, including a CT scan of the chest and abdomen, a bone marrow biopsy, a percutaneous liver biopsy, a lower limb lymphangiogram (LAG), and an exploratory laparotomy may be done if there is evidence of lymph node involvement below the diaphragm, hepatomegaly or abnormal liver function, extension of the lymphoma to mediastinal lymph nodes, or splenomegaly. Positive results on these tests often mean a stage IV disease. (pp. 1297, 1298, and Table 43-2, p. 1300)

7.  **The answer is d.** For HD, prognosis is most closely related to stage. Age and the total number of lymph node groups involved (independent of stage) are other prognostic factors, whereas for NHL, prognosis is most closely related to histologic type. (pp. 1299–1300)

8.  **The answer is a.** Patients with stage IIB disease may receive total or subtotal nodal radiotherapy if laparotomy is negative. Otherwise they should receive chemotherapy. Chemotherapy may include either MOPP or ABVD regimens. Either regimen produces complete remission in more than half of the patients who have recurrent disease after treatment with the other regimen. (p. 1301)

9.  **The answer is a.** Most patients with NHL present to their physicians with advanced disease (stage III or IV), reflected by painless, generalized lymphadenopathy. Systemic B symptoms (fever, night sweats, and/or weight loss) are the initial complaint in as many as 20% of cases. (p. 1304)

10.  **The answer is b.** CHOP appears to be the best treatment for intermediate-grade and high-grade NHL. (p. 1312)

11.  **The answer is d.** Toxic effects include acute and chronic pericarditis, along with a spectrum of symptoms ranging from cough and chest pain to edema, paradoxical pulse, cardiac tamponade, and hemodynamic compromise. Coronary artery disease and cardiomyopathy are also seen following extensive mediastinal radiation. (p. 1314)

# Chapter 44     Multiple Myeloma

## INTRODUCTION

- In multiple myeloma, the malignant cell is the plasma cell, the functional mature cell that differentiates and develops from the B lymphocyte. Multiple myeloma, the most common malignant plasma cell disorder, can affect the hematologic, skeletal, renal, and nervous systems.

## EPIDEMIOLOGY

- Within the United States, multiple myeloma represents 1% of all hematologic malignancies.

## ETIOLOGY

- The exact etiology of multiple myeloma is unknown.
- Chronic antigenic stimulation, such as recurrent infections and drug allergies, may be part of the medical history in individuals who develop multiple myeloma. Occupational exposure to low-dose ionizing radiation, wood, textile, rubber, metal, petroleum products, and chemicals used as herbicides has been associated with the development of multiple myeloma.

## NORMAL PHYSIOLOGY

- Chronic antigenic stimulation, such as recurrent infections and drug allergies, may be part of the medical history in individuals who develop multiple myeloma. Occupational exposure to low-dose ionizing radiation, wood, textile, rubber, metal, petroleum products, and chemicals used as herbicides has been associated with the development of multiple myeloma.
- In adults, IgG constitutes the largest proportion of immunoglobulin, followed by IgA and IgM.

## PATHOPHYSIOLOGY

- The plasma cell is derived from the B lymphocyte and is the functionally mature cell producing immunoglobulins; it has been thought to be the identifiable malignant cell in multiple myeloma.
- Regardless of the exact location of the malignant change in multiple myeloma, there is abnormal overproduction of one immunoglobulin called the M protein; the *M* refers to monoclonal antibody, myeloma protein, or malignant protein.

### The Role of Cytokines in the Pathogenesis of Multiple Myeloma

- The exact site of the malignant transformation that causes multiple myeloma remains unknown.
- Interleukin-6 (IL-6) has been identified as one of the major growth factors involved in the development of multiple myeloma.

## DIAGNOSIS AND STAGING

- Once symptoms are present, untreated individuals with multiple myeloma have a median survival of seven months. This can be extended with standard therapy to a median survival of two to three years.
- Once symptoms occur, systemic therapy becomes necessary.

- The most frequent symptom at presentation is bone pain. The clinical course of the disease is complicated by pathological fractures, pain, hypercalcemia, spinal cord compression, anemia, fatigue, thromboctyopenia, recurrent bacterial infection, and renal failure.
- The diagnosis of multiple myeloma can be confirmed by bone marrow biopsy with histological confirmation of increased (> 10%) numbers of plasma cells.
- The diagnostic workup for multiple myeloma is designed to determine the extent of involvement of other organs (Table 44-2, text page 1322).
- The Durie/Salmon system for use in staging multiple myeloma (Table 44-3, text page 1322) integrates clinical and laboratory findings associated with multiple myeloma.

## CLINICAL MANIFESTATIONS

### Skeletal Involvement

- Symptoms assicated with osteolytic lesions include hypercalcemia (20%–40% of patients), pathological fractures with acute and chronic pain, decreased mobility, and an inability to fully participate in activities of daily living.
- Bone lesions can be of three distinct types: (1) a solitary osteolytic lesion, (2) diffuse osteoporosis, and (3) multiple discrete osteolytic "punched-out" or "cannonball" lesions. The pathophysiology of the bone destruction is thought to be myeloma cell production of osteoclast-activating factor (OAF).
- OAFs have been identified as a class of bone-resorbing factors (cytokines) produced by lymphocytes and monocytes.
- Myeloma-associated bone lesions occur as a result of increased osteoclast activity and are most readily diagnosed by roentgenograms or bone surveys. Magnetic resonance imaging (MRI) is the test of choice for evaluating and diagnosing spinal cord compression. If untreated, myeloma-induced osteolytic lesions can lead to compression fractures of the spine with irreversible neurological sequelae, refractory hypercalcemia compromising renal function, and possibly death.

### Infection

- A number of mechanisms have been identified as responsible for the immunosuppression and infection associated with multiple myeloma. These include a deficiency in the normal amount and function of immunoglobulins, neutropenia associated with plasma cell replacement in the bone marrow, qualitative defects in neutrophil and complement system functioning, and decreased physical activity as a result of symptoms and syndromes caused by the disease.

### Bone Marrow Involvement

- A normocytic, normochromic anemia clinically manifested by fatigue and weakness occurs in over 60% of patients at initial diagnosis. The anemia is initially caused by the excessive replacement of erythrocyte precursors with plasma cells in the bone marrow.
- A multifactorial model for multiple myeloma-associated anemia has been postulated (Table 44-4, text page 1323).

### Renal Insufficiency

- At initial diagnosis, renal insufficiency is present in 29% of patients with multiple myeloma.
- Multiple myeloma can cause intrinsic renal lesions as well as renal failure precipitated by the sequelae of the disease (infection, hypercalcemia, and dehydration). "Myeloma kidney" is the principal type of lesion associated with renal failure. In myeloma kidney, the renal tubules are filled with damaging, dense casts surrounded by multinucleated giant cells. These large, dense, tubular casts lead to the formation of precipitates in the tubules that can obstruct and rupture the tubular epithelium.

## Sequelae

- Untreated hypercalcemia in multiple myeloma patients can precipitate renal insufficiency.
- Hyperuricemia occurs as a result of a large tumor burden with an increased rate of cell death. Uric acid-induced nephropathy is caused by precipitation and crystallization of uric acid in the distal tubules.
- Infection is the leading cause of death in multiple myeloma patients.

## Hyperviscosity Syndrome

- Although rare, hyperviscosity syndrome can occur in individuals with IgM myeloma and occasionally in those with IgA, IgG1 and IgG3 myeloma. It is caused by a high concentration of proteins that increase serum viscosity and result in vascular sludging.
- Initial clinical signs (blurred vision, irritability, headache, drowsiness, confusion) may indicate neurological impairment.

## Peripheral Neuropathy

- Peripheral neuropathies have been recognized as part of the clinical sequelae associated with multiple myeloma.

## ASSESSMENT

- Physical examination findings may include bone pain, with or without a decrease in range of motion, an inability to bear weight, or signs and symptoms of spinal cord compression.
- Individuals with multiple myeloma may present with changes in mental status.
- Routine laboratory values may be significant for elevations in blood urea nitrogen (BUN), creatinine, uric acid, and calcium.
- Serum protein immunoelectrophoresis (SPEP) can confirm the monoclonal spikes, and immunoelectrophoresis (IPEP) can also confirm the presence of M protein in the urine.
- Individuals may show evidence of anemia on peripheral blood counts and evidence of plasmacytosis on bone marrow biopsy.
- A number of negative prognostic factors have been identified in Table 44-5, text page 1325.

## TREATMENT
### Chemotherapy

- With the onset of symptoms (anemia, bone pain, and hypercalcemia), systemic antineoplastic therapy consisting of melphalan and prednisone is the first line of therapy.
- Patients are monitored closely for signs of renal impairment (increased BUN and creatinine, proteinuria), and the dose of melphalan may need to be reduced based on the severity of renal toxicity. It is also important to closely monitor serial blood counts because the bone marrow-suppressive effects of melphalan may be cumulative in older patients.
- 30% to 40% of myeloma patients will not respond to first-line therapy, while those who initially respond will eventually relapse.
- The most consistently effective second-line therapy, resulting in a 70% response rate with projected survival greater than one year, is the combination of vincristine, doxorubicin, and dexamethasone.

### Interferon

- Alfa-interferon has been proposed as a strategy to prolong remission duration and survival in multiple myeloma patients who initially respond to cytotoxic therapy.
- The dose-reduction schedule and plan to discontinue interferon are dependent on the individual's response to the severity of the toxicity.

## Radiation

- Radiation therapy has been effective in arresting local bone disease prior to the point of fracture, but it does not lead to bone repair and healing.
- Hemibody irradiation has been used in individuals with refractory or advanced multiple myeloma.
- It allows for the potential treatment of both halves of the body sequentially in doses that are higher than could be delivered with total-body irradiation.

## Bone Marrow Transplantation

- Bone marrow transplantation (syngeneic, allogeneic, autologous) and peripheral stem cell support have been attempted in the treatment of multiple myeloma.
- A number of questions remain unanswered regarding the appropriate use of transplantation in the treatment of multiple myeloma.

## Long-Term Sequelae

- Clinicians must monitor multiple myeloma patients for evidence of acute leukemia.
- Secondary acute leukemia can be refractory to treatment. Treated patients have a dismal median survival of four to eight months.

## NURSING MANAGEMENT

- A symptom management approach to nursing care with a review of systems is useful in organizing assessments and interventions (Table 44-7, text page 1330).

## Neurological

- The most frequent symptom that myeloma patients present with is pain. Bone destruction from the myeloma results in osteoporosis and pathological fractures of long bones or vertebrae.
- Acute pain is characterized by a specific trauma (fracture) and is of short duration (less than six months), whereas chronic pain has no specific obvious initiation point and may occur over a protracted period.
- Mental status changes can be an initial sign of hypercalcemia, hyperviscosity syndrome, or drug toxicity.

## Protective Mechanisms

- Infection is the leading cause of death in patients with multiple myeloma.

## Respiratory

- The respiratory system is the most frequent site of infection in myeloma patients.
- Due to the underlying defect in humoral immunity patients should be instructed not to receive vaccines with live organisms or be in close contact with others who may have received live organism vaccines that may be shedding organisms.

## Gastrointestinal

- Multiple myeloma patients are at risk for constipation as a result of decreased physical activity due to bone pain/pathological fractures, treatment of pain with narcotic analgesics, dehydration, and the use of vincristine.

## Genitourinary

- Renal insufficiency or failure can be exacerbated as a result of the primary disease, fluid and electrolyte abnormalities, dehydration, and/or infection.

# PRACTICE QUESTIONS

1. Regardless of the exact location of the malignant change in multiple myeloma, there is abnormal overproduction of one immunoglobulin called the M protein. The *M* refers to:
   a. monoclonal antibody.
   b. myeloma protein.
   c. malignant protein.
   d. all of the above.

2. Although the exact etiology of multiple myeloma is not known, certain factors increase one's risk. Which of the following have been associated with an increased incidence of multiple myeloma?
   a. chronic low-level exposure to radiation.
   b. chronic antigenic stimulation.
   c. chronic high dose vitamin intake.
   d. a and b.

3. Mrs. Otis has been diagnosed with multiple myeloma and has recently exhibited symptoms of anemia, bone pain, and hypercalcemia. Systemic therapy consists of which of the following?
   a. melphalan and prednisone
   b. the VAD regimen
   c. alfa-interferon
   d. b and c

4. As treatment begins, you will monitor Mrs. Otis closely for adverse drug effects such as:
   a. decreased BUN and creatinine.
   b. hypercalcemia and bone pain.
   c. bone marrow-suppressive effects.
   d. all of the above.

5. Multiple myeloma is a cancer of which of the following cell types?
   a. B lymphocyte
   b. plasma cell
   c. monoclonal lymphocyte
   d. a and b

6. Diagnosis of multiple myeloma is confirmed by:
   a. sterrotactic biopsy.
   b. bone marrow biopsy with > 10% plasma cells.
   c. serum Iga.
   d. serum Igm.

7. The anemia associated with multiple myeloma is due to:
   a. the effects of radiation.
   b. a normochromic iron deficiency.
   c. the replacement of erythrocyte precursors with plasma cells.
   d. erythrocyte destruction by WBCs.

8.  Multiple myeloma is associated with renal failure precipitated by numerous factors. Which of the following contributes most to renal failure in multiple myeloma?
    a.  infection
    b.  hypercalcemia
    c.  dehydration
    d.  any of the above

9.  Mrs. Mura has chronic myeloma and has recently begun to complain of blurred vision, headache, drowsiness, and occasional confusion. These symptoms may be caused by which of the following?
    a.  a high concentration of proteins that increases serum viscosity
    b.  chronic effects of steroid use
    c.  hyperviscosity syndrome
    d.  a and c

## ANSWER EXPLANATIONS

1.  **The answer is d.** Regardless of the exact location of the malignant change in multiple myeloma, there is abnormal overproduction of one immunoglobulin called the M protein; the M refers to the monoclonal antibody, myeloma protein, or malignant protein. (p. 1321)

2.  **The answer is d.** Chronic low-level exposure to radiation and chronic antigenic stimulation are associated with increased incidence of multiple myeloma. (p. 1320)

3.  **The answer is a.** With the onset of symptoms (anemia, bone pain, and hypercalcemia), systemic antineoplastic therapy consisting of melphalan and prednisone is the first line of therapy. The VAD regimen (vincristine, doxorubicin, and dexamethasone) is gaining widespread acceptance for resistant or refractory myeloma, but it is still the most consistently effective second-line therapy. Alfa-interferon has been proposed as a strategy to prolong remission duration in those who initially respond to cytotoxic therapy. (p. 1325)

4.  **The answer is c.** Patients are monitored closely for signs of renal impairment (increased BUN and creatinine, proteinuria), and the dose of melphalan may need to be reduced based on the severity of renal toxicity. It is also important to closely monitor serial blood counts because the bone marrow-suppressive effects of melphalan may be cumulative in older patients. Hypercalcemia and bone pain are symptoms of the disorder itself rather than adverse effects. (p. 1325)

5.  **The answer is d.** In multiple myeloma, the malignant cell is the plasma cell, the functional mature cell that differentiates and develops from the B lymphocytes. (p. 1320)

6.  **The answer is b.** The diagnosis of multiple myeloma can be confirmed by bone marrow biopsy with histological confirmation of increased (> 10%) numbers of plasma cells. (p. 1322)

7.  **The answer is c.** A multifactorial model for multiple myeloma-associated anemia has been postulated, including the replacement of erythrocyte precursors with plasma cells. (Table 44-4, p. 1323)

8.  **The answer is d.** Infection, hypercalcemia, and dehydration are all possible contributing factors to the renal failure associated with multiple myeloma. (p. 1324)

9.  **The answer is d.** The patient's symptoms could be caused by hypersensitivity syndrome, a rare occurrence in myeloma patients caused by a high concentration of proteins that increases the serum viscosity. (p. 1324)

# Chapter 45      Prostate Cancer

## EPIDEMIOLOGY

- Prostate cancer is the most commonly diagnosed cancer in American males and the second-leading cause of cancer-related deaths.
- The incidence of prostate cancer is 37% higher for black men than for white men. Japanese males have the lowest incidence and mortality rates from prostate cancer.
- Two of the events that may be important are diet and serum testosterone levels. Japanese living in Japan consume a mostly vegetarian diet. The vegetarian diet reduces serum testosterone levels. Serum testosterone levels are on average 15% higher in black males than in white males.

## ETIOLOGY

- The cause of prostate cancer is unknown. Risk factors relate primarily to lifestyle, age, and heredity.
  - Lifestyle factors include nutrition and exposure to carcinogens.
- Body fat composition may predispose one to prostate cancer development.
- Exposure to carcinogens such as cigarette smoking, cadmium, or zinc may play a role in prostate cancer development.
- The use of vasectomy for birth control may increase the risk of prostate cancer. The risk appears to be greater for men who had a vasectomy more than 20 years ago.
- Prostate cancer is clearly a disease of the older male.
- Hereditary prostate cancer is characterized by an early onset and the presence of an autosomal dominant pattern of inheritance.
- Several oncogenes have been identified in prostate cancers, including the c-*erbB-2* oncogene.

## PREVENTION, SCREENING, AND EARLY DETECTION

- Because the etiology of prostate cancer is unknown, specific recommendations regarding prevention cannot be made. Rather, based upon the known risk factors, several suggestions can be made. These include the following: consuming a low-fat, high-fiber diet; maintaining normal weight for height; obtaining one's vitamins and trace minerals from vegetable sources; avoiding known carcinogens; and considering alternative methods of contraception.
- Screening for prostate cancer involves the use of digital rectal exam (DRE), analysis of prostate-specific antigen (PSA) level, and, if appropriate, evaluation of the gland using transrectal ultrasound (TRUS).
- DRE involves palpation of the prostate gland and is the most commonly performed screening exam for prostate diseases.
- PSA is a glycoprotein found in normal prostatic tissue.
- Anything that destroys the natural tissue barrier allows PSA to enter the bloodstream, where it can be collected and evaluated in a laboratory.
- Conditions other than prostate cancer can give rise to elevated PSA levels.
- TRUS is used to follow up abnormal DRE or elevated PSA levels. Its role in screening programs is not yet defined. The test can evaluate prostate volume and identify suspicious areas for biopsy.

## PATHOPHYSIOLOGY

- The prostate gland is composed of three major sections: the central zone, the peripheral zone, and the transitional zone.
  - Peripheral zone is the most common site for cancer.

### Cellular Characteristics

- The vast majority of prostate cancers are adenocarcinomas.
- Two types of prostatic proliferative lesions have been identified. One is described as "atypical adenomatous hyperplasia" or "adenosis."
- The second is "prostatic intra-epithelial neoplasia" (PIN).
- Prostate tissue specimens are subjected to a type of pathological scoring based on cellular architecture known as Gleason's grade.
- Tumors graded 1–3 are considered well-differentiated and those 4 or greater are considered poorly differentiated carcinomas. (See Table 45-2, text page 1338.)
- Prostate cancers can also be divided into those that are clinically important and those that are clinically unimportant. Clinically important cancers include features such as large tumor volume, Gleason grade 3–5 (moderate to poor differentiation), an invasive, proliferative pattern of growth, elevated PSA, and origination in the peripheral zone. These cancers threaten the patient's life because they progress to fatal metastatic cancers.
- Indolent cancers comprise the vast majority of prostate cancers.

### Progression of Disease

- Prostate cancer is characterized by a slow pattern of growth.

## CLINICAL MANIFESTATIONS

- An annual DRE is the most effective method of early detection. Patients may present with urinary tract obstructive symptoms similar to benign prostatic hypertrophy (BPH), such as frequency, hesitancy, nocturia, and urgency.
- Other symptoms may include a change in erectile capability.
- Advanced prostate cancer is evidenced by the appearance of ureteral obstruction caused by ureterovesical junction compression.
- Hydronephrosis can then ensue.
- Back pain may reveal the presence of vertebral body metastases with the potential for spinal cord compression. There may also be local pain due to the presence of the cancer in the prostate gland and referred pain to the legs and abdomen. Bone pain can be problematic.

## ASSESSMENT

### Patient and Family History

- The nurse should evaluate the patient's voiding pattern and ask if the patient has problems with dysuria, frequency, nocturia, hematuria, and other signs of bladder outlet obstruction. (See Table 45-3, text page 1339.)

### Physical Exam

- The patient is examined for evidence of local and distant metastases. Inguinal nodes are palpated, and the patient is asked about bone pain, specifically back pain.

## Diagnostic Studies

- Once a presumptive diagnosis of prostate cancer is made, the patient will have a PSA level drawn and a DRE performed if these tests have not previously been performed.
- PSA level may be drawn before and after therapeutic interventions and then periodically to monitor the status of the cancer. Additional blood tests include serum chemistries, urinalysis, (CT) scans of the abdomen and pelvis, and bone scan.
- TRUS may be used to assist in evaluating the extent of localized prostate cancer.

## Prognostic Indicators

- Unfortunately, not all prostate cancers produce PSA, and other diagnostic studies, such as CT scan, may be needed to monitor disease status.
- PSA levels should be normal 3 to 18 months after completion of therapy. Failure of PSA to normalize often reflects localized disease recurrence.

## CLASSIFICATION AND STAGING

- The most commonly used staging system for prostate cancer is the American Urologic Association (AUA) System.
- A tumor-node-metastasis (TNM) system was developed by the American Joint Committee on Cancer (AJCC).
- See Table 45-4, text page 1340, for a comparison of the two staging systems.

## THERAPEUTIC APPROACHES AND NURSING CARE

- A patient may be offered watchful waiting (periodic observation), surgery, radiation therapy, hormonal manipulation, chemotherapy, or investigational drugs.

### Watchful Waiting or Periodic Observation for Early Stage Prostate Cancer (Stages A and B)

- Prostate cancer is a heterogenous disease.
- Clinically diagnosable prostate cancer, untreated, will continue to grow and threaten the life of the patient. Latent or clinically unimportant cancers do not threaten the patient's life. Of men aged 50 or older, approximately one-third will have malignant cells in their prostate.
  - However, only 3% of men who develop malignant cells in their prostate will die of the disease.
- For patients over 70, watchful waiting may be an appropriate option.
- Prostate cancer may behave in a more aggressive manner because of higher grade tumors in younger men, and for this reason alone, treatment is offered.
- Standard therapy with surgery or radiation therapy will be offered to patients with localized prostate cancer.

### Surgery

#### Transurethral resection of the prostate (TURP)

- Prostate cancer is not cured by TURP. Rather, it is used to treat symptoms of bladder outlet obstruction and in some patients, provides pathological evidence that a cancer, previously unsuspected, is present.
- See Table 45-5, text pages 1342–1344, for management of the TURP patient.

### Radical prostatectomy

- The increasing use of radical prostatectomy is related to the use of PSA to screen asymptomatic men.
- Radical prostatectomy is usually done on patients staged with A or B disease. With stage C disease, it may be more difficult to obtain tumor-free margins.
- There is potential for postoperative incontinence and impotence. Up to 15% of men remain incontinent six months postoperatively.
- Surgery may damage or sever the nerves that control erectile function.
- The nerve-sparing procedure is recommended for patients with stage A or B disease who are eligible to undergo radical prostatectomy.
- If disease is more advanced and there is involvement of the prostatic capsule or seminal vesicles at the time of surgery, resection may involve removal of or damage to the nerves.
- Men who have undergone treatment for localized prostate cancer are more likely to have problems related to sexual, urinary, or bowel function.
- Hematuria and clots are common for the first three to four postoperative days.
- Urinary incontinence guidelines provide an in-depth discussion of incontinence and its management. (See Table 45-6, text page 1346.)
- See Table 45-7, text page 1347, for "Helpful Hints for Men Starting Sexual Activity After Prostate Surgery."

## Radiation Therapy

- External beam radiation therapy (XRT) may be administered in curative doses to treat men with early prostate cancer (A2, B1, B2) confined to the gland itself. Young men with A1 disease usually are also offered treatment rather than periodic observation. Radiation therapy is an option available if a patient wishes to avoid surgery or is not a surgical candidate.
- The dose of radiation administered is based on disease stage.
- Radiation is also useful in managing complications of advanced prostate cancer including hematuria, urinary obstruction, ureteral obstruction, and pelvic pain.
- Radiation therapy side effects include impotence, urinary incontinence, bone marrow depression, lower extremity edema, cystitis, urethral strictures, diarrhea, proctitis, and rectal bleeding.

### Brachytherapy

- Prostatic brachytherapy involves the placement of radioactive seeds directly into the prostate.
- After insertion of the source, the principles of time, distance, and shielding should be used as Iodine-125 emits gamma radiation. Hospitalization lasts until decay of the source is reduced to 30 millicuries or less.
- The patient poses no danger as a radioactive source; the patient and his family must understand this concept before discharge to avoid issues related to self-imposed isolation for fear of exposing others to radiation.

## Hormonal Therapy

- Advanced prostate cancer is frequently managed by altering the patient's hormonal status. Three different cell populations comprise both normal and malignant prostate tissues: hormone dependent, hormone sensitive, and hormone independent.
- Androgen is the hormone on which hormone-dependent and hormone-sensitive cells are dependent.
- The goal of hormone therapy for prostate cancer is to reduce the level of circulating androgens, causing the death of hormone-dependent cells and inhibiting the growth of hormone-sensitive cells, thereby reducing tumor size. Hormonal manipulation is not curative therapy, but can provide many patients with symptom palliation.

- There are surgical and medical approaches to reducing serum testosterone levels. Bilateral orchiectomy quickly reduces testosterone levels as 90%–95% of testosterone is produced by the testicles.
- LHRH agonists initially increase testosterone levels, but after several days of therapy, testosterone levels fall to castration level. The surge of testosterone production after initiation of an LHRH agonist is called a "flare." During a flare, patients need to be aware that symptoms can worsen and require prompt medical intervention.
- Flutamide, an antiandrogen, prevents the binding of testosterone to receptors on prostate cells.
- Combining antiandrogenic therapy with an LHRH agonist, such as leuprolide or goserelin, is called total androgen ablation.
- All hormonal manipulations have the potential to produce side effects. The most common ones are hot flashes, impotence, and decreased libido.
- Patients will respond well to hormonal therapy 70%–89% of the time and responses can be several years in duration.

## Chemotherapy

- For a patient with hormone-refractory prostate cancer, antineoplastic therapy may be an option.
- The most effective single agents available for treating prostate cancer are vinblastine, trimetrexate, mitoquazone, and estramustine.
- The most effective drug combination consists of vinblastine and estramustine.
- Suramin may be a useful chemotherapeutic drug in the treatment of prostate cancer. A complex polysulfated polysaccharide with the ability to inhibit multiple unrelated enzymes. Suramin's ability to block growth factor receptors may play a role in its antineoplastic activity. Dose-limiting toxicities have been coagulopathies and neurotoxicities.
- Additional side effects include anaphylaxis, pancytopenia, infection, hyperglycemia, rash, elevated BUN and serum creatinine, adrenal insufficiency, and myopathy.

## SYMPTOM MANAGEMENT AND SUPPORTIVE CARE

- Advanced prostate cancer patients require management of bone pain with narcotic analgesics, nonsteroidal antiinflammatory drugs (NSAIDs), and laxatives and stool softeners to control narcotic-induced constipation. Bladder outlet obstructive symptoms may require catheterization and subsequent TURP to remove the obstructing tissue.
- These men and their families need to be aware that worsening back pain, weakness of the lower extremities, or sensory deficits require immediate medical attention. Radiation therapy will be administered in most cases to control tumor impingement on the spinal cord.

# PRACTICE QUESTIONS

1.  Byron is being assessed for possible presence of prostate cancer. Which of the following is *least* likely to be a risk factor?
    a.  promiscuity
    b.  body fat composition
    c.  vasectomy as birth control
    d.  hereditary

2.  _____ is the most commonly performed screening exam for prostate disease.
    a.  Analysis of prostate-specific antigen (PSA) level
    b.  Digital rectal exam (DRE)
    c.  Evaluation of the gland using transrectal ultrasound (TRUS)
    d.  Urinalysis

3.  The *least* threatening prostate cancers are those that:
    a.  feature large tumor volume.
    b.  have a Gleason grade of 3–5.
    c.  originate in the peripheral zone.
    d.  are indolent.

4.  Byron is diagnosed with prostate cancer. After diagnosis, he will receive:
    a.  CT scans of the abdomen.
    b.  bone scan.
    c.  urinalysis.
    d.  all of the above.

5.  Which of the following patients with prostate cancer is most likely to be given "watchful waiting" as a treatment choice?
    a.  Frank, who is 37, recently married, and still hopes to have children
    b.  Harold, who is 76 and enjoying an active retirement with his wife
    c.  Byron, who is 56 and has poorly differentiated localized disease
    d.  Phil, who is 40 and has a high grade tumor

6.  A new patient, Charles, receives transurethral resection of the prostate (TURP). He asks if this will cure the disease. You explain that:
    a.  TURP is sometimes found to cure prostate cancer, but the chances diminish with patient age and tumor involvement.
    b.  TURP is used to treat symptoms of bladder outlet obstruction.
    c.  TURP provides pathological evidence that a cancer, previously unsuspected, is present.
    d.  b and c

7.  Which of the following patients is *least* likely to respond well to radical prostatectomy?
    a.  Alex, who has stage A disease
    b.  Bill, who has stage B disease
    c.  Chuck, who has stage C disease
    d.  a and b

8. External beam radiation therapy (XRT) may be administered in *curative* doses to treat men who:
   a. have A2, prostate cancer.
   b. have advanced prostate cancer with hematuria and urinary obstruction.
   c. are not surgical candidates.
   d. a and c.

9. Hank has had seeds of Iodine-125 inserted in prostatic brachytherapy. Which of the following would not be included as part of your patient education plan for Hank and his family?
   a. Hank must remain hospitalized until the source that emits gamma radiation has completely decayed so that he is not a source of radiation to those around him.
   b. Hank's hospitalization will last until decay of the source is reduced to 30 millicuries or less.
   c. A condom should be worn during intercourse for two months after implantation.
   d. a and c.

10. Alex is undergoing hormone therapy. You explain to him that the goal of hormone therapy for prostate cancer is to:
   a. increase the level of circulating androgens, causing the death of hormone-dependent cells.
   b. inhibit the growth of hormone-sensitive cells.
   c. provide curative therapy.
   d. all of the above.

11. Daniel is administered an LHRH agonist to reduce his serum testosterone levels. Almost immediately, Daniel's pain worsens and he shows symptoms of bladder outlet obstruction. The physician will not tell Daniel's family that:
   a. after several days of therapy, Daniel's testosterone levels will fall to castration level.
   b. these worsening symptoms are a temporary increase in testosterone levels and are referred to as a "flare."
   c. treatment must be discontinued immediately, and the worsening symptoms and heightened testosterone "flare" given prompt medical attention; in light of this "flare" reaction, surgery is now the only option for Daniel.
   d. a and b.

12. Michael has hormone-refractory prostate cancer and is soon to undergo antineoplastic therapy, using a drug combination. Knowing this, you prepare a patient education plan that centers around the use and effects of:
   a. vincristine and trimetrexate.
   b. vinblastine and estramustine.
   c. estramustine and mitoquazone.
   d. vincristine and aminoglutethimide, followed by hydrocortisone.

13. Mark is being sent home from the hospital. His prostate cancer involves some bone metastasis. Which of the following developments would be likely to indicate a need for radiation therapy?
   a. worsening back pain
   b. weakness of the lower extremities
   c. sensory deficits
   d. all of the above

14. Which of the following statements is *not* true regarding prostate-specific antigen?
   a. PSA is elevated only in men who have prostate cancer.
   b. When tumor destroys the natural tissue barrier, PSA enters the blood stream.
   c. PSA levels are used as a screening test for prostate cancer.

15. Suramin may be a useful chemotherapeutic drug in the treatment of prostate cancer. Which of the following statements is true regarding suramin?
    a. It acts primarily by inhibiting enzyme activity and blocking growth factor receptors.
    b. Dose-limiting toxicities are coagulopathies and neurotoxicities.
    c. Other toxicities include rash, adrenal insufficiency, and myopathy.
    d. all of the above.

# ANSWER EXPLANATIONS

1. **The answer is a.** Body fat composition, exposure to carcinogens, vasectomy as birth control, and advancing age may predispose one to prostate cancer development. Hereditary prostate cancer is characterized by an early onset and the presence of an autosomal dominant pattern of inheritance. (p. 1335)

2. **The answer is b.** Screening for prostate cancer involves the use of digital rectal exam (DRE), analysis of prostate-specific antigen (PSA) level, and if appropriate, evaluation of the gland using transrectal ultrasound (TRUS). DRE involves palpation of the prostate gland and is the most commonly performed screening exam for prostate disease. (p. 1336)

3. **The answer is d.** Clinically important cancers include features such as large tumor volume; Gleason grade 3–5; an invasive, proliferative pattern of growth; elevated PSA; and origination in the peripheral zone. These cancers threaten the patient's life because they progress to fatal metastatic cancers. The vast majority of prostate cancers do not threaten the patient's life and are termed *indolent*. (p. 1339)

4. **The answer is d.** Once a presumptive diagnosis of prostate cancer is made, the patient will have a PSA level drawn and a DRE performed if these were not performed beforehand. A urinalysis, CT scans of the abdomen and pelvis, bone scan, and TRUS are frequently performed as part of the staging and evaluation of metastasis. (p. 1340)

5. **The answer is b.** For patients over 70, watchful waiting may be an appropriate option. Research has yet to demonstrate that for those with stage A or B cancer, treatment is more beneficial than watchful waiting. For men under 70, a physician may often be reluctant to offer watchful waiting, and there is evidence that for younger men with moderately or poorly differentiated localized prostate cancer, treatment may offer a survival advantage. (p. 1341)

6. **The answer is d.** Prostate cancer is not cured by TURP. Rather, it is used to treat symptoms of bladder outlet obstruction and in some patients, provides pathological evidence that a cancer, previously unsuspected, is present. (p. 1342)

7. **The answer is c.** Radical prostatectomy is usually done on patients staged with A or B disease. With stage C disease, it may be more difficult to obtain tumor-free margins. (p. 1344)

8. **The answer is d.** External beam radiation therapy (XRT) may be administered in curative doses to treat men with early prostate cancer (A2, B1, B2) confined to the gland itself. Young men with A1 disease usually are also offered treatment rather than periodic observation. Radiation therapy is an option available if a patient wishes to avoid surgery or is not a surgical candidate. (pp. 1345 and 1347)

9. **The answer is a.** After insertion of the source, hospitalization lasts until decay of the source is reduced to 30 millicuries or less. A condom should be worn during intercourse for two months after implantation, but the patient poses no danger as a radioactive source. (p. 1348)

10. **The answer is b.** The goal of hormone therapy for prostate cancer is to reduce the level of circulating androgens, causing the death of hormone-dependent cells and inhibiting the growth of hormone-sensitive cells, thereby reducing tumor size. Hormonal manipulation is not curative therapy but can provide many patient with symptom palliation. (p. 1348)

11. **The answer is c.** LHRH agonists initially increase testosterone levels, but after several days of therapy, testosterone levels fall to castration level. The surge of testosterone production after initiation of an LHRH agonist is called a "flare." During a flare, patients need to be aware that symptoms can worsen and require prompt medical intervention. (p. 1349)

12. **The answer is b.** For a patient with hormone-refractory prostate cancer, antineoplastic therapy may be an option. The most effective drug combination for treating prostate cancer consists of vinblastine and estramustine. (p. 1349)

13. **The answer is d.** All patients with bone metastasis are at risk for spinal cord compression. Worsening back pain, weakness of the lower extremities, or sensory deficits require immediate medical attention—usually radiation therapy to control tumor impingement on the spinal cord. (p. 1350)

14. **The answer is a.** Conditions other than prostate cancer can give rise to elevated PSA levels. (p. 1336)

15. **The answer is d.** All of the statements are true concerning suramin. (pp. 1349–1350)

# Chapter 46    Skin Cancers

## INTRODUCTION

- Cancers of the skin consist of basal cell carcinoma (BCC), squamous cell carcinoma (SCC), and malignant melanoma. BCC and SCC are often grouped together and referred to as *nonmelanoma skin cancer* (NMSC). Most melanomas are cutaneous (CM).
- NMSCs have a higher incidence but have a low metastatic potential and mortality rate.
- Conversely, melanoma has a much lower incidence rate but a mortality rate triple that of the NMSC.

## EPIDEMIOLOGY

- BCC is the most common form of skin cancer; it generally occurs in adults over age 55.
- Although CM represents only about 4% of skin cancers, it accounts for an estimated 7200 cancer deaths annually.

## ETIOLOGY AND RISK FACTORS

- Ultraviolet radiation (UVR) is the probable cause of most skin cancers.
- Types of UVR harmful to the skin are UVB and UVA.
- The incidence of both CM and NMSC is higher in latitudes closer to the equator.
- See Table 46-1, text page 1358, for examples of etiologic factors for basal cell carcinoma, squamous cell carcinoma, and cutaneous melanoma.
- A persistently changed or changing mole or presence of irregular pigmented precursor lesions (dysplastic nevi, congenital nevi, lentigo maligna) represents a major high-risk situation for CM.
- Skin pigmentation is clearly important in the etiology of skin cancers.
- Whites with red hair and fair complexions who tend to sunburn or freckle easily have higher relative risks for all skin cancers.
- Other possible risk factors for CM include age, hormonal factors, immunosuppression, a previous history of melanoma, and a family history of CM. No conclusive evidence exists regarding the use of oral contraceptives.

## NONMELANOMA SKIN CANCERS
### Basal Cell Carcinoma
#### Pathogenesis

- BCC, also called basal cell epithelioma, is the least aggressive type of skin cancer.

#### Assessment

- Common classifications include nodular (also called nodulo-ulcerative), superficial, pigmented, morpheaform, and keratotic (Table 46-2, text page 1359). Nodular BCC is the most common type.
- Clinically, nodular BCC begins as a small, firm, well-demarcated, dome-shaped papule. The color can be pearly white, pink, or skin-colored.
- Superficial BCC is the second most common type, histologically exhibiting islands of irregular proliferating tumor tissue attached to the undersurface of the epidermis.

- Pigmented BCC is less common and may be nodular or superficial with a brown, black, or blue color that can be clinically mistaken for melanoma.
- Morpheaform BCC is the rarest type.

## Squamous Cell Carcinoma

### Pathogenesis

- SCC is more aggressive than BCC.

### Assessment

- SCC appears as a flesh-colored or erythematous raised, firm papule.
- SCC is usually confined to areas exposed to UVR.
- With the exception of the lower lip site, SCC on these areas is less likely to metastasize than lesions located on areas not exposed to UVR.

## Treatment of Nonmelanoma Skin Cancers

- Standard treatment for NMSC includes surgical excision, Mohs' micrographic surgery, curettage and electrodesiccation, radiation, cryotherapy, and topical chemotherapy.
- Choice of treatment is affected by such factors as tumor type, location, size, and growth pattern, and whether the tumor is primary or secondary.

### Surgical excision

- The advantages of surgical excision as a treatment are rapid healing, the fact that an entire specimen for histological examination can be obtained, and favorable cosmetic results. Disadvantages are that the procedure is time-consuming and requires a skilled physician.
- A skin graft or flap may be performed as an adjunct to surgical excision.

### Mohs' micrographic surgery

- Mohs' micrographic surgery (also called chemosurgery) involves horizontal shaving and staining of tissue in thin layers.
- Mohs' microsurgery is most often used as a first line of treatment for cancers in high-risk areas such as the nose and nasolabial folds, the medial canthus, and pre- and postauricular locations. It is also used for lesions with unclear margins, recurrent lesions, aggressive tumors, and extensive lesions.

### Curettage and electrodesiccation

- Curettage and electrodesiccation (also called *electrosurgery*) treatment is used only for BCC skin cancers that are small (< 2 cm), superficial, or recurrent because of poor margin control.
- Electrodesiccation maintains hemostasis and softens normal tissue so a safe margin can be curettaged.

### Radiotherapy

- Radiotherapy generally is recommended only for lesions that are inoperable; lesions located in sites such as the corner of the nose, eyelid, lip, and canthus; and those greater than 1 cm but less than 8 cm.
- The treatment is not recommended for younger patients (less than age 45).

## Cryotherapy

- Cryotherapy involves tumor destruction by using liquid nitrogen to freeze and thaw tumor tissue.
- Cryotherapy can be used for small to large primary tumors, for certain recurrent lesions such as those in areas of prior radiation, for multiple superficial BCC, and for lesions needing palliative treatment. Only lesions with well-defined margins benefit from this treatment.

## Chemotherapy

- Topical 5-fluorouracil (5-FU) applied to BCC for several weeks produces an inflammatory response that prevents DNA synthesis and cellular reproduction.

## MELANOMA

## Cutaneous Melanoma

### Pathogenesis

- CM arises from melanocytes, which are cells specializing in the biosynthesis and transport of melanin.
- Three specific precursor lesions of CM that have been well studied are dysplastic nevi, congenital nevi, and lentigo maligna.

### Dysplastic nevi (DN)

- Also known as *atypical moles*, DN may be familial or nonfamilial.
- DN are absent at birth. An early clinical indication may be the presence of an increased number of histologically normal nevi between the ages of 5 and 8 years, with dysplastic changes occurring after puberty.
- DN generally have one or more of the clinical features of CM (i.e., asymmetry, border irregularity, color variegation, and a diameter greater than 6 mm).
- DN appear on the face, trunk, and arms but also may be seen on the buttocks, groin, scalp, and female breast. Pigmentation is irregular.

### Congenital nevi

- Congenital nevi are present at birth or shortly thereafter.
- The color of a congenital nevus ranges from brown to black, and lesions may be slightly raised, with an irregular surface and a fairly regular border.

### Assessment

- A thorough patient history and physical examination are essential to identify individuals at high risk and for early detection of CM and suspicious lesions.
- Physical recognition of CM by practitioners and those at risk can be initiated by using the "ABCDE" rule. In this rule, A = asymmetry, B = border irregularity, C = color variation or dark black color, D = diameter greater than 0.6 cm (pencil eraser size), and E = elevation.
- Melanoma can metastasize to virtually every organ in the body, and individuals with the diagnosis should undergo the recommended examinations for metastatic disease.

### Classification

- Melanoma has been classified into several types: lentigo maligna (LMM), superficial-spreading (SSM), nodular, acral lentiginous (mucocutaneous).
- The four major types of CM are described in Table 46-3 on text page 1363.
- LMM is the least serious type. It occurs on body areas heavily exposed to UVR.

- LMM are large and are primarily tan with different shades of brown throughout (Figure 46-6—Plate 24).
- SSM accounts for approximately 70% of CM. In men this lesion is most commonly seen on the trunk, and in women, on the legs. SSM usually arises in a preexisting nevus.
- Nodular melanoma constitutes 15%–30% of CM. This lesion appears as a raised, dome-shaped blue-black or red nodule on areas of the head, neck, and trunk that may or may not be exposed to the sun. Ulcerations and bleeding may be present. It is more aggressive than the other melanoma types.
- Acral lentiginous or mucocutaneous melanoma is the most frequent type of CM in people of color but accounts for less than 5% of CM in whites. This lesion occurs on the palms, soles, nail beds, and mucous membranes. Acral lentiginous melanoma exhibits both a radial and a vertical growth phase.

## Staging and prognostic factors

- *Microstaging* is a term used to describe the level of invasion of the CM and maximum tumor thickness. Two systems are used in assessing the depth of invasion of melanoma (Figure 46-10). The first is the anatomic level of invasion, or the Clark level, and the second is the thickness of tumor tissue, or the Breslow level.
- The traditional three-stage system (Table 46-4, text page 1365) is still used, even though it does not include important disease criteria such as tumor thickness. The American Joint Committee on Cancer (AJCC) four-stage system for CM is preferable because it divides patients more evenly and allows for more consistent exchange of information (Table 46-5, text page 1366).
- As CM thickness increases, survival rates decrease.
- Younger patients and women have a somewhat better prognosis.
- Lesions on the hands, feet, and scalp may have a poorer prognosis.

## Treatment

### Surgery

- The initial surgical procedure for suspected CM is a biopsy. An excisional biopsy that removes a few millimeters of normal tissue surrounding the lesion is preferable.
- An incisional biopsy can be used for lesions located in cosmetically sensitive areas or for large lesions.
- For stage I CM the standard treatment is a wide excision.
- Elective lymph node dissection (ELND) has a high degree of morbidity, and use of this procedure is debatable when no clinical evidence of nodal involvement exists.
- Standard surgical therapy of clinical stage II (clinical, but not histological, evidence of draining lymph node involvement) disease includes excision of the primary lesion, along with surgical dissection of the involved nodes.
- Surgery is also useful for palliation of disease and symptomatic involvement.

### Chemotherapy

- Metastatic malignant melanoma is highly resistant to systemic chemotherapeutic agents, indicating the need for further research in this area. Dacarbazine (DTIC) is the most active agent for disseminated melanoma.

### Radiotherapy

- Radiotherapy is most effective when tumor volume is low and when a high dose per fewer fractions radiation level is used.
- Hyperthermia may enhance the effect of radiation.

### Hormonal therapy

- A hormonal influence on melanocyte and melanoma cell proliferation has been suggested by the usual occurrence of CM following puberty, increased incidence during menopause, and increased or decreased CM growth during pregnancy or after parturition.

### Immunotherapy

- Immunotherapy is a recent form of melanoma treatment with the rationale for use paralleling the natural history of CM, indicating that immunologic intervention by the host may alter the growth pattern of CM.
- Immunotherapy is currently being investigated as adjuvant therapy and as treatment for metastatic disease.

### Gene transfer therapy

- Now becoming known as the fifth modality for cancer treatment, gene therapy is being studied for its effect on CM.

### Other treatments

- Topical 5-FU has shown desirable results for extensive facial LMMs. In lentigo maligna CM with poor prognosis, preoperative treatment with topical 5-FU has been improving surgical results.

## PREVENTION

## Primary Prevention

- Many skin cancers can be prevented by reducing exposure to avoidable risk factors, particularly exposure to excessive UVR.
- Specific sun protection behaviors are discussed on text page 1368, Col. 2.
- People who work with substances known to cause skin cancer should wear protective clothing and use protective equipment to reduce their exposure.

## Chemoprevention

- Retinoids (vitamin A and its derivatives) used as biological treatment agents have shown some effect as chemopreventive agents in persons with BCC, actinic keratosis, keratoacanthoma, epidermodysplasia verruciformis, and dysplastic nevi.

## Screening

- Most changes on the skin are easily visible and can be detected early, thereby improving chances for cure.
- Figure 46-11, text page 1369, is an example of a patient education poster that describes these early changes.

## NURSING MANAGEMENT

## Interview

- Nurses who are trained in pedigree assessment can complete a family pedigree to ascertain family history of skin cancers. The history and exposure to risk factors will determine how detailed a skin assessment should be.

## Skin Assessment

- The location and descriptive characteristics of suspicious lesions should be recorded on an anatomic chart. Warts, moles, scars, vascularities, and birthmarks should also be documented.

## Education

- Education for those at high risk for or diagnosed with skin cancers begins with an initial assessment of their knowledge deficit related to skin cancers.

## Posttreatment Management

- Surgical excision is still the most common treatment for skin cancers, and postoperative nursing management is determined by the extent of the procedure.
- Nursing management of patients receiving chemotherapy, radiotherapy, or immunotherapy is determined by the specific treatment regimen administered.
- Patients need to understand the importance of follow-up visits and testing and of informing the physician or nurse of any physical or mental changes that occur.

# PRACTICE QUESTIONS

1. The most common form of skin cancer is:
   a. basal cell carcinoma (BCC).
   b. squamous cell carcinoma (SCC).
   c. malignant melanoma.
   d. superficial spreading melanoma (SSM).

2. High-risk factors for cutaneous melanoma (CM) include all of the following *except*:
   a. skin pigmentation.
   b. a persistently changed or changing mole.
   c. the presence of a precursor lesion such as dysplastic nevi.
   d. oral contraceptives.

3. One way that basal cell carcinoma (BCC) is distinguished from squamous cell carcinoma (SCC) is by its:
   a. common occurrence on the head and hands.
   b. lower incidence.
   c. slower growth rate.
   d. less well-demarcated margins.

4. A 60-year-old female reports a flesh-colored, raised, firm papule on the top of her nose. It is examined and found to be a squamous cell carcinoma (SCC). How do SCCs differ from most BCCs?
   a. They tend to be less aggressive than BCCs, even though they have faster growth rates.
   b. Their margins are well demarcated, as compared to those of the BCCs.
   c. They tend to have greater metastatic potential.
   d. a and c.

5. A graft or flap is most often used in the surgical treatment of a nonmelanoma cancer when:
   a. the lesion is large or located in an area with insufficient tissue for closure.
   b. risks of bleeding are high and vasculature must be maintained.
   c. the actual extent of the tumor must be accurately assessed and margins are relatively unclear.
   d. the lesion is small, superficial, or recurrent.

6. Which of the following statements about dysplastic nevi (DN) is incorrect?
   a. DN may be familial or nonfamilial.
   b. Most persons affected by DN have about 25–75 abnormal nevi.
   c. DN develop from precursor lesions of CM known as congenital nevi.
   d. A distinctive feature of DN is a "fried egg" appearance with a deeply pigmented papular area surrounded by an area of lighter pigmentation.

7. Physical recognition of CM by practitioners and those at risk can be initiated by using the "ABCDE" rule. In this rule, *C* stands for:
   a. change in symmetry.
   b. crusting or bleeding.
   c. color variation or dark black color.
   d. cause.

8. The phase of CM tumor growth that is characterized by focal deep penetration of atypical melanocytes into the dermis and subcutaneous tissue is the:
   a. radial phase.
   b. vertical growth phase.
   c. nodular phase.
   d. acral lentiginous phase.

9. Of the following factors related to CM prognosis, the one most closely correlated with decreased survival rates in patients with stage I CM is:
   a. anatomic level of tumor invasion.
   b. tumor location.
   c. Clark level.
   d. tumor thickness.

10. The preferred initial surgical procedure for suspected CM is:
    a. excisional biopsy.
    b. incisional biopsy.
    c. wide excision.
    d. curettage and electrodesiccation.

11. Which of the following statements about primary prevention of skin cancers is false?
    a. UV radiation is strongest during the mid-part of the day.
    b. For most people, sunscreen is not required on overcast days.
    c. Certain medications (e.g., oral contraceptives) can make individuals photosensitive.
    d. Surfaces such as sand and water can reflect more than one-half of the UV radiation onto the skin.

## ANSWER EXPLANATIONS

1. **The answer is a.** BCC is the most common form of skin cancer in whites and outnumbers SCC by a ratio of 3:1. Nonmelanoma skin cancers, including BCC, have a higher incidence but a lower metastatic potential and mortality rate than malignant melanoma. Malignant melanoma has a much lower incidence but a mortality rate that is triple that of the nonmelanoma cancers. Increased mortality is directly related to its high potential for metastasis. (p. 1356)

2. **The answer is d.** Multiple etiologic and risk factors are associated with skin cancers. High-risk factors for CM include a persistent changed or changing mole and the presence of irregular pigmented precursor lesions, including dysplastic nevi, congenital nevi, and lentigo maligna. Other possible risk factors for CM include UV radiation, age, hormonal factors, immunosuppression, and a previous history of melanoma. There is not conclusive evidence regarding the use of oral contraceptives and the increased risk of CM. High-risk factors for nonmelanoma cancers include ultraviolet (UV) radiation, especially UV-B and UV-A, and skin pigmentation. (p. 1358)

3. **The answer is c.** BCC is the least aggressive type of skin cancer and has its origins in either the basal layer of the epidermis or in the surrounding dermal structures. It is most commonly found on the nose, eyelids, cheeks, neck, trunk, and extremities. It grows slowly by direct extension and has the capacity to cause major local destruction. Metastasis is rare and most often occurs in the regional lymph nodes. SCC, on the other hand, may arise in any epithelium. It is most commonly found on the head and hands. It is more aggressive than BCC, as it has a faster growth rate, less well-demarcated margins, and a greater metastatic potential. Metastatic disease is usually first noted in the regional lymph nodes. (p. 1358)

4. **The answer is c.** SCC is more aggressive than BCC as it has a faster growth rate, less–well-demarcated margins, and a greater metastatic potential. SCC appears as a flesh-colored or erythematous raised, firm papule. It is usually confined to areas exposed to UVR. (p. 1359)

5. **The answer is a.** A graft or flap is indicated when a lesion is large or located in an area where insufficient tissue for primary closure would result in deformity, for example, after excision of large carcinomas of the eyelid and lip. Function is preserved in this manner. A skin flap consists of skin and subcutaneous tissue that are transferred from one area of the body to another. A flap contains its own blood supply, whereas a graft is avascular and depends on the blood supply of the recipient site for its survival. (p. 1360)

6. **The answer is c.** DN are precursor lesions of cutaneous melanoma (CM) that develop from normal nevi, usually after puberty. It has been reported that 50% of CM evolve from some form of DN. They may be familial or nonfamilial, with the risk of CM in a family member with DN approaching 100% in melanoma-prone families. DN are often larger than 5 mm and can number from 1–100, with most affected persons having 25–75 abnormal nevi. They appear typically on sun-exposed areas, especially on the back, but also may be seen on the scalp, breasts, and buttocks. Pigmentation is irregular, with mixtures of tan, brown, and black or red and pink. A distinctive feature is a "fried egg" appearance. (pp. 1361–1362)

7. **The answer is c.** Physical recognition of CM by practitioners and those at risk can be initiated by using the "ABCDE" rule. In this rule, $A$ = asymmetry, $B$ = border irregularity, $C$ = color variation or dark black color, $D$ = diameter greater than 0.6 cm, and $E$ = elevation. (p. 1362)

8. **The answer is b.** Melanoma has been classified into several types, including lentigo maligna (LMM), superficial spreading (SSM), nodular, and acral lentiginous. Each type is characterized by a radial and/or vertical growth phase. In the radial phase, tumor growth is parallel to the skin surface, risk of metastasis is slight, and surgical excision is usually curative. The vertical growth phase is marked by focal deep penetration of atypical melanocytes into the dermis and subcutaneous tissue. Penetration occurs rapidly, increasing the risk of metastasis. (Table 46-3, p. 1363)

9. **The answer is d.** Microstaging describes the level of invasion of the CM and maximum tumor thickness. The two parameters that are used in assessing the depth of invasion are the anatomic level of invasion or the Clark level and the thickness of tumor tissue or the Breslow level. The prognosis for patients with metastatic disease at the time of diagnosis is poor, with most dying within 5 years. As CM thickness increases, survival rates decrease. Thus, the Breslow level has consistently proved to be a significant prognostic variable in stage I CM. (p. 1364)

10. **The answer is a.** Biopsy is the initial surgical procedure for suspected CM. Because it provides a definitive diagnosis along with microstaging information, an excisional biopsy that entails removal of a few millimeters of normal tissue surrounding the lesion is preferable. An incisional biopsy can be used for lesions in cosmetically sensitive areas or for large lesions. Electrocoagulation, curettage, shaving, and burning are never used to remove a suspicious mole. (pp. 1364–1365)

11. **The answer is b.** Sunscreen should always be applied on overcast days because 70%–80% of UV radiation can penetrate cloud cover. (p. 1368)

# Chapter 47 Testicular Germ Cell Cancer

## INTRODUCTION

- Testicular cancer is a relatively rare cancer, yet it is the most common cancer in men aged 15 to 35.

## EPIDEMIOLOGY

- Testis cancer most commonly affects those in the 20- to 30-year-old age group. It occurs less frequently in adolescents and in men over 40 years of age.
- As a group, testicular germ cell cancers are comprised of seminomas and nonseminomatous cell types. Nonseminomatous germ cell tumors include teratoma, yolk sac, embryonal (endodermal sinus tumor), choriocarcinoma, or mixed combinations.
- The most common tumor is embryonal.

## ETIOLOGY

- Testis cancer is more likely to occur in men with a history of an undescended testicle.
- First-degree male relatives of men with testicular cancer have an overall greater incidence of cyptorchidism, inguinal hernias, hydroceles, and testicular cancer. These data suggest that some genetic predisposition and/or in utero environmental event(s) may result in several urothelial developmental abnormalities.
- A specific cytogenetic abnormality located on chromosome 12 is associated with testicular cancer and extragonadal tumors.
- The use of exogenous estrogens during pregnancy in the mothers of men with testicular cancer has been analyzed by several investigators.

## PREVENTION, SCREENING, EARLY DETECTION

- Up to 80% of males with testicular cancer will be oligospermic at the time of diagnosis.
- Men experiencing fertility problems should be evaluated for testicular cancer.
- Males are encouraged to perform monthly testicular self-examinations (TSE) by age 15.

## PATHOPHYSIOLOGY

- Testicular cancer has a remarkably high tumor cell doubling-time, which unlike other cancers, is a factor in the favorable response to treatment.
- Approximately 90% of men diagnosed with testicular cancer will be cured. Advanced disease at diagnosis is rare.
- Alpha-fetoprotein (AFP) and beta human chorionic gonadotropin (BHCG) are meaningful tumor markers for testicular cancer.

## CLINICAL MANIFESTATIONS

- The most common sign of testicular cancer is a small hard mass in the scrotum. However, a dragging sensation, swelling, dull aching, or pain in the scrotal area also may be presenting symptoms.
- Germ cell tumors are often mistaken for epididymitis as well as other benign causes of testicular symptoms. (Table 47-2, text page 1377).

- Frequently a complaint of low back pain is a presenting symptom indicating that the cancer has spread into the retroperitoneal lymph nodes.

## ASSESSMENT

### Physical Exam

- A physical exam should include an examination of the neck for supraclavicular adenopathy, lungs, breast for gynecomastia, the abdomen for retroperitioneal masses, and the testicles. Any testicular mass found on clinical exam should be transilluminated.

### Diagnostic Studies

- Ultrasound is obtained to identify scrotal masses.
- Inguinal orchiectomy remains the standard approach for definitive pathological diagnosis. A biopsy or a transcrotal approach orchiectomy can cause possible spread of tumor.
- Both a fine needle biopsy and a transcrotal approach are contraindicated.
- Chest x-rays and chest scans, together with serum tumor markers consisting of the beta subunit of human chorionic gonadotropin (BHCG) and alpha-fetoprotein (AFP), can be useful in the staging of testicular cancer, but also in documenting disease recurrence, as well as in monitoring response to treatment. (See Table 47-1, text page 1377.)

### Prognostic Indicators

- Most men with seminoma limited to the testis at the time of diagnosis receive radiotherapy.
- Overall 95% or more of men diagnosed with stage I and II nonseminomatous germ cell tumors will survive their disease.

## CLASSIFICATION AND STAGING

- The most common clinical staging systems used for seminoma and nonseminomatous germ cell tumors are from Royal Marsden Hospital (Table 47-3, text page 1378). Indiana University Hospital has developed an exclusive staging system used for only disseminated disease (Table 47-4, text page 1378).

## THERAPEUTIC APPROACHES AND NURSING CARE

### Nonseminomatous Germ Cell Tumors

#### Stage I

- A retroperitoneal lymph node dissection (RPLND) has been the time-honored approach to the treatment of testicular cancer confined to the testis. Recently, however, this approach for patients with early-stage nonseminomatous germ cell tumors has been challenged. Treatment options following orchiectomy include surgery with RPLND or a nonoperative approach.
- The rationale for surgery is well-grounded. RPLND in low-volume testis cancer is useful for staging.
- Surgery alone provides cure to approximately 90% of patients with pathological stage I testis cancer with less than 1% chance of local recurrence.
- RPLND is advantageous for two reasons, for staging and as a therapeutic modality.
- The major objection to RPLND has been the fertility consequences.
- Males who undergo full bilateral lymphadenectomy universally lose emission and the ability to ejaculate with resultant loss of fertility.
- Unilateral RPLND preserves the contralateral sympathetic efferent nerves and normal ejaculatory function in 75%–100% of males with testicular cancer.

- Selection for surveillance must be considered carefully for individuals with clinical stage I testicular cancer. Individuals must have normal serum BHCG and AFP following orchiectomy, plus normal x-rays and scans.
- Individuals selected for this approach must be highly motivated and able, logistically and psychologically, to comply with consistent lifelong follow-up.

## Pathological stage II A/B

- Individuals who are thought to have clinical stage I testis cancer, but are found at RPLND to have metastasis to the retroperitoneum are considered to have pathological stage II disease with either microscopic (II A) or gross (II B) involvement.

## Clinical stage II B

- Chemotherapy alone will provide 98% of individuals with a complete remission, with less than one-fourth requiring RPLND postchemotherapy for residual disease or because of persistent serum marker elevation.

## Disseminated disease

- A palpable abdominal mass with lymph nodes <5 cm or involvement of more than five lymph nodes is designated as stage II C disease. Abdominal disease of this magnitude will prohibit initial surgical resection.
- Approximately 70% of men with stage III disease will achieve a complete remission.
- Chemotherapy is the mainstay of treatment. Following orchiectomy, initial cisplatin-based chemotherapy is recommended for cytoreduction and potential cure. The most widely used frontline regimen is BEP (see Table 47-5, text page 1379), consisting of bleomycin, etoposide, and cisplatin.
- Research has shown that in men presenting with minimal to moderate disease, three cycles of BEP is the chemotherapy regimen of choice (Table 47-5, text page 1379).
- Intensification of therapy has included both high-dose cisplatin as well as administering all five active agents within the same regimen (i.e., VIP/VeB—etoposide, ifosfamide, cisplatin, vinblastine, bleomycin). Other intensification has included high-dose carboplatin and etoposide with either bone marrow transplantation or peripheral stem cell rescue.
- Thirty percent of men who present with disseminated disease will require surgery postchemotherapy. A postchemotherapy RPLND (PC RPLND) is indicated if a residual mass remains.
- Side effects of PC RPLND include pulmonary toxicity from the combination of bleomycin and anesthesia; temporary rise in serum creatinine and tachycardia from necessary fluid restrictions; noncardiogenic pulmonary edema; and ileus.

## Late relapse testis cancer

- Most relapses occur within two years following completion of therapy.
- Late relapse in testicular cancer is thought to be a recurrence after greater than a 24-month disease-free interval.
- The presence of teratoma in the original pathology may be a statistically significant predictor of late relapse.

## Seminomas Germ Cell Tumors

- Pure seminomas account for approximately 47% of all germ cell tumors of the testicles. With the use of effective chemotherapy and radiotherapy, the overall cure rate for all stages is above 90%.

- Both stage I and stage II A/B are treated with external-beam irradiation. Chemotherapy is the primary treatment of bulky stage II C and disseminated disease.

### Stage I and II A/B

- Although surveillance may be an option following orchiectomy for stage I seminoma, excellent results with minimal side effects and morbidity make radiation the treatment of choice.
- Long-term survival of more than 95% of men diagnosed with stage I disease is expected.

### Stage II C

- Treatment of bulky, localized retroperitoneal disease is controversial.
- A viable option may be to use chemotherapy for individuals with retroperitoneal disease >5 cm and radiation as a front-line, single modality treatment for those individuals with <5 cm retroperitoneal disease, retaining chemotherapy for the 30%–40% that will eventually relapse.

### Stage III and IV

- Stage IV, extranodal disease of the bone, lung, liver, or central nervous system, has a cure rate of 60%–80% with chemotherapy. Bleomycin, etoposide, and cisplatin for three to four cycles, in identical doses to those used in nonseminomatous germ cell tumors, are standard treatment (Table 47-5, text page 1379).

## Salvage Therapy in Recurrent Disease

- Testicular cancer is one of the few cancers where second-line chemotherapy offers a chance of cure.

### Salvage chemotherapy

- Occasionally individuals will be misdirected for salvage chemotherapy based on misleading radiographic evidence or rising serum markers (AFP, BHCG) that appear to demonstrate progressive disease.
- The combination of cisplatin, vinblastine (or etoposide, if not included in initial chemotherapy), and ifosfamide (VeIP) is the recommended front-line salvage regimen for recurrent disease when initial induction therapy was composed of cisplatin, etoposide (or vinblastine), and bleomycin.
- Phase I and II trials are in progress investigating agents for use in third-line chemotherapy.

### Surgical salvage

- Individuals with persistently elevated serum markers, indicative of persistent viable disease following salvage chemotherapy, may be candidates for surgery.
- Approximately 20% of carefully selected individuals achieve long-term survival with salvage surgery.

## High-Dose Chemotherapy with Rescue

- Individuals who recur following salvage chemotherapy or do not respond to first-line cisplatin therapy are incurable by standard chemotherapy. Autologous bone marrow and/or peripheral blood stem cell rescue in conjunction with high-dose chemotherapy have been and continue to be investigated in this population.

## Sanctuary Sites

- In advanced testis cancer the central nervous system (CNS) and contralateral testicle are the most common sanctuary sites.

- Chemotherapy poorly penetrates the blood-brain barrier. Whole-brain radiation therapy in combination with chemotherapy for systemic disease is recommended for individuals with CNS metastasis and disseminated disease.
- Those individuals relapsing with a single CNS focus without evidence of systemic relapse undergo resection followed by radiotherapy and two postoperative cisplatin-based chemotherapy regimens.
- It is questionable whether chemotherapy penetrates the testicle.
- Normally the testis primary tumor is surgically resected prior to treatment. However, in the presence of advanced disseminated disease and positive tumor markers, chemotherapy may be initiated prior to a tissue diagnosis. At the completion of chemotherapy the involved testis is removed.

## SYMPTOM MANAGEMENT AND SUPPORTIVE CARE

### Surgery

- An inguinal orchiectomy performed to establish a histological diagnosis is an outpatient procedure.
- Men need to understand that neither sexual function nor fertility will be impaired or changed.
- RPLND is associated with specific side effects, namely adult respiratory syndrome with pulmonary fluid overload, ileus, and fertility issues.

#### Pulmonary complications

- Men who have received bleomycin at a cumulative dose of greater than 200 mg/m$^2$ are at greater risk of pulmonary edema with subsequent respiratory failure.
- Rigid fluid restrictions imposed during surgery and a reduction in inspired oxygen to an FiO$_2$ of 0.24 has been shown to prevent mortality.
- As a result of fluid restrictions, transient elevations of the serum creatinine and sinus tachycardia may occur.

#### Gastrointestinal complications

- Ileus, a common side effect of abdominal surgery in general, may be prolonged for two to four days after an RPLND depending on the extent of the abdominal resection and length of time under anesthesia.

#### Fertility

- The traditional bilateral RPLND results in the loss of antegrade ejaculation with resultant infertility from retrograde ejaculation. The ability to experience a normal orgasm is not impaired.
- Sperm banking prior to initiation of treatment may be an option depending on the stage of disease and sperm count at diagnosis.

### Radiation

#### Gastrointestinal complications

- Unlike radiation to other parts of the body, nausea and vomiting are not unusual with the first radiotherapy treatment.

#### Fertility

- Radiotherapy does not effect libido or potency but can lead to impairment of spermatogenesis.

#### Myelosuppression

- Radiation to the para-aortic lymph nodes and the pelvis often produces myelosuppression.

## Chemotherapy

- The side effects of chemotherapy are specific to the drug combinations and the dosages administered.
- Nursing management can best be approached with awareness and anticipation of potential side effects (See Table 47-6, text page 1386, for nursing care and emotional needs of patients receiving chemotherapy for testicular cancer.)

## CONTINUITY OF CARE: NURSING CHALLENGES

- The shift from inpatient to primarily outpatient chemotherapy, the role of managed health care, continued shortening of inpatient hospitalization following surgery, and the increasingly important role of home care has affected how care is provided to the individual with testicular cancer.

## PRACTICE QUESTIONS

1. Based on what is currently known regarding the epidemiology of testicular germ cell cancer, which of the following patients would be considered at greater risk for developing testis cancer?
   a. 18-year-old Todd, who is very athletic
   b. Todd's great-grandfather
   c. 26-year-old Eric, who is an accountant
   d. Frank, who just had his 50th birthday

2. The most common presenting symptom of testicular cancer is:
   a. a small, hard mass in the scrotum.
   b. a dragging sensation.
   c. swelling.
   d. dull aching or pain in the scrotal area.

3. During the initial work-up Mr. Smith, who has testicular cancer, complains of low back pain that has been present for about 1 month. This may indicate:
   a. metastatic disease to the lumbar spine.
   b. the cancer has spread to the prostate.
   c. the cancer has spread into the retroperitoneal lymph nodes.
   d. a and c.

4. Which of the following procedures is considered the standard approach for definitive pathological diagnosis?
   a. biopsy
   b. fine needle biopsy
   c. transcrotal approach orchiectomy
   d. inguinal orchiectomy

5. Mr. Allen has an embryonal cell nonseminomatous testicular carcinoma confined to the testis. He is scheduled for surgery with a unilateral retroperitoneal lymph node dissection (RPLND). Your teaching would emphasize which of the following?
   a. This procedure is curative, but Mr. Allen will need to be monitored on a monthly basis for markers.
   b. Although the treatment is curative, the surgery will likely leave him without the ability to ejaculate.
   c. The surgery helps to stage his cancer and remove lymph nodes in the retroperitoneum.
   d. a and c.

6. Two weeks following orchiectomy and RPLND, Mr. Jones was found to have elevated serum BHCG and AFP. Why is this important?
   a. It means he will not be sterile.
   b. It means the lymph nodes were not removed completely.
   c. It means cancer remains in his body and chemotherapy is necessary.
   d. It does not mean anything because it takes a month for markers to be normal.

7. Richard has advanced disseminated disease and receives an orchiectomy. Which treatment will be the most likely choice for cytoreduction and potential cure?
   a. a platinum-based regimen to follow up the orchiectomy
   b. cisplatin, etoposide, and bleomycin
   c. radiation plus chemotherapy
   d. radiation alone

8. Mr. James has been told by his physician that he has a seminoma of the testis that is high grade—meaning it has a high tumor cell doubling time. Mr. James is confused about what this means in terms of his prognosis. Your explanation would include which of the following?
   a.  High-grade tumors generally carry a poor prognosis.
   b.  Tumors with a high tumor cell doubling time typically become resistant to chemotherapy.
   c.  A high tumor cell doubling time means the disease has likely metastasized.
   d.  A high tumor cell doubling time means he has a favorable prognosis.

9. Mario has a stage I seminoma. What follow-up treatment is most appropriate?
   a.  external-beam irradiation
   b.  surveillance
   c.  BEP
   d.  a and c

10. Ron has stage IV, extranodal testicular cancer involving the lung. Standard treatment will involve:
    a.  external-beam irradiation.
    b.  vinblastine, ifosfamide, and cisplatin.
    c.  oral etoposide.
    d.  bleomycin, etoposide, and cisplatin (BEP).

11. Alpha-fetoprotein (AFP) and human chorionic gonadotropin (BHCG) are measured primarily for which of the following reasons?
    a.  staging of testis cancer
    b.  documenting disease recurrence
    c.  monitoring response to treatment
    d.  all of the above

12. In cases of advanced testis cancer, the most common sanctuary sites include:
    a.  the lung and CNS.
    b.  the brain and lymphatic system.
    c.  the contralateral testicle and the CNS.
    d.  the lung, skin and bone.

13. Eliot has relapse in advanced disease and demonstrates CNS metastasis and disseminated disease. What is the recommended response?
    a.  whole-brain radiation therapy in combination with chemotherapy
    b.  chemotherapy alone
    c.  resection followed by radiotherapy
    d.  two postoperative cisplatin-based chemotherapy regimens

14. Your patient with disseminated testis cancer has just completed BEP treatment and is scheduled for surgery to remove a residual retroperitoneal mass. Which of the following would be appropriate to emphasize in your teaching of this patient?
    a.  Bleomycin-induced pulmonary toxicity is a potential side effect.
    b.  This treatment is designed to be curative.
    c.  This treatment is not curative but will significantly increase his survival.
    d.  a and b.

15. The traditional bilateral RPLND results in:
    a. the loss of antegrade ejaculation.
    b. infertility from retrograde ejaculation.
    c. impaired ability to experience a normal orgasm.
    d. a and b.

# ANSWER EXPLANATIONS

1. **The answer is c.** Testis cancer most commonly affects those in the 20- to 30-year-old age group. It occurs less frequently in adolescents and in men over 40 years of age. (p. 1375)

2. **The answer is a.** The most common sign of testicular cancer is a small, hard mass in the scrotum. However, a dragging sensation, swelling, dull aching, or pain in the scrotal area also may be presenting symptoms. (p. 1376)

3. **The answer is c.** Frequently a complaint of low back pain indicates that the cancer has spread into the retroperitoneal lymph nodes. (p. 1376)

4. **The answer is d.** Inguinal orchiectomy remains the standard approach for definitive pathological diagnosis. A biopsy or transcrotal approach orchiectomy can cause possible spread of tumor. Both a fine needle biopsy and a transcrotal approach are contraindicated. (p. 1377)

5. **The answer is d.** This procedure is curative, but he will need to be monitored on a monthly basis for markers. The surgery helps to stage his cancer and remove lymph nodes in the retroperitoneum. (p. 1379)

6. **The answer is c.** It means cancer remains in his body and chemotherapy is necessary. (p. 1379)

7. **The answer is b.** Chemotherapy is the mainstay of treatment in men with advanced or bulky disease. Following orchiectomy, initial cisplatin-based chemotherapy is recommended for cytoreduction and potential cure. The most widely used front-line regimen is BEP. (p. 1380)

8. **The answer is d.** A high tumor cell doubling time means he has a favorable prognosis. (p. 1376)

9. **The answer is a.** Both stage I and stage II A/B are treated with external-beam irradiation. Chemotherapy is the primary treatment of bulky stage II C and disseminated disease. (p. 1381)

10. **The answer is d.** Stage IV—extranodal disease of the bone, lung, liver, or CNS—has a cure rate of 60%–80% with chemotherapy. Bleomycin, etoposide, and cisplatin for three to four cycles are standard treatment. (p. 1382)

11. **The answer is d.** Chest x-rays and chest scans, together with serum tumor markers consisting of the beta subunit of human chorionic gonadotropin (BHCG) and alpha-fetoprotein (AFP), can be useful in the staging of testicular cancer, but also in documenting disease recurrence, as well as in monitoring response to treatment. (Table 47-1, p. 1377)

12. **The answer is c.** In advanced testis cancer, the CNS and contralateral testicle are the most common sanctuary sites. (p. 1383)

13. **The answer is a.** Chemotherapy poorly penetrates the blood-brain barrier. Whole-brain radiation therapy in combination with chemotherapy for systemic disease is recommended for individuals with CNS metastasis and disseminated disease. Those relapsing with a single CNS focus without systemic relapse undergo resection followed by radiotherapy and two postop cisplatin-based chemotherapy regimens. (p. 1383)

14. **The answer is d.** Men who received bleomycin at a cumulative dose of greater than 200 mg/m$^2$ are at greater risk of pulmonary edema with subsequent respiratory failure. Treatment is curative. (p. 1380)

15. **The answer is d.** The traditional bilateral RPLND results in the loss of antegrade ejaculation with resultant infertility from retrograde ejaculation. The ability to experience a normal orgasm is not impaired. (p. 1384)

# Chapter 48   Psychosocial Responses to Cancer

---

## INTRODUCTION
### The Need For Psychosocial Care

- Persons with cancer are confronted with a series of stressors: including diagnosis and treatment of their disease, long-term physiological alterations, fears of relapse and death, dependence on caregivers, survivor guilt, and negative effects on families.
- Cancer affects the entire family unit and forces them to adjust their routines and basic functions including eating, sleeping, working, and communicating with each other. No family emerges unchanged.
- Families who are able to share their feelings and the work of caregiving may have less difficulty coping with the changes than families who function in isolation from each other.

### A Model of the Stress and Coping Process

- The stress and coping model of Lazarus and Folkman provides the clinician with a useful framework for understanding the complex psychosocial problems of individuals and families when an individual has cancer.

#### The appraisal-coping process

- Central to the model is the appraisal-coping process.
- Appraisal is a person's evaluation of the problem.
- Coping refers to the cognitive and behavioral strategies used to manage the stressful situation.
- Coping serves two basic functions. Problem-focused coping efforts are directed at managing or altering the problem causing the stress, while emotion-focused coping strategies are directed at regulating emotional responses to the stressful situation.
- Problem-focused coping also includes strategies for reducing environmental pressures or barriers, information-seeking, and learning new skills or behaviors.
- Emotion-focused coping includes strategies with the direct intent of reducing the emotional distress caused by the stressful problem.
- The success of a coping strategy is determined by its outcome or intended outcome. The behavior of denial is "value neutral," meaning that it is not inherently adaptive or maladaptive. Its adaptiveness is determined by what it can or does achieve.

#### Adaptational outcomes

- An outcome is commonly defined as a relevant end result. The principal psychosocial outcomes of the appraisal and coping process are the maximization of (1) physical health, (2) functioning in work and social living, and (3) psychological well-being.
- To the extent that the appraisal-coping process fosters one or more of these outcomes, it is adaptive; when it does not, it is maladaptive.

#### Professional interventions

- Professional interventions may include preparatory information, teaching cognitive or behavioral skills, or providing supportive care.

## ASSESSMENT OF THE APPRAISAL-COPING PROCESS

- Professional nursing assessment is indicated at two junctures: (1) the initial contact (baseline assessment), and (2) when the nurse observes a breakdown in the effectiveness of the appraisal-coping process.
- The individual's perception of a problem is a major component of his or her appraisal.
- An important aspect of the individual's perception of the problem is his or her feelings about it.
- Another important aspect of appraisal is the individual's perception of the resources her or she has for dealing with the problem.

## FACTORS THAT INFLUENCE THE APPRAISAL-COPING PROCESS

### Person-related Factors

#### Cultural background

- Values, beliefs, and norms are culture-bound ideals that guide thinking, decision making, and actions and explain many differences in behavior.
- Communication may be a problem if there are discrepancies between the nurse and patient with regard to language or their conceptions of health and illness, space, time, social organization, use of family resources, religious affiliation, health-seeking and sick role behaviors.

#### Socioeconomic status

- Differences in culture may be compounded by differences in socioeconomic status.
- Minorities in the United States often have fewer financial and educational resources.
- Individuals with low annual incomes are three to seven times more likely to die of cancer than those with high annual incomes.

#### Age

- Age is a sociodemographic factor that is predictive of psychological adjustment to cancer.
  - Younger people report greater adjustment difficulties in comparison to their older counterparts.
  - Younger people often undergo more aggressive therapy with greater threats to their quality of life.

#### Psychological coping styles

- Beliefs are personally formed or culturally shared cognitive ideas about reality that determine what is fact and shape the individual's understanding of reality. Traits are relatively stable and enduring ways in which one individual differs from others and that exert generalized effects on behavior.
- Individual differences in stable coping styles serve as buffers in stressful situations.

### Illness-related Factors

- A history of previous psychiatric diagnosis and the presence of other comorbid conditions when cancer is diagnosed also seem to heighten the individual's risk for psychological problems.
- Individuals with comorbid chronic illnesses have poorer social and role functioning, poorer mental health, and perceptions of poorer health than individuals without comorbid conditions.
- Severity of disease has also been associated with poorer psychological adjustment.

## PSYCHOSOCIAL INTERVENTIONS

- Crisis intervention and brief therapy models of intervention both use similar approaches with regard to early assessment, present-day focus, limited goals, counseling direction, and prompt interventions.

## Education

- Education assists the individual with cancer to reduce his or her sense of helplessness and inadequacy.

## Counseling

- The individual who is depressed or has difficulty coping with the disease is best managed with consistent emotional support and counseling within the context of a trusting relationship.
- Counseling optimizes past strengths, supports past coping efforts, and mobilizes resources.

## Storytelling

- Storytelling can be an effective method of communicating with individuals for whom more direct methods of communication are ineffective.
- Metaphor is easily taken in and is less likely to trigger a defensive response.

## Relaxation

- Progressive muscle relaxation is helpful in dealing with nausea, anxiety related to stressful situations and physiological arousal. Relaxation techniques distract oneself and increase one's sense of control.

## PSYCHOSOCIAL OUTCOMES

## The Importance of Outcomes

- Articulation of intended outcomes helps the oncology nurse and the patient and family set the direction and course for their work together.
- The effectiveness of any medical intervention is evaluated with regard to its effect on "cure" and survival rates.
- Nurses need to be able to identify and quantify nursing's effect on patient outcomes in order to define their worth and position in patient care.

## What Outcomes Are Important

- Quality of life (QOL) is the appraisal of and level of satisfaction with one's current state of well-being.
- Four dimensions that are typically represented include physical, functional, psychological, and social well-being.

### Physical well-being

- The physical dimension of QOL refers to perceived bodily dysfunction or disruption.

### Functional well-being

- Functional status refers to the ability to perform activities related to one's personal care and role responsibilities.

### Psychological well-being

- This domain refers to emotional state, including both positive and negative moods.

### Social well-being

- Social well-being includes social support, family functioning, and intimacy.

# COMMON PROBLEMS OF THE INDIVIDUAL/FAMILY WITH CANCER

## Making Decisions About Treatment

- There are two issues the oncology nurse must consider: role preference in treatment decision making and desire for information.
- Three different role preferences have been identified among individuals with cancer: active role in making the final selection of treatment; passivity; collaboration with the physician in making decisions.

## Dealing with Uncertainty

- Uncertainty interferes with the formation of a realistic appraisal of stressful problem.
- Appraisal in a situation of uncertainty involves the processes of inference and illusion. When using inference, the individual bases his or her appraisal on general knowledge and past experience.
- Illusions—beliefs constructed in the absence of knowledge—can be valuable in protecting the individual when information is unavailable or when information is available but difficult to accept.
- The most common means of reducing uncertainty is to provide preparatory information about the specific aspects of the cancer experience faced by the individual.

## Managing the Side Effects of Treatment

- Preparatory information prevents or alleviates treatment-related symptoms.
- The ability to anticipate side effects assists the individual in planning daily activities.
- Stress reduction and distraction including relaxation, music, self-hypnosis, and massage have been effective for nausea and vomiting or pain. Physical remedies have also been used: exercise or oral ginger for nausea and vomiting; extremity wraps for shivering and oral care for mucositis.

## Responses of Families and Caregivers

- The overwhelming demands and complexity of care for the individual with cancer can result in caregiver burden.
- The oncology nurse plays a critical role in informing the patient and spouse of the diagnosis and in deepening the spouse's understanding of the situation from the patient's perspective.
- The nurse can help them adopt a terminology for describing disease phenomena and referring to aspects of the situation. This process of patient and spouse education may help the parties to initiate a dialogue between them.
- Research has identified other important supportive roles for the oncology nurse: twenty-four hour accessibility and availability of the hospice nurse was identified by family caregivers as critical in reducing their anxieties about caregiving.

## Changes in Sexual Functioning

- Sexual dysfunction in cancer patients may be related to a variety of biological, psychological, or social factors: diseases that affect the sexual organs, pelvis, or breasts; invasive or disfiguring surgery; hormonal changes including ovarian failure can result in loss of desire as well as problems with arousal; nausea and vomiting as well as hair loss affect body image and feelings of attractiveness; concurrent medical conditions and/or treatments such as diabetes and the use of antihypertensive drugs; negative moods, loss of personal control, cancer worries, relationship difficulties (such as poor communication or fear of rejection), and past psychiatric problems (including alcohol abuse).
- The nurse who conducts a nonthreatening and nonjudgmental sexual history at the beginning of cancer treatment can do a lot to prevent and reduce the anxiety and guilt that can surround sexual concerns and problems.

- Interventions for changes in sexual health generally combine education and counseling.

## Problems of Cancer Survivors

- Even after definitive cure, cancer survivors are less certain about living a long life and have greater anxiety and mood changes.
- Survivors often experience stress during reentry into the "well role."
- Employment-related problems include denial of insurance or other benefits, not getting job offers, conflict with supervisors or coworkers, and termination of employment.

## PROFESSIONAL RESPONSES TO CANCER

- Nurses may find themselves avoiding certain situations or responding to them irrationally. In turn, they hide feelings of embarrassment, shame, guilt, and anger focused at themselves for their weaknesses.
- Two concepts, distancing and caring, can be examined from the standpoint of being "value neutral" forms of coping. Either strategy employed to excess can have negative consequences.
  - Distancing can be helpful in allowing the patient and family to try out their own problem-solving skills in a controlled situation.
  - Distancing becomes "unsuccessful" when it occurs over a long period of time and results in increased loneliness and isolation in those for whom one is caring.
- Professionals also use caring as a response to cancer.
  - Caring is communicated by accepting the patient and respecting thoughts, feelings, and needs. It implies access.
  - A boundary is a psychological term referring to one's sphere of influence. Boundaries can be rigid, diffuse, or clear (Figure 48-4, text page 1407).
  - When psychological boundaries are clear, they touch another's but do not get mixed up with the other person's priorities or goals. This is when caring is therapeutic.
- Nurses need to understand themselves and the dynamics of their family of origin; seek balance between their personal and professional lives; seek the counsel of their managers, peers, families, friends, or a mental health professional; take the time to recognize limitations and vulnerabilities; and let go of the illusion of controlling the whole situation.

# PRACTICE QUESTIONS

1. A patient who has just been diagnosed with lung cancer is denying the diagnosis and refusing to hear about it. The patient's behavior of denial is:
   a. adaptive.
   b. maladaptive.
   c. value neutral.
   d. none of the above.

2. Individuals with low annual incomes:
   a. are three to seven times more likely to die of cancer than those with high annual incomes.
   b. rarely experience a definable difference in survivorship or treatment outcome based solely on their economic status
   c. are twice as likely to experience recurrence, treatment failure, or death as those with higher annual incomes.
   d. none of the above.

3. You have two patients with the same stage II lymphoma diagnosis. One is 26; the other is 58. Younger patients report:
   a. less confusion about prognosis and treatment options than their older counterparts.
   b. fewer adjustment difficulties in comparison to their older counterparts.
   c. greater adjustment difficulties in comparison to their older counterparts.
   d. a and b.

4. One dimension that is not as frequently represented in QOL is _____ well-being.
   a. psychological
   b. functional
   c. spiritual
   d. social

5. The QOL dimension of social well-being includes:
   a. family functioning and intimacy.
   b. religious practices.
   c. positive and negative moods.
   d. all of the above.

6. The most common means of reducing uncertainty for the patient is:
   a. providing prepatory information and education.
   b. referring him or her to a professional therapist.
   c. protecting the individual from all negative information.
   d. a and c.

7. Nausea and vomiting have been effectively treated with:
   a. massage
   b. exercise.
   c. oral ginger.
   d. all of the above.

8. Two basic approaches to nursing intervention for alterations in sexual health of cancer patients are:
    a. education and counseling.
    b. screening and role playing.
    c. affective therapy and role modeling.
    d. enhancing reality surveillance and reinforcing personal power.

9. Which of the following statements about employment among cancer survivors is correct?
    a. Approximately 40% of cancer patients return to work after being diagnosed.
    b. The work performance of cancer survivors differs little from others hired at the same age for similar assignments.
    c. "Job-lock" refers to the situation in which cancer survivors are reluctant to accept new jobs that might involve increased responsibilities.
    d. Most federal and state laws specifically include cancer survivors among the "handicapped or disabled."

10. In a recent article, a colleague, Richard, writes about the emotional aspects of dealing with a very unique patient he worked with last year. In describing the kinds of psychological boundaries he established with this patient, you notice that he has drawn a diagram in which his and the client's boundaries are touching. You realize that his boundaries with this patient were:
    a. rigid; the patient's boundary was not allowed to intersect, or overlap, with Richard's.
    b. clear; he was accessible, but did not get mixed up with the patient's personal priorities or goals.
    c. diffuse; Richard became enmeshed with the patient and overinvolved.
    d. diffuse; his boundaries made a limited intersection with those of the patient, yet Richard managed to keep a "professional" distance.

## ANSWER EXPLANATIONS

1. **The answer is c.** The success of a coping strategy is determined by its outcome or intended outcome. The behavior of denial is "value neutral," meaning that it is not inherently adaptive or maladaptive. Its adaptiveness is determined by what it can or does achieve. Also, since this patient has "just been diagnosed," we may assume that not enough time has passed for us to determine if the denial is adaptive or maladaptive. (p. 1395)

2. **The answer is a.** Individuals with low annual incomes are three to seven times more likely to die of cancer than those with high annual incomes. (p. 1396)

3. **The answer is c.** Age is a sociodemographic factor that is predictive of psychological adjustment to cancer. Younger people report greater adjustment difficulties in comparison to their older counterparts. (p. 1397)

4. **The answer is c.** Four dimensions that are typically represented in QOL include physical, functional, psychological, and social well-being. (p. 1400)

5. **The answer is a.** The QOL dimension of social well-being includes social support, family functioning, and intimacy. Psychological well-being refers to emotional state, including both positive and negative moods. (p. 1400)

6. **The answer is a.** Education assists the patient in reducing his or her sense of helplessness and inadequacy. The most common means of reducing uncertainty is to provide preparatory information about the specific aspects of the cancer experience faced by the individual. Preparatory information also prevents or alleviates treatment-related symptoms. (p. 1402)

7.  **The answer is d.** Nausea and vomiting have been effectively treated with stress reduction and distraction methods, exercise, and oral ginger. (p. 1403)

8.  **The answer is a.** Recent studies have indicated the effectiveness of education and counseling as approaches to treatment of changes in sexual health. One problem with respect to such interventions is that effectiveness is often measured in terms of resumption of sexual intercourse rather than effect of the intervention on self-concept or on relationships with others. Another problem is that patients are generally not screened for participation. Screening would increase the probability of identifying those patients and partners with preexisting problems that may require more intensive therapy. (p. 1405)

9.  **The answer is b.** Up to 80% of cancer patients return to work after being diagnosed, and their performance differs little, if any, from others hired for similar assignments. "Job-lock" refers to survivors' fear of losing medical coverage were they to change jobs. Only a few states explicitly protect those with a history of cancer. (p. 1406)

10. **The answer is b.** When psychological boundaries are clear, they touch another's but do not get mixed up with the other person's priorities or goals. This is when caring is therapeutic. (p. 1407)

# Chapter 49    Physical, Economic, and Social Adaptation of the Cancer Survivor

## INTRODUCTION

- Cancer rehabilitation concerns any aspect of the individual's quality of life that is affected by the disease or its treatment.
- Four main considerations affect the adult cancer survivor's ability to achieve optimal physical, social, and psychological function: developmental considerations, disease trajectory considerations, physical function and cosmesis, and socioeconomic considerations.

## DEVELOPMENTAL CONSIDERATIONS FOR ADULT CANCER SURVIVORS

### Young Adulthood

#### Employment

- The shift of cancer treatment from inpatient to ambulatory and home care settings has enabled many patients undergoing active treatment for some tumors to continue working successfully.
- The Americans with Disabilities Act (ADA) prohibits discrimination against individuals with serious illnesses.

#### Insurance coverage

- Federal legislation passed in 1996 has mandated that, as of July 1997, insurance companies can no longer deny coverage for or impose restrictive waiting periods on individuals with preexisting illnesses such as cancer.

#### Parenting

- Cancer in a parent of young children may be more disruptive to the family than cancer in a young child.

#### Fertility

- Reproductive organs are the fourth most common cancer site, and treatment of nonreproductive cancers can result in infertility and premature menopause.

#### Sexuality

- Sexuality is an important issue for cancer rehabilitation at any age.
- The nurse should never assume that someone else has discussed these issues with the patient.
- Sperm should be banked and stored before treatment or early in treatment.

### Middle Adulthood

- In middle age (45–64 years) cancer incidence rates begin to rise, and the more common cancers such as lung, breast, ovarian, and colorectal cancers begin to occur in larger numbers.
- Important considerations for middle-aged adults are career advancement; job security; financial security; sexuality/body image and physical appearance; interpersonal relationships; sick role behaviors;

being a member of the "sandwich generation" with caregiving responsibilities for aging parents as well as children; and the well-being of children.

- Concerns about job security may negatively affect a middle-aged adult's ability to optimize treatment.

## Older Adulthood

- Hard-won financial security may be threatened by cancer. Health insurance is less of a problem once Medicare coverage begins at age 65.
- Cancer rehabilitation efforts may be hampered by the presence of other chronic conditions and age-related physiologic changes.
- Social networks provide three types of support: emotional, instrumental, and informational.
  - The social networks of elderly persons are frequently compromised as a result of death, disease, or disability, and may not be able to provide the amount or type of support an elderly cancer patient needs.
- In the elderly, fragmentation of care is common because older individuals frequently see several different health providers for different problems.
- Caregiving often demands changes in established roles and interpersonal relationships within a family, resulting in severe emotional strain for all involved.
- Important but often neglected aspects of caring for the elderly concern sexuality and body image.

## DISEASE TRAJECTORY CONSIDERATIONS

- Wells conceptualized cancer rehabilitation as having three levels, depending on the presence or absence of disfigurement or disability and life expectancy. Table 49-1, text page 1417, summarizes the three levels and rehabilitation goals and considerations for each level.
- Advanced stage at diagnosis is the most powerful predictor of cancer survival.

## SOCIOECONOMIC CONSIDERATIONS

- Cancer imposes inordinate financial demands, regardless of socioeconomic status. For the very poor, government assistance programs such as Supplemental Security Disability Insurance or Medicaid are available but difficult to access. For the elderly, Medicare and Medicare supplemental insurances are not designed to deal with long-term care or chronic disease needs. There is little help available for the "working poor," who often have no insurance benefits or job security.
- For middle- and upper-class families with adequate health insurance and relatively secure jobs, out-of-pocket expenditures for deductibles, copayments, and gaps in insurance coverage can still drive a family into poverty.

# PRACTICE QUESTIONS

1. Your new position in a cancer clinic gives you the opportunity to counsel cancer survivors. You are aware that the adult cancer survivor's ability to achieve optimal physical, social, and psychological function can be most significantly affected by:
   a. socioeconomic considerations.
   b. disease trajectory considerations.
   c. physical function and cosmesis.
   d. all of the above.

2. Mrs. Henderson is thirty years old, married, with no children. She is concerned about how her cancer will affect her fertility. Which of the following are true regarding cancer and infertility?
   a. Reproductive organs are the second most common cancer site.
   b. Premature menopause resulting from a nonreproductive cancer has been proved to be nothing more than a popular myth.
   c. Treatment of certain nonreproductive cancers can result in infertility.
   d. All of the above.

3. _____ at diagnosis is the most powerful predictor of cancer survival.
   a. Advanced disease
   b. Changes in appearance or body function
   c. Comorbid physical or mental conditions
   d. a and b

4. Middle- and upper-class families with adequate health insurance and relatively secure jobs:
   a. can still be excessively burdened by out-of-pocket expenditures for deductibles and copayments.
   b. now can expect no gaps in insurance coverage.
   c. represent the only segment of the population with no serious concerns about health expenses.
   d. b and c.

# ANSWER EXPLANATIONS

1. **The answer is d.** Four main considerations affect the adult cancer survivor's ability to achieve optimal physical, social, and psychological function: developmental considerations, disease trajectory considerations, physical function and cosmesis, and socioeconomic considerations. (p. 1413)

2. **The answer is c.** Reproductive organs are the fourth most common cancer site, and treatment of nonreproductive cancers can result in infertility and premature menopause. (p. 1414)

3. **The answer is a.** Advanced disease at diagnosis is the most powerful predictor of cancer survival. (p. 1417)

4. **The answer is d.** For middle- and upper-class families with adequate health insurance and relatively secure jobs, out-of-pocket expenditures for deductibles, copayments, and gaps in insurance coverage can conceivably drive a family into poverty. (p. 1418)

# Chapter 50    Spiritual and Ethical End-of-Life Concerns

## INTRODUCTION
### Definitions

- *Spirituality* refers to that dimension of being human that motivates meaning-making and self-transcendence—or intra-, inter-, and transpersonal connectedness.
- Spirituality prompts individuals to make sense of their universe and to relate harmoniously with self, nature, and others—including any god/s (as conceptualized by each person).
- Religion is the representation and expression of spirituality.
- *Ethics* involves reflecting systematically about right conduct and how to live as a good person.

### Spirituality and the Cancer Experience

- Individuals surviving cancer characteristically become more aware of their spirituality. This increased awareness may be experienced as painful and negative, and/or positive and pleasant.

### The Relationship between Spirituality and Imminence of Death

- There is evidence of a direct relationship between spirituality and imminence of death; that is, the closer to death an individual with cancer gets, the more she or he will become aware of and concerned with personal spirituality.
- Significant losses and changes can cause individuals to search for meaning, as a way of trying to make sense of such a negative experience.
- Table 50-1, text page 1423, lists possible contributors to increased spiritual awareness for cancer patients facing imminent death.
- The experiences of suffering and dying also frequently contribute to isolation and loneliness.
- No one can share the personal experience of irreversible death with a dying individual. Furthermore, the fear and denial of death prevalent in our society causes people to distance or remove themselves from those who are dying.

## FUNDAMENTAL "END-OF-LIFE" QUESTIONS
### How Shall I Die?

- *Suicide* is the intentional taking of one's own life. *Euthanasia* refers to the act of assisting or enabling a sufferer's death, preferably without pain. Because suffering is thereby relieved by death, euthanasia is often called "mercy killing"; euthanasia is sometimes referred to as assisted suicide or assisted death.
- Active euthanasia refers to direct intervention causing death, whereas passive euthanasia refers to letting a sufferer die by withholding or withdrawing life-sustaining care.

### Nurses' perspectives on end-of-life issues

- In 1996, a resolution recognizing factors that interfere with provision of humane end-of-life care and affirming oncology nurses' commitment to quality end-of-life care was proposed to the ONS membership.

### Illness-related factors influencing end-of-life decisions

- Compared with the general population, cancer survivors have been found to have a higher suicide rate. Numerous factors contribute to a cancer survivor's desire to end life with suicide or euthanasia: these factors include medical, social, psychological, and spiritual concerns.
- Pain and other symptom distress are the most frequently addressed factors contributing to cancer-related suicide or euthanasia.

### Ethical considerations

- The spiritual urge to be and do right is reflected in the debate about what the ethical response is to end-of-life decisions.

## How Shall I Live Before I Die?

- Two primary end-of-life challenges that cancer patients often deal with are spiritual and ethical in nature: (1) how to ascribe meaning to their life, illness, and death; and (2) how to relate to themselves and others (which might include a deity or other spiritual beings).

### Meaning making

- Perhaps the most frequent approach to meaning making is attempting to attribute a cause to the cancer.
- Another aspect of meaning making is construing benefit or ascribing a positive significance to the negative experience of cancer.
- Table 50-2, text page 1427, identifies 12 attitudes toward personal suffering by which individuals explain theodical issues.

### Relating

- Dependent cancer patients often perceive that they are "being a burden."
- Activities that can allow a person to return the gifts of love to others include: praying for others, listening to others, sharing personal wisdom gained from the cancer experience with others, creating legacy gifts such as poems, prose, taped oral histories, or crafts as functional ability permits.
- While individuals' relationships with others may change as a result of the cancer experience, so also may their relationship with their deity or spiritual beings.
- Relational experience with a deity may range from intensity and closeness to apathy and distance.

## APPROACHES TO MAKING SPIRITUAL AND ETHICAL END-OF-LIFE DECISIONS

- When caring for a person confronted with any end-of-life decision, the goal of nursing care is to facilitate and promote informed decision making by: (1) encouraging activities that increase the individual's sense of meaningfulness, self-awareness, and spiritual sensitivity; (2) offering a caring relationship and openness to dialogue; and (3) providing information about decision making and the issues confronted.
- Various religious beliefs regarding death are summarized in Table 50-3, text page 1428.

## Dedication to a Mission or Cause

- One way to create a sense of meaningfulness and purpose is to dedicate oneself to a cause or mission. This mission may be sociopolitical, artistic, or scientific in nature.

## Leaving a Legacy

- Those who question how to confront mortality may find comfort and meaning in activities that leave a legacy.

## Storytelling

- Encouraging people to tell their stories allows them to organize their thoughts and experiences, to reflect on their past, and to make sense of their life. Storytelling also allows them to share and connect with the listener, promoting intimacy. Finally, storytelling allows the individual to transmit values and leave a legacy.

## Prayer, Meditation, and Journal Writing

- Regardless of one's beliefs about religion, prayer (liberally defined) can be a resource to all; conversational and meditative types are usually more directly correlated with spiritual well-being than petitionary and ritualistic approaches.
- In addition to the content of prayer reflecting end-of-life issues, individuals' prayers may change form.

## Spiritual Mentoring

- A spiritual mentor can assist with spiritual issues and provide comfort, encouragement, and companionship, as well as guidance and prodding.

## Cognitive Strategies

- When individuals' assumptions about the world are shattered, they will work to reconstruct their world view so that it includes assumptions that are maturer and wiser, encompassing the trauma.
- This work of reconstructing a world view involves a process of balancing thinking about the painful subject with avoiding painful thoughts (approach versus avoidance).
- Using therapeutic techniques such as clarification and summarization, the nurse can assist a person in identifying and appreciating cognitive strategies that provide comfort and meaning.

## Confronting the Reality of Death

- Recognizing the function and multifaceted nature of denial will assist the nurse in addressing death at an appropriate level.
- Table 50-4, text page 1431, offers Bresnitz's typology of denial with examples from the context of cancer-related death.

## Advance Directives

- Most state statutes support two types of advance directives (ADs). An AD "is a statement made by a competent person that directs their medical care in the event that they become incompetent." A Directive to Physician, or Living Will, allows individuals to state their wishes regarding medical treatment in the event they become unable to do so. A Durable Power of Attorney for Health Care allows an individual to designate an agent who will make health care decisions on his or her behalf in the event he or she becomes incompetent.
- ADs provide the following: clarification of individual's wishes and values, guidance for family members concerning patients' choices, direction for the health care team, and protection of patients' assets from depletion caused by futile, high-cost care.
- Patients can confuse what a Living Will means; it does not specify disbursement of assets.
- ADs do not address all possible medical situations.

- The words "artificial" and "extraordinary" are often used in an AD; however, these words can be interpreted differently.
- A directive may not always be honored and implemented; technicalities can arise such as questions about the patient's competency when the AD was signed or the inability of medicine to determine the terminality of the patient's condition
- An AD is a one-person statement, not a legally binding contract.

## PRACTICE QUESTIONS

1. Spirituality refers to that dimension of being human that:
   a. represents and expresses one's life principle.
   b. prompts individuals to make sense of their universe and to relate harmoniously with self, nature, and others.
   c. involves reflecting systematically about right conduct and how to live as a good person.
   d. all of the above.

2. Active euthanasia refers to:
   a. the intentional taking of one's own life.
   b. direct intervention causing death.
   c. letting a sufferer die by withdrawing life-sustaining care.
   d. all of the above.

3. The most frequently addressed factors contributing to cancer-related suicide or euthanasia are:
   a. pain and other symptom distress.
   b. advanced illness and poor prognosis.
   c. family history of suicide or personal suicide history.
   d. hopelessness and loss of self-esteem or control.

4. Regardless of one's beliefs about religion, some individualized form of _____ prayer is known to be directly correlated with spiritual well-being.
   a. petitionary
   b. ritualistic
   c. conversational
   d. none of the above

5. The work of reconstructing a world view to include new, wiser assumptions in response to trauma involves a process of balancing:
   a. clarification and summarization.
   b. approach versus avoidance.
   c. identifying and appreciating cognitive strategies.
   d. none of the above.

6. The primary goal of the Patient Self-Determination Act is to:
   a. facilitate a systematic process of eliciting and honoring patient wishes.
   b. control health care costs in the last 6 months of life.
   c. require health care institutions to notify patients on admission of their rights under the law to execute an advance directive.
   d. facilitate a responsible use of technological intervention.

7. A patient of yours makes some comments about a Living Will that lead you to conclude that the patient needs more information. You will know that he understands what a Living Will is when he says it:
   a. specifies disbursement of assets.
   b. addresses all possible medical situations.
   c. may not always be honored and implemented.
   d. all of the above.

8. Which of the following statements about Living Wills and Advance Directives is true?
   a. A Durable Power of Attorney gives advance directives for the final period of terminal illness.
   b. The underlying principle of any advance directive is the prevention of suffering and the opportunity to state one's wishes regarding medical treatment while still competent.
   c. A Living Will identifies a specific person who can express the wishes of the individual should she or he become incompetent or ill.
   d. In some states, the Living Will is also called a Durable Power of Attorney.

9. A mentally competent 71-year-old patient receiving chemotherapy treatment for her newly diagnosed breast cancer expresses her worry that she will receive treatments at the end of her life that prolong her suffering. She is not married and has no children. Although she has nieces and nephews, they live across the country and are not involved in her care. She considers the woman with whom she has shared a house for the past 25 years her closest "relative." In providing counseling to her regarding her concern, you would:
   a. discuss the meaning of a DNR order and the Patient Self-Determination Act.
   b. encourage her to consider a Living Will.
   c. explore her wishes and preferences about end-of-life decisions, and provide information about a Durable Power of Attorney.
   d. contact her physician so that he or she can discuss DNR with the patient.

## ANSWER EXPLANATIONS

1. **The answer is b.** Spirituality refers to that dimension of being human that motivates meaning-making and self-transcendence—or intra-, inter-, and transpersonal connectedness. Spirituality prompts individuals to make sense of their universe and to relate harmoniously with self, nature, and others—including any god/s (as conceptualized by each person). Religion is the representation and expression of spirituality. Ethics involves reflecting systematically about right conduct and how to live as a good person. (p. 1422)

2. **The answer is b.** Suicide is the intentional taking of one's own life. Euthanasia refers to the act of assisting or enabling a sufferer's death, preferably without pain. Active euthanasia refers to direct intervention causing death, whereas passive euthanasia refers to letting a sufferer die by withholding or withdrawing life-sustaining care. (pp. 1424–1425)

3. **The answer is a.** The most frequently addressed factors contributing to cancer-related suicide or euthanasia are pain and other symptom distress. (p. 1425)

4. **The answer is c.** Regardless of one's beliefs about religion, prayer (liberally defined) can be a resource to all; conversational and meditative types are usually more directly correlated with spiritual well-being than petitionary and ritualistic approaches to prayer. (p. 1429)

5. **The answer is b.** The work of reconstructing a world view to include new, wiser assumptions in response to trauma involves a process of balancing thinking about the painful subject with avoiding painful thoughts (approach versus avoidance). Using therapeutic techniques such as clarification and summarization, the nurse can assist a person in identifying and appreciating cognitive strategies that provide comfort and meaning (p. 1430)

6. **The answer is c.** The Patient Self-Determination Act may also serve to control health care costs in the last 6 months of life and to facilitate a responsible use of technological intervention. However, these are not the primary goals of the act. The act does not necessarily facilitate a systematic process of eliciting and honoring patient wishes. (p. 1430)

7. **The answer is c.** Patients can confuse what a Living Will means: it does not specify disbursement of assets. ADs do not address all possible medical situations. The words "artificial" and "extraordinary" are often used in an AD; however, these words can be interpreted differently. A directive may not always be honored and implemented; an AD is a one-person statement, not a legally binding contract. (p. 1431)

8. **The answer is b.** The principle underlying any advance directive is the prevention of suffering and the opportunity to state one's wishes regarding medical treatment before (and in the event that) the patient becomes incompetent. A Durable Power of Attorney, not a Living Will, gives another person authority to make health care decisions for an individual who becomes incompetent to do so. A Living Will is a much more limited document than the Durable Power of Attorney. The Living Will gives advance directives for the final period of terminal illness, interpreted to mean the last few weeks of a person's life. The Living Will and the Durable Power of Attorney are not the same. (p. 1431)

9. **The answer is c.** Although part of the counseling process to address this patient's concerns might include discussing DNR, such a discussion may not be comprehensive enough to address the patient's presenting concerns since DNR is concerned essentially with the withholding of cardiopulmonary resuscitation. Discussion of the Patient Self-Determination Act is only a launching point for an exploration of the patient's wishes and preferences regarding end-of-life decisions and for discussion of the concept of a Durable Power of Attorney, which names an individual who will speak for the patient when the patient is incompetent to make decisions about health care. A Living Will tends to be a more limited document covering only the terminal phase of an illness. Discussion with the physician about DNR orders may or not be appropriate, depending on the nurse's discussion with the patient about her wishes. (p. 1431)

# Chapter 51    Cancer Programs and Services

## INTRODUCTION

- Fully integrated, full-service cancer care programs span the continuum of cancer care: prevention, detection, genetic counseling, diagnosis, multidisciplinary treatment, supportive care, lifetime follow-up, research, rehabilitation, and hospice services.
- These programs also are uniting the various caregivers and settings to offer combined pricing and services to health care consumers and payers.

## FORCES AFFECTING CANCER CARE DELIVERY

### Forces in Health Care

- The shifts in health care are a direct result of economic pressures from payers.
- Table 51-1, text page 1438, identifies shifts in health care delivery.
- The overall cost of cancer care in the nation reached $104 billion in 1990. Cancer potentially could represent 15%–20% of the country's health care expenditures in the future.
- Factors influencing accelerated growth of managed care include the following: the presence of a national employer, state initiatives to capitate Medicaid recipients, provider overcapacity, presence of PHO structures, a strong presence by Blue Cross-Blue Shield, emerging HMO companies, and the areas' demographics.

### Demographic Factors

- Three unprecedented demographic variables will affect U.S. health care services: the senior boom; the birth dearth; and the aging baby boomers.

### Mission, Market, and Margin

- There are clear mission, margin, and marketing reasons for developing and expanding cancer care services.
- Three motivators for developing outpatient cancer centers are (1) economic incentives toward more profitable outpatient care, (2) establishment of a market niche, and (3) meeting patient demand for cancer care that is convenient and accessible.
- Currently, cancer accounts for the largest population of patients and the highest rate of reimbursement on a per-case basis from Medicare.
- The hospitals that are the most profitable offer radiation therapy.
- Cancer care services, like cardiac services, often exhibit a "halo effect."
  - The halo effect manifests the public's assumption that an institution with an outstanding reputation for cancer care must deliver excellent care for other (perhaps less-feared) diseases and conditions.

### Networks, Mergers, Affiliations

- Consolidation of providers is taking place in three major forms: (1) hospitals are forming networks and other collaborations; (2) hospitals and physicians are integrating; and (3) small medical practices are consolidating into larger groups.

- Much of the integrating of hospitals and physicians is driven by managed care entities that dictate close collaborations between providers; for example, physician-hospital organizations (PHOs), management service organizations (MSOs), foundation models, or integrated health organizations (IHOs).
- Table 51-3, text page 1441, shows ten characteristics critical to successful integration.
- There are two critical elements that will hold together physician-hospital alliances and make them profitable: (1) the operating system to which the parties agree, and (2) the financial incentives.
- The current models for oncology practice alignment include the multispecialty network (including primary care physicians and specialists), larger-group, single-specialty practice (either medical or radiation oncologists), and oncology specialty practice groups (including all relevant oncological specialties).

## CANCER PROGRAM DEVELOPMENT

### Defining Cancer Programs

- The NCI classifies cancer centers as comprehensive, clinical, basic science, or consortium programs.
- The Cooperative Group Outreach Program (CGOP) led to the initiation of the Community Clinical Oncology Program (CCOP) in 1983 to provide support for physicians to enter community-based patients into clinical research protocols.

### Strategic Planning

- A strategic plan spans three to five years and sets out the major initiatives that will require the bulk of human and financial resources over the specified time frame.
- The planning process involves three phases: (1) clarify values and aspirations, (2) analyze information, and (3) develop a strategy to create the image. The central focus of a strategic plan relies upon shared values.
- An organization undertaking a strategic planning process begins by evaluating and, perhaps, revising its mission.
- The next stage of strategic planning is to identify the service lines that will be the cornerstones of future development.
- Identifying who will be involved in the planning process and who will serve as interim and final decision makers is imperative.
- One well-utilized framework for data gathering is the SWOT analysis to identify Strengths, Weaknesses, Opportunities, and Threats.
- A careful evaluation must be conducted with the financial department regarding present workload, payer mix, cost, charges, and revenue for all areas and sites where oncology care is delivered.
- An assessment is made of the present cancer market in the service area, demographics, the number of patients, where they are treated, and by whom.
- Projections for future workload and revenue are imperative and include the following: anticipated changes in practice patterns, potential mergers or networking, reimbursement policies of third-part payers, technology, personnel policies, shifts to managed care and capitation, and changes in physicians practicing at the facility.
- The strategic plan defines the long-range target and the sequence of development.
- To realize the strategic goals, specific programs may be developed. These specific plans are referred to as *business plans*.

### The Business Plan

- After a list of potential business plans has been developed from the strategic plan's goals, it is wise to establish a small working group to design very specific business plans.

- Business plans generally have a time frame of one year or less and are specific in terms of financial projection, milestones for development, and evaluation criteria.
- A sample business plan outline is shown in Table 51-4, text page 1445.

## Improving Quality, Outcomes, and Cost Effectiveness

- The emerging business of health care systems is to conserve clinical resources and engineer value into the provision of care.
- Value may not be equal to, but is at least proportional to, quality divided by cost. (Value = Quality ÷ Cost). As we increase the quality while maintaining costs, we increase the value; as we reduce costs to provide services, we increase the value as long as the quality remains unchanged.
- Integrated cancer programs have an excellent opportunity to take the lead in establishing quality outcomes and cost-effectiveness for cancer care.

### Quality and outcome measurements

- Outcomes and quality have become important to patients, payers, and providers.
- Specific items that a cancer program may consider reporting to interested parties are included as Table 51-5, text page 1445.
- The care of a person with cancer offers special challenges to practitioners to ensure that care over the illness trajectory is not just a series of discrete events, thus patients expect and should receive highly coordinated continuity of services and convenient access to services.

### Clinical care paths

- The key to ensuring continuity of care is coordinated communication.
- One excellent tool is the clinical care path, critical path, or care Multidisciplinary Action Plan (MAP).
- The benefits to developing paths are many: clearly stated goals to which both patient and provider agree, coordinated sequencing of treatment and services, outcome or variance analysis, and a scientifically-based practice.

### Case management

- The case manager spans the continuum of care by coordinating services and information between hospital, outpatient diagnostic and treatment settings, home care, hospice, and social support groups and organizations.
- Case management systems include: patient self-care teaching, a documented plan shared by patients and caregivers, and a backup communication system when the patient is in physical or psychosocial stress.

## Organization and Structure
### Standards for programs

- The Joint Commission on Accreditation of Healthcare Organizations (JCAHO) provides general delivery of care standards and scoring guidelines that can apply to oncology care.
- Several clinical indicators relate directly to oncology patients. These measure the use of multi-modality therapy for female patients with stage II pathological lymph node-positive breast cancer, and track specific clinical events to assess surgical care for lung cancer.
- The ACCC standards deal with inpatient, outpatient, hospice, and home care. They also relate to a wide variety of services in those settings.

- The American College of Surgeons' (ACoS) Commission on Cancer is currently the only agency in the United States that accredits or approves cancer programs.
- Another organization currently involved in external review and accreditation is the National Committee for Quality Assurance (NCQA).
- NCQA's goals are to improve quality of care and to provide quality information to purchasers of managed care systems.
- The Oncology Nursing Society (ONS) publishes many useful resources to assist managers in planning and monitoring individual programs.

## Structure for oncology program development

- In the integrated health system, hospitals are cost centers; inpatient units are small; and the majority of cancer patients are not only ambulatory but are served in a variety of outpatient settings as part of an organized network.
- Organizing the cancer program as a business with an adequate infrastructure will be vital and includes the following: a program director, a medical director, a program board, case management, quality and outcomes management, uniform records and financial systems, strategic and financial objectives, coordinated planning and strategy development.

### Product line management model

- In product line management (PLM), a single administrator is responsible for strategy formulation; coordination of resources; monitoring of production; and marketing, budgeting, and measuring results for the product line.
- Figures 51-2, 51-3, and 51-4, text pages 1448–1450, illustrate three different PLM structures for oncology programs.
- In the absence of a product line manager, and often as an initial organizing step, a clinical manager or nurse manager will take the role of cancer program coordinator. This role differs from the product/service line manager primarily in the diminished scope of service components.

### Program leadership

- Cancer programs that achieve their goals do so because leaders provide the vision, strategy, motivation, and organization to support the multidisciplinary cancer care team members, as they achieve their objectives.
- Ideally, program leadership is shared by a physician director and an administrative director.
  - The administrative director is charged with coordination and direction and serves as the leader and facilitator of a group of professionals typically representing departments or delivery sites.
  - The medical director is responsible for ensuring treatment of patients, coordinating clinical care among distinct oncology specialties, and helping to align physician and hospital incentives.
  - See Table 51-7, text page 1450, for a list of administrative director responsibilities.
  - See Table 51-8, text page 1451, for a list of medical director responsibilities.

## Financial Analysis

- A primary goal of business is to sustain positive revenues and control costs while providing a high-quality product or service.
- The cancer program's strategic plan sets overall goals for volume and income growth.
- To assess cost containment, actual costs must be available for all inpatient and outpatient services.

- Table 51-9, text page 1451, details a list of parameters to be collected and reviewed periodically.
- Inpatient data are usually more easily attainable than outpatient data. Both are needed.
- The most effective method for maximizing revenues is negotiating favorable contracts with payers.
- The most successful strategy for controlling costs is appropriate use of resources.
- Irregularities in the Medicare payment systems presently reward some programs with cost-based reimbursement.

## COMPONENTS OF A CANCER PROGRAM

- Table 51-10, text page 1456, lists some of the hundreds of components program designers may consider.
- A vast array of strategic initiatives should be considered when choosing the components for a specific program.
- A cancer program's strategic plan should clearly dictate components.

### Support Services

- Table 51-11, text page 1457, is a list of potential supportive and continuing care services.
- Studies suggest that the primary reasons patients have unmet needs is (1) the lack of information and awareness that supportive care services exist and/or (2) the patient's inability to negotiate complex bureaucracies to obtain services in a timely manner.

### Rehabilitation

- Rehabilitation addresses the issues of function, quality of life, and independence in life routines.
- Rehabilitation opportunities to be evaluated are recommended on text page 1457.
- Table 51-11, text page 1457, lists suggested supportive care services.

### Screening and Education

- *Unless limited to high-risk individuals*, screening for cancer costs more than therapy.

## RESOURCE ALLOCATION

- The challenge in resource allocation is the desire to implement new services as they emerge without reducing present services.
- Table 51-12, text page 1458, is a simple method of initially prioritizing new service ideas.

### Physical Facilities

- The decision to develop or renovate is based upon the need for new space to meet projected volume of patients, the need to accommodate new technology being introduced, or the need to consolidate present services in contiguous space.
- As functions within spaces become defined, integration of some services may be considered. Functional issues to address are listed in Table 51-13, text page 1459.

### Equipment and Technology

- The most expensive components in an oncology program are still the capital investments necessary for radiation therapy equipment and diagnostic equipment (PET scanners, genetics laboratories) and the human and technical resources for bone marrow transplant programs.
- A simple process of evaluating new technology has five basic steps: (1) determining decision makers, (2) oncology team evaluation, (3) oncology team recommendations, (4) business planning, and (5) organizational approval.

## Human Resources

- Cross-training of staff throughout oncology can provide variable staffing and continuity of care between inpatient and outpatient areas.
- The key to redesign among RNs and unlicensed assistive personnel (UAPs) is to maintain the RN's critical functions and to teach RNs how to manage UAPs.
- UAPs should not be used in those situations where the patient's disease or response are unpredictable or where specialized knowledge, judgment, or skills are necessary such as chemotherapy, pain management, symptom management plans, grading of toxicity, and unstable patient assessment.
- It is important for the oncology leadership to involve staff in planning and implementing redesign that meets the outcome and satisfaction needs of patients and the professional satisfaction needs of the staff.

## CANCER PROGRAM MARKETING AND CONTRACTING

### Marketing

- Marketing is recognized as a needed management function in a highly competitive environment characterized by an excess capacity of inpatient beds and an oversupply of medical specialists.
- Successful marketing includes a well-designed product or service, appropriate pricing, communication methods, and a system for distributing the products/services.
- The cancer program leadership needs to develop a marketing plan by determining the needs and wants of target markets and then designing, communicating, pricing, and delivering appropriate and competitively viable products and services.
- Health status indicators vary by community, and typically reflect the community's definition of health.

### Contracting

- Today a wide variety of contracting opportunities are available: discounted charge-basis, per diem rates, per visit or stay rates, global pricing, and capitation rates.
- To remain competitive in the marketplace and maintain cancer program prominence, skillful contracting is necessary.
- Most per diem, per visit, or per stay rates are negotiated for an entire hospital organization.
- The risk the hospital accepts in per diem or per stay rates is that the population covered will maintain present illness and wellness patterns.
- A much greater risk is accepted by the organization that engages in managed-care contracts involving *global pricing* and *capitation*. *Global pricing* is an all-inclusive price for the delivery of a discrete set of services. This pricing strategy can be applied to a specific procedure (e.g., breast biopsy) or a course of treatment (e.g., diagnosis through one year of treatment for early-stage breast cancer).
- *Capitation* refers to the per capita payment amount managed care organizations or providers are paid to provide an enrollee (or member) with a specified package of medical services. The capitation payment rate is expressed on a per member per month (PMPM) basis.

## PRACTICE QUESTIONS

1. The hospitals that are the most profitable offer:
   a. the PLM concept.
   b. radiation therapy.
   c. nuclear medicine.
   d. teaching facilities.

2. Alliances between hospitals and physicians are referred to as:
   a. PHOs.
   b. MSOs.
   c. IHOs.
   d. all of the above.

3. As an organization is involved in a strategic planning process, which of the following should be considered as projections for future workload and revenue?
   a. changes in physicians practicing at the facility
   b. reimbursement policies of third-party payers
   c. shifts to managed care and capitation
   d. all of the above

4. As we increase the quality of any service while maintaining costs, we:
   a. decrease its value.
   b. lose profitability.
   c. increase the value.
   d. none of the above.

5. In today's market, the most effective method for maximizing revenues is:
   a. negotiation of favorable contracts with payers.
   b. close control of medical records coding through cost optimization techniques.
   c. the use of charge accumulation and reconciliation methods.
   d. appropriate utilization of resources.

6. The most expensive components in an oncology program are still the capital investments necessary for:
   a. radiation therapy equipment.
   b. diagnostic equipment (PET scanners, genetic labs).
   c. the human and technical resources for BMT programs.
   d. all of the above.

7. You are working in an oncology center that has just hired UAPs. Their training and supervision will be conducted by RNs, but it is your responsibility to lay the basic guidelines for use of UAPs. You establish that UAPs may provide:
   a. treatment assessment.
   b. direct patient care.
   c. symptom management planning.
   d. all of the above.

8. Greater risk is accepted by the organization that engages in managed-care contracts involving:
   a.  global pricing.
   b.  per diem rates.
   c.  capitation.
   d.  a and c.

9. Capitation is:
   a.  the per capita amount to provide an enrollee with a specified package of medical services.
   b.  paid on a per stay basis.
   c.  paid on a per member per day basis.
   d.  a and c.

## ANSWER EXPLANATIONS

1. **The answer is b.** The hospitals that are the most profitable offer radiation therapy. (p. 1439)

2. **The answer is d.** Alliances between hospitals and physicians are usually physician-hospital organizations (PHOs), management service organizations (MSOs), foundation models, or integrated health organizations (IHOs). (p. 1441)

3. **The answer is d.** All of these factors should be detailed as footnotes to market projections during strategic planning. (p. 1443)

4. **The answer is c.** As we increase the quality of any service while maintaining costs, we increase the value. (p. 1444)

5. **The answer is a.** The most effective method for maximizing revenues is negotiating favorable contracts with payers. (p. 1452)

6. **The answer is d.** The most expensive components in an oncology program are still the capital investments necessary for radiation therapy equipment and diagnostic equipment (PET scanners, genetic labs), and the human and technical resources for BMT programs. (p. 1459)

7. **The answer is b.** UAPs may provide direct patient care. They should not be used in those situations where the patient's disease or response are unpredictable, or where specialized knowledge or skills are needed, such as chemotherapy, pain management, symptom management plans, toxicity grading, and unstable patient assessment. (p. 1460)

8. **The answer is d.** The risk the hospital accepts in per diem or per stay rates is that the population covered will maintain present illness and wellness patterns. However, a much greater risk is accepted by the organization that engages in managed-care contracts involving global pricing and capitation. (p. 1461)

9. **The answer is a.** Capitation refers to the per capita payment amount that managed care organizations or providers are paid to provide an enrollee or member with a specified package of medical services. The capitation payment rate is expressed on a per member per month (PMPM) basis. (p. 1461)

# Chapter 52    Ambulatory Care

## AMBULATORY CARE OVERVIEW

- Ambulatory care is synonymous with outpatient care and includes services such as diagnostic testing; treatment modalities; patient and family education; rehabilitation; nutritional support; psychosocial intervention; symptom management; and survivor services.
- Advances in cancer treatment and technology and the influences of economics and quality-of-life issues have promoted ambulatory services as a method for providing cancer patient and family care.
- It is estimated that 80%–90% of all cancer care is delivered in outpatient settings.

### Ambulatory Care Settings

- A wide variety of ambulatory care settings are available, including comprehensive cancer centers, community cancer centers, freestanding cancer centers, 23- to 24-hour clinics, chemotherapy and infusion centers, day surgery centers, physicians' offices, outreach and network programs, and other specialty centers that focus on screening, rehabilitation, and symptom management.
- Comprehensive cancer centers, authorized by the National Cancer Act of 1971 and designated by the National Cancer Institute (NCI), are dedicated to conducting clinical research, training physicians in oncology subspecialties, maintaining data for new diagnoses, and providing clinical care to cancer patients.

#### Freestanding centers

- A freestanding cancer center (FSCC) may be a facility separate from an existing medical care delivery center such as a hospital, or it may be contiguous with or within a hospital facility. Freestanding centers may be joint ventures between health care providers or may be corporately owned and operated.
- The movement toward FSCCs resulted from the shift in medical care delivery from inpatient to outpatient settings and from patient demand for sophisticated therapies in the local community. FSCCs are usually based within the community, do not incorporate training of oncologists, and are not involved with on-site basic research.
- Affiliations of community programs with university-based cancer centers are occurring.

#### Twenty-three– and twenty-four–hour clinics

- The need for ambulatory services on a continuous basis has precipitated the development of a number of 24-hour services across the country.
- Even though the centers may not be open 24 hours a day initially, health care professionals are on call to meet the needs of patients seeking therapy during nontraditional hours.
- Such settings are specifically designed to deal with side effect management and unpredictable changes in the patient's condition following therapy.
- Twenty-three–hour clinics usually refer to a maximum length of stay for individuals rather than to the hours of operation.
- Individuals classified as 23-hour observation patients are on an inpatient unit of a hospital for this 23-hour stay.

## Day surgery

- Many types of cancer-related surgical procedures are performed in an ambulatory setting.
- Advantages of ambulatory surgery include reduced cost, fewer complications, less disability, more individualized attention, and less anxiety for the individual undergoing the procedure.
- Disadvantages include situations in which individuals have not followed proper preoperative instructions, and difficulty with transportation home and with appropriate aftercare.

## Outpatient clinics and treatment centers

- Clinics may specialize in treatment of specific disease sites, such as lung or breast, with highly specialized physicians and nurses. Individuals may also seek second opinions from clinicians in these settings.
- Another trend that continues is the development of site-specific cancer centers, such as breast clinics or centers.
- Table 52-1, text page 1468, highlights the operational and programmatic components.
- Two styles of breast centers are commonly seen: diagnostic breast centers and comprehensive breast centers. Diagnostic centers offer a variety of imaging services, education about breast self-examination, and clinical examination by a physician. In contrast, comprehensive centers offer these services as well as a full range of treatment and rehabilitative services in one setting with a multidisciplinary team approach.

## Outreach and satellite centers

- Since individuals often want to remain in their own communities to receive cancer treatment, linkages between tertiary and rural hospitals are being developed.
- Through this program, patients are treated by oncologists at a tertiary setting and then return to rural or community hospitals for continued treatment.
- Many community oncologists also perform outreach services through satellite centers in clinics within 20–100 miles of their base practice.
- The use of telemedicine to bring physicians and/or patients together through two-way interactive video conferencing has great potential for future rural health care settings and learning opportunities.

## Office practices

- Many office practices administer chemotherapy and provide a number of other care services for patients, including laboratory, x-ray, nutritional counseling, education, and support groups.
- Increasingly, care of the bone marrow transplant patient is being provided in the office setting. This may include actual delivery of high-dose chemotherapy prior to the transplant as well as post-transplant care.

## Other ambulatory centers (screening, rehabilitation, genetic)

- The basic focus of these programs is to provide low-cost cancer detection services.
- Among the factors contributing to a successful screening center are convenience and visibility, adequate volume to keep the cost affordable, and an approach directed at screening programs outside the usual programs.
- A realignment of financial incentives is encouraging practitioners to prevent illness or detect it earlier, and thus there is increased support for cancer prevention and early detection programs.

## Planning Issues

- Detailed discussions about planning ambulatory care services and facility design are available in the literature.
- Table 52-3, text page 1471, describes an external and internal analysis utilizing a multidisciplinary planning process prior to beginning clinic planning.

# THE ROLE OF THE NURSE IN AMBULATORY CARE

## Overview

- Three challenges commonly encountered by ambulatory oncology nurses are (1) the use of the telephone in successful delivery of patient care, (2) the time frame for conducting assessments and meeting patient needs, and (3) assisting with patient transition from one setting to another.

### Standards of care

- The American Academy of Ambulatory Care Nursing (AAACN) is a professional organization whose members believe that ambulatory care nursing is essential.
- Table 52-4, text page 1472, provides a summary of the nine standards developed by the AAACN.

### Responsibilities of the nurse

- Multiple roles and responsibilities for nurses in ambulatory care settings, include that of staff nurse, nurse manager (head nurse), clinical nurse specialist, nurse practitioner, nurse data manager or research nurse, and cancer program director.
- Oncology nurses reported most frequent involvement in (1) health care maintenance activities, followed by (2) counseling and (3) communication.
- Table 52-5, text page 1473, describes dimensions of the current staff nurse role in ambulatory care.
- Significant factors that attract and retain nurses in ambulatory care are client and family contact, hours and schedules, the challenging nature of the job, seeing the outcomes of care, and autonomy. A lack of time, lack of support staff, excessive paperwork, and administrative blocks to clinical practice were identified as barriers.
- The role of the oncology nurse in the office practice has expanded greatly with the shift of health care to the ambulatory setting; it now encompasses a variety of roles, including clinical, administrative/business, academic, and consultative.
- Nurse practitioners and oncology clinical nurse specialists are increasingly assuming roles in the radiation oncology setting.

## Nursing Process

- Nursing care delivered in the ambulatory setting follows the constructs of the nursing process and includes patient assessment, patient and caregiver teaching, telephone management, and documentation.

### Admission and assessment

- The first visit can be utilized to give important logistical details about parking facilities, how to find the department, the routine at the time of the visit, and how long to plan to be there.
- Many settings provide patient education material and support groups. A "questions and concerns form" may also be helpful for patients to use to record any of their concerns between appointments.
- Once the assessment has been completed, a discussion with the patient about the financial implications of the treatment plan is initiated and appropriate referrals are made.

### Planning and evaluation

- Planning and evaluation include activities such as development of the nursing care plan, use of nursing diagnoses, and evaluation of patient outcomes.

### Documentation

- Documentation includes the nursing process, fulfills legal requirements, describes the nursing care delivered, and reflects the quality of nursing care.

#### Self-report tools

- Another approach to documentation is patient self-report. Patients are usually asked to complete the tool at home and bring it on the day of treatment. The nurse then reviews the self-assessment, identifies concerns, and discusses interventions.

#### Computerized patient record

- Use of point-of-care computer terminals has the potential for simplifying documentation. These systems enable the nurse to immediately enter data into the computer, thus decreasing documentation time and improving accuracy.
- Voice-activated systems are increasingly utilized in the medical setting.

## Technical Procedures

- Technical procedures can involve educational as well as physical preparation of the patient, being present and offering support during the procedure, and actually performing the procedure.
- Among the many types of care settings, community hospital outpatient nurses had the highest frequency of performance of technical procedures.
- Nurses in ambulatory oncology settings are more likely to be performing high-tech procedures such as complex chemotherapy/biotherapy administration, blood and blood product administration, monitoring patients before and after procedures such as bone marrow biopsy and aspiration, lumbar punctures, stereotactic radiosurgery, and high-dose brachytherapy.

## Teaching and Advocacy

- Patient education is a key component of the nurse's role in the ambulatory setting.
- It is important to assess the patient's desired method of learning rather than use the same approach for all patients. Some patients prefer to see a demonstration, while others prefer a one-to-one teaching approach. Still others may benefit from a videotape.
- Nurses should be involved with the planning, development, and testing of educational materials.
- Strategies for meeting information needs of families are described in Table 52-7 on text page 1478.
- Education can be accomplished only after the patient has achieved symptom relief.
- Group classes provide opportunities for patients to interact with each other and share common experiences.

## Telephone Communications and Management

- Triaging phone calls appropriately and efficiently is a major and time-consuming role. Telephone activities include assessing patients' responses to the treatment given, providing information about prevention of side effects and symptoms, and evaluating patient outcomes.
- Patient care–oriented calls can have multiple purposes: communication of changes in the care plan, reassurance of the patient and family about side effects, instructions to lessen the severity of the side effects, and assessment of supportive services.

- Another use of the telephone in ambulatory oncology care is the "hot line," a toll-free 800 number that patients can call to make appointments or ask questions.
- Follow-up phone calls after treatment provide an excellent opportunity for patient assessment and further self-care instructions.

## Care Coordination

- The development and implementation of critical pathways and guidelines will have a significant impact on cost and outcomes in cancer care.
- Critical paths consist of a series of interventions specific to a group of patients with common attributes that are designed to promote the attainment of specific patient outcomes within a specific time frame.
- Trends can be identified that affect length of stay, resource consumption, or patient outcomes.
- Variances direct revisions necessary.
- The use of benchmark comparisons to improve services in health care is relatively new.

## NURSING ISSUES
### Models of Nursing Care Delivery

- A model of care delivery is a generic term to describe a method of organizing resources for the provision of patient care.
- Models of care proposed include primary prevention, primary health care, primary nursing, case management, and paired partners. *Primary prevention* includes activities that either promote health in general or prevent the occurrence of diseases or injuries.
- A *primary health care* model constitutes the first level of contact of individuals, the family, and the community with the health system.
- *Primary nursing*, distinctly different from primary prevention or primary health care, is a model for nursing care delivery designed to improve the quality of nursing care; recognize the patient and family as the unit of care, with the care designed accordingly; improve coordination of care between specialties; and ensure continuity of care between settings.
- *Case management* is loosely defined as a means of organizing care throughout the episode of illness, regardless of location.
- A *paired-partners approach* implies that the RNs work closely with their partners, including hiring, orienting, coaching, evaluating, and even firing them.

## Productivity and Classification Systems

- Patient classification systems are a method of sorting individuals into levels for the purpose of predicting the demand for nursing care time.
- In the outpatient setting, classification systems are typically used for retrospective analysis of patient characteristics, justification of resources, use of monitored trends for program planning, nursing workload analysis, patient care charges, validation of the nursing care provided, and quality assurance.

## Quality and Outcomes

- The National Committee on Quality Assurance has joined the JCAHO in developing standards for accreditation.
- Key principles include measuring what is done; measuring what is important to the customers; measuring what is feasible to collect and report and is meaningful to clinicians; and assuring that the measures selected are operational and concrete.
- Table 52-9, text page 1489, provides sample indicators for the oncology ambulatory setting.

- Patient satisfaction should be integrated with other quality measures to improve service.

## Occupational Hazards

- Oncology nurses working in ambulatory settings face occupational hazards—specifically, the safe handling of antineoplastic agents, radioactive materials, and blood and body fluids. Guidelines for protection in handling antineoplastic agents were revised by the Occupational Safety and Health Administration (OSHA) in 1995. The ONS has also published guidelines and recommendations for practice related to chemotherapy. Unfortunately, wide variations in practice still exist. Ambulatory oncology nursing administrators are challenged to establish protective measures in their settings.
- The growth of continuous infusion administration of chemotherapy in the home setting necessitates considering these same issues for the home.
- Implementation of a facility-wide chemotherapy and radiotherapy task force is recommended to establish standards, protocols, procedures; recommend protective equipment purchases; and evaluate compliance with the accepted standards.

## Continuity of Care

- The oncology nurse in the ambulatory setting frequently maintains continuity of care with the patient and family.
- To achieve a continuity of care that is integrated and comprehensive, several key components are highlighted in Table 52-10 on text page 1490.
- The technical capability of the computer to integrate information from multiple sources, store, and then later transmit the data to another location is especially advantageous for care of patients with cancer.
- Another approach to enhancing continuity of care is through multidisciplinary patient care conferences.
- The patient and family must clearly understand who should be called and when to call.
  - Another method for ensuring improved continuity of care is a daily morning conference.

## Research

- Research protocols are commonly offered to patients in outpatient settings and mandate that ambulatory nurses are familiar with the careful documentation essential to the clinical trials.
- Nursing research in the ambulatory setting is now more common and is expected to be a major focus of future research efforts.
- Table 52-11, text page 1492, details research-related roles and expectations of staff nurses in a comprehensive cancer program.
- Table 52-12, text page 1492, is a listing of ambulatory care nursing research problems that nurses may want to consider pursuing.

## PATIENT-RELATED ISSUES

### Self-Care

- Transition of patient care from the hospital to ambulatory and home settings has resulted in a shift in responsibility for family members caring for patients receiving treatment.
- *Self-care* is defined as how individuals care for themselves or alter conditions or objects in their environment in the interest of their own lives, health, or well-being.
- A self-care diary is effective for obtaining patients' reports of the side effects experienced and the usefulness of self-care activities.

- Cancer resource libraries are another method of empowering cancer patients and encouraging self-care.
- Self-care teaching and written guidelines for patients and families about care of venous access lines, administration of parenteral fluids, and symptom management are critical to effective management of these patients in an ambulatory environment.
- For optimal self-care behavior, patients and families need to be adequately taught about the specific treatment modality and side effect management.

## Ethical Issues

- Ethical issues encountered in ambulatory care are similar to those that arise in other settings.
- Two ever-present issues are (1) whether patients are making informed decisions and (2) how best to provide high-quality care.
- Open and honest professional dialogue is usually an effective approach.
- As reimbursement becomes more limited, health care providers will face increasingly difficult decisions about who and how to treat, when to stop treatment, the aggressiveness of treatment, who is making decisions about treatment, and so on.

## Economic Issues

- Direct reimbursement for nursing services continues to be a goal within nursing.
- The *nurse complement model* is defined as a model in which the nurse complies with the medical directives and functions as a complement to the oncologist.
- The *nurse substitute model* is one in which the oncology nurse is in a collaborative relationship with the oncologist and regularly acts as a physician substitute.
- In the substitute model, care normally provided by the oncologist is performed by the nurse.

## PRACTICE QUESTIONS

1.  Ambulatory oncology services have increased over the past decade or so for all of the following reasons *except:*
    a.  economic pressures.
    b.  developments in cancer treatment.
    c.  innovation in cancer technology.
    d.  decreased patient acuity.

2.  Freestanding cancer centers (FSCCs):
    a.  are usually based within the community.
    b.  incorporate training of oncologists.
    c.  are involved with on-site research.
    d.  all of the above.

3.  Among the many types of care settings, _____ nurses have the highest frequency of performance of technical procedures.
    a.  emergency room
    b.  community hospital outpatient
    c.  surgical unit
    d.  a and b

4.  Critical paths consist of:
    a.  emergent oncological care based on triage techniques followed by categorization or classification and individualized treatment plans.
    b.  methods used to conquer oncology care problems through critical thinking models.
    c.  a series of interventions designed to promote the attainment of specific patient outcomes for a very specific group of patients within a specific time frame.
    d.  all of the above.

5.  Primary nursing is a model for:
    a.  promoting health in general or preventing the occurrence of diseases or injuries.
    b.  the first level of contact of individuals, the family, and the community with the health system.
    c.  recognizing patient and family as the unit of care and improving continuity of care between settings and specialties.
    d.  none of the above.

6.  Applying the definition of self-care to oncology, an example of self-care actions initiated by patients would be:
    a.  to keep a diary of their side effects and the efficacy of their efforts to control the side effects.
    b.  to entrust their loved one with the care of their venous access device.
    c.  to trust that their care providers would provide total care.
    d.  to have their significant other review the patient education material for them.

7.  You are asked to set up a program to teach self-care to patients who receive follow-up care in the ambulatory care setting after major cancer treatments, such as bone marrow or peripheral stem cell transplant patients. Which of the following will you be sure to include?
    a.  care of venous access lines.
    b.  administration of parenteral fluids.
    c.  symptom management.
    d.  all of the above.

# ANSWER EXPLANATIONS

1. **The answer is d.** Advances in cancer treatment and technology, the influences of economics, and quality-of-life issues have promoted ambulatory services as a method for providing cancer patient and family care. With shortened hospitalizations driven by reimbursement changes, patients are being discharged quicker and sicker; therefore, the patient acuity is actually higher. (p. 1466)

2. **The answer is a.** Freestanding cancer centers (FSCCs) are usually based within the community, do not incorporate training of oncologists, and are not involved with on-site research. (p. 1466)

3. **The answer is b.** Among the many types of care settings, community hospital outpatient nurses have the highest frequency of performance of technical procedures. (p. 1476)

4. **The answer is c.** Critical paths consist of a series of interventions specific to a group of patients with common attributes that are designed to promote the attainment of specific patient outcomes within a specific time frame. (p. 1483)

5. **The answer is c.** Primary nursing is a model for nursing care delivery designed to improve quality, recognize patient and family as the unit of care, improve coordination of care between specialties, and ensure continuity of care between settings. Primary prevention includes activities that either promote health in general or prevent the occurrence of diseases or injuries. A primary health care model constitutes the first level of contact of individuals, the family, and the community with the health system. (p. 1485)

6. **The answer is a.** Maintaining a diary with recorded side effects, severity of each, and the recorded efficacy of self-care activities is an example of self-care actions. Any action initiated by the patient and family to prevent, detect, and manage side effects of radiation or chemotherapy can be defined as self-care. (p. 1493)

7. **The answer is d.** Self-care teaching and written guidelines for patients and families about care of venous access lines, administration of parenteral fluids, and symptom management are critical to effective management of these patients in an ambulatory environment. (p. 1493)

# Chapter 53    Home Care

## OVERVIEW OF HOME HEALTH CARE

- Home health care is one of the most rapidly growing and changing fields in health care.
- Precipitous growth occurred after revisions in the *Medicare Home Health Agency Manual* (HAM) in 1989 expanded eligibility and coverage of home health services.
- As defined by insurance eligibility guidelines, care at home can be preventive, diagnostic, therapeutic, rehabilitative, or long-term maintenance care.
- A physician oversees the care and the nurse is a primary provider and care manager through collaboration.

## Home Care Services

- The goals of home health care are to promote, maintain, or restore health; to minimize the effects of illness and disability; or to allow for a peaceful death.
- The traditional services covered by Medicare reimbursement and provided by certified home health agencies include nursing, physical therapy, speech and language pathology, medical social work, occupational therapy, home health aide services, and nutrition therapy.

### Nursing

- Nursing is the foundation of home health care.
- The nurse is the coordinator of all home care provided to the patient. Home care nursing responsibilities include assessment, direct physical care, evaluation of patient progress, patient and family teaching, supervision and coordination of patient care, and provision of psychosocial support.
- Home health care nursing differs from private duty nursing in that care is provided on an intermittent basis rather than daily or for extended time periods.

### Homemaker-home health aide

- The availability of homemaker-home health aide service is often the factor that determines whether a patient and family can opt for home care.
- Responsibilities of the home health aide include assistance with personal hygiene and homemaking tasks.
- Under the direction of the nurse, the home health aide may assist the patient and family to perform treatments (e.g., wound care or ambulation exercises).

### Physical therapy

- Physical therapists provide therapy for patients at home to treat their illness or injury or for restoration or maintenance of function that has been affected by the illness or injury.
- The physical therapist also instructs patients and caregivers in implementation of maintenance therapies.

### Occupational therapy

- Occupational therapists assist patients to achieve their highest functional level and to be as self-reliant as possible. They can teach patients adaptive techniques to improve their level of independence in activities essential to daily living, provide preprosthetic and prosthetic training, and assist in the selection or construction of splints to correct or prevent a deformity.

### Speech and language pathology

- A major treatment goal is to facilitate maximum speech and language recovery and to enable patients to achieve a higher level of communicative abilities.

### Social work

- Social workers in the home care setting have traditionally been considered referral agents and counselors and patient advocates.

### Nutrition services

- Direct care is often secondary to consultation and staff education because few third-party insurers will reimburse for direct patient counseling by the nutritionist at home.

### Additional care services

- In addition to the traditional services provided by certified home health agencies, a diverse assortment of services for the patient in the home are provided.
- Some supplemental services may require payment by the individual requesting them. However, some may be available from community service organizations at a reduced rate.

## Types of Home Care Agencies

- Selection of the most appropriate type of home care agency is based primarily on: patient and family needs; the patient's financial arrangement or type of health insurance coverage; availability of family and community support; the type of home care services available in the patient's community.
- Three classifications of agencies provide home care services: the official agency of the public health departments, Medicare-certified home health agencies, and private duty agencies.

### Official public health agencies

- Official agencies are organized and administered within city, county, or multicounty health departments. The major focus of official health agencies has been preventive health care and infectious disease control.
- Home nursing care consists of biweekly or monthly home visits for patient teaching and supervision rather than direct physical care.

### Medicare-certified home health agencies

- Home health agencies, structured and operating within the specific guidelines may be certified to participate in the federal health insurance program.
- Medicare-certified home health agencies may be facility-based, freestanding, public, proprietary, or private nonprofit.

### Private duty agencies

- Private duty agencies provide nursing care in the home by registered nurses, licensed practical nurses, home health aides, or companions for specific periods of time.

- Services may be contracted and paid by the patient or family or arranged through a case manager from the patient's health insurance company.

### Other agencies

- Durable medical equipment (DME) companies provide medical equipment and supplies, including respiratory equipment, ostomy appliances, and parenteral feedings and supplies.
- Infusion therapy agencies provide parenteral medications (e.g., antibiotics, antineoplastics), total parenteral nutritional feedings, parenteral solutions, infusion devices, and equipment.

## Continuity of Care

- The most frequently used processes to ensure a comprehensive multidisciplinary approach to patient care are case management and discharge planning.

### Case management

- Case management has been defined as a health care delivery process with the goals of providing quality health care, decreasing fragmentation, enhancing the patient's quality of life, and containing cost.
- The benefits of case management in the inpatient setting are a decrease in length of stay, coordination of resources for discharge, and facilitation of communication among the disciplines.

### Discharge planning

- Discharge planning centers on the family or significant other to facilitate the transition of the patient from one level of care to another, usually from the hospital to the home.
- In the current health care environment, patient and family involvement is essential for developing a plan for posthospital care and the successful implementation of posthospital treatment.
- Palliation of symptoms and pain control are major home care issues.
- The potential for success in home care is increased if the types of home health services necessary to assist with the supervision and management of the patient and adequate informal support are available.
- The degree of informal support available also affects the family's ability to manage home care, such as friends, neighbors, and church groups.

### Unique Characteristics of the Home

- In the home the patient and family determine when and how the patient's plan of care will be implemented.
- The patient and family are encouraged to assume responsibility for the care of the patient; this is the overall goal of home care.
- Greater personal control over an individual's life is associated with higher levels of self-esteem, lower self-reported anxiety, and more purpose in life.
- It is critical that the home health nurse evaluate the physical and financial conditions to support the care required by the patient at home.

## ROLE OF THE NURSE IN HOME HEALTH

- The advances in treatment of disease and changes in reimbursement of health care services have shifted the focus of home care nursing in the 1990s to one that emphasizes care of the acutely ill patient in the home.

## The Patient and Family as the Unit of Care

- For home health nursing care to be successful, the nurse assesses the family's structure and processes, develops a plan of care that is congruent with the family's values and lifestyle, and includes the patient and family in the decision-making process.
- Three types of family units are supportive, ambivalent, and hostile.
- The way a family functioned in the past is generally the way it will confront the current crisis of cancer.
- Family behavior can be described in terms of cohesion, adaptability, and communication. *Family cohesion* is the emotional bonding that members have with one another. *Family adaptability* is the ability of the system to change its power structure, role relationships, and relationship rules in response to situational and developmental stress. *Family communication* is a facilitator; it can enhance or restrict movement on the cohesion and adaptability dimensions.

### Family assessment

- Assessment of the family begins with the patient's family of origin to obtain a history of family functioning: ages, geographic location, socioeconomic status, cultural and ethnic background, roles, relationship to patient, developmental level, major stressors, alliances, and frictions.
- Assessment includes patterns of authority, level of family development, values, behavior, coping ability, health and functional status, stressors, support systems, and knowledge of the illness and health practices.
- The following topics should be addressed during assessment of the family: structure, pattern of authority; level of family development; values; behavior; coping ability; health and functional status; stressors; support systems; and knowledge of illness and health practices.

### Demands on caregivers

- Most caregivers reported that the patient's daily physical needs were being met by immediate relatives and close friends.
- The problems most often identified were a lack of knowledge in management of the patient's physical symptoms and psychological needs as well as measures to assist the caregiver in coping with his or her role.
- Caregivers have reported a decrease in their abilities to cope when changes occur in the patient's health status. In addition, feelings of despair, isolation, vulnerability, and helplessness often negatively affect their coping abilities.
- The financial burden on the family of a patient with cancer has increased significantly as patient care shifts from the acute care setting to the home setting.
- To enhance the family's ability to care for a patient at home, the home health nurse must function in two significant areas: nursing care that contributes to the physical well-being of the patient and nursing care that provides the patient and family with reassurance and practical and emotional support.
- Nursing interventions that foster cohesion of the family and strengthen interaction, communication, cooperation, and emotional involvement will decrease isolation and enable the family to increase its autonomy and stability.

## Implementation of the Nursing Process
### Assessment

- The assessment of health problems in the home setting includes the patient's actual and potential health problems as well as relevant characteristics of the family and the environment (social, economic, and physical).

- The parameters for assessment of patients with cancer and their families at the time of admission to home care are listed in Table 53-3, text page 1509.

### Planning

- The high-incidence problem areas defined in the ANA/ONS *Standards of Oncology Nursing Practice* provide the framework.
- Problem areas for assessment and planning include comfort, nutrition, protective mechanisms, mobility, elimination, sexuality, ventilation, and circulation.
- Special care requirements are listed in Table 53-4, text page 1510.

### Nursing interventions

- Nursing interventions in home health assist the patient and family by providing direct care and treatment, supervision of patient care, health and disease management teaching, counseling, and coordination of health care services.
- The typical interventions, functions, and activities of the nurse in a cancer home health agency are listed in Table 53-5, text page 1511.

### Evaluation

- Outcome measures can be used to assess the quality of nursing care in specific areas based on predictable results (i.e., adequacy of patient teaching, improvement in physiological status, improvement in functional status, improvement in compliance with treatments, and satisfaction with care as reported on patient and family surveys).

## Coordination of Services

- A multidisciplinary group of health care professionals from a variety of health care institutions and community service agencies may be involved with the home care of the person with cancer.
- The nurse can provide reassurance to the patient and family by explaining the purpose of each service and coordinating the visits. The nurse also maintains and shares an awareness of the goals for rehabilitation for each patient in order to provide direction to the service providers.
- Incorporating case management into the role of the home health nurse will achieve better patient care.

## Documenting Nursing Care

- Legal responsibilities of the home health oncology nurse include knowledge of and compliance with the nursing role as defined in the state Nurse Practice Act, the regulations that govern home health, and the standards of nursing practice for the nurse's community. The best evidence that the nurse has complied with these regulations and standards is the documentation of patient care.
- Documentation must be complete, clear, accurate, objective, and timely to fulfill federal and state certification requirements and Medicare and third-party reimbursement requirements.
- Principles of documentation include a comprehensive, accurate, and objective description of assessments, nursing actions, and the responses of the patient, family, and caregivers to interventions.

## Rehabilitation Nursing

- The goal of cancer rehabilitation is to improve the quality of life by maximizing functional ability and independence regardless of life expectancy and, when appropriate, reintroduction into the socioeconomic life of the community.
- Effective intervention requires the participation of the family in planning and implementing care.

- The greatest needs of patients with cancer and their caregivers have been found to be primarily psychological and informational. Teaching stress reduction methods, communication and problem-solving skills, and information on disease process and care principles may facilitate patient and family coping.
- Encouraging the patient and family to develop networks and supports in the community fosters independence and facilitates patient discharge from the home health agency.
- The discharge plan provides information on community agencies and services; the patient's health insurance coverage and contact persons; transportation services; vocational rehabilitation programs; and support groups.
- As the disease advances and the ability to maintain activities for independent functioning wanes, it is important to recognize that cancer patients are likely to need services such as personal care, meal preparation, shopping, housekeeping, and transportation. Failure to obtain these services may precipitate a family crisis.

## Role of the Advanced Practice Nurse (APN)

- The nursing activities of the APN in homecare include education, consultation, research, and administration, with the APN providing direct patient care and psychotherapy, developing nursing care protocols, teaching and consulting with health care professionals, and coordinating quality improvement activities.

### Practitioner role

- Direct care activities provided by the APN in home health care include advanced services and skills not usually available from the general nursing staff.
- The APN is particularly adept in management of complex physical and psychological care requirements such as infusion therapy, extensive wounds, parenteral nutrition, intractable pain, and counseling and problem solving.

### Educator role

- The APN has expertise in developing and implementing staff orientation, continuing education programs for the agency and community, and presenting patient care conferences to enhance staff knowledge and improve patient care.

### Consultant role

- Consultation may include assisting staff with managing difficult cases or providing information to improve their skills, knowledge, self-assurance, or objectivity.

### Researcher role

- Research activity for the APN varies from the basics of interpreting, evaluating, and communicating research findings to caregivers to the advanced level of research collaboration and actively generating or replicating research projects.

### Case management role

- The activities of the APN case manager in home care include assessment of patients with high acuity, complex care requirements, or high-risk status, and assessment of their family, environment, and health insurance benefits; establishment of nursing diagnosis; development of a multidisciplinary plan of care; implementation of the plan of care including delegation of specific interventions to the multidisciplinary team, coordination of services provided; collaboration with the multidisciplinary team and the health insurance worker; referral to community resources; and evaluation of outcomes.

### Evaluation of the APN role

- APNs have provided education and support to staff nurses and have produced revenues through home visits; participated in revisions of policies, procedures, and documentation forms; developed and conducted nursing process audits; served as home health liaisons; and participated in professional oncology nursing activities in the community.

## ECONOMIC ISSUES

### Financing Home Health Care

- Home health nurses need to be familiar with reimbursement guidelines defined by each reimbursement source, obtain the necessary approvals for care, and complete the required forms.
  - Medicare eligibility requirements state that the beneficiary must be homebound and require skilled nursing, physical therapy, or speech and language pathology services ordered by a physician. *Homebound* means that leaving the home requires considerable effort.
  - Services must be provided on a part-time, intermittent basis. *Part-time* currently is defined as nursing and home health aide time totaling less than 8 hours per day or 35 hours per week. *Intermittent* currently is defined as services required at least every 60 days and daily visits limited to 21 consecutive days or having a predictable and finite end if daily visits extend beyond 21 days.
- Medicare reimburses at the lower end of reasonable cost or agency charge, on a per visit basis.
- Medicaid funding for home health services is a joint federal-state assistance program for the poor of all ages.
- States receive matching funds for their expenditures and are allowed extensive flexibility in determining eligibility, services, and reimbursement.
- Private insurance carriers vary significantly in their coverage for home health services.

### Documentation for Reimbursement

- Accurate descriptive documentation of home health nursing care is vital to reimbursement and continuation of home health services.

### Home Care for the Socially Disadvantaged

- More than one-third of the population has minimal or no health care insurance protection.
- Because home health reimbursement by payers is based on cost, most home health agencies have limited funds available for services to persons without home health insurance.
- The Medicare home health benefit does not cover long-term or chronic care.
- A growing number of elderly persons with cancer with functional limitations and chronic health problems live alone or with a spouse or sibling who may also be frail and elderly.
- When a patient has a limited income, the social work home care staff are faced with the problem of locating a community service agency that provides follow-up monitoring and support services for personal care or homemaking without cost.
- The 1989 HCFA revisions to the *Medicare Home Health Agency Manual* recognized "management and evaluation of a beneficiary's plan of care" as skilled nursing care and thus reimbursable. This benefit expanded reimbursable home health services to include assessment, monitoring, teaching, and revisions of the plan of care for persons whose conditions have stabilized but who are at risk for complications or require frequent unskilled care from caregivers.

## ETHICAL CONCERNS

- The increased complexity of home health care have generated an increase of ethical concerns unique to the home care setting.
- Personal lifestyle, financial means, possessions, routines, and family structures may not be conducive to the provision of health care in the home.
- The most frequently cited ethical problems are (1) patient decisions regarding treatment and health care that conflict with the health care provider's goals, (2) truth telling that reveals patient confidences or would lead to denial of needed patient care, and (3) provisions of health care benefits that are based on insurance reimbursement rather than patient need.
- Home health nurses are usually familiar with the ethical principles of advocacy for patient autonomy and the patient's right of self-determination to refuse treatment when incapacitated.

### Moral Values

- The values of the patient, family, and caregiver are not usually known when a patient is admitted to home care and not easily assessed during the initial visit.
- Their values have sometimes been formulated by cultural and societal beliefs that are different from those held by the nurse.
- Ongoing assessment of the values of the patient, family, and caregivers is essential to identify potential ethical conflicts and to plan for nursing care that is compatible with their needs and values.

### Ethical Principles

- The ANA *Code for Nurses* identifies six principles that the nurse should use as moral guides to action: autonomy, beneficence, justice, veracity, confidentiality, and fidelity.
  - *Autonomy* is the principle that gives patients the right to determine their actions based on their own decisions.
  - The principle of *beneficence* directs the nurse to do good, to promote the welfare or well-being of others.
  - The principle of *justice* guides the nurse to treat all persons equally and to give individuals what is owed to them by another person or society.
  - The principle of *veracity* obligates the nurse to be truthful with the patient, peers, and other professionals.
  - The principle of *confidentiality* requires the nurse to respect and hold confidential all information shared by the patient. However, when innocent parties are in jeopardy, public law requires disclosure of this information.
  - Finally, the principle of *fidelity* requires the nurse to be faithful to his or her commitments and profession.

### Ethical Decision Making

- A decision-making process can be used to assess the problem and potential courses of action and to consider what is right or good based on the values of the persons involved and ethical principles. Guidelines developed to assist the nurse are listed in Table 53-6, text page 1517.

## INFUSION THERAPY IN THE HOME

- Infusion therapy is one of the most rapidly growing segments of home care.
- In addition to cost reduction, home infusion therapy reduces the risk of complications from nosocomial infections, is convenient for patient and caregiver, and provides psychological benefits to patients who desire the comfort of their homes.

- The disadvantage to home infusion therapy is the burden placed on caregivers to learn and comply with treatment schedules and procedures.
- Advanced technology has produced an array of long-term central venous access devices (VADs) and infusion pumps that simplify parenteral administration of drugs in the home and have less risk for complications.
- The most frequently used central VAD for cancer therapies in the home are venous access ports.
- The peripherally inserted central catheter (PICC) is used frequently in the home because it can be inserted by a nurse who is certified in the procedure. Because the PICC is biocompatible and flexible, it can often remain in place for weeks or months.
- PICC lines require frequent flushing with heparin and dressing changes every three to seven days.
- Caregiver education focus is on caring for the patient and family rather than on management of the equipment.
- Communication between the infusion therapy personnel and the home health nurse for coordination of services and delineation of responsibilities will also decrease patient and family confusion and anxiety.
- An Infusion Therapy/Home Health Coordination Record (Table 53-7, text page 1519) can be helpful in decreasing confusion and false expectations.
- If risk of exposure to blood or other potentially infectious materials occurs during care of the patient receiving infusion therapy in the home, the nurse must comply with universal precautions.

## Chemotherapy Administration

- Currently, continuous infusion of chemotherapeutic agents through an ambulatory infusion pump is the most frequently used deliver system in the home.
- Continuous infusion and regional infusion of antineoplastic drugs increase exposure of tumor cells to higher total dose of drug, theoretically increasing tumor cell kill. Nursing responsibilities may include changing the pump cassette containing the antineoplastic drugs, reprogramming the infusion pump, and monitoring and evaluating side effects of the therapy.

### Criteria for patient selection

- See text page 1518 for specific criteria for intermittent, bolus administration of chemotherapy in the home.

### Policies for chemotherapy administration

- Home health agencies that offer chemotherapy as a service must develop specific policies and procedures. A typical list is shown on text page 1518.
- Some agencies limit approved antineoplastic agents given at home to those that are nonvesicant or noncaustic.
- Home infusion therapy companies may administer antineoplastic drugs that require hydration and infusion over several hours.
- Specific hematologic parameters must be designated at which chemotherapy will or will not be administered.

### Staff education

- The nurse administering chemotherapy or caring for the person receiving continuous infusion chemotherapy must have the theoretical knowledge base and technical skills necessary to ensure the safety of the patient.
- Knowledge required to administer chemotherapy at home is listed on text page 1520.

## Safety considerations

- Potential hazards associated with the administration of antineoplastic agents have prompted the Occupational Safety and Health Administration (OSHA) to set guidelines for compounding, transporting, administering, and disposing of toxic chemotherapy agents.
- More specific safety considerations are discussed on text page 1520 and include: transport of drugs, preparation of drugs, spills, patient care, and disposal.

## Patient and family responsibilities

- Some agencies require a caregiver to be present on the day(s) chemotherapy is administered to observe for problems and assist the patient in managing side effects.
- Written information about potential side effects is provided along with the descriptions of symptoms that need to be reported immediately to the physician or nurse.
- The patient and family is educated regarding management of side effects and self-care measures.
- Reimbursement for chemotherapy administration in the home varies according to the reimbursement policies of the third-party payers.

## Home Parenteral Nutrition

- The administration of parenteral nutrition, one of the more complex therapies given in the home, is a rapidly growing option for cost-effective therapy for the malnourished patient with cancer.

## Criteria for patient selection

- Recommended criteria for acceptance of a patient into an HPN program are listed on text page 1521 and include the patient's physical status, a central venous access device (VAD), good vision and manual dexterity, care requirements, availability of adequate resources, and conducive home environment.
- The patient and family must assume primary responsibility for the administration of HPN.
- The financial costs of HPN vary according to locale and patient needs.
- Reimbursement from third-party payers has been inconsistent and restrictive.

## Initial home assessment

- The initial visit by the home care nurse should occur soon after the patient's arrival at home and should coincide with the arrival of supplies, equipment, medication, and home infusion therapy company personnel.
- It is essential that agencies administering HPN provide 24-hour service.
- The initial assessment includes the following:
  1. the type and status of the VAD
  2. the patient's and family's knowledge
  3. evaluation of the home environment for safety and cleanliness factors required for HPN

## Nursing management

- Twice-a-day home nursing visits are usually required initially.
- The nurse starts the infusion of HPN in the evening and discontinues it in the morning.
- The patient and family are instructed to record the date, time, and results of the following:
  - time of initiation/completion of HPN infusion
  - daily temperature, pulse, respirations
  - weight
  - urine fractionals

- intake (HPN, additional IV fluids, oral fluids)
- output
- medications added to HPN; other medications given
- catheter care (heparin flush, cap change, dressing change)
- blood draws for laboratory tests

## Intravenous Antimicrobial Therapy

- Antimicrobial therapy is the most commonly used IV therapy at home.
- It is the most appropriate therapy for infectious diseases that require either prolonged, repeated, or short-term antimicrobial agents with infrequent administration of drugs that are relatively safe.

### Criteria for patient selection

- Criteria for patient selection for HPAT are listed on text page 1523.

### Nursing management

- Infusion therapy agencies with pharmacies will prepare and deliver the antibiotics and the supplies on schedule.
- During the active treatment phase, nursing visits may vary in frequency from three times a day to once a week.
- Although the patient may prepare, store, and administer the HPAT, the home care nurse is responsible for ensuring that specific pharmaceutical guidelines are followed during the course of therapy (e.g., storage and mixing of drugs).
- By far the simplest and least costly drug delivery system is gravity infusion adapted to the home.
- Factors such as dosing interval or adverse effects profile are important in selecting a drug. The antimicrobial agent of choice for home administration would be the safest, most effective, cost-efficient, and easily administered antimicrobial agent available.
- Patient education is the key to safe administration of antimicrobial agents in the home.
- Content areas include venous access site care, signs and symptoms of drug side effects and recurrent infection, proper drug preparation procedures, drug administration techniques, catheter flushing and care, infusion pump operation (if applicable), and identification and resolution of problems.
- Reimbursement for HPAT has been inconsistent and varies according to the reimbursement policies of the individual third-party payer.

## Pain Management

- Principles of pain management in the home setting are listed on text page 1524.
- Oral analgesics are preferable for long-term cancer pain management for a number of reasons: effectiveness, ease of administration, increased compliance, allowance of uninterrupted sleep, no restriction of movement, and no equipment requirement.
- Intermittent or continuous infusion therapy for pain is given in the home setting via a variety of routes: subcutaneous, intravenous (IV), epidural, and subarachnoid.
- For continuous infusions, use of ambulatory infusion pumps offers unimpeded mobility.
- Patients and families are taught preparation and administration procedures, dressing change procedures, and catheter site care.
- Patient-controlled analgesia (PCA) is an IV drug delivery system that delivers continuous dosing and allows patients to administer intermittent predetermined doses of analgesic.
- Difficulty in obtaining narcotics for home use must be considered; therefore, analgesic requirements must be anticipated and methods of obtaining prescriptions planned.

- Physicians may be reluctant to prescribe adequate doses of pain medication for patients in the home setting because of restrictive controlled substance laws in some states. If this situation occurs, the home care nurse will send references supporting adequate pain management approaches to physicians. If needed, a referral to a pain clinic will be requested or other physicians who have provided care can be contacted for assistance in managing the patient's pain.
- Measures to decrease pain other than narcotic analgesics may be more effective in the comfort of the patient's home: behavioral coping strategies and noninvasive techniques.
- Assessment of pain is ongoing. A change in the location, severity, or type of pain may indicate an acute problem that requires other interventions.
- Patients and caregivers often negatively influence the treatment of pain as a result of their fears or beliefs about pain and potent narcotics. They may increase the dose interval, withhold doses, or refuse certain medications or certain routes of administration as they attempt to prevent dependence, addiction, somnolence, or sedation.
- Dose usually increases over time, indicating the development of tolerance. Addiction is a phenomenon rarely seen in cancer pain management. This information is helpful to share with patients and families as they struggle to manage cancer pain at home.

## DISCHARGE FROM HOME HEALTH CARE

- The overall goal of home health care is to facilitate the patient's and family's independence in managing daily life within the constraints imposed by the malignant disease.
- Home health services are discontinued or modified when the level of care required by the patient decreases; the family is willing, able, and knowledgeable in managing the patient's care; and the identified outcomes developed by the nurse, patient, and family have been achieved.
- Patients will also be discharged when an exacerbation of the disease process produces symptoms that require management in an inpatient setting or when service needs change.
- Another reason for discharge occurs when the person's health status declines so that family members are physically, mentally, or emotionally unable to provide care at home.
- When evaluating the discharge process, important points to consider and document are (1) the patient's status on discharge, (2) evidence of planning for discharge, and (3) timeliness of the decision to discharge.

## QUALITY IMPROVEMENT IN HOME CARE

- Standards that are pertinent to home care for persons with cancer include the ANA and Oncology Nursing Society's *Standards of Oncology Nursing Practice* and the ANA's *Standards of Home Health Nursing Practice*.
- Credentialing organizations have developed models for continuous quality improvement in home health agencies.
- A quality improvement resource group with members from senior management and key departments can facilitate implementation of a quality improvement program.
- The process of service delivery is routinely evaluated by most home health agencies in quarterly utilization review committees, periodic process audits, and routine clinical record review by supervisors.
- With quality improvement, processes of agency operations and service delivery that are essential to improving and achieving quality are targeted.
- The National Association for Home Care has developed a uniform minimum data set of items of information with uniform definitions and categories that involve specific dimensions of home care services to guide health agencies in the collection of meaningful information.
- A sampling of quality indicators is listed in Table 53-10, text page 1526.

# PRACTICE QUESTIONS

1.  The potential for success in home care is increased by the:
    a.  support received by friends and family.
    b.  degree of complexity of care.
    c.  age of the patient.
    d.  need for colostomy.

2.  *Homebound* is defined as:
    a.  being able to leave one's home only with great difficulty.
    b.  being confined to a wheelchair.
    c.  requiring home care for over 35 hours per week.
    d.  requiring intermittent care.

3.  The family assessment in home care is *least* likely to include which of the following questions?
    a.  What is the pattern of authority at home?
    b.  What is the functionality of the caregiver?
    c.  How many fire exits are available?
    d.  What other support systems are there?

4.  In the nurse's planning of home care, which of the following measures is most important?
    a.  Schedule extra visits during the working stage.
    b.  Avoid upsetting the family by discussing possible emergency situations.
    c.  Wait until discharge to order materials and supplies.
    d.  Be realistic about expected outcomes.

5.  One of the nurse's roles in home parenteral nutrition (HPN) is to:
    a.  keep records of times of infusion, intake, and output.
    b.  deliver all supplies, equipment, and medicines to the patient.
    c.  evaluate the patient, the home environment, and the family's ability to manage HPN.
    d.  perform all infusion regimens at home.

6.  Accurate and timely documentation is crucial to the solvency of a home care agency since it is required for:
    a.  reimbursement.
    b.  continued referrals
    c.  medical consultations
    d.  access to hospital records.

7.  Upon conducting a family assessment, the home health care nurse identifies conflict among the family members caring for the patient. Upon inquiry, the nurse learns that the conflict is "not new" and has existed "for years." Using this information, the home health care nurse establishes a plan of care that:
    a.  attempts to change the behavior among the family members since the patient is upset by the conflict.
    b.  involves having psychological services counsel the "conflicting members."
    c.  schedules family meetings about how the conflict is affecting the patient and what can be done to resolve it.
    d.  is sensitive to the feelings of the members in conflict but does not attempt to treat the causes of the conflict.

8. A major advantage of the peripherally inserted central catheter (PICC) is that:
   a. it does not require frequent flushing because of the one-way valve.
   b. dressing changes are simpler and more cost-effective.
   c. it can be inserted at home by a certified nurse.
   d. it has a separate designated port for blood withdrawal.

9. The overall goal of home care is:
   a. to provide complete and holistic care for the patient.
   b. to assist the patient in a peaceful death with dignity.
   c. to provide palliative care.
   d. for patients and families to assume responsibility for the care.

10. Guidelines for the handling of antineoplastic agents in the home are in accordance with those established by:
    a. the Food and Drug Administration.
    b. the Occupational Safety and Health Administration.
    c. the American Nurse's Association.
    d. the Health Care Financing Administration.

11. Which of the following activities or facts is the home health care nurse most likely *not* to teach the patient and/or family in order to ensure safe antibiotic administration in the home?
    a. at what temperature to store the medication
    b. what signs/symptoms of drug side effects to report
    c. how to withdraw heparin from a vial
    d. how to prepare and mix the antibiotic

12. Upon a return visit to a man with metastatic prostate cancer to the ribs, the home health nurse notes that he is in pain and has not been receiving the morphine at the increased frequency prescribed 48 hours earlier. The wife is visibly upset at his discomfort yet is concerned about his increased lethargy when the drug interval was first changed. The nurse's interventions at this point would be directed at:
    a. explaining to the wife that increasing the frequency of the drug is what probably gave him some pain relief and his sleep was a sign that he was comfortable.
    b. empathizing with the wife over her concerns that the decreased drug interval was a sign that her husband was becoming addicted.
    c. congratulating the wife for being astute enough to recognize that the drug was building up in his system.
    d. changing the pain regimen to include a different narcotic.

## ANSWER EXPLANATIONS

1. **The answer is a.** It is important to the family and the caregiver to be able to draw on other people and institutions for support at this time. Success in home care requires that the services needed be available, but the degree of informal support from family, friends, neighbors, church groups, and the like is critical. (p. 1505)

2. **The answer is a.** The homebound status is necessary for insurance and Medicare coverage, and it has to be established and documented by the health care nurse. *Homebound* means that leaving the home requires considerable effort. (p. 1514)

3.   **The answer is c.** A detailed family assessment is important, particularly with regard to the status of the caregiver. Families are categorized as supportive, ambivalent, or hostile, and they generally continue to act in this crisis as they reacted to other crises in the past. (Table 53-3, text page 1509)

4.   **The answer is d.** Evaluation of care is based on patient outcomes. Potential limitations must be considered when outcome measures are used. Expected outcomes should be realistic and achievable so that the patient, caregiver(s), and health care providers are able to provide good care and to feel a sense of satisfaction and accomplishment. The family should know what is realistic and achievable from the start. Choice **b** would be a serious problem—families are better off if they know how to deal with emergencies. (p. 1508)

5.   **The answer is c.** Home care assessment for HPN begins with a visit coincidental with the arrival of equipment. The nurse should review orders for HPN with the supplying agency. The assessment should include the type and status of the venous access device, the patient and family's knowledge of the management of HPN, and an evaluation of the home for safety factors. Adequate refrigeration should be available in the home for a 2–3 week supply of solutions. An electric infusion pump with a battery backup is normally part of the equipment. Choices **a** and eventually **d** are handled by the family; **b** is done by the home infusion therapy company personnel. (p. 1522)

6.   **The answer is a.** Accurate, descriptive documentation of home health nursing care is vital to reimbursement and continuation of home health services. It has been postulated that the rise in health care expenditures, including those for home health care, has led the government and fiscal intermediaries to enact regulations requiring specific documentation and has increased focused review in an effort to decrease costs by denial of payment for services designated by the reviewer as "noncovered." (pp. 1509 and 1515)

7.   **The answer is d.** Family units can be identified as supportive, hostile, or ambivalent with behavior described in terms of cohesion, adaptability, and communication. When crisis occurs or families are faced with the serious and difficult implications of cancer and its treatment, their behavior usually does not change and in some cases can intensify. Therefore, if a family was dysfunctional, hostile, or in conflict, it is very likely that the behavior will continue. The home health care nurse's primary concern is to support and care for the patient. The chances are high that the home health care nurse would be unable to change the behavior of the family members in conflict. (p. 1512)

8.   **The answer is c.** The PICC catheter does require daily flushing and central line dressing changes as frequently as every 3–7 days. Although some PICC catheters have more than one lumen, any lumen can be used for blood withdrawal. The major advantage is that the catheter can be placed by specially trained nurses in the home without the patient's needing to go to the hospital or doctor's office. (p. 1517)

9.   **The answer is d.** Although care does consist of holistic and direct physical care, the ultimate goal is to enable the family and/or patient to provide the care. Choices **b** and **c** apply more to hospice care and not necessarily to home care. The patient and family are encouraged to assume responsibility for the care of the patient. (p. 1505)

10.   **The answer is b.** Potential hazards associated with the administration of antineoplastic agents have prompted the Occupational Safety and Health Administration (OSHA) to set guidelines for compounding, transporting, administering, and disposing of toxic chemotherapy agents. (p. 1520)

11.   **The answer is d.** It is important for the patient and/or family to know at what temperature to store the medication because consideration needs to be given to the stability of the drug. Signs and symptoms are important to know because the nurse will not be present at most infusions. Withdrawal of heparin and heparin administration are required following drug administration in order to keep the VAD patent. Infusion therapy agencies with pharmacies will prepare and deliver the antibiotics and the supplies on schedule. (p. 1523)

12. **The answer is a.** The husband is not becoming addicted but might be experiencing some degree of drug tolerance. This is normal, and it is not uncommon for drug doses to increase over time. He also might be having increased bone metastasis or other sites of pain; further assessment is required. Sleep is often the first sign of pain relief because patients may have been unable to rest comfortably with pain. Patients and caregivers often negatively influence the treatment of pain because of their fears about potent narcotics. They may increase the dose interval, withhold doses, or refuse certain medications or certain routes as they attempt to prevent dependence, addiction, somnolence, or sedation. The wife needs education regarding cancer pain and relief methods, as well as a great deal of support. (p. 1525)

# Chapter 54    Hospice Care

## INTRODUCTION
### Development of the Hospice Concept

- Developers of the hospice concept recognized that allowing a "natural death" requires preparation of the patient and family, changes in medical practice, and redesign or circumvention of some aspects of the existing health care system.
- When hospices first began to appear as organized programs, they were commonly volunteer programs.
- The ideas for the American hospice were adapted directly from the English model at St. Christopher's Hospice, the world's first hospice, developed by Dame Cicely Saunders in 1968.
- Today, hospice care is specialized care for terminally ill people. Hospice care is a medically directed, interdisciplinary team-managed program of services that focuses on the patient/family as the unit of service. Hospice care is palliative rather than curative.

### Role of Nurses in the Development of Hospice

- Dame Cicely Saunders, medical director and founder of St. Christopher's Hospice, developed many of the current concepts in palliative care, including oral narcotic administration on a regular rather than on an as-needed basis.
- In 1984 the Joint Commission on Accreditation of Hospitals (JCAH) published its first standards manual for hospice programs.
- Another factor influencing the development of palliative care was the groundbreaking work in the 1960s of Elisabeth Kübler-Ross, a psychiatrist at the University of Chicago. Dr. Kübler-Ross helped to demystify the dying process by devising the radical teaching technique of interviewing dying patients in front of a group of health care professionals.

## PALLIATIVE CARE APPROACHES

- Palliative management involves a shift in treatment goals from curative toward providing relief from suffering.

### Principles of Palliative Care

- The overall goal of treatment is to optimize quality of life; that is, the hopes and desires of a patient are fulfilled. Death is regarded as a natural process, to be neither hastened nor prolonged.
- Diagnostic and invasive procedures are minimized, unless likely to result in the alleviation of symptoms.
- When using narcotic analgesics, the right dose is the dose that provides pain relief without unacceptable side effects. The patient is the "expert" on whether pain and symptoms have been adequately relieved.

### Palliative versus Acute Care

- In an acute care situation, a patient will have diagnostic studies to determine the etiology of the problem.

- When the goal of care is palliation, the etiology generally is either already known or could be unimportant if the patient has a short time to live.

## Patient Criteria for Hospice Care

- For a patient to qualify for the Medicare Hospice Benefit, two physicians must certify that he or she is terminally ill and has less than six months to live. This latter criterion is controversial: accurate predictions of time of death cannot be made.
- It has proven to be even more difficult to predict prognosis in noncancer end-stage patients.
- At the urging of the Health Care Finance Administration (HCFA), guidelines were revised in 1996 with more comprehensive criteria for eight categories of non-cancer, end-stage illness: heart, pulmonary, and liver disease; dementia; and HIV.
- The patient must sign a consent form or election statement declaring that hospice and palliative care are their choice of treatments and that they have the right to elect out of hospice at any time.
- Additional criteria required by most hospice programs include:
  - The patient must have a primary caregiver.
  - The patient needs to reside in the hospice program's geographic area.
  - The patient must desire palliative, not curative, treatment.

## HOSPICE CARE IN THE PRESENT

- Federal guidelines that define the Hospice Medicare Benefit Plan include cost incentives for encouraging home hospice care rather than hospitalization and cost control via a financial cap for all hospice care provided.

## Models of Hospice Care

- The present models for hospice care vary greatly in their size and the means by which they provide care.
- While 40% of all hospices are independent, community-based programs, others are owned by hospitals or operated as part of a home health agency. A small percentage are coalition programs or operated in a nursing home setting. Coalition programs are usually a negotiated care service contracted between long-term care facilities and hospice.
- According to Medicare guidelines, at least 80% of an individual hospice's aggregate patient days of care under the Hospice Benefit must be provided at home.
- If the maximum aggregate inpatient ratio of 20% is exceeded, the hospice can be denied reimbursement for the excess days.
- Medicare guidelines dictate that a full-service hospice be a medically directed program that incorporates home nursing care, social services, home health aid care, dietary counseling, occupational therapy, physical therapy, speech therapy, and counseling, along with trained volunteers to complete the nucleus of core services.
- The Medicare Hospice Benefit is the only federally funded health care program mandating the use of volunteers.
- Nursing and physician services, as well as medications, must be available 24 hours a day. In addition, the hospice must provide bereavement follow-up to the patient's family after death.

## Reimbursement and Funding Methods

- Hospice care was a prototype for what is now commonly referred to as *case management*. Consistent with this case management approach is the Medicare Hospice Benefit's capitated per diem reimbursement structure that pays a flat daily rate for all services provided rather than paying for individual services or items on the traditional fee-for-service basis.

- The per diem for the Medicare Hospice Benefit is reimbursed on four levels, as defined by the HCFA: (1) a routine rate, (2) a continuous rate for home care, (3) an inpatient rate for acute care, and (4) an inpatient rate for respite care.
- Recertification of the patient's appropriateness for hospice care is required three times under the benefit.
- Eighty-nine percent of current hospices are operated not for profit.

## Patient Population

- Of the patients who received hospice care in 1992, 78% were diagnosed with cancer, 4% had AIDS, 10% had end-stage heart disease, 1% had Alzheimer's disease, and 1% had renal diagnoses. The remaining 6% had "other" terminal conditions.
- Tables 54-1 and 54-2 demonstrate some of the unique challenges presented by a young patient whose care follows the multidisciplinary care management hospice model.

## NURSING AND HOSPICE CARE

### Nurse's Role

- It is imperative that the nurse be an experienced practitioner who develops skill in the specialized area of symptom management and support of the terminally ill.
- The nurse works cooperatively and communicates effectively within a multidisciplinary framework to actively promote holistic palliative care for hospice patients and their families.
- The education and experience required for hospice nurses vary among hospice programs.
- The ability of the nurse to foster a relaxed, warm, personal relationship with the patient, family, and other team members helps to promote confidence in achieving the goals of care.

### Management of Care Issues

- The nurse provides basic nursing care and assesses the patient response to current care approaches and generally determines what and when changes need to be made.
- See Tables 54-3 and 54-4 for a summation of selected principles and approaches for symptom management in palliative care.
- Ongoing assessment of pain is an activity best accomplished with a formal assessment tool. Some hospice programs use a pain-intensity scale numbered 0–5, with 0 indicating no pain and 5 denoting maximum pain.
- Effective physical assessment skills can make a difference in identifying a potential problem early enough for timely intervention to occur.
- A nurse on the hospice team is available to the patient on call 24 hours, 7 days a week, to address questions or concerns that develop between visits by the team. A physician also is available on a 24-hour basis to assist in consultation on medical issues.
- The nurse instructs the patient and family in the skills needed to provide safe and comfortable home care.
- Teaching tools should include written material to be left in the home whenever possible.

## DEATH IN THE HOME

- It is common for patients and families to respond initially to the idea of death at home with fear and anxiety.
- Patients' overriding concerns about death at home often revolve around being a burden to their family.
- For most families, the ability to provide care for a home death will require teaching them about the death event itself, immediate signs of death, how to relieve symptoms and suffering, and how to access professional help when needed.

## Advantages of Home Death

- Loss of control may be the most overwhelming and distressing feeling.
- Terminal care and death at home can afford the patient and family control over their environment, as well as the comfort of being in the midst of familiar surroundings.
- Rather than being protected from the illness and death, children can benefit from being involved in very concrete ways to better understand the dying process and facilitate their own grief.
- Being cared for at home can afford the opportunity for an alert patient to maintain his or her family role.
- At home, unwanted medical intervention is much less likely to occur than for a patient in a hospital or nursing home setting.

## Disadvantages of Home Death

- Caregivers, particularly those lacking social outlets or family support, may find the physical and emotional task of home care and home death too difficult.
- Although most anticipated deaths occur quietly without physical distress, the occasional patient may have symptoms too difficult to manage at home; hospitalization may be the better option.
- An initial psychosocial assessment of the patient and family in the home environment, together with the nursing assessment of the patient, provides the basis for planning care and determining patient and family needs.
- At each subsequent home visit, the hospice staff must reevaluate the patient/family situation and revise plans as necessary.

## Preparation of the Patient and Family

- Once home death has been established as a desired goal, an individualized home care plan is developed with the patient and family.
- The primary caregiver is continually and carefully assessed to determine what he or she wants to do and is capable of doing for direct care.

### Knowledge and preparation for the death event

- Families need to be prepared for the actual time of patient's death and the time immediately preceding it. The most difficult aspect of preparation is that each patient is an individual and each death occurs in a way that may not be completely predictable.
- Table 54-5, text page 1542, is an example of a patient and family instruction sheet that lists many of the common signs seen in patients who are imminently dying.

### Funeral arrangements

- In most situations a home death will go more smoothly if the patient and/or family chooses a funeral home before the death occurs.
- The hospice team should be a resource to families as to different types of funeral homes available in their area.
- The hospice team needs to be a resource to ensure that the family is aware of local ordinances or laws surrounding an expected home death.

## Availability of the Hospice Team

- Of utmost importance in supporting families through a patient's home death is instructing them on how to access the hospice team at any time.

- Families should be encouraged to call about any changes in the patient's status or for what may seem like minor questions to them.

## Facilitating Grief

- As family members prepare for the death of a loved one at home, they are also preparing themselves for the loss. This is often referred to as *anticipatory grief.*
- It may be helpful to explore with family members previous losses and coping mechanisms used. The family is encouraged to identify and discuss unresolved issues with the dying person.
- Preparing family members for the death of their loved one often means discussing issues the nurse assesses they may not yet be ready to hear.

## BEREAVEMENT CARE

- Bereavement support is a required component of hospice care under Medicare and most state licensing regulations.
- Grieving is a normal reaction to loss, with a wide variety of physical and emotional manifestations, such as loss of appetite, sleeplessness, heart palpitations, lack of energy, sadness, and anger.
- Four tasks necessary for the normal grief process to progress include:
  1. to accept the reality of the loss
  2. to experience the pain of grief
  3. to adjust to the environment in which the deceased is missing
  4. to withdraw emotional energy and replace it in another relationship
- The goal of bereavement care or counseling is to assist and support survivors to move through the loss and toward resolution.
- Hospice programs generally follow survivors for one year, the usual time frame in which the most acute grief occurs, not the period in which mourning is completed.
- Methods of bereavement care commonly include a bereavement assessment, contact of survivors at regularly scheduled intervals, and, as necessary, additional referrals for professional counseling for those with complicated or abnormal grief reactions.

## Abnormal Grief

- Survivors unable to progress through the tasks of mourning will develop some form of abnormal or complicated grief.
- Generally, complicated grief will manifest itself in one of three ways: prolonged; masked in behavioral or physical symptoms; or exaggerated expressions of normal grief reactions, such as excessive anger, sadness, or depression.
- Because unresolved grief has been associated with multiple physical and emotional illnesses, including increased risk of suicide, facilitation of anticipatory grieving and bereavement can be viewed as preventive health care for survivors.

## STRESS AND THE HOSPICE NURSE

- Staff attitudes toward death can be greatly influenced by unresolved grief issues in their own personal or professional lives.
- Stress can be increased due to unrealistic expectations of ourselves, our coworkers, or the therapy we use to manage symptoms.
- Caregivers with high-stress jobs who cope successfully are able to recognize when signs of stress are developing within themselves, acknowledge their own limits, and initiate self-help techniques or seek the help of others.

## LEGAL AND ETHICAL ISSUES SURROUNDING HOSPICE CARE

### Advance Directives

- The federal Patient Self-Determination Act, enacted in December 1991, requires hospices, hospitals, and other health care agencies to provide patients, on admission, with written information about two key areas: (1) their right to accept or refuse treatment under state law and (2) ways to execute advance directives such as a living will and a durable power of attorney for health care.
- Hospice team members provide whatever information is needed to assist the patient in making an informed decision, especially when it affects the patient's decision not to have CPR, intravenous fluids, or tube feedings.
- Hospice patients and families may need reassurance that their focus on comfort and quality of life is being reinforced by their decision not to have CPR. This same approach holds true when the decision not to have intravenous fluids or tube feedings is challenged.
- Fluid depletion has the following benign effects on quality of life:
  - Urine output is decreased, so there is less incontinence.
  - Gastric secretions lessen; therefore, episodes of vomiting decrease.
  - Pulmonary secretions lessen, resulting in less congestion.
  - Peripheral edema secondary to tumor subsides, resulting in decreased pain from nerve compression.
  - Although the sensation of dry mouth and thirst may increase, this can be relieved by good mouth care and small amounts of oral fluids.
- Life-and-death decisions depend on the availability of written evidence of the patient's wishes.
- In general, the power of attorney for health care is more useful than the living will. A living will is applicable only when it pertains to a terminal illness but not for a patient whose health is declining for medical reasons other than those that can be classified as terminal or if the patient is in a permanent vegetative state.
- Through the power of attorney for health care, the patient chooses an agent to act on the patient's behalf if the patient is no longer competent to make decisions.

### Euthanasia and Suicide

- Euthanasia has come to mean the intentional taking of the life of a terminally ill person for purposes of compassion.
  - Active euthanasia is achieved by "doing something."
  - Passive euthanasia can be described as "not doing something" that would preserve life, yet without being significantly burdensome.
  - Pain medication or other symptom management measures that are used in unusual quantity to improve comfort but could lead to an early death should not be considered euthanasia. The operative and distinguishing concept is intent. If the intent is to relieve pain or manage symptoms and not to cause death, then the unintentional hastening of death by such care is not euthanasia.
- The NHO has taken a formal and firm position against physician-assisted suicide.
- When someone asks about, or expresses the desire for, euthanasia, the appropriate initial response from an individual nurse is a listening and caring attitude, followed by careful exploration of the patient's or family member's concerns or fears.

## FUTURE TRENDS AND CHALLENGES FOR HOSPICE CARE

### Underserved Populations

- African-American and Hispanic populations historically have been underserved by health care agencies and hospice.

- Both of these minority populations are under-represented or totally lacking among hospice staff and volunteers.
- Children represent another underserved population in the United States.
- Patients with AIDS represent a tremendous challenge to hospice.
- AIDS patients utilize more resources than have been the norm for hospice patients. Their care is more complex and requires longer and more frequent nursing and social work visits. Patients with AIDS may require more attendant or custodial care.
- Medications and supplies used are more varied and expensive.
- The course of AIDS is less predictable than that of most cancers, making prognostication within the six-month criterion difficult.

## Research Issues

- Existing research focuses on pain and symptom management and psychosocial care. Areas least studied are volunteerism and spiritual care, the features most unique to hospice.
- Both hospice models and hospice patient populations inherently make research difficult. Limited funding and the relative lack of hospice and palliative care programs associated with academic institutions provide additional barriers to research.

## Integration into Health Care Practices

- Terminal care should be integrated into all health care practice, particularly in the areas of oncology, geriatrics, and AIDS.
- Hospice now needs to integrate and adapt to the challenges facing our ever-changing health care system such as the following:
  - health insurance plans promoting hospice as a cost-effective care approach
  - accessing hospice care earlier
  - delivering cost-effective care
  - contracting with HMOs and managed care

# PRACTICE QUESTIONS

1. The basic medical and nursing approach toward patients in a hospice program is:
   a. acute care.
   b. curative care.
   c. palliative care.
   d. euthanasia care.

2. When caring for the patient in a hospice setting, who is the "expert" on whether pain and/or symptoms have been adequately relieved?
   a. The primary caregiver
   b. The attending physician
   c. The primary nurse
   d. The patient

3. The hospice nurse may decide in the initial interview that patient criteria for hospice care will not be met because:
   a. the patient's spouse expresses his wish to be involved in his wife's care.
   b. the patient has entered a clinical trial through the National Cancer Institute.
   c. the patient's home is 5 minutes from the hospice offices.
   d. the patient does not wish to be resuscitated if she stops breathing at home.

4. The husband of a woman with end-stage breast cancer is concerned that his wife is sleeping more and is not even waking to eat or drink. The hospice nurse would explain to the husband that:
   a. these are signs of approaching death.
   b. the pain medication has reached a high blood level and needs to be reduced.
   c. there is no reason to be concerned.
   d. her oncologist should be called in order to obtain some direction for her care.

5. Which of the following grief reactions of an elderly woman who has lost her husband of 40 years would prompt the hospice nurse to suggest counseling?
   a. She takes out 40 years' worth of photograph albums and wants to review her marriage and life with her deceased husband with the hospice nurse.
   b. She refuses to let her sister and brother-in-law into her home anymore, blaming them for buying her husband cigarettes "all those years."
   c. She plans her husband's funeral by herself, listens to all his favorite classical music pieces and chooses passages from his bible.
   d. She delegates all the responsibility for disposition of her husband's belongings to the children.

6. Which of the following "directions" provides patients who are at risk for loss of decision-making ability the best chance of having their health care wishes carried out?
   a. Power of attorney for health care
   b. Verbal instructions to the attending physician
   c. A living will
   d. A do-not-intubate/ventilate order on admission

## ANSWER EXPLANATIONS

1. **The answer is c.** Hospice care pivots around the idea of palliative medical management. Palliative management involves a shift in treatment goals from curative toward providing relief from suffering. Euthanasia means active interventions to hasten a person's death and this is NOT the philosophy of hospice care. (p. 1533)

2. **The answer is d.** The patient is the "expert" on whether pain and symptoms have been adequately relieved. This is a principle of palliative care. (p. 1533)

3. **The answer is b.** Clinical trials are experimental medical trials often developed to see if there is any disease response to a new antineoplastic regimen. Patients and their families often turn to an experimental procedure when there are limited, if any, options remaining that might halt their disease progress. This choice suggests that the patient has not agreed to palliative care and is still pursuing curative treatment. Further assessment is indicated here to make sure this is not the case, because a patient criteria for hospice care is that the patient is agreeable to palliative and not curative care. The remaining three options are actually patient criteria for hospice care: the patient has a primary caregiver; the patient resides in the hospice program's geographic area; and some programs require that the patient has a DNR status prior to admission to the hospice program. (p. 1533)

4. **The answer is a.** The hospice team's goal is to help the family prepare for their loved one's death. Families need to be prepared for the actual time of the patient's death and what universal signs they can anticipate. Increasing sleep, a gradual decrease in need for food and drink, increased confusion or restlessness, decreasing temperature of extremities, and irregular breathing patterns may occur. Calling the oncologist would be indicating the need for intervention, when in fact the goal of care is purely palliative. The pain relief regimen should not be altered if the patient is comfortable, even if the patient is sleeping more and death is approaching. (Table 54-5, p. 1542)

5. **The answer is b.** Abnormal grief may manifest itself in exaggerated or excessive expressions of normal grief reactions, such as excessive anger, sadness, or depression. For most hospice programs, therapy for abnormal grief extends beyond the scope of the bereavement care services provided. The hospice program staff should be able to identify and recommend competent referrals for abnormal grief syndromes. It is therapeutic to review a person's life with their loved one. Listening to a family member share stories of their life with the loved one honors the meaning of their relationship and their life together. Funeral planning can be therapeutic and facilitate someone's loss as they do one last thing in a special way for their loved one. Delegating responsibilities that can be overwhelming or too painful might actually be an indicator of the grieving party being aware of their limitations and calling on their resources and support systems. (p. 1544)

6. **The answer is a.** A living will may be applicable only when it pertains to a terminal illness but not for a patient whose health is declining for medical reasons other than those that can be classified as terminal or if the patient is in a vegetative state. In general, the power of attorney for health care is more useful than the living will. The living will does not identify another person who can act as the agent for a disabled patient. Verbal instructions are of little value if a family member or anyone else chooses to argue against what has been reportedly verbally communicated. Written instructions are necessary. An order that instructs not to intubate does not address any other interventions that might be suggested. (p. 1546)

# Chapter 55    Impact of Changing Health Care Economics on Cancer Nursing Practice

**This chapter corresponds to Chapter 56 in *Cancer Nursing: Principles and Practice*, Fourth Edition.**

## INTRODUCTION

- Multiple internal and external forces have converged to transform the health care industry.
- Nursing is moving from a profession focused on caring for patients in the hospital to one concerned about the health of communities.
- Change began in the 1980s with the advent of prospective payment models from government payers.

## CHANGING HEALTH CARE ECONOMICS

### Prospective Payment Model

- Diagnostic related groups (DRGs) were initiated by the federal government in the 1980s.
- The payment model is a "case rate" in which providers are reimbursed a predetermined amount based on a given illness or incident.
- Health maintenance organizations (HMOs), preferred provider organizations (PPOs), and independent practice associations (IPAs) have risen in numbers at significant cost savings.

### Health Care Delivery Models

- Managed care health plans reduce costs. The major models are HMO, PPO, point of service (POS), and physician-hospital organization (PHO), which are differentiated by structure, provider risk-sharing, and degree of consumer choice of services, locations, and providers.

#### Health maintenance organization (HMO)

- HMOs (the oldest and largest type of managed care) contract to provide health care at a prenegotiated rate on a "per member per month" basis. The early success of HMOs was related to two major factors: the assumption of financial risk by physicians and the combining of the costs of all services (hospitals, ambulatory services, and physicians) into one charge.
- The basis of the HMO model is primary care physician (PCP) who is selected by the participant. All care must be authorized by this physician (frequently referred to as the "gatekeeper"), who is paid a fixed amount per patient to coordinate the care.
- HMOs can be divided into three types based upon the relationship between the physician and health care facility: staff model, group model, and network models.
- In a staff model HMO, all physicians are employed and salaried by the HMO.
- In a group model HMO plan, the physicians are not salaried, but have a contractual arrangement. The physician is compensated through the private practice.
- Both staff and group models are referred to as "closed models" due to the inability of community physicians to participate, with the care being rendered only by the HMO-designated physicians.
- The third plan, the network model, requires that physicians contract directly with the HMO, but the physicians continue to deliver care in their own private offices and also to treat non-HMO patients.
- This plan is referred to as an "open model" and is becoming a very popular option.

- Information about how various HMOs compare is available from Health Plan Employer Data and Information Set (HEDIS).

### Preferred provider organization (PPO)

- In a PPO, contractual arrangements are negotiated between payers and health care providers (hospitals and/or physicians) to render care at a predetermined discounted amount.
- Members of PPOs have a greater variety of choices.

### Point of service (POS) plans

- The POS plan allows members to access out-of-plan providers but imposes strict utilization strategies.

### Physician-hospital organization (PHO)

- In a PHO, there is a contractual relationship between physicians and the hospital to accomplish several goals: to increase the opportunity to obtain managed-care contracts, to align the organizational structure with the financial incentives found in capitation, and to measure quality of care through outcomes.

### Integrated delivery systems (IDSs)

- PHOs often organize into integrated delivery systems (IDSs) to provide care more efficiently. IDSs can be both vertically and horizontally integrated.
- Vertical integration means that services such as inpatient, outpatient, radiation therapy, home care, physician office, and hospice oncology services are capable of being provided within the same system.
- Horizontal integration is when these services are provided at different sites in the community.
- The strength of a vertically and horizontally integrated system is not in ownership of facilities and services and large corporate offices, but rather in the ability to provide the optimal delivery method of care for the patients.

## Impact of Managed Care

- The differences among HMOs, PPOs, and fee-for-service (indemnity) plans have begun to fade.
- The public sector has demonstrated interest in promoting managed-care risk products for both Medicare and Medicaid programs in order to decrease their costs.

## Payment Models

- Financial incentives change behavior more effectively than stringent utilization management strategies.
- Thus the payment model selected will have a more significant impact on reducing costs than any other variable.

### Indemnity plans

- Prior to the advent of DRGs, over 90% of all Americans were covered under indemnity plans (also referred to as "fee-for-service"); there were no financial incentives to conserve resources by either the hospital or physician.

## Discount from charges

- Discount from charges is a modification of the fee-for-service model. The underlying premise of reimbursement for each service tendered remains unchanged, but a discount is negotiated from the provider.

## Per diem payments

- Per diem payment programs reimburse for each day of hospitalization; this strategy has led to increased length of stay (LOS), as there are no incentives to shorten stay in acute-care settings.

## Capitation

- Capitation is an established dollar amount "per member per month," regardless of the services rendered by the providers; thus, providers have an incentive to keep enrollees healthy and prevent utilization of all services.
- Capitation generally includes both specialist and primary care services (full capitation) to prevent cost shifting to a noncapitated component.
- Full capitation has raised ethical concerns regarding quality of care as a result of data indicating significant reductions in referrals to specialists.
- Instruments such as HEDIS and NCDQ accreditation standards will assist in objectively evaluating quality of care.

## Case rates

- *Case rates* provide the institution with a set amount of money per procedure or service. Case rate is the model used for the Medicare DRG system.
- *Global rate* is a case rate that encompasses both the physician component and hospital costs for specific incidents. The global rate prevents cost shifting from physicians to the hospital.
- *Churning* refers to the practice of increasing procedures and visits to enhance revenue as fees are discounted. *Upcoding* occurs when physicians report a more complex level of care or diagnosis to enhance reimbursement. Both of these practices are unnecessary with a capitated model.

## Determining Cost of Service

### Charges/cost

- The first step in analyzing cost of service is to determine the costs of the specific diagnoses being examined. It is important not to confuse charge with cost. The charge is simply the price that is set initially for the service, while the cost is the actual dollar amount it takes to deliver the service

### Net revenue

- Payers are now routinely negotiating discounts from providers; thus net revenue (discounts subtracted from the charges) is the primary number to review when revenue is examined.

### Direct/indirect costs

- Costs are classified from two different perspectives: behavior in relation to volume and ability to trace the service to a patient. The latter is separated into two categories: direct and indirect.
- Direct costs can be traced clearly to a specific patient or service. Indirect costs frequently are referred to as overhead costs.

### Variable/fixed costs

- Variable costs change in relation to the number of patients cared for. The fixed costs remain stable as the number of patients changes.

### Net operating income

- Once the net operating revenue is determined (by subtracting the discount negotiated by the payer from the charges), total operating costs can be subtracted to obtain the net operating income. By dividing net operating income into the net revenue, the profit margin percent ratio can be obtained.

## INDUSTRY RESPONSE TO THE ECONOMIC ENVIRONMENT

### Move to Outpatient Care

- By the year 2000, a multispecialty group of 40 physicians will be capable of performing in its offices 80%–90% of the procedures currently performed in a 300-bed community hospital.
- Excess inpatient capacity in many markets is leading to brutal, unrelenting price competition and the necessity for massive downsizing.

### Implementation of Case Management

- Case management is a collaborative process that promotes quality care for the individual and cost-effective results or outcomes for the health care coverage provider.
- Typically, case managers are registered nurses who are responsible for managing care for patients with complex and potentially costly diseases such as cancer.
- Case managers act as advocates for both the patient and the program.

### Development/Utilization of Critical Pathways and Guidelines

- The development of critical pathways results in a plan of action that delineates the critical components or key indicators necessary to achieve a given outcome at the most efficient cost.

### Implications for Nursing

- Personnel costs, especially costs of professional caregivers, have been the target of cost-cutting efforts.
- Nursing positions have been replaced with lesser-trained individuals.

## NURSING APPROACHES TO THE CHANGING HEALTH CARE ENVIRONMENT

### Partnering with MDs

- Physicians have moved from being a customer of nursing to being a partner of nursing.
- Some hospitals have physician and nursing leaders as partners in providing day-to-day operational direction to specific service lines such as cancer.

### Benchmarking

- Benchmarking identifies "best practice" in relation to current performance. There are several indicators that are extremely helpful to benchmark: skill mix, nursing hours per patient day (NHPPD), cost per case, and length of stay.

### Productivity Standards/Skill Mix

- Defining NHPPD for the specific units is critical to achieving financial targets and can be essential for a hospital's survival.

- Involving the staff in collecting the benchmark data on the NHPPD promotes acceptance of the validity of the data more effectively than a "top-down" approach.
- Quality indicators are being developed by multiple professional organizations to begin measuring the impact of changes in registered nurse ratios and NHPPD upon care of the patient.

## Outcome Measurements

- In response to aggressively managed guidelines by HMOs and the advent of outcomes research, a new field has emerged: disease management. The underlying premise is that chronic diseases such as cancer or diabetes can be managed more effectively long term (lower costs and increased quality of life) by protocol-driven actions along the continuum of care.

## SPECIFIC ECONOMIC ISSUES IN CANCER CARE

- In September 1994 the National Cancer Advisory Board (NCAB) Subcommittee to Evaluate the National Cancer Program identified six major issues to be addressed if we are to prevail in our war on cancer. These are listed on p. 1596.

## Oncology Networks

- The concepts of *oncology networks* and *integrated systems* have emerged to respond to economic changes.
- The key components of value in integrated delivery systems include:
  1. Competitive position
  2. Standardized diagnostic/treatment protocols
  3. Measurable, documented quality patient outcomes and survival rates

### Hospital alliances

- A simple alliance model aligns cancer programs at separate hospitals and retains separate day-to-day management of the two cancer programs.
- A second structure identified as a "feeder" system aligns smaller hospitals offering fewer cancer services with larger centers that offer more specialized care.
- The third model features a strong, centralized ownership of facilities.
- The fourth model links a hospital or provider of care with an oncology "carve-out" organization. In effect, the carve-out takes charge of all cancer care provided to alliance members.
- See Table 56-1, text page 1597, for more on models for hospital alliances.

### Physician/hospital alliances

- Numerous services typically provided by a network through its participants or through ancillary provider contracts in a capitated environment are listed on pages 1596 and 1597, showing office-based, hospital-based, and ancillary provider-based services.

### Physician networks

- One of the fastest-growing methods for grouping together physicians of varying specialties is a physician practice management group, or PPM.

### Academic center alliances

- A number of alliances have occurred both among academic institutions and among academic institutions and community organizations.

## Clinical Trials

- Trials sponsored by drug companies generally do not pose a financial concern for oncology programs.
- A major barrier for both patients and institutions to participation in national studies is that third-party payers do not cover experimental treatment, which includes all research trials.
- From a community program perspective, the benefit to participation in clinical trials is the ability to provide patients access to state-of-the-art therapies for cancer treatment, control, and prevention.
- Insurers have developed various criteria for defining the experimental status of medical treatments and procedures that relate to one or more of the following categories: scientific criteria, research criteria, and professional criteria.
- Of primary concern is whether oncology programs will be able to financially support participation in cancer prevention and control trials in the future. The NCI clearly is committed to research to prevent cancer as well as to improve the quality of life for those who develop cancer.

## Cancer Drugs and Managed Care

- Two major concerns exist regarding cancer drugs in the managed-care environment. The first is whether or not new drug research will be slowed as the snowballing influence of managed care intensifies. The second is the long-standing need for approval of off-label usage of chemotherapeutic agents.

## Critical Pathways/Care Guidelines

- A number of national-level efforts to develop cancer treatment guidelines are underway.
- Critical pathways usually describe a protocol specific for a particular organization or for a detailed patient management plan for a specific procedure.
- A clinical algorithm clearly defines decision points in the care process and provides explicit directions to the caregiver.
- Future guideline development will require definition of care across the continuum.

## Continuum of Care

- A number of initiatives hold promise for improvements in the provision of care and consumer outcomes:
  1. Oncology care has long emphasized the diagnostic and treatment segments of the continuum of care with a recent shift to the left of the continuum with emphasis on prevention and keeping people healthy.
     - HMOs and third-party payers are including clauses in their policies that allow different levels of coverage based upon the insured's health habits.
     - The National Cancer Institute is placing greater emphasis on cancer prevention clinical trials.
  2. Initiatives are expected to grow for screening of those cancers for which early diagnosis benefits patient outcomes.
  3. Diagnostic workup and treatment planning will become more efficient with the increase in the number and availability of multispecialty clinics in the community setting.
  4. Efficient movement of the patient across the continuum will continue and improve as case management becomes refined.
  5. As care shifts to the outpatient setting, home care and hospice services will become more fully integrated into the care-planning and guideline-development process.

## ONCOLOGY NURSING: POSITIONING FOR THE FUTURE

- Within the nursing profession, several values and assumptions must be reassessed to meet the future demands of health care systems. These are reflected in the following four paradigm shifts:

1. Our practice must evolve from a needs-driven model of care to one that is sensitive to limited resources.
2. Nurses believe that there is a direct correlation between manpower and quality. The true correlation is between critical thinking and quality.
3. Standardization and routines for patient care will be replaced by individualization and creativity.
4. Accountability, responsibility, and authority for clinical decision making will evolve from the manager to the practitioner, in partnership with the patient.

## Nursing Roles

- The diminishing role of hospitals within the health care continuum means the real future for nurses may lie elsewhere: in HMOs, ambulatory surgery centers, home care, nursing homes, etc.
- Table 56-2, text page 1602, lists ten major forecasts for cancer in the twenty-first century. As this table reflects, new "hybrids" of oncology nurses will emerge.
- McCaffrey-Boyle et al project the following changes:
  1. Nurses will take on the role of health care broker (case manager), matching patient needs to finite resources. They will have admitting privileges.
  2. Nurses' work focus will include an intense orientation to wellness, and they will render health-prescriptive services at the worksite.
  3. Critical care oncology nurses of the future will have prescriptive capabilities, including titration of biologics and supervision of complex ventilator weaning and extubation.

## Advanced Practice Roles

- The Oncology Nursing Society (ONS) endorses the title *advanced practice nurse* (APN) to designate clinical nurse specialist (CNS) and nurse practitioner (NP) roles in oncology nursing. The ONS notes that the term advanced practice nurse does not imply the merger of the CNS and NP roles, nor does it exclude other master's prepared nurses in education, administration, or research roles.
- Nurses in advanced practice roles can make major impacts in the following areas:
  1. Provision of direct patient care, as a physician extender
  2. Assisting the staff nurse to develop critical thinking skills, raising the level of assessment
  3. Monitoring and evaluating outcomes of care.

## Setting Ethical Standards

- The American Nurses' Association outlined the precepts that form a values base for the entire nursing profession in the ANA's *Code for Nurses*. This code delineates the fundamental ethical mandates that apply to all nursing roles and transcend varied practice settings and changing clinical realities.
- The Oncology Nursing Society's five core values of *respectful care*, *quality of life*, *competence*, *collegiality*, and *fairness* speak from the shared experience of oncology nurses and provide a context for applying the *Code for Nurses* in oncology nursing practice.

## A CONTROVERSIAL ISSUE IN CANCER CARE
## Use of Unlicensed Personnel

- Budgetary constraints and the effects of the nursing shortage of the late 1980s—early 1990s have caused a restructuring of the delivery of nursing care in acute care hospitals by the addition of unlicensed assistive personnel (AP) as a clinical support service to the professional nursing staff.
- There are widely diverse opinions regarding the use of unlicensed personnel and the implications for both nursing practice and the quality of patient care.
- Until nurses are able to clearly define the value of the professional caregiver, there will always be less expensive personnel available to perform tasks.

- In March 1996, the Oncology Nursing Society presented a position paper entitled *Assistive Person-nel: Their Use in Cancer Care.* ONS proposes "the oncology nurse who assesses, plans, implements, monitors, intervenes, evaluates, and coordinates the patient's plan of care, regardless of the patient's disease status or the setting in which care is provided, is accountable and responsible for all nursing care tasks delegated by her/him to an AP." This paper states:
- Patient care activities may be delegated to APs when the patient is stable, has a predictable disease trajectory, controlled symptoms and side effects, and predictable care outcomes. Activities that may be delegated with appropriate supervision include:
  - Activities of daily living
  - Vital signs
  - Measuring intake and output
  - Non-nursing tasks such as clerical work, stocking supplies, and errands
  - Other limited, routine, patient care activities
- Patient care activities should not be delegated to APs when the patient's condition is not stable or when care outcomes are not predictable. These situations include, but are not limited to:
  - Complex patients with multiple, interrelated problems (e.g., patients with acute leukemia not in remission or superior vena cava syndrome)
  - Patients who are symptomatic due to critical lab values
  - Patients who are undergoing bone marrow transplant
  - Patients who are critically ill or medically unstable (e.g., patients with sepsis or DIC)
  - Patients with uncontrolled or poorly controlled pain
  - Patients with or who are exhibiting early signs/symptoms indicative of oncologic emergencies
  - Patients with complex disease processes and poorly controlled symptoms and treatment-related side effects
- Finally, the Oncology Nursing Society states that the following list of nursing care functions, although neither exhaustive nor all inclusive, should be performed by oncology registered nurses (with appropriate education and experience) and should not be delegated to APs:
  - Antineoplastic and biotherapy administration and management
  - Assessment and management of patients receiving brachytherapy
  - Pain assessment and management
  - Wound assessment and management
  - Symptom assessment, management, and toxicity grading
  - Extravasation assessment and management
  - Medication administration, assessment, and management
  - Assessment and management of patient and family psychosocial needs
  - Disease, treatment, and survivorship-related patient and family education
  - Clinical trials education, administration, and documentation
  - Assessment, management, and troubleshooting of intravenous catheters; venous, arterial, peri-toneal, and intraventricular access devices; and ambulatory pumps (routine site care may be delegated)
  - Assessment and management of long-term survivor issues
  - Assessment and management of end-of-life care (components of care and/or comfort measures may be delegated)
  - Facilitation of advanced directives
  - Communication with multidisciplinary team members
  - Development, assessment, and evaluation of patient care plans and discharge planning (in collaboration with others)

## PRACTICE QUESTIONS

1. The early success of HMOs was related to:
   a. the assumption of financial risk by physicians.
   b. the combining of the costs of all services into one charge.
   c. the ability to gain access to a wide variety of care without the need for a "gatekeeper."
   d. a and b only.

2. Jean works in a clinic where the physicians are not salaried, but have a contractual arrangement. Each physician is compensated through the private practice. The HMO Jean's clinic works with is operating on the:
   a. staff model.
   b. group model.
   c. network model.
   d. open model.

3. The hospital in your community approaches a number of physicians and meets with them, campaigning to form a contractual relationship to increase the opportunity to obtain managed-care contracts and align the organizational structure with the financial incentives found in capitation. Such an arrangement is referred to as a:
   a. physician-hospital organization.
   b. preferred provider organization.
   c. health maintenance organization.
   d. none of the above.

4. Rebecca's health plan committee at work has reviewed complaints from employees about their lack of ability to access care outside the present plan if they require a treatment found only in one of their city's two research hospitals. In response, the company switches to a plan that allows members to access out-of-plan providers but imposes strict utilization strategies. This is most likely a(n):
   a. point of service (POS) plan.
   b. health maintenance organization (HMO).
   c. physician-hospital organization (PHO).
   d. preferred provider organization (PPO).

5. A Chicago PHO is organized into an integrated delivery system that uses different sites in the community to provide a wide variety of services. This is referred to as:
   a. vertical integration.
   b. horizontal integration.
   c. depth of services.
   d. none of the above.

6. As part of the plan under which your clinic operates, providers are paid an established dollar amount "per member per month," regardless of the services rendered. This can be described as a(n) _____ model.
   a. case rate
   b. discount from charges
   c. capitation
   d. per diem

7. A physician is accused of reporting a more complex level of care or diagnosis to enhance reimbursement. This practice is referred to as:
   a. upcoding.
   b. churning.
   c. using case rates.
   d. instituting a global rate.

8. The head nurse or clinical nurse specialist on staff in a program is an example of a:
   a. variable direct labor.
   b. overhead.
   c. fixed indirect labor.
   d. fixed direct labor.

9. A small hospital in your community aligns itself with a larger center that offers more specialized cancer care. This alliance is sometimes referred to as a(n):
   a. simple alliance.
   b. "feeder" system.
   c. consolidation.
   d. carve-out model.

10. A major barrier for both patients and institutions to participation in national studies is that:
    a. trials sponsored by drug companies pose a financial burden for most oncology programs.
    b. the NCI rarely is committed to research to prevent cancer since success is fairly limited; thus, it only consistently supports research to improve the quality of life for those who develop cancer.
    c. third-party payers do not cover experimental treatment, which includes all research trials.
    d. b and c.

11. Which of the following do(es) not reflect the recent paradigm shifts that have occurred in response to future demands of health care systems?
    a. Our practice must become sensitive to limited resources.
    b. We need to recognize a direct correlation between manpower and quality.
    c. Accountability, responsibility, and authority for clinical decisions will evolve from the manager to the practitioner, in partnership with the patient.
    d. Standardization and routines for patient care will be replaced by individualization and creativity.

12. The Oncology Nursing Society (ONS) endorses the title advanced practice nurse (APN) to designate:
    a. clinical nurse specialist (CNS) and nurse practitioner (NP) roles in oncology nursing.
    b. the merger of the CNS and NP roles.
    c. exclusion of other master's prepared nurses in education, administration, or research roles.
    d. all of the above.

13. What responsibilities should be carried out only by oncology nurses as opposed to APs?
    a. measuring intake and output
    b. vital signs
    c. extravasation assessment and management
    d. a and c

# ANSWER EXPLANATIONS

1. **The answer is d.** The early success of HMOs was related to two major factors: the assumption of financial risk by physicians and the combining of the costs of all services (hospitals, ambulatory services, and physicians) into one charge. The basis of the HMO model is a primary care physician (PCP) who is selected by the participant and who then authorizes all care, thus acting as a "gatekeeper" for coordinated care. (p. 1589)

2. **The answer is b.** In a staff model HMO, all physicians are employed and salaried by the HMO. In a group model HMO plan, the physicians are not salaried, but have a contractual arrangement. The physician is compensated through the private practice. The network model requires that physicians contract directly with the HMO, but the physicians continue to deliver care in their own private offices and also to treat non-HMO patients. This plan is referred to as an "open model." (p. 1590)

3. **The answer is a.** In a PHO, there is a contractual relationship between physicians and the hospital to accomplish several goals: to increase the opportunity to obtain managed-care contracts, to align the organizational structure with the financial incentives found in capitation, and to measure quality of care through outcomes. (p. 1590)

4. **The answer is a.** A POS (point of service) plan allows members to access out-of-plan providers but imposes strict utilization strategies. (p. 1590)

5. **The answer is b.** Horizontal integration occurs when a PHO is organized into an integrated delivery system that uses different sites in the community to provide a wide variety of services. Vertical integration means that these services are capable of being provided within the same system. Vertical integration is sometimes referred to as depth of services, and horizontal integration, as breadth of services. (p. 1591)

6. **The answer is c.** Capitation is an established dollar amount "per member per month," regardless of the services rendered by the providers. Case rates provide the institution with a set amount of money per procedure or service. Discount from charges is a modification of the fee-for-service model; and per diem payment programs reimburse for each day of hospitalization. (p. 1592)

7. **The answer is a.** Upcoding occurs when physicians report a more complex level of care or diagnosis to enhance reimbursement. Churning refers to the practice of increasing procedures and visits to enhance revenue as fees are discounted. Case rates provide the institution with a set amount of money per procedure or service. Global rate is a case rate that encompasses both the physician component and hospital costs for specific incidents. (p. 1592)

8. **The answer is d.** Direct costs can be traced clearly to a specific patient or service; indirect costs frequently are referred to as overhead costs and cannot be assigned directly to a specific patient, but need to be spread across all patients. Variable costs change in relation to the number of patients cared for, while fixed costs remain stable as the number of patients changes. Fixed direct labor includes the head nurse or clinical nurse specialist. On the other hand, staff nurses represent variable direct labor. (p. 1593)

9. **The answer is b.** A "feeder" system aligns small hospitals offering fewer cancer services with larger centers that offer more specialized care. A simple alliance model aligns cancer programs at separate hospitals and retains separate day-to-day management of the two cancer programs. The consolidation features a strong, centralized ownership of facilities. The carve-out model links a hospital or provider of care with a second firm or organization that takes charge of all cancer care provided to alliance members. (pp. 1596–1597)

10. **The answer is c.** A major barrier for both patients and institutions to participation in national studies is that third-party payers do not cover experimental treatment, which includes all research trials.

Trials sponsored by drug companies generally do not pose a financial concern for oncology programs. The NCI clearly is committed to research to prevent cancer as well as to improve the quality of life for those who develop cancer. (p. 1598)

11.  **The answer is b.** The reassessing of our values and assumptions to meet the future demands of health care systems are reflected in the following four paradigm shifts: (1) Our practice must evolve from a needs-driven model of care to one that is sensitive to limited resources; (2) We need to shift from making a direct correlation between manpower and quality to identifying a true correlation between critical thinking and quality; (3) Standardization and routines for patient care will be replaced by individualization and creativity; and (4) accountability, responsibility, and authority for clinical decisions will evolve from the manager to the practitioner, in partnership with the patient. (p. 1603)

12.  **The answer is a.** The Oncology Nursing Society (ONS) endorses the title *advanced practice nurse* (APN) to designate clinical nurse specialist (CNS) and nurse practitioner (NP) roles in oncology nursing. The ONS notes that the term *advanced practice nurse* does not imply the merger of the CNS and NP roles, nor does it exclude other master's prepared nurses in education, administration, or research roles. (p. 1603)

13.  **The answer is c.** Although patient care activities, like vital signs and measuring intake and output, may be delegated to APs when the patient is stable, certain nursing care functions, like extravasation assessment and management, should be performed by oncology registered nurses and should not be delegated to APs (p. 1605)

# Chapter 56    Ethical Issues in Cancer Nursing Practice

This chapter corresponds to Chapter 57 in *Cancer Nursing: Principles and Practice*, **Fourth Edition.**

## INTRODUCTION

- In addition to the many physical and emotional challenges faced by oncology nurses, many different ethical issues arise in caring for patients with cancer.

## GENERAL ETHICAL ISSUES

### Autonomy

- Autonomy is a principle that compels us to respect the self-command of the individual. It is part of what makes us moral. Autonomy is more than the patients' rights or even the freedom to choose. The core of what it means to be a person is moral responsibility to oneself and to others. This is freedom to take responsibility for one's own actions and their consequences.
- Caregivers have a duty to respect the moral origins of the person, not just to respect the choices the person makes.
  - For centuries, health care practitioners practiced a form of paternalism, acting in the best interests of others without asking their preferences, or even explicitly acting against their preferences.
  - Caregivers are often reluctant to accept the wishes of individuals with serious disease, especially if they think something still might be done to improve either longevity or quality of life. This can create a conflict between the caregiver's sense of duty to protect and prolong life and the autonomy and privacy rights of the individual patient.

### Beneficence

- *Beneficence* is the principle of altruism, that is, to act in the best interests of others.
  - The principle creates an expectation in patients and in society as a whole that health professionals have promised and will take exceptional steps to place their patients' interests above their own.
  - Beneficence does not rule out trying to persuade patients and even sometimes to almost coerce them to overcome their fears and to help them choose what is in their best interests. It is unethical to act against the wishes of patients if they continue to refuse the offerings of modern health care.
  - It is frequently hard to determine what is in the patient's best interest. There may be conflicting courses of treatment, or only statistical or epidemiological information that may or may not apply to the circumstances.

### Nonmaleficence

- When caregivers find that there is confusion or disagreement about what is in the patient's best interest, they must fall back on the principle of nonmaleficence, "To help, or at least to do no harm."
- Nonharm is a minimalist beneficence position. Respecting the personhood of the patient requires an attempt to honor autonomy *and* to act in his or her best interest. At the very least, it means never harming intentionally. The problem is to define harm.

## Justice

- The principle of justice requires that we give each person his or her due.
- There are competing opinions of how to measure what is due. Some argue for taking from the rich and giving to the poor; others argue that egalitarian methods are more appropriate (everyone is entitled to exactly the same treatment); Libertarians argue that justice requires a fundamental respect for autonomy and that one cannot alter the social situation without the consent of the governed.
- Different views of justice have little bearing on clinical decisions at this time, although they do influence various proposals for access to care.

## Alternative Ethical Theories

- The difficulty in clinical ethics is rooted in the tendency of ethics to refine abstract thought versus the concrete, individual problems encountered by professionals who must make quick decisions about complex matters in order to benefit their patients.
- Health professionals must do ethics on the run.
- *Hermeneutics* means interpreting the case in its whole context—the individual's life plans and values, the family's values, social and cultural factors, and the like.
- *Ethics as story* relies upon concrete narrative to ferret out the interests and values in each instance, especially with relationship to caregivers themselves.
- *Virtue theory* means no principle could be implemented without the commitment of caregivers or patients to the good as they perceive it.
- Relying solely on the virtuous caregiver and patient, without a set of objective moral guidelines or principles, leads to opportunity for abuse.
- There is the need for a relation between objective standards and the virtue of the nurse.

## Reconciliation Efforts

- Pellegrino and Thomasma proposed that the goal of health care ought to be "beneficence-in-trust", wherein the caregiver holds in trust the values of the patient in making joint decisions with the patient about best interests.
- No matter what approach is taken, it is important that individual moral commitments are not separated from ethical decision making.

### Casuistry

- Casuistry is the theory that each case is unique, and from that case certain norms are developed that may or may not be applicable in analogous cases.
- The goal of casuistry is to establish the paradigm case, in which most analysts would agree that a certain norm predominates. Other cases are then related to this one and analyzed for the extent to which they "match" or "do not match" the paradigm case.

### Contextualism

- Casuistry neglects the importance of theory and of the nexus of values that ethical theory seeks to protect.
- The contextual grid theory rests on two distinctions.
    - The first is the distinction between primary, secondary, and tertiary care settings—a standard distinction in medicine that forms one set of coordinates of the grid.

- The second distinction is that made between the individual and the number of persons affected by the problem. The moral significance of this distinction is based on the increasing complexity that occurs when we must consider the values of different persons affected by the outcome of the case; it is also based on our increased tendency to protect the common good, the greater the number of persons affected.

## Ethical Workup

- See text page 1613 for the Ethical Workup Guide.

## NURSING ETHICAL ISSUES

### The Virtue of Compassion

- The community traditionally supported compassionate care of individuals by enabling individuals who were sick to be surrounded by those who loved them the most and knew their values. Decisions about health care were made within a context of compassion and respect for the values of the patient. Such care was impervious to marketplace economics.
- Today the community seems more concerned about the resources the sick divert from other projects. Rationing care appears to be more valued than providing it. The most vulnerable—the infants, the mentally ill—are the ones who will suffer the most from rationing.
- For health professionals and the family or surrogates, compassion is the quality that keeps them from operating solely on the basis of objectivity and rationality.
- Compassion enables decision makers to assist in healing.
  - True healing and appropriate decision making can only take place when all of the particulars and values of the individual and all the parties involved in the process of caring for the sick person are taken into account.
  - Compassionate care also means that the patient who cannot be cured by medical sciences may still be "healed" if we help him or her to express the meaning of a life in the final days of that life by respecting, insofar as possible, the patient's values and commitments.

### Clinical Ethics and the Relation to the Patient

- The nexus between clinical judgment and clinical ethics can help reveal structures of good decision making in patient care that are not simple products of contractual models of the provider-patient relationship.
- Leon Kass suggests that the reason we are compelled to put animals out of their misery is that they are not human and thus demand from us some measure of humaneness. By contrast, human beings demand from us our humanity itself.
- We are tempted to employ technology rather than one's personhood in the process of healing.
- A responsible use of technological intervention with and for the sake of a patient requires not only rational analysis but also sensitivity to the particularities of the case and the emotional content of value commitments of the parties involved.
- The responsible use of power is a clinical ethics judgment about the best balance of interventions and outcomes.
- The virtue of compassion requires an awareness of the physical condition of the patient (to assess outcomes), as well as an awareness of the values of patients or of those speaking for them (to assess the quality of those outcomes measured against the patient's values).

## The Patient Self-Determination Act

- The Patient Self-Determination Act requires all health care institutions, including home care and hospice, to notify patients upon admission to the institution or service of their rights under state law to execute an advance directive.
  - Other provisions include asking patients whether they have issued an advance directive or wish to do so, asking for a copy if they have, putting that copy prominently in the patient record, and notifying the patient of the institution's commitment to honor the patient's wishes.
  - Part of the reason for the Act was surely to underscore the importance of patients' rights, but also to control costs of health care, particularly during the last six months of a patient's life.
  - Difficulties arise when the wishes expressed do not anticipate future events.
  - Many health professionals are concerned that advance directives will artificially tie their hands in treatment decisions. In such cases an ethics consult or patient-care discussion is recommended.

## Compassionate Analysis

- Advances have occurred in emphasizing the rights of patients not only to determine the treatments they desire and do not desire during the dying process but also to choose treatments at any time during life, not just while dying.
  - The underlying principle is to increase the role of compassion in decisions about life-prolonging technology.
- A living will gives advance directives for the final period of terminal illness. In most states where it has been approved, the living will covers only the terminal phase of an illness, interpreted to mean the last few weeks of a person's life. Consequently, the living will is a limited instrument.
- Much more favored is the durable power of attorney. This instrument gives another person authority to make health care decisions for an individual who becomes incompetent to do so. Not only would this person know the patient's wishes, but also he or she could communicate with the caregivers to discern the best treatment or nontreatment options during the course of temporary or permanent incompetency.
  - The durable power, unlike the living will, covers any treatment decisions, formally anticipated or not, and at any stage in life, not just in a terminal situation.

## CANCER ETHICAL ISSUES

### The Dynamics of Cancer

- The *dynamics of cancer* refers to the spiritual struggle of the patient to come to terms with the diagnosis of cancer.
  - The spiritual realm is often neglected in daily life because external matters and concerns so easily obscure it.
- The dynamics of cancer has its own structure.
- At first, patients may feel guilty. Later, patients come to see that they are not usually responsible for their cancer.
  - Depending on age and habits of resiliency, patients may choose to fight the cancer.
  - Guilt reemerges when individuals decide not to continue against the odds. This guilt is attached to the patient's worries about loved ones.
- The likelihood of participating in research therapies for cancer treatment may decline in elderly cancer patients due to lowered life span expectations; poorer prognosis due to more advanced stages of the disease; the body's inability to cope with the collateral effects; and, a value hierarchy that places other factors, like the grandchildren's college education, over one's own continued life.

## Cancer and Autonomy

- Patients are engaged with at least three struggles:
  1. with the body, often leading to physical exhaustion
  2. with the environment, family, community, job, nursing home, etc.
  3. with their own values, including their life plans, expectations, the hierarchy of their values, and so on
- While the cancer dynamic continues, the patient identifies autonomy with reshuffling a hierarchy of values.
  - By respecting this hierarchy we can best protect against paternalistic overtreatment against a patient's wishes and any biased undertreatment of cancer patients.
  - Finding out patients' values is part of the process of respecting them as persons and is a guiding principle in constructing a therapeutic plan.

## Cancer and Suffering

- The first source of suffering is the bifurcation of the person into an ego, often isolated and alone, and the body that has betrayed that person, the object taken over by the disease.
- There is a documented disparity between patient and physician evaluation of the quality of life.
  - Concern for patient values, both making the effort to discover them and using them to design a humane treatment plan, is fundamental.
  - The biggest danger a cancer patient faces is that of being stripped of his or her values in the face of the panoply of interventions we have available.
- The primary task of caregivers is to aid in synthesis as much as possible. Some recommendations are:
  - Minimize suffering, not only through pain control efforts but also by confronting one's own blockages to meeting the suffering person as a person.
  - Make every effort to understand the patient's value system.
  - Implement the care plan as a means to minimize suffering.
  - Respect his or her values so that the person he or she was, despite the current condition, is nonetheless respected.

## Termination of Treatment

- Each instance concerning termination of treatment must be judged on its own characteristics.

### Withholding and withdrawing

- Most caregivers today seem more willing to withhold and withdraw major interventions deemed "heroic," but their reasons appear somewhat confused.
- Two possible lines of reasoning exist:
  - the goal of bringing about the patient's death (death induction)
  - the goal of removing treatments that prolong the patient's suffering, while not intending the patient's death
- The distinction in intent between aiming at the patient's death and aiming at reducing suffering originally was used to distinguish between active and passive euthanasia.
- There is no moral difference between withholding and withdrawing on the one hand and actively bringing about death on the other, if the intent is that the patient's death would be a good thing.

- If our intent in withdrawing care is to bring about death, then other more direct forms of euthanasia may seem much more appropriate.
- Currently Americans are hotly debating whether to legalize active euthanasia, aid in dying, and physician-assisted suicide.
- Having more dialogue about values will honor and support dying cancer patients. Use an interview format around values assessment, but do not confine the process to a single conversation.
- Of major concern is allowing physicians to kill patients out of mercy in the context of a society that has so little respect for human life in other areas.

### Control of dying and life support

- Undertreatment occurs when the "bottom line" predominates over benefit to the patient. Only a national health coverage plan would eliminate this injustice.
- Overtreatment occurs through the technological enthusiasms of caregivers, the fear of "letting go," or appeals for unreasonable treatments from patients.
- Only institutional policies about appropriate treatment decisions coupled with compassionate analysis, as suggested earlier, will answer these problems.

### Nutrition and hydration

- Patients have a common-law right and probably a constitutional right to refuse treatment even if they are not dying.
- Patients may request aid in dying on the grounds that death is a good thing and others have a duty out of compassion to bring about such a good. "Bringing it about" does not necessarily entail active, direct euthanasia, or even physician-assisted suicide. But it does require that all interventions, including fluids and nutrition, be examined for their impact on the desired goal of treatment.
  - Those who support withholding or withdrawing fluids and nutrition think if an earlier and less painful death, with less suffering for the patient, is the desired goal, then how does it make sense to provide medically delivered food and water unless the patient specifically requests it?
  - Those who oppose the withdrawal of nutrition and hydration argue that such withdrawing or withholding leads directly to the death of the patient as much as does an injection, since the patient dies not of the underlying disease process but from starvation and dehydration.
  - Some ethicists think that only objective criteria (medical indications presumably)—not the context, life plans, or values of the individual—can be used in all withholding and withdrawing decisions.
  - Ethicists also argue that nothing else can be used to bring about death in patients who have made no advance directives or who have left only vague statements about not using heroic measures to prolong their lives.

### The role of the family

- The role of the family in speaking for patient values is confused. It is very important to obtain advance directives from all patients, especially seriously ill ones.
- The preferred instrument in most states is the Durable Power of Attorney for Health Care, which names ahead of time an individual who will speak for the patient when the patient is incompetent to make decisions about health care.
- Despite the cautions noted by the Supreme Court about family surrogacy, most persons feel comfortable about naming a family member to make decisions, since such a person knows them and their values best.

## Access to care

- Some argue that when patients are competent and can speak for themselves about medical care, that their options be limited past 80 years of age and that some interventions no longer be considered.
  - This point should not be set by ageist limits but rather by the limits of medicine to provide any meaningful change in the outcome for patients during their last years.
  - It may not be necessary to set limits on the basis of age if we first try to respect a patient's value system.
  - Elderly persons will usually choose highly technical interventions less often than will younger cancer patients.
  - Patients over 80 are more accustomed to thinking that they will soon die anyway.
  - The post-80 syndrome may lead patients to give up too early on their care when they could achieve a significant quality of life, or it may lead to age bias in offering and withholding care.
- Other important issues regarding access to cancer care are the problem of the rights of all persons to expensive interventions, the right to request experimental therapy, allocating scarce resources, large-scale distribution of health care among competing health needs, and the distribution of funding for other human needs versus health care needs.

## Playing God

- Modern medical technology empowers individuals beyond their normal capacities and it tempts us to exceed the bounds of temperance. This leads to a kind of paternalism in which an individual comes to believe that he or she knows best what is good for another person due to superior technical knowledge.
- It is important for health care that providers understand the risks and benefits of the technological interventions they propose.

## Euthanasia

- The problem of euthanasia involves the question of dominion over life.
  - Our technology makes the temptation to take control over life itself almost overwhelming.
  - It is important to distinguish between objective evaluation of interventions and outcomes on the well-being of the patient and subjective quality-of-life judgments in which the physician and other caregivers judge that the life the patient is now living is not worthwhile for that person.
  - The danger is the economic sphere, in which it may be easier to dispatch those persons whose care costs too much or who are now considered to be a burden on society, than to address their suffering.
  - The issue focuses attention on the importance of maintaining compassionate respect for human life in our society.
  - For some, actions to eliminate burdensome life, even if requested by the patient him- or herself, are a form of "privatizing life," denying its social and communal dimensions as both a private and public good.
  - Others argue that euthanasia and assisted suicide are appropriate and important forms of caring for persons whose lives, by their own assessment, have become too burdensome to continue.

## CONCLUSION

- The duty to protect a patient's life lies primarily in protecting his or her autonomy and value hierarchy. Strategies for ensuring this in the future include the following:
  - Discover the patient's value system through a values assessment interview and through constant discussion with the patient and the family throughout the course of treatment.

- Require advance directives before one receives the first retirement check, enter that advance directive on a central computer, and update it whenever one enters a health care institution, nursing home, or hospice in accordance with current Patient Self-Determination Act procedures.
- Develop teaching guides for all health care professionals to train them in the processes of implementing patient advance directives, since resistance to these directives is still encountered.
- Change the current default mode of health care delivery (in which it is assumed that everyone desires technological support of their life) to the opposite assumption—unless the patient has issued advance directives to the contrary.
- Use a process like the Ethical Workup Guide to analyze and discuss cases that arise in one's service.

## PRACTICE QUESTIONS

1. Which of the following principles can be used as a basic model for how good decisions emerge in health care?
   a. No principle could be implemented without the commitment of caregivers or patients to the good as they perceive it.
   b. Competent patients are entitled to make their own choices.
   c. Caregivers cannot charge paying patients and their insurance companies more for cancer care than non-paying patients.
   d. Each case is unique and serves as a paradigm to which other cases are compared.

2. The Ethical Workup Guide requires health caregivers to:
   a. construct an exhaustive list of possibilities and relevant interests.
   b. take a position on ethical theory.
   c. decide on a course of action and defend it with ethical values.
   d. make decisions based on more than one ethical value.

3. The Patient Self-Determination Act (December 1991) requires:
   a. caregivers to decide on the treatment plan when their patients cannot.
   b. all health care institutions to notify patients upon admission to the institution or service of their rights under state law to execute an advance directive.
   c. caregivers to respect individuals' moral centers.
   d. institutions to advise patients to avoid advance directives and let the doctor decide.

4. Which is preferable, the durable power of attorney or the living will, and why?
   a. The living will is preferable because it prevents more suffering.
   b. The durable power of attorney is preferable because it only covers terminal situations.
   c. The durable power of attorney covers not only decisions in a terminal situation, but any treatment decisions, and therefore is preferable.
   d. The living will is better because health care providers are concerned about the ethical issues in active, direct euthanasia.

5. Which one of the following is not a potential problem with policies regarding the post-80 syndrome?
   a. It may lead to age bias in offering and withholding care.
   b. It may lead caregivers to sell patients a "bill of goods" that may bankrupt other patient values.
   c. It may lead patients to give up too early on their care when they could achieve a significant quality of life.
   d. all of the above

6. Euthanasia involves one individual making judgments about the value of another person's life. Therefore the responsible individual must distinguish several possible results. Which of the following should this person not consider?
   a. the objective evaluation of interventions
   b. the outcomes on the well-being of the patient
   c. the economic consequences of prolonging the patient's life
   d. the subjective quality-of-life judgments

# ANSWER EXPLANATIONS

1.  **The answer is d.** Casuistry can be used as the basic model for how good decisions emerge in health care. Casuistry is the theory that each case is unique, and from that case are developed certain norms that may or may not be applicable in analogous cases. (p. 1611)

2.  **The answer is c.** The Ethical Workup Guide requires caregivers to come up with an ethically justifiable course of action for their patient. They can use one or more of the ethical values in their decision. (p.1613)

3.  **The answer is b.** The Patient Self-Determination Act requires all health care institutions, including home care and hospice, to notify patients upon admission to the institution of their rights under state law to execute advance directives. Other provisions include asking patients whether they have issued an advance directive or wish to do so, asking for a copy if they have, putting that copy prominently in the patient's record, and notifying the patient of the institution's commitment to honor the patient's wishes. (p.1615)

4.  **The answer is c.** The durable power of attorney is preferable. A living will gives advance directives for the final period of terminal illness, while the durable power of attorney covers any treatment situations at any stage in life. This document names ahead of time an individual who will speak for the patient when the patient is incompetent to make decisions about health care. (p.1616, 1620)

5.  **The answer is d.** All three are problems with the post-80 syndrome. (p. 1620)

6.  **The answer is c.** It is important to distinguish between objective evaluation of interventions and outcomes on the well-being of the patient and subjective quality-of-life judgments in which the physician and other caregivers judge that the life the patient is now living is not worthwhile for that person. (p. 1621)

# Chapter 57    Alternative Methods of Cancer Therapy

This chapter corresponds to Chapter 58 in *Cancer Nursing: Principles and Practice*, **Fourth Edition.**

## INTRODUCTION

- Each year thousands of cancer patients and many others who merely fear they might develop cancer will devote countless hours and invest billions of dollars in the use of alternative cancer remedies outside the realm of mainstream medicine.
- Alternative treatments range from those that are both fraudulent and dangerous to those that are hazardous mainly to the pocketbook.
- Often, these treatments offer individuals a chance to participate in their own care, reflecting the naturalistic approaches so popular with the public today.
- The American Cancer Society (ACS) has defined *alternative therapies* as unproven or disproven methods, whereas *complementary therapies* are supportive therapies that are used to complement standard mainstream therapy.
- Alternative methods of cancer management include diagnostic tests or therapeutic methods that have not shown activity in animal tumor models or in scientific clinical trials but are promoted for general use in cancer prevention, diagnosis, or treatment. Such methods may not be safe.

## HISTORICAL PERSPECTIVES

### Legislation

- Before the Food and Drug Act of 1906, thousands of unproven treatments were promoted to the American public.
- In 1906 President Theodore Roosevelt signed into law the Pure Food and Drug Act, which forbade misleading or false statements on the labels of remedies.
- In 1912 Congress passed the Sherley Amendment, which made it a crime to make false or fraudulent claims regarding the therapeutic efficacy of a drug.
- In 1962 Congress added that drugs must demonstrate efficacy in addition to safety.

### Past Unproven Methods

- Examples of unorthodox approaches are identified in Table 58-1, text page 1627.

#### Koch antitoxin therapy: 1940s–1950s

- Koch antitoxin therapy was a popular unproven cancer treatment during the 1940s and 1950s. The treatment consisted of pure distilled water mixed with one part per trillion of a chemical called glyoxylide, which is merely glyoxylic acid with water removed.

#### Hoxsey method: 1950s

- Hoxsey maintained that cancer was a result of a chemical imbalance in the body that caused healthy cells to mutate and become cancerous and that this therapy restored the chemical environment and killed the cancerous cells. Hoxsey's Herbal Tonic consisted of several different formulas.

662

- No legitimate case of a cure was discovered. In 1960 a federal court injunction declared sale of the treatment illegal.

## Krebiozen: 1960s

- Krebiozen was developed from blood extracted from horses.

## Laetrile: 1970s

- Laetrile is a general term for a group of cyanogenic glucosides, derived from several different seeds, also known as amygdalin and "vitamin $B_{17}$."
- Laetrile does not fulfill the requirements of a vitamin, because no disease state exists in its absence. Evidence suggests that laetrile has toxic effects.
- Laetrile has been the most extensively tested unproven method of all time.
- Laetrile's use as an anticancer drug has not ended. Proponents are combining it with vitamins, enzymes, or so-called metabolic therapy.

## POPULAR ALTERNATIVE METHODS OF TODAY

- Alternative methods of cancer treatment during the 1980s and the 1990s are primarily related to lifestyle, and as such cannot be regulated by the FDA. Many of the unproven methods place responsibility for a healthy lifestyle on the patient and have an aura of respectability in relation to conventional scientific medicine that is concerned with diet, environmental carcinogens, lifestyle, and the relationship between emotions and physiological responses.
- Nutritional therapy represents a major type of alternative cancer treatment.

## Dietary Therapy/Metabolic Therapy

- The goals of alternative dietary therapy overlap the goals of conventional nutritional support for cancer patients.
- However, alternative dietary methods go beyond scientifically accepted nutritional measures in that they claim to reverse the course of disease.
- The concepts of metabolic therapy are based on the theory that cancer is a result of impaired metabolism that causes a buildup of toxins in the body. According to this theory, detoxification and manipulation of diet can remove these toxins, to accomplish cure.

### Gerson regimen

- The Gerson treatment is the original "metabolic" therapy. It proposes that constipation or inadequate elimination of wastes from the body interferes with metabolism and healing. Cure can be achieved through manipulation of diet and "detoxification," or purging the body of so-called toxins.
- The Gerson Institute claims are not supported by data or statistics. The program's repeated enemas and purgatives are more likely to lead to metabolic imbalance than to correct it, and its coffee enemas have killed people.

### Manner metabolic therapy

- The "Manner cocktail" consists of an intravenous solution of dimethyl sulfoxide (DMSO), and massive doses of vitamin C, vitamin A, and laetrile.
- There is no objective evidence that the metabolic therapy of Harold Manner has any benefit in the treatment of cancer.

### Macrobiotic diets

- Today, the macrobiotic diet probably is the most popular, both for curing cancer and for preventing cancer. This diet has its origin in Zen mysticism, which proposes two antagonistic and complementary forces, yin and yang, that govern all things in the universe. Each food is classified as yin or yang, whereas each tumor is classified as being caused by an imbalance of either yin or yang. The diet is matched to the tumor to restore the balance.
- With adequate planning, vegetarian diets may be nutritionally sound; however, macrobiotic therapy can result in malnutrition and cause a variety of serious health problems. Of special note, cancer patients who follow the macrobiotic regimen should ensure adequate intakes of vitamins $B_{12}$ and D.

## Pharmacological and Biological Approaches

### Antineoplaston therapy

- Antineoplastons were developed by Stanislaw R. Burzynski, MD, in the late 1960s. Burzynski claims that antineoplastons are natural peptides and amino acid derivatives that cause cancer cells to change to normal cells, inhibit the growth of malignant cells, and are also useful in diagnosing cancer.
- To date, prospective, controlled clinical studies of antineoplastons have not taken place.
- In November of 1995, Burzynski was indicated on 75 counts of mail fraud and violation of federal medical regulations.

### Cancell

- Cancell, also known as Entelev, Jim's Juice, Croinic Acid, and Sheridan's Formula, is a mixture of synthetic chemicals created for their electrical properties.
- According to Sopack, the formula reacts with the body electrically and lowers the voltage of the cell structure. Because cancer cells are weak, they convert directly to waste material when the voltage is lowered by Cancell, and the body then eliminates this waste material. The cancer cells are replaced with normal cells, and the cancer no longer exists.
- The FDA obtained a permanent injunction prohibiting the distribution of Cancell in interstate commerce.

### Dimethyl sulfoxide (DMSO)

- The use of a 50% solution of DMSO for bladder instillations is the only FDA-approved use of this agent in humans.
- A review of the literature by the American Cancer Society revealed no evidence that DMSO results in objective benefit in the treatment of cancer patients.

### Live-cell therapy

- Live-cell therapy—fresh-cell therapy, or cellular therapy—is the injection of cells from animal embryos or fetuses. The type of cells given supposedly matches the diseased tissue or organ in the patient.
- Serious side effects (brucellosis, encephalomyelitis, anaphylactic shock) have resulted from this treatment.

### Megavitamins

- The use of supplemental vitamins is another unproven approach that has been promoted as a treatment for cancer.
- Excessive vitamin intake is useless against cancer and, more important, may be toxic.

## Vitamin C

- Megadose vitamin C probably is the most popular self-administered vitamin supplement.
- Megadoses of vitamin C can cause severe kidney damage, release cyanide from laetrile, and may cause death if administered intravenously.

## Vitamin A

- Megadoses of vitamin A have also become popular for the treatment of cancer.
- Doses as low as five times the RDA may be toxic and have no clear value.

## Pangamic acid ("vitamin B$_{15}$")

- Pangamic acid is not a vitamin.
- There is evidence that the chemicals in products labeled "B$_{15}$" or "pangamate" may promote the development of cancer.

# Oxymedicine

- Promoters claim that oxygen treatment stimulates immunity, oxidizes toxins, and kills bacteria and viruses.
- Oxidizing agents can be harmful, causing oxygen emboli and death.

# Shark cartilage

- Proponents claim that shark cartilage is a protein that inhibits angiogenesis; however, no well-designed clinical trials have been done. The molecules of the active ingredients in the shark cartilage sold in health food stores are too large to be absorbed and the ingested product decomposes into inert ingredients.

# Herbal remedies

- Herbal concoctions are not examined for safety and efficacy by the FDA, and they can be harmful.

# Immunologic Approach: Immunoaugmentative Therapy (IAT)

- IAT is based on the theory that stimulation of the immune system will enable the body's normal defenses to destroy tumor cells.
- Scientific documentation of this therapy is lacking.
- Safety concerns have arisen over the years. IAT remains a hazardous approach to the treatment of cancer, with no documented clinical activity or scientific rationale.

# Behavioral and Psychological Approaches

## Mind body interventions

- Although the scientific and medical communities support the notion that a positive mental attitude can increase patient comfort and promote a sense of control and well-being, the mind body methods may be harmful, in that individuals may be made to feel guilty because their particular personality type was responsible for the development of cancer.
- These approaches suggest that those patients who do not survive may not have been strong enough or had a good attitude. The ethical implications of these approaches should be a major concern.

## ALTERNATIVE TREATMENT FACILITIES

- Unorthodox clinics are flourishing in Tijuana, Mexico, which has become a haven for promoters who treat cancer patients with alternative cancer therapies.
- Most therapies are metabolic in nature, but combinations of numerous approaches exist.
- Table 58-2, text page 1634, provides information on the major Tijuana clinics.

## PROMOTERS AND PRACTITIONERS OF ALTERNATIVE METHODS

### Strategies Used by Promoters

- It is a paradox that highly motivated and better-educated individuals are more likely to turn to questionable methods because of the promise that "you control your disease."

## WHO SEEKS ALTERNATIVE CANCER TREATMENTS, AND WHY

### Motivations and Reasons for Use

- There are a variety of reasons why cancer patients pursue questionable therapy: fear of pain or risk of side effects from conventional treatment; desire for self-control rather than passive inclusion in treatment; isolation/antiestablishment; and social pressures from family and friends.

## CONTROL OF ALTERNATIVE METHODS

- Recently, the National Institutes of Health (NIH) were congressionally mandated to establish the NIH Office of Alternative Medicine (OAM).
- The federal and state governments participate in the regulation of alternative treatment methods via the FDA, the Federal Trade Commission (FTC), and the U.S. Postal Service.

## ROLE OF NURSES/NURSING INTERVENTIONS

- Table 58-3, text page 1636, lists sources of information on questionable cancer remedies.
- Behavioral methods are of major interest to nurses.
- The responsible position requires that nurses avoid simplistic clichés and deal realistically with the complexities and limitations of modern cancer care as well as the subtlety and seductiveness of the alternative cancer treatment industry. The following four specific steps will assist in this difficult task.

### Identification of Alternative Therapies (Legitimate vs. Fringe Care)

- The Subcommittee on Unorthodox Therapies of the American Society of Clinical Oncology has listed ten questions to ask in making a decision as to whether a treatment should be suspected of being questionable (Table 58-4, text page 1637).

### Assessment of Communication Channels and Patient Motivations

- Communication patterns between the patient and family must be evaluated. The family may become preoccupied with seeking different therapies as a means of coping with stress. Such a situation may be intense enough to cause the family to exclude the patient from the decision-making process.

### Maintenance of Positive Communication Channels

- Table 58-5, text page 1638, identifies some potential questions to ask in order to assess a patient's risk and possible motivations for seeking alternative methods of cancer therapy.
  - A nonjudgmental attitude facilitates the assessment of the patient's and family's motivations for wanting to try an unproven method.

## Maintenance of Patient Participation in Their Health Care

- It is important for patients and family to participate in health care. Patients will be less likely to seek questionable cancer remedies if such needs are met. Patient education can increase patient satisfaction, increase patient knowledge, and enhance self-care.

## PRACTICE QUESTIONS

1. Which of the following does the federal government insist on before a drug can be marketed?
   a. the safety of the drug only
   b. the efficacy of the drug only
   c. the safety and the efficacy of the drug only
   d. the safety, efficacy, and long-term value of the drug

2. One of the principal appeals of most alternative methods of treatment to the cancer patient is their:
   a. perceived absence of risks and side effects.
   b. ready availability and modest costs.
   c. level of acceptability to family and friends.
   d. high degree of efficacy and safety.

3. Which of the following reasons is *least* likely to explain a decision by a cancer patient to explore an alternative method of treatment?
   a. a desire for greater control over the treatment process
   b. pressure from family and friends
   c. valid data on the efficacy of the method
   d. resentment toward an impersonal medical system

4. One problem that may arise in the mind body cancer treatment techniques is that:
   a. these techniques exclude standard cancer therapies.
   b. patients may be made to feel that their mental attitude cased their cancer.
   c. the long duration of the treatment causes patients to lose faith in its therapeutic value.
   d. other aspects of patient care, notably nutrition, are overlooked.

5. Which of the following questions would a nurse be *least* advised to ask the cancer patient or family member who desires to use an alternative treatment method?
   a. "What do you know about this method?"
   b. "How do you think this method will help you [or your loved one]?"
   c. "Have you [as a family member] discussed this method with your loved one?"
   d. "Are you aware of the potential dangers of this treatment?"

## ANSWER EXPLANATIONS

1. **The answer is c.** The Food and Drug Act of 1906 called for the truthful labeling of ingredients used in drugs but did not ban false therapeutic claims on drug labels. The Sherley Amendment in 1912 made it a crime to make false or fraudulent claims regarding the therapeutic efficacy of a drug, but proof of intent to defraud the customer was needed. Finally, in 1962, Congress added that drugs must demonstrate efficacy in addition to safety before they can be marketed, and a process was created by which a substance can become approved for prescription use. (p. 1627)

2. **The answer is a.** Individuals use alternative methods for a variety of stated reasons, such as "I have nothing to lose" or "If it won't hurt me, why not try it?" Often they are confused by conflicting reports of cure rates of standard treatments and frightened by treatment risks and possibly side effects. Many unproven methods promise no side effects and draw on the patient's fantasy of cure involving "the body's natural defenses." By using an unconventional therapy, the patient hopes for an unconventional cure. (p. 1635)

3. **The answer is c.** In theory, valid data on the efficacy of an alternative method would be the best reason for a patient to choose that method, but then the method would no longer be "alternative." The fact remains that none of the various alternative methods discussed in this chapter has stood up to scientific scrutiny, especially the requirement of proven efficacy in human subjects. The reasons stated in the other choices are among the most likely to motivate the cancer patient to seek an alternative therapy. (p. 1635)

4. **The answer is b.** Mind body techniques are based on the idea that a positive mental attitude can improve an individual's physiologic responses, resulting in improved response to standard therapies. Patients are taught to use mental imagery and relaxation techniques to visualize cancer cells as weak and sick and to imagine body defenses as a strong army that attacks and eliminates cancer cells. Patients are encouraged to continue conventional treatment, however. Besides the problem of patient guilt, other problems with this method are that objective benefits have yet to be documented by clinical studies, and individuals may become overly reliant on the method to the exclusion of standard medical therapy. (p. 1633)

5. **The answer is d.** The first job of the nurse is to assess the underlying motivations of a patient or family member who wishes to discuss an unproven method. This can be done by asking questions such as those in choices **a–c**. The individual is usually aware that such techniques are not likely to be approved by the professional. Asking questions such as those in choices **a–c** may help the professional to discover unmet needs of the patient and family and to assess their understanding of the therapies that have been administered. A nonjudgmental attitude on the part of the professional also may make the patient and family more receptive to the information provided by the caregiver. A question such as that in choice **d**, on the other hand, may be regarded by the patient as negative and judgmental, and it may serve to cut off further discussion. (p. 1638)

# Chapter 58    Patient Education and Support

This chapter corresponds to Chapter 59 in *Cancer Nursing: Principles and Practice*, **Fourth Edition.**

## A DEFINITION OF PATIENT EDUCATION

- *Patient education* is "a planned learning experience using a combination of methods such as teaching, counseling, and behavior modification techniques that influence patients' knowledge and health behavior."
- Patient education involves *planned* learning experiences. It is not haphazard or accidental.
- The goal of patient education is to *effect some change in the learner.*

## PATIENT SUPPORT

- There is a distinction between psychotherapy groups—which seek to effect individual change through personal exploration and reflection, though done within the context of a group—and social support groups, which seek to help the group members find meaning and a sense of belonging through participation in the group.

## UNDERSTANDING THE PURPOSES OF PATIENT EDUCATION

- Five rationales or perspectives supporting the need for patient education have been identified: patients' rights, professional standards, legal and agency mandates, benefits to patients, and benefits to society and/or health care agencies. Of these, two are traditional views supporting patient education: providing benefits to patients and satisfying professional standards.

### Patients' Rights

- The idea of patients' rights as a basis for patient education flows from philosophical principles recognizing individual autonomy and the right to self-determination.
- In 1972 the American Hospital Association developed its formal statement on the rights of patients.
  - These include rights to information about diagnosis, treatment, prognosis, procedures and their medical consequences, and other areas.
- In 1989 the National Coalition for Cancer Survivorship developed a statement of the rights of cancer survivors, *The Cancer Survivor's Bill of Rights.* This statement includes areas that have direct implications for patient education.
  - The first section discusses responsibilities of health care professionals, but the statement also deals with issues of employment opportunity, insurability, and the personal expectations and pressures often placed upon cancer survivors.

### Professional Standards

- Clear guidelines regarding patient education responsibilities as part of professional standards are relatively new.
- Current guidelines provide descriptive criterion statements organized around five areas: the responsibilities and qualifications of the oncology nurse; patient and family educational resources; the content

of patient and family education; the teaching-learning process and application of theory; and the anticipated learning outcomes for patients and family.

## Legal and Accreditation Requirements

- States are responsible for establishing guidelines for professional practice through state law.
- A specialized issue in legal responsibility for patient education is the area of informed consent.
- In 1993 the Joint Commission for the Accreditation of Healthcare Organizations (JCAHO) reorganized its standards for accreditation to bring stronger focus to the area of patient and family education.
- The Health Care Financing Administration (HCFA), which regulates Medicare and Medicaid reimbursement, mandates discharge planning and the patient and family education this implies.

## Patient Benefits

- A major focus of much patient education and of most support programs is improving psychological status by reducing anxiety, relieving depression, and maintaining self-concept of self-esteem. The ultimate goal is that education and support can contribute to improved physical status, defined in various ways when confronting an illness with high mortality rates.
- Much of the literature on patient outcomes for education and support interventions deals primarily with aspects of psychosocial status.
  - For example, a group program providing both psychosocial support and training in coping skills resulted in improved mood status and enhanced quality of life. A group psychotherapy program for cancer patients experiencing depression helped to reduce anxiety and maladaptive somatic preoccupation as well as reducing depression. An inpatient education and support program that included informational, emotional, and spiritual components increased knowledge of symptom management, decreased anxiety, reduced patients' sense of isolation, and increased their sense of control and comfort.
- Educational programs clearly serve to increase patient knowledge regarding self-care, symptom management, and monitoring and reporting changes in health status.

## Benefits to Society and to Health Care Organizations

- Benefits accruing to organizations or individuals beyond the patient and family include reduced hospital stays, reduced use of health care materials and resources, and reduced absenteeism from school or work.

# THE TEACHING-LEARNING PROCESS: THEORY AND PRACTICE

## The Health Belief Model

- Several proposed models draw from a value expectancy perspective; that is, an individual's actions are shaped or determined by expectations of outcomes and the value placed upon those expected outcomes.
- The Health Belief Model is based on several simple principles
  - First, the individual must perceive a threat.
  - Second, there must be an expectation that something can be done regarding the threat. The expectation includes three components:
    - that a behavior change or an action taken will be beneficial in reducing either the severity of or the susceptibility to the threat;
    - that benefits of the behavior change or action to be taken outweigh barriers or negative outcomes; and
    - that one can accomplish the behavior change or action required.

## The PRECEDE Model

- The PRECEDE Model (the acronym is derived from Predisposing, Reinforcing, and Enabling Causes in Educational Diagnosis and Evaluation) attempts to provide a comprehensive consideration of factors predisposing, reinforcing, and enabling targeted health behaviors.
- Predisposing factors may be positive or negative.
- Reinforcing factors support the continuation of the intended health behavior or reinforce resistance to the targeted behavior.
- Enabling factors are resources within an individual's environment that may impact the target health behavior, enabling or facilitating or, conversely, inhibiting the intended behavior.

## Control Theory

- The primary underlying perspective of control theory is an individual's perception or belief that specific outcomes are contingent upon the individual's own action or, alternately, other sources. Social learning theory, or self-efficacy theory, is one widely used control theory.
- A sense of self-efficacy derives from four sources of information: personal mastery, vicarious experiences, verbal persuasion, and physiological feedback.
- Another theoretical perspective in the general area of control theory is locus of control, that is, a view that behavior is a function of expectancy and reinforcement, with expectancy defined along an internal control-external control continuum.

## Coping Theory

- Coping involves behavioral and/or cognitive responses to perceived stressors or threats intended to mediate or manage those stressors or threats.
- Miller identified two coping styles for dealing with cancer or other major health threats—monitoring and blunting—that have implications for patient teaching.
  - *Monitors* are individuals who give high levels of attention to threatening health information. They tend to seek a great deal of information, to be more active in understanding their health condition, and to seek greater participation in decisions.
  - *Blunters* are individuals who avoid information that presents threatening health information. They tend not to seek additional information and take less responsibility for health decisions.
  - The monitor-blunter coping style framework may be helpful to the health professional in guiding how to react to individual patients, how to best provide information that is most helpful to the individual.

## Adult Learning Theory

- Much of adult education in recent years has been influenced by the work of Malcolm Knowles and the principles of *andragogy*, or adult education, that he proposed.
- Adult learning theory emphasizes task- or problem-oriented learning relevant to the needs and interests of the learner.
- Table 59-1, text page 1649, provides a summary of Knowles's four assumptions regarding adult learners and their implications for patient education.

## Guidelines for Patient Teaching Practice

- Techniques for patient teaching that can assist the nurse in thinking about effective ways of meeting patients' needs are presented in Table 59-2, text page 1650.
- Basic steps for conducting patient education include assessing educational needs, planning the teaching process, implementation, and evaluation.

- Effective needs assessment must involve the patient, seeking to identify needs as seen from the patient's perspective.
- The care provider needs to be attentive to indications of knowledge gaps expressed by patients, to be ready to ask questions, and to give patients ample time to think through their concerns and questions.
- Assessing patient needs must be an ongoing process, recognizing that information often needs to be repeated and that new needs and questions will arise as the individual progresses through treatment.
- Once needs are identified, plans for patient teaching activities to meet these needs can be developed. Planning allows for selection of resources and identification of specific activities to address all of the needs identified.
- Evaluation is ongoing, a part of the teaching-learning process.

## CONTINUITY ACROSS CARE SETTINGS

- The concept of continuity of care includes not only coordination and consistency across multiple settings but also the ongoing availability of or access to care services.
- There are a variety of models available for strengthening continuity of care.

## DEVELOPING PATIENT EDUCATION AND SUPPORT MATERIALS AND PROGRAMS

- Material and program development has been described as a six-step process that should continually repeat itself; that is, evaluation of the implemented program should provide feedback that can then be used to refine the program, progressing again through the development steps. The process described here has been adapted from the developmental process presented by the National Cancer Institute Office of Cancer Communication.
- This process is shown graphically in Figure 59-1, text page 1653.

### Step 1: Planning and Strategy Selection

- This is the basic planning stage for educational materials development. Several key issues are included in this stage:
  1. Clearly identify the issues, problems, or patient education goals.
  2. Identify the target audience.
  3. Identify the intended outcomes.
  4. Identify constraints placed upon the development process.

### Step 2: Selecting Processes and Materials

- This is the stage in which the purposes, characteristics of the audience, and constraints identified in Step 1 will guide decisions about the types of materials or programs structure that will be used.

### Step 3: Developing Materials and Pretesting

- At this stage the process moves from planning to development. The work of drafting and producing the actual materials must be done, with ongoing testing throughout the process.

#### Serving special populations

- If the materials are being developed for use with a specific target audience, care must be taken to ensure that elements of the audience's standards and practices are properly presented and respected.
- Cultural differences may affect many aspects of the interaction between health care professionals and their clients.

- Strategies for effective culturally sensitive approaches to patient education and support are varied. Health care professionals need to make linkages with key members of the target community, involving members of the community in the development of educational materials, programs, and community outreach strategies.

### Readability

- A fifth-grade reading level has been identified as the minimum reading level for making good use of basic written materials.
- The ACS and the NCI, as well as many other organizations that provide cancer patient education materials, are actively addressing problems with the level of literacy required for comprehending their materials.
- Tables 59-4 and 59-5, text page 1656, provide guidelines for both reducing the reading difficulty and enhancing comprehension through design, illustrations, and other visual effects.

### Pretesting

- Individual interviews, focus groups, surveys, and pilot testing of materials are all mechanisms that can be used for pretesting.
- It is important at this stage to use feedback from health care professionals who will use the materials.

## Step 4: Implementation

- Close monitoring of the implementation, especially in the early stages, is important.

## Step 5: Assessing Effectiveness

- The primary question to be addressed is whether the program or materials met the objectives.

## Step 6: Program Refinement

- The final step is to use the results of the evaluation to revise and refine the materials or program. The development cycle in effect becomes a spiral, with the evaluation findings of one cycle being used as the starting point.

## RESOURCES FOR PATIENT EDUCATION AND SUPPORT

- The growth in resources and programs reflects the success in treatment of cancer and the resulting change in perspective, from viewing cancer as a fatal illness to a chronic illness.
- Public demand for information and support programs also reflects a growth in a consumer-oriented perspective and increased awareness of the need for information.
- Effective patient teaching is dependent not only upon process but also upon content.

### American Cancer Society

- The ACS is a nationwide, community-based organization that offers a wide range of programs and services focused on public understanding about cancer; research on treatment, prevention, and early detection of cancer; and education and support for both health professionals and cancer patients and their families.
- In addition, the ACS provides direct information to individuals through two primary inquiry routes: the Resources, Information and Guidance (RIG) system operated by the division or local unit offices of the ACS, and the Cancer Resource Service (CRS) provided by the national ACS office.

- The CRS and the RIG are complementary services, with the national service focused primarily on access to a wide variety of specialized informational materials and the local service intended to make links to the many direct services and programs available at the local level.

### "I Can Cope"

- "I Can Cope" is an eight-session, 12-hour structured patient education program originally developed by oncology nurses with support from a local ACS office.

### "Reach to Recovery" and "CanSurmount"

- "Reach to Recovery" and "CanSurmount" are similar programs offered by the ACS. Through these programs, cancer patients are put in contact on a one-on-one basis with ACS volunteers with similar backgrounds who are survivors of cancer.

### "Look Good . . . Feel Better"

- This national program is designed to help women undergoing cancer treatment to address ways of maintaining grooming and appearance.

## National Cancer Institute

- Two offices within the NCI are especially assigned research and information responsibilities—the Office of Cancer Communication (OCC), and the International Cancer Information Center (ICIC).

### Physician Data Query

- Developed in 1984, Physician Data Query (PDQ) is the NCI's most up-to-date source of cancer information. PDQ provides three types of information: cancer information summaries, clinical trial and standard protocols, and directories.

### Cancer Information Service

- The Cancer Information Service (CIS) is a national network of 19 regional offices funded and coordinated by the NCI's OCC.
- The CIS is responsible for three types of services; the first is to provide up-to-date information in response to inquiries.
- In addition, each center in the network is responsible for maintaining a directory of cancer-related services and programs in the region it serves.
- Finally, each center's staff includes an outreach coordinator who is responsible for an outreach program designed to serve as a catalyst for cancer education initiatives in the region and for providing technical assistance for activities related to those initiatives.

### CancerLit

- CancerLit is a comprehensive bibliographic database of published cancer research.

### Cancer Patient Education Network

- The Cancer Patient Education Network is a network of patient education specialists to improve communication among health care professionals on cancer education needs and advances.
  - This network has three prime goals: (1) to increase cancer patient educators' access to the materials, services, and technical expertise; (2) to encourage networking and sharing of information and resources; and (3) to provide PES staff with a direct link to the issues and concerns of cancer patients.

## Combined Health Information Database

- The Combined Health Information Database (CHID) is a computer-based bibliographic database developed and maintained cooperatively by several health-related federal government agencies.
- The database includes bibliographic citations and abstracts for a variety of special reports, pamphlets, audiovisuals, product descriptions, "hard-to-find information sources," and health promotion and education programs at state and local levels.

## Advocacy and Support Groups

- Specialized organizations focus on providing education and support programs for cancer patients and their families, particularly in the area of cancers affecting women.
- There are many such groups, some of national prominence, some with more regional impact. Some of these groups are discussed on text page 1661.

## New Technologies and the Growth of Patient Education and Support

- Nurses need to keep informed about new resources and how these might be used in their clinical practice.
- It is also important to be aware of the resources available to patients and families who seek information on their own.
- The increasing availability and use of information drawn from electronic networks, and of talk groups as a source of nonprofessional information and support, raise a variety of questions regarding impact, the potential for benefit but also for misinformation and nonbeneficial contact, and changes that may result in the role of health care professionals in patient education.

## FUTURE CONSIDERATIONS FOR PATIENT EDUCATION AND SUPPORT

### Demographic Patterns and Their Implications

- Demographic patterns, in conjunction with changing socioeconomic patterns—themselves caused in part by demography—have implications for patient support structures and economic factors affecting education and support opportunities.

### Changes in Technology

- Special challenges in the area of using technology will be keeping pace with new developments, assisting those who find use of computers or other electronic equipment stressful or perplexing, and simply finding ways to assess, select, and manage the vast amount of resources that become available.

### The Changing Patterns of Health Care Delivery Systems

- The changing health care delivery system presents two major challenges from a patient education and support perspective.
  - First, nurses need to be alert to the need to be advocates for strong education and support programming.
  - Second, particular attention is needed to ensure continuity in patient education and support services across the diverse components of the delivery system.

### Demonstrating Effectiveness of Patient Education and Support

- Patient education and support must be shown to be essential elements of the health care system, and the system must be built in a way that will ensure the time, the resources, and the financial support for these critical elements.

# PRACTICE QUESTIONS

1. The Health Belief Model is based on the principle that:
   a. the individual must perceive a threat.
   b. one can accomplish the behavior change or action required.
   c. benefits of the behavior change outweigh barriers or negative outcomes.
   d. all of the above.

2. Two coping styles for dealing with cancer include monitoring and blunting. Blunters are individuals who:
   a. give high levels of attention to threatening health information but whose stress levels blunt their ability to respond to conventional patient education interventions.
   b. seek excessive participation in treatment decisions, thereby blunting the health professional's greater effectiveness.
   c. avoid information that presents threatening health information.
   d. a and b.

3. In the development of patient education materials and resources, pretesting is used primarily during which phase(s)?
   a. planning and strategy selection
   b. implementation
   c. assessing effectiveness
   d. all of the above

4. Strategies for designing effective culturally sensitive patient education programs include which of the following?
   a. consulting with key members of the cultural community in designing the program
   b. limiting involvement of members of the community in program development
   c. presenting the program to the community leaders for their support
   d. teaching educational programs in high school

5. The purpose of the Cancer Patient Education Network is to:
   a. create a database that is readily accessible to cancer patients through any local or regional ACS office, with the eventual goal of database access from any clinic or physician's office in the United States.
   b. improve communication among health care professionals on cancer education needs and advances.
   c. provide an outreach program from a variety of local or regional offices to serve as a catalyst for cancer education initiatives in these regions and for providing technical assistance for activities related to those initiatives.
   d. a and c.

# ANSWER EXPLANATIONS

1. **The answer is d.** The Health Belief Model is based on the principles that the individual must perceive a threat and that something can be done about it. This second expectation has three components: that a behavior change or action will reduce either the severity of or the susceptibility to the threat; that one can accomplish the behavior change or action required; and that benefits of the behavior change outweigh barriers or negative outcomes. (p. 1647)

2. **The answer is c.** Blunters are individuals who avoid information that presents threatening health information. (p. 1648)

3. **The answer is a.** In the development of patient education materials and resources, pretesting is used primarily in the following phases: planning and strategy selection; selecting processes and materials; and developing materials and pretests. (p. 1653)

4. **The answer is a.** Make linkages with key members of the target community, involving members of the community in the development of educational materials, programs, and community outreach strategies. (p. 1653)

5. **The answer is b.** The purpose of the Cancer Patient Education Network is to improve communication among health care professionals on cancer education needs and advances. (p. 1660)

# Chapter 59    Advancing Cancer Nursing Through Nursing Education

**This chapter corresponds to Chapter 60 in** *Cancer Nursing: Principles and Practice*, **Fourth Edition.**

## HISTORY OF CANCER NURSING EDUCATION

- Specialized education in oncology nursing began in the 1940s.
- Continuing education (CE) has been the most widely used method to increase the knowledge and skill of nurses.
- The ACS was an early provider of educational programs for practicing nurses.

## IMPORTANT INFLUENCES ON CANCER NURSING EDUCATION

### Organizations

- Several very important cancer organizations have had a powerful impact on education in cancer nursing. They include the ACS, the Oncology Nursing Society (ONS), the NCI, and the Association of Pediatric Oncology Nurses (APON).

#### American Cancer Society

- The ACS professorship program was established to improve the care of the patient and the quality of nursing education in cancer.

#### Oncology Nursing Society

- The ONS mission today is to promote excellence in oncology nursing by setting standards, studying ways to improve oncology nursing, encouraging nurses to specialize in oncology nursing, fostering the professional development of oncology nurses, and maintaining an organizational structure responsive to the needs of its members.
- The Education Committee of the ONS has been active over the years in developing standards of education that have had a significant impact on cancer nursing education.

#### National Cancer Institute

- The NCI has made major contributions to oncology nursing education in a number of ways, including educational programs, work-study programs, fellowship programs, funding for research, predoctoral and postdoctoral research training grants, publications, and providing access to current reliable information through the Cancer Information Service (CIS).

#### Association of Pediatric Oncology Nurses

- Association of Pediatric Oncology Nurses (APON) objectives are to promote excellence in the care of children with cancer, provide communication for nurses, disseminate information about care of patients, encourage publication in professional and lay literature, and support research in pediatric oncology.

## Scholarships

- In 1981 scholarships for master's-level preparation were established by the ACS, and in 1986 scholarship support at the doctoral level began.
- The ONS also offers scholarships at both the bachelor's and the master's levels.
- The NCI offers fellowships at the predoctoral, doctoral, and postdoctoral levels.
- Many hospitals have tuition reimbursement programs.

## Certification

- The mission of the Oncology Nursing Certification Corporation (ONCC) is to advance oncology nursing through the certification process. Ultimately, the goal of certification is to promote the health and well-being of those diagnosed with or at risk for experiencing cancer.
- In 1984 the ONCC contracted with the Educational Testing Service (ETS) to develop a test to assess the general oncology knowledge of the professional nurse.
- The certification examination is open to nurses who have the following:
  - a current license
  - two and one-half years of experience as a registered nurse over the 5-year period prior to application
  - at least 1000 hours of oncology nursing practice within two and one-half years prior to application
- Oncology-certified nurses have the opportunity to renew their certification at four-year intervals.
- The first Advanced Oncology Nursing Certification examination was offered in 1995 to nurses with a master's or higher degree and experience in administration, education, practice, or research.
- In a number of states, Advanced Oncology Nursing Certification is recognized for the licensure of advanced practice nurses.

## CANCER NURSING EDUCATION TODAY

### Conceptual Framework

- Central to oncology nursing practice is the individual-family concept. The health-illness concept is the adaptation of the individual and family along a continuum. The practice of cancer nursing occurs in the health care system. The community-environment concept provides the resources and support necessary for individuals with cancer.

### Standards of Oncology Nursing Education

- The *Outcome Standards for Cancer Nursing Education at the Fundamental Level* were first published in 1982. The ultimate outcomes of the standards are to enhance the quality of oncology nursing education and to improve the health care for the public.
- In 1987 the *Scope of Advanced Oncology Practice* was developed and laid the foundation for the development of *Standards for Oncology Nursing Education: Advanced Level*.
- The purpose of the standards is to provide guidelines to:
  - plan and evaluate generalist education encompassing diploma, associate, and baccalaureate programs
  - plan and evaluate advanced education at the master's, doctoral, and postdoctoral levels;
  - plan and evaluate continuing education programs at all levels; and
  - assess individual knowledge of oncology nursing care.
- At both the generalist and specialist levels, five categories of standards with general descriptive statements relate to faculty, resources, curriculum, the teaching-learning process, and the learner.

### Generalist level

- The generalist level of cancer nursing, originally referred to as the fundamental level, provides a core of knowledge, skill, and attitudes for beginning practice in cancer nursing. Although the generalist level encompasses diploma, associate, and baccalaureate educational programs, the literature deals only with baccalaureate education.

### Advanced level

- The advanced level of cancer nursing education encompasses graduate education. Education at this level is concerned with the development of a broader scope of practice, coordination, continuity, and evaluation of care.

## Continuing Education

- Nurses should participate in CE to maintain and enhance special knowledge and skills unique to oncology nursing.
- The ONS has a responsibility to provide CE to its members to help them acquire the knowledge and skills necessary for competent practice.

## CRITICAL ISSUES AND CHALLENGES

## Invitational Conference on the Clinical Nurse Specialist Role

- There are a number of critical issues and challenges in cancer nursing that educators must consider.
- Two invitational conferences on the role of the oncology clinical nurse specialist were held. These are reviewed on text pages 1672–1673.

## State-of-the-Knowledge Conference on Advanced Practice in Oncology Nursing

- Participants at this invitational conference, held in 1994, discussed titling, reimbursement, documentation, prescriptive authority, education, licensure, certification, and credentialing. Their recommendations are listed on text page 1673.

## Continuing Education

- Because baccalaureate and master's educational programs do not always have the time or the flexibility to include all things, continuing education must be relied on to provide some of the content that cannot be dealt with within the confines of a curriculum.

## Recruitment of Students

- Because admissions to nursing programs at both the undergraduate and graduate levels have decreased over the past few years, effort must be made to try to attract the traditional as well as the older, nontraditional student—an often untapped source. Recruitment of minority nurses is crucial.

## Prevention and Early Detection

- More emphasis must be placed on prevention, risk reduction, and early-detection activities.
- It is estimated that one in four individuals could be saved through early detection.
- Nurses can have a powerful impact on patients in prevention and early-detection activities for the major sites of cancer.

### Practitioner or Specialist

- Advanced practice nurses with clinical nurse specialist, nurse practitioner, or blended roles are essential to meet future challenges.
- The roles of the APN are diverse and are expanding and evolving rapidly.

### Standards and the Curriculum

- Faculty should be familiar with the recommended curriculum and follow the guidelines set forth in the *Standards*.
- While still in school, students should be encouraged to share their knowledge, skills, and expertise with others through publishing and public speaking.
- Students should be encouraged to participate in local and national ACS and ONS activities or, if in pediatrics, APON activities. Participation should be mandatory, particularly at the graduate level.
- The opportunities to network with others, share ideas, and interact with the leaders in oncology nursing abound in these organizations and can enhance one's career.

### Teaching Approaches

- Adult learning concepts—including problem-centered approaches to teaching, immediate application of knowledge, recognition of individual experience, flexible scheduling, and self-directed learning—must be incorporated into educational offerings. In addition, computer-assisted instruction (CAI) needs to be incorporated into curricula.

### Faculty Competence

- Faculty at all levels need to be prepared in oncology nursing. In addition, faculty need to be both knowledgeable in the latest trends and clinically competent as both clinical specialists and nurse practitioners.
- The clinical doctorate (DNS and DNSc) is not a solution to clinical competence unless the graduates of these programs find ways to keep their skills and expertise current.
- New and different ways to ensure competency must be explored, including:
  - new forms of collaboration between faculty and clinical staff;
  - a faculty consultation service in clinical sites; and
  - joint research projects.

### Program Evaluation

- The outcomes of the advanced practice nurse must be evaluated.

### Preceptors and Clinical Facilities

- Nursing educators must continue to nurture clinical preceptors to act as role models for students in clinical agencies.
- It is essential to recognize the contributions made by preceptors.
- Close cooperation between teachers and clinicians is essential to dispel the old dichotomy between education and practice.

### Doctoral Education

- Doctorally prepared oncology nurses are needed to ensure high-quality education, research, and practice in the future.

## Complex Care

- It is estimated that nearly 90% of cancer care is delivered in the outpatient setting. Patients cared for in the home today are far sicker, with many more complex needs, than hospital patients of yesterday. This calls for changing roles and responsibilities of nurses.

## Certification and Recertification

- The question of recertification may need to be explored further to determine whether reexamination is the best alternative for keeping the knowledge and practice of the membership current.

## Care of the Elderly

- Curricula in schools of nursing must include information on how to plan programs to incorporate healthy behaviors into lifestyles, and information specific to teaching and providing care to the elderly.

## Health Care Reform

- *Restructuring* is dedicated to reducing waste while cutting costs. *Reengineering* is involved with examining the process of what things are accomplished and how. *Redesign*, or decision making about who does what, should ensure that the most appropriately trained and educated nurses are doing the work they are best suited to do.
- Registered professional nurses have been replaced with unlicensed and ill-trained personnel who are performing skills at the bedside, hospital staff are being cross-trained to streamline care, and new graduates are having difficulty obtaining positions.

## Meeting New Health Care Challenges

- We can never become complacent about what we do in cancer education or practice, for new challenges continually arise, requiring innovative solutions and application of new knowledge and skills.

## PRACTICE QUESTIONS

1. Which group has been the *most* active over the years in establishing standards of cancer nursing practice as well as guidelines for cancer education?
   a. the Oncology Nursing Society (ONS)
   b. the American Cancer Society (ACS)
   c. the National Cancer Institute (NCI)
   d. the American Nurses' Association (ANA)

2. Within the conceptual framework for cancer nursing education developed in accordance with the Outcome Standards for Cancer Nursing Practice, which of the following concepts is central to oncology nursing practice?
   a. community-environment
   b. health care system
   c. individual and family
   d. health-illness

3. Which of the following generally applies only to the advanced level of nursing education and not to the generalist level?
   a. a baccalaureate degree
   b. a broader scope of practice
   c. clinical experience
   d. conceptual knowledge and skills

4. The *best* teaching approach to enable the cancer nurse to keep up with the changing health care environment, treatment modalities, and the nurse's numerous roles and responsibilities is:
   a. didactic lecture.
   b. hospital training with minimal lecture.
   c. self-directed learning.
   d. structured, inflexible coursework.

5. Faculty consultation in clinical sites, faculty-clinical staff research projects, and faculty-clinical staff manuscript preparation are all examples of efforts to:
   a. identify new research topics.
   b. maintain faculty clinical competence.
   c. increase academic and hospital revenue.
   d. recruit students.

6. Which of the following is *not* required for use of the designation oncology certified nurse (OCN)?
   a. two and one-half years experience as an RN within the last 5 years
   b. a baccalaureate degree with credits toward a master's degree
   c. a minimum of 1000 hours of cancer nursing practice within the last two and one-half years
   d. a passing score on the ONCC certification examination

# ANSWER EXPLANATIONS

1. **The answer is a.** The ONS has been promoting excellence in oncology nursing by setting standards, studying ways to improve oncology nursing, encouraging nurses to specialize in oncology nursing, and fostering the professional development of oncology nurses. In addition, the Education Committee of the ONS has been active over the years in developing standards of education that have had significant impact on cancer nursing education. (p. 1668)

2. **The answer is c.** Central to cancer nursing practice is the individual-family concept. The health-illness concept is the adaptation of the individual and family along a continuum. The practice of cancer nursing occurs in the health care system. The community-environment concept provides the resources and support necessary for individuals with cancer. (p. 1669)

3. **The answer is b.** Cancer nursing is practiced by both nursing generalists and nursing specialists. Nursing generalists have conceptual knowledge and skills acquired through basic nursing education, clinical experience, and professional development and updated through continuing education. They meet the concerns of individuals with cancer and provide care in a variety of health care settings. Nursing specialists have substantial theoretical knowledge gained through preparation for the master's degree. They meet diversified concerns of cancer patients and their families and function in a broader scope of practice. (p. 1671)

4. **The answer is c.** Adult learning concepts, including problem-centered approaches to teaching, immediate application of knowledge, recognition of individual experience, flexible scheduling, and self-directed learning, must be incorporated into educational offerings. (p. 1674)

5. **The answer is b.** Faculty need to be prepared in oncology nursing and need to be both knowledgeable in the latest trends and clinically competent. In addition to joint appointments, new and different ways to ensure competence must be explored. (p. 1675)

6. **The answer is b.** The Oncology Nursing Certification Corporation (ONCC) administers a certification program for cancer nurses. A certification examination is offered twice yearly. Nurses with an RN license, $2\frac{1}{2}$ years' experience as a registered nurse within the last 5 years, and a minimum of 1000 hours of cancer nursing practice within the last $2\frac{1}{2}$ years are eligible to take this examination. Certification is valid for 4 years. Renewal of certification involves a process similar to the initial certification process. Candidates must meet the same criteria as before, and an examination will constitute the requirements for recertification. (p. 1669)

# Chapter 60    Advancing Cancer Nursing Through Nursing Research

This chapter corresponds to Chapter 61 in *Cancer Nursing: Principles and Practice*, **Fourth Edition.**

## TRENDS IN HEALTH CARE AND ONCOLOGY

- Oncology care is currently more politicized and under greater public scrutiny than at anytime in history.
- The ability to forecast potential cancers in entire populations of healthy people will revolutionize cancer prevention, screening, and detection activities; systems for monitoring people with a positive genetic profile for cancer; and health care ethics.
- The magnitude, scope, and pace of scientific discovery is pushing oncology nursing practice beyond the edge of existing theory.

## TOPICS AND PRIORITIES FOR ONCOLOGY NURSING RESEARCH

- Topics for research can be identified from the results of research priority surveys and by looking at the types of studies conducted by other cancer researchers, at databases of currently funded projects and new grants, and by looking at the small grants funded by the Oncology Nursing Foundation.
- Topics continuously ranked among the top ten research priorities from 1981 to 1994 include stress, coping, and adaptation; pain; patient education; prevention and early detection; and cost containment and economic issues. Quality of life emerged as a leading research priority in both the 1991 and 1994 surveys.
  - Three topics were ranked in the top ten priorities for the first time in the 1994 survey: risk reduction and screening, neutropenia and immunosuppression, and ethical issues.

## OUTCOMES FOR NURSING RESEARCH

- There is an urgent need to link caring behaviors, care pathways, and guidelines for practice to measurable, biopsychosocial outcomes of nursing care.
- Studies of nursing outcomes must include system and organizational variables as well as outcomes that may be influenced more by other care providers or by the family.
- Table 61-2 on text page 1682 lists some of the common outcomes previously used for nursing research and quality assurance studies, nursing effectiveness studies, and cancer-related quality of life.

## MECHANISMS FOR ONCOLOGY NURSING RESEARCH
### Research Conducted by Nurse Clinicians and Advanced Practice Nurses

- Table 61-3 on text page 1683 identifies some of the ways nurses can participate in research depending on their level of education, formal research preparation, and the willingness of their employer to support research.
- Research occurs within a context of critical inquiry. A climate for research can be fostered by initiating different activities that raise the level of critical thinking.

## How to make a project feasible

- The investigator should make sure that the specific aim of the project is narrow, focused, and attainable in a realistic time period and that the timeline for completing the study is realistic and flexible.
- Sometimes it is more efficient to tag a small study onto an existing protocol than to initiate a new project. Research nurses who manage projects for physician researchers often add a nursing component to an existing medical protocol. This type of adjunct study is called a companion study.
- Figure 61-1 on text page 1684 identifies the major components of a research protocol and grant application.

## Research consultation

- Expert consultation from colleagues, a nurse scientist, and a statistician is essential. The consultant should read and critique the proposal or grant application in the early, formative stages.
- Another source of research consultation is a local chapter of the Oncology Nursing Society.
- Other sources of consultation include the research committee of the state nurses' association, local chapters of nursing specialty organizations, and the faculty of local schools of nursing.

## Tips for grant preparation

- Identify your strengths and weaknesses as a researcher. Find ways to overcome deficiencies.
- If you do not have a track record, get one or more consultants to improve your competitive edge.
- The grant application and instructions are the road map. Follow the rules and suggested guidelines carefully.
- Do not propose a full-scale study if a feasibility study is more appropriate. Pilot studies are useful to determine feasibility of a research design; to pretest an instrument; and to evaluate the risk, side effects, and compliance with a new nursing therapy.
- Try to anticipate how the reviewer will respond to your application.
- Never assume the reviewers will understand your proposal as well as you do.
- Use an editor.
- Use the appendices to support your application rather than as a catch-all.
- Support letters should be written specifically for the proposal and project.
- Budgets should never be inflated.
- Check the application for any fatal flaws.
- Check the overall integrity and logical consistency of the application by drawing a diagram that shows the interrelationships among the specific aims, design, sample, variables, instruments, and analysis plan.

## Funding for research

- A good fit between your study and the goals of the funding agency is essential to successful funding.
- The American Nurses' Foundation, a subsidiary of the American Nurses' Association, funds approximately 20 small grants each year for new researchers or researchers entering a new area of study.
- If you are seeking funding from a national or local pharmaceutical company, be sure to find out whether the funding is unrestricted or whether the company requires you to study one of their products or the side effects associated with the use of a product.
- Other sources of funding often can be found in the investigator's agency or local community.
- Chapters of the Oncology Nursing Society or other nursing specialty organizations are additional sources of local funding.
- It is important to be aware of the various funding bulletins published.

## RESEARCH CRITIQUE

- Using a systematic tool or set of guidelines to evaluate the scientific merit of a study will allow the nurse to gauge the value of the study's findings for practice.
- Oncology Nursing Foundation criteria are geared more for quantitative research designs than for qualitative designs.

## Components of Research Critique

### Qualifications of investigators and staff

- What are the qualifications of the principal investigator, consultants, and project staff?

### Abstract

- Does the abstract accurately reflect the proposed research?

### Specific aims

- Are the aims clear and understandable?

### Significance of study

- Is the study relevant to oncology nursing practice?

### Background and review of literature

- Is the conceptual or theoretical framework for the study identified? Is the review succinct, focused, and current?

### Design and methods

- There are several components to this section of a research proposal, including the following: design; sample and setting; experimental variables; instruments and measurement; data collection schedule and procedures; data analysis; study limitations; and protection of human participants.

### Statement of scientific integrity

- Procedures for maintaining the accuracy of data, adhering to IRB guidelines, ensuring the confidentiality of data, and the standardization of data collection should be described. Moreover, data entry and coding, analysis, and reporting issues should be discussed.

### Additional sections

- The proposal should also contain a reference list, time table for accomplishing the study, and letters of support from agency personnel and consultants.

## SCIENTIFIC AND ETHICAL CONDUCT OF RESEARCH

- Monitoring the scientific integrity of a project is an integral aspect of all nursing research.
- Research misconduct is any "significant misbehavior that improperly appropriates the intellectual property or contributions of others, that intentionally impedes the progress of research, or that risks corrupting the scientific record or compromising the integrity of scientific practices."
- Misappropriation refers to an intentional or reckless act of plagiarism or a violation of the confidentiality associated with the review of scientific manuscripts or grants.
- Misrepresentation is defined as a deliberate attempt to deceive or commit a reckless disregard for the truth by stating or presenting a falsehood, omitting facts, or the fabrication of data and findings.

- Other examples of research misconduct may include intentionally enrolling certain types of participants in a study to bias the findings, entering participants that fail to meet eligibility criteria, administering an experimental treatment despite severe adverse reactions, fabricating data, reporting findings of a study that was never conducted, or substituting falsified data for legitimate data.

- The principal investigator is ultimately responsible for establishing procedures to monitor the scientific integrity of a specific project.

- Table 61-4 on text page 1689 lists the types of generic activities that are needed to monitor scientific integrity and the ethical conduct of research.

## FUTURE DIRECTIONS FOR RESEARCH

- Leading the transformation of cancer care, oncology nurses will set the research agenda on cancer-related women's health, access to affordable and comprehensive care by a diverse population, the assessment of symptom distress, and the management of disease symptoms and regimen-related toxicities.

- Moreover, nurses will be the preeminent clinical researchers in the areas of cancer pain, quality of life, spirituality, cancer-related fatigue, families' responses to cancer, and caregiver issues.

- Models that synthesize the personal, environmental, and genetic risks for cancer are needed to guide research. Efforts must be made to synthesize several divergent literatures: (1) studies of cancer prevention, detection, screening, and diagnosis; (2) research on cultural beliefs about cancer; and (3) studies of the decision-making processes used by people undergoing traditional, experimental, or alternative therapy.

- With the advent of the genetics revolution, models are urgently needed to guide holistic research and practice.

- Other types of studies are needed to examine systems of care and models of nursing care delivery (e.g., advanced practice and certification issues and the care given by generalists, specialists, and unlicensed personnel).

- New mechanisms for conducting research must be established to gather data that are trustworthy and generalizable to large segments of cancer survivors.

## PRACTICE QUESTIONS

1. Three topics ranked in the top ten priorities for the first time in the ONS 1994 survey included:
   a. stress, coping, and adaptation.
   b. cost containment and economic issues.
   c. ethical issues.
   d. quality of life.

2. Of the topics listed below, the one most frequently funded by the Oncology Nursing Foundation from 1984 to 1996 was:
   a. pain.
   b. biophysical variables.
   c. quality of life.
   d. ethical issues.

3. Common outcomes appropriate to a study of quality of life might include such issues as:
   a. activities of daily living.
   b. cognitive status and will-to-live.
   c. patient acuity.
   d. all of the above.

4. Harriet, Ellen, and Min are all part of the same research team. As the only team member with a BSN, Harriet is most likely to be involved in:
   a. conducting pilot/feasibility studies with assistance of a research mentor.
   b. acting as research mentor to staff nurses and providing research critique.
   c. generating concept definition and theory development.
   d. providing expert testimony for health policy formation and funding priorities.

5. Pete is a research nurse who manages projects for a physician researcher. As a new study begins this time, Pete adds a nursing component to the existing medical protocol. This practice is called:
   a. a dependent pilot study.
   b. a companion study.
   c. misappropriation.
   d. misrepresentation.

6. Pilot studies are useful to:
   a. assess the feasibility of a research design.
   b. pretest an instrument.
   c. evaluate the risk, side effects, and compliance with a new nursing therapy.
   d. all of the above.

7. Which of the following researchers would be most likely to find Oncology Nursing Foundation criteria helpful for evaluating a study?
   a. Ed, who is conducting a pilot study
   b. Marian, who is conducting a qualitative study
   c. Kim, who is conducting quantitative research
   d. none of the above

8. If Ann is guilty of misappropriation in the course of conducting her research, she has most likely:
   a. misused the research funds entrusted to her through a grant.
   b. committed plagiarism.
   c. tagged her study onto an existing protocol rather than initiating a new project.
   d. deliberately omitted fact or fabricated data and findings.

---

## ANSWER EXPLANATIONS

1. **The answer is c.** Three topics were ranked in the top ten priorities for the first time in the ONS's 1994 survey: risk reduction and screening, neutropenia and immunosuppression, and ethical issues. The other choices have already been leading research priorities in past surveys. (p. 1680)

2. **The answer is c.** Some of the topics most frequently funded by the Oncology Nursing Foundation from 1984 to 1996 include the following (beginning with the most frequently funded): stress, coping, and adaptation; breast cancer; intervention studies; and quality of life. (Table 61-1, p. 1681)

3. **The answer is a.** Common outcomes appropriate to a study of quality of life might include such issues as physical functioning (activities of daily living, sexuality, etc.); family function and social support; symptoms; spirituality (religiosity, self-transcendent experiences, etc.); emotional functioning; and economic status. (Table 61-2, p. 1682)

4. **The answer is a.** Nurses with a BSN may typically participate in research by acting as study monitors, data collectors, and project managers; helping develop and review feasibility of projects; conducting pilot/feasibility studies with assistance of research mentor; participating in journal clubs; conducting electronic literature searches; and preparing research-based guidelines for practice and care pathways. (Table 61-3, p. 1683)

5. **The answer is b.** A companion study is a type of adjunct study in which a small study is tagged onto an existing protocol rather than initiating a new project. Research nurses who manage projects for physician researchers often add a nursing component to an existing medical protocol. (p. 1683)

6. **The answer is d.** Pilot studies are useful to determine the effective size of an intervention; to assess the feasibility of a research design; to pretest an instrument; and to evaluate the risk, side effects, and compliance with a new nursing therapy. (p. 1684)

7. **The answer is c.** Oncology Nursing Foundation criteria are geared more for quantitative research designs. Criteria for evaluating qualitative studies can be found elsewhere. (p. 1686)

8. **The answer is b.** Misappropriation refers to an intentional or reckless act of plagiarism or a violation of the confidentiality associated with the review of scientific manuscripts or grants. (p. 1688)

# Chapter 61      Cultural Diversity Among Individuals with Cancer

*This chapter corresponds to Chapter 62 in* Cancer Nursing: Principles and Practice, *Fourth Edition.*

## INTRODUCTION

### Overview

- Ethnic minority populations are growing at rates that are surpassing the rest of the population. This trend is not matched in the composition of health care professionals.
- A fundamental challenge for health care providers is that the health care beliefs and practices of many ethnic groups may not be congruent with mainstream medicine.
- See Table 62-1 on text page 1693 for definitions of selected terms.

### Epidemiology

- From the latest available national data, there are obvious differences in cancer incidence, mortality, and survival rates when data are compared across all ethnic groups.
- Age-adjusted incidence rates (overall and selected cancer sites) for 1988–1992 are based on SEER data and are provided in Table 62-2 on text page 1694.
- Mortality rates, age-adjusted for the same time period, are shown in Table 62-3 on text pages 1696–1697 and are based on cancer deaths for the entire U.S. population.
- Table 62-4 on text page 1698 shows five-year relative survival rates for 1975–1984 based on data from the NCI Special Populations Studies Branch.
- There are limitations in the SEER data because (1) SEER data does not reflect the total U.S. population; (2) cancer rates in smaller populations are less precise than rates in larger populations; (3) the native American population is represented by two separate groups: Alaska native and American Indian; and (4) individuals who classify themselves as being of Hispanic ethnicity may be of any race, resulting in some overlap.
- However, the SEER data are helpful in identifying general ethnic patterns of cancer.
- Possible factors that contribute to variations in cancer incidence and mortality in different ethnic groups include environmental and/or socioeconomic factors; access to health care; cultural values, beliefs, and health practices; and genetic predisposition. These factors are often interdependent and interrelated. Table 62-5 on text page 1699 provides a brief summary.

## TRANSCULTURAL NURSING AND ASSESSMENT

### Transcultural Nursing

- The aim of transcultural nursing is to understand and assist diverse cultural groups and members of such groups with their nursing and health care needs.
- A nurse must carefully identify his or her personal cultural beliefs and values to separate them from the patient's beliefs and values.
- Cultural relativity, the attempt to view or interpret the behavior of culturally different individuals within the context of their own culture, is the nurse's goal.
- Transcultural nursing is concerned with shared meanings and the degree to which the nurse and patient agree or disagree about the cultural symbols of health, healing, illness, disease, and caring.

## Cultural Assessment

- Giger and Davidhizar's Transcultural Assessment Model, outlined in Figure 62-1 on text page 1700, identifies six essential cultural phenomena that the nurse considers in providing culturally competent nursing care. These phenomena include communication, space, social organization, time, environment control, and biological variations.

### Communication

- Communication is the means by which culture is transmitted and preserved.
- The most obvious cultural difference among people is language.
- The meaning of silence varies among cultural groups.
- Nonverbal behavior may repeat, clarify, contradict, modify, emphasize, or regulate the flow of communication.
- To communicate effectively with culturally diverse patients, the nurse needs to be aware of what nonverbal behaviors mean to the patient and what specific nonverbal behaviors mean in the patient's culture.
- Strategies for effective communication are outlined in Table 62-6 on text page 1702.

### Space

- The relationship between the individual's own body, the objects, and people within the space is learned and influenced by one's culture.
- In Western cultures, spatial distances are defined as the intimate zone, the personal zone, and the social and public zones.
- Personal space is the area that surrounds a person's body and includes space and objects within the space. Spatial behavior most often is described as a universal need for territoriality.
- Territoriality is a state characterized by possessiveness, control, and authority over an area of physical space.
- Nurses move through all spatial zones; thus, the nurse must be sensitive to patients' reactions to movement toward them.
- Objects in the environment may affect communication differently in different cultures.
- Certain clothing or objects may be worn, reflecting cultural beliefs.
- Patients may wish to arrange their space differently and control the placement of objects on their bedside cabinet or over-bed table.

### Social organization

- Significant components of social organization include knowledge of family structure and organization, religious values and beliefs, and how ethnicity and culture relate to role and role assignment within group settings.
- The family is the basic unit of society.
- The value placed on children and elderly is also culturally determined.
- Gender roles are often culturally determined.
- The extent of the family's involvement in a hospitalized patient's care may be dictated by the culture.
- Religions have an influence on the lifestyles of most cultures and may affect health care practices.

### Time

- Time orientation refers to an individual's focus on the present or the future.
  - The American focus on time tends to be directed to the future, emphasizing planning and schedules.

- The present-oriented perspective is that time is flexible and events will begin when the person arrives.

### Environmental control

- Environmental control refers to the ability of members of a particular cultural group to plan activities that control nature or direct environmental factors.
- Herberg describes three health belief views.
  - In the magico-religious health belief view, health and illness are controlled by supernatural forces.
  - The scientific or biomedical health belief view is that life and life processes are controlled by physical and biochemical processes that can be manipulated by humans.
  - The holistic health view is that the forces of nature must be in balance or harmony. Human life is one aspect of nature and must be in harmony with the rest of nature.
    - The four aspects of the individual's nature—the physical, the mental, the emotional, and the spiritual—must be in balance for the individual to be healthy.
- Folk medicine is defined as those beliefs and practices relating to illness, prevention, and health that derive from cultural traditions rather than from modern medicine's scientific base. Folk medicine is thought to be more humanistic.

### Biological variations

- Biological variations include differences in skin, eye, and hair color; facial characteristics; the amount of body hair; and body size and shape. Some cultural groups are more susceptible to certain diseases.
- Table 62-7 on text page 1705 outlines a brief cultural assessment tool based on the Transcultural Assessment Model.

## Heritage Consistency

- The heritage consistency theory views acculturation on a continuum and aids in assessing the degree to which people identify with the dominant or traditional cultures.

## Self Assessment

- Figure 62-3 on text page 1708 provides a simple tool for nurses to use in exploring their anticipated responses to types of individuals representing five general categories: ethnic/racial, social issues/problems, religious, physically/mentally handicapped, and political.

## ETHNICITY AND CANCER

- Spector has summarized data for four major ethnic minority groups using the six cultural phenomena of the Transcultural Assessment Model. (See Table 62-8 on text page 1710.)
- There are many subgroups within the four major ethnic groups (African-American, API, Hispanic, and native American).

## African-Americans

- In general, the overall cancer incidence rate for African-American males is about 16% higher than that for Caucasian males. Among the different ethnic groups, African-Americans have the highest incidence and mortality rates for cancers of the esophagus, larynx, pancreas, and prostate, and for multiple myeloma.

- African-American women have the highest mortality rate for cervical cancer, and African-American men have the highest incidence and mortality rates for lung cancer.
- African-American women experience significantly more cervical cancer and early-age breast cancer than Caucasians.

### Health beliefs and practices

- The health beliefs of African-Americans include a tendency to categorize events as either desirable or undesirable.
- There is a strong relationship between faith and healing.
- Another belief among some African-Americans is that everything has an opposite.
- African-Americans tend to be less knowledgeable about cancer than Caucasians and tend to underestimate the prevalence of cancer and the significance of the common warning signs for cancer.
- African-Americans are often more fatalistic about cancer and are less likely to believe that early detection or treatment can make a difference in the outcome of the disease.
- African-Americans are more likely than Caucasians to prefer not to know their own cancer diagnosis.
- African-Americans may choose not to seek care if they perceive that values will be compromised.

### Healing practices

- A variety of folk healers are used by African-Americans. These healers are well-respected individuals and can be a powerful resource to the health care team. Religion is incorporated as part of therapy and is a means to a cure.
- A treatment plan that is congruent with the patient's own beliefs has a better chance of being successful.

### Social organization

- The African-American family is often oriented around women, and the wife or mother generally is charged with the responsibility for protecting the health of family members.
- Some families have large social networks that are very supportive during times of illness.
- Many African-Americans find it impossible to separate religious beliefs from health beliefs. The most common and frequently cited method of treating illness remains prayer.

### Communication

- The use of standard English versus black English varies among African-Americans and is sometimes related to educational level and socioeconomic status. Black English is a unifying factor for African-Americans in maintaining their cultural and ethnic identity. It is not uncommon for some African-Americans to speak standard English when in a professional capacity or when socializing with Caucasians, and then revert back to black English when in African-American settings.
- For more effective communication, the nurse who works with African-Americans must understand as much of the context of the dialect as possible.

### Space and time

- Many African-Americans have a "today" or "present" health orientation and their approach to the prevention of cancer may be to work out problems as they occur, rather than trying to prevent them from occurring.

## Death and dying issues

- In African language the primary time frames are past and present. No word exists for the distant future, as it has not yet happened. Consequently the future and the past are merged into the present. Life is viewed as cyclical.
- The strong family network of African-Americans is called into action when a family member is seriously ill.
- Death may be viewed as a passage from the evils of this world to another state. It is a "going home" to be reunited with loved ones.

## Biological variations

- A major biological variation in African-Americans is skin color. Some African-Americans may erroneously believe this darkness protects them from burning from the sun and from skin cancer.
- The diet of many African-Americans contains little fresh produce, is highly seasoned, and includes frequent use of smoked and fatty meats as seasoning for vegetables and soups.
- Lactose intolerance affects 75% of African-Americans.
- Alcoholism is a major health problem in the African-American community and a risk factor for cancer of the mouth, larynx, tongue, esophagus, lung, and liver.

# Asian/Pacific Islanders

- APIs are the fastest growing ethnic minority group in the United States.
- Approximately 95% of APIs are Asian Americans compared to 5% who are Pacific Islander Americans.

## Health beliefs and practices

- Many APIs believe that a balance between hot and cold elements is essential for good health. In the Chinese, Japanese, and Korean cultures, in particular, this balance is defined as *yin* (cold) and *yang* (hot).
- The Chinese believe that the human body, illnesses, and foods possess *yin* or *yang* characteristics and treatment is aimed at reestablishing the balance. For example, cancer is a *yin* or cold illness and would be treated with foods, herbs, and healing ceremonies that possess "hot" properties.
- There exists a widespread belief among some API groups that suffering is part of life.
- Many APIs believe that blood is a life force that cannot be replaced or, if taken, will disrupt the body's balance causing weakness and even death.

## Healing practices

- APIs practice the use of herbal medications, seek traditional healers, and perform healing ceremonies.
- Traditional healers among the API are often consulted before Western medical practitioners.
- Healing ceremonies or practices vary considerably across API groups. Some of these practices include moxibustion, cupping, acupuncture, massage, and skin scraping or coining.
- In the native Hawaiian culture, healing includes special rituals, prayers, and chants as well as the use of special herbs and plants.

## Social organization

- The APIs have very strong, family-centered systems. In many API groups, patrilineal authority along with filial piety and respect for elders often means that the eldest son or male head of the clan is the spokesperson for the patient.
- API family members are more likely to actively participate in the patient's daily care.

## Communication

- In many API groups, communication patterns are influenced by values that emphasize politeness, respect for authority, and avoidance of shame. These values prevent many APIs from asking health professionals questions or challenging a proposed diagnostic workup and/or treatment plan.
- In communicating with some API groups, Western practitioners may need to avoid or limit engaging in direct eye contact, because such eye contact may be perceived as being rude, challenging, or just culturally unacceptable.
- Many APIs prefer limited or no physical contact.

## Space and time

- APIs value privacy and many are also very modest. When physical examinations or procedures necessitate exposure of the body, exposure should be minimized by revealing only that part of the body that needs to be examined.
- The concept of time varies among the API groups. The Japanese, who are present and future oriented, are usually prompt and adhere to fixed schedules. On the other hand, Chinese are more present oriented, do not necessarily adhere to fixed schedules, and may be late for appointments. Filipinos are past and present oriented and may disregard health-related matters.

## Death and dying issues

- Bioethics, truth telling, patient's right to know, and advance directive decisions may not be culturally acceptable or valued.
- The initiation and continuation of life-support measures also may vary from group to group.
- Conflict may arise between the value in Western medicine of open disclosure of a terminal illness and the value shared by many API groups that "to tell someone he or she is dying is not only rude but dangerous."
- Although hospice care discussions may not always be encouraged, some APIs prefer to die at home rather than at the hospital.

## Biological variations

- The incidence rate for liver cancer is exceptionally high in API groups, particularly the southeast Asian groups. This increased rate for liver cancer is linked to the high incidence of hepatitis B infection in these groups.
- Japanese, Koreans, and Vietnamese all have high rates of stomach cancer.
- Lactose intolerance is also common in APIs.
- The physical characteristics of APIs may necessitate adjusting the dosage of certain medications.
- A distinguishing yellow cast to skin can make the recognition of jaundice more challenging.
- See Table 62-9 on text page 1717 for comparative percentages of participation among the different ethnic groups.

# Hispanics

- *Hispanic* is an umbrella term for several subgroups in the United States including people of Mexican, Puerto Rican, Cuban, Caribbean, and Central and South American origin.
- Generally, the cancer incidence rate among Hispanics ranks in the middle when compared with other ethnic groups.
- The largest concentrated population of Hispanics in the United States lives in Los Angeles. In this group there is a high risk of gallbladder, cervical, and stomach cancers.

- There appears to be a genetic predisposition and higher incidence of gallbladder cancer among Hispanic men and women in New Mexico. A similar pattern was found for biliary cancer in Hispanics in Los Angeles County.

## Health beliefs and practices

- Health is often believed to be the result of good luck or a reward from God for good behavior.
- There is often a fatalistic belief that one is at the mercy of the environment and has little control over what happens.
- Hautman identifies several categories of disease in the Hispanic culture.
  - The concept of hot and cold imbalance resembles the *yin* and *yang* in the Chinese culture. An equilibrium exists between hot and cold elements in a healthy body.
  - Another common health disorder is believed to be caused by the dislocation of organs.
  - Another group of illnesses is believed to be caused by magical interventions.
  - In Hispanic culture, there are two types of emotional diseases: mental and moral illnesses.
  - The last category includes scientific diseases that cannot be treated by traditional health practices and must be diagnosed and treated by the Western health care system.
- Cancer is seen fatalistically as God's will, and it goes against principle to aggressively treat the disease.
- Hispanic individuals may believe that there is no need to see a physician unless a person is very ill. Hospitals are seen as places where people die.
- Many Hispanics fear that because of their economic status and ethnicity, they may receive inferior care in the U.S. medical system. Some believe they should receive only health care they can afford.
- Hipanics often believe that it is not appropriate to question those giving care because of the fear of retaliation.
- Because some Hispanics believe that physical touch can promote healing, if Western providers do *not* touch during their visit, some Hispanics may believe that they did not derive any benefit from that visit.
- Suggestions for assimilating Hispanic individuals to the U.S. health care system are listed on text page 1718.

## Healing practices

- Home remedies are the first line of treatment. To cure a hot or cold imbalance, the opposite quality of the causative agent is applied.
- There is usually a family folk healer, someone respected for her knowledge of folk medicine. The healing practices are passed down in the family from mother to daughter.
- The Cuban population may seek medical help from a *santero*, a medicine man who works with the spirits of good within a system to promote wellness. A *jerbero* is a healer that uses herbs and spices for prevention of illness and for healing. A *brujo* uses witchcraft for healing illnesses that may be related to jealousy or envy (*envida*). If these fail, then Western physicians may be sought for help.

## Social organization

- The nuclear family is the foundation of the Hispanic community. Men are the breadwinners, they assume the dominant role in Hispanic families, and they are considered big and strong (*macho*). Women have always been the primary caretakers. The extended family is valued and the family's needs supersede those of the individual members. The family should be used to help with the patient's care.
- The patient may turn to religious practices to help overcome the illness; allowing time and providing privacy for the family to carry out these religious practices will be helpful to many Hispanics.

## Communication

- Spanish is the primary language with many dialectal differences. The traditional Hispanic approach to communication requires the use of diplomacy and tactfulness. Politeness and courtesy is highly regarded.
- Body language may be dramatic when expressing pain or emotion. Hispanics in pain may groan and moan to let those around them know they are uncomfortable and suffering.

## Space and time

- Adult Hispanics may be described as tactile in their relationships but there is a high degree of modesty.
- They generally do not like being touched by others or having to touch themselves and are not comfortable being examined by health care professionals of the opposite sex. Embarrassment is a common reaction to invasive procedures or body exposure during an examination.
- Hispanics generally have a relaxed concept of time—a present orientation—and may be late for appointments.

## Death and dying issues

- The afterlife of heaven and hell exists in the Hispanic culture. Because many Hispanics are Catholic, religious practices like baptism of the dying and the administration of the sacrament of the sick are important.
- As expected, the family serves as a protective network for helping the dying and their survivors handle the emotional problems associated with death.
- Public expression of grief is expected.

## Biological Variations

- The traditional Hispanic diet is high in fiber and carbohydrates from staples such as rice, beans, and corn. It contains few leafy green vegetables. The use of lard and the common practice of frying foods contribute to the high fat content of the Hispanic diet.
- Among the high-risk behaviors in the Hispanic population are obesity, alcohol consumption, and sexual practices.
- Obesity is a common problem among Hispanics in the United States due to their diet and lack of physical activity.
- Hispanic men tend to drink at younger ages and consume larger amounts of alcohol more often than do Caucasians.
- There is a high risk for cervical cancer because of male sexual promiscuity and infrequent use of condoms, predisposing females to sexually transmitted diseases.

## Native Americans

- The native Americans include natives of the continental United States, Aleuts, and Alaskan Eskimos. They are a very diverse group consisting of many tribes and over 400 federally recognized nations, each with its own traditions and cultural heritage.
- Reservations have a high percentage of very young members and a growing number of members over 55 years of age. Because the reservation land cannot support a growing and increasingly concentrated population, poverty and welfare dependency are common.
- Nearly two-thirds of all native Americans live in non-reservation communities.
- Cancer is ranked as the third leading cause of death among native Americans, preceded by accidents and heart disease. Native Americans (American Indians) also have the lowest cancer incidence and rank mid to low in mortality rates of all U.S. minority populations.

- Incidence rates are the highest for cancers of the kidney and renal pelvis in native American men, and of the ovary in native American women. Low rates of cancer of the lung, breast, and colon/rectum are evident in native Americans.
- Because native Americans are younger than the majority population and have a shorter life expectancy, they often do not live long enough to develop cancer.
- This group has high rates of obesity and diseases associated with alcohol and tobacco use that are risk factors for many types of cancers.
- The increased incidence of cervical cancer primarily among older native American women is a result of infrequent or no history of Pap smear screening and lack of follow-up for abnormal results.
- Gallbladder cancer and gallbladder diseases are common in native Americans.
- At least one-third of the native American population live in extreme poverty.
- Although health care is available through the Indian Health Service, barriers for native Americans to access it include poverty and the lack of transportation. Native Americans believe in living day-to-day rather than in planning for the future, and most do not have savings or insurance to pay for health care.

## Health beliefs and practices

- Tribes vary in their beliefs about health and illness, but most tribes link health beliefs and religion. To the native American, religion is something that surrounds an individual at all times and has a profound influence on the entire being.
- Health reflects living in harmony with nature, and humans have an intimate relationship with nature.
- Unwellness is caused by the disharmony of mind, body, and spirit. Natural unwellness is caused by the violation of a sacred or tribal taboo.
- Illness may be caused by witchcraft.
- All causes of illness or disease are believed to have supernatural aspects.
- Diseases of object intrusion refer to the invasion of the body by a worm, snake, insect, or small animal. This may be a result of witchcraft.
- Many native Americans believe that they are responsible for their own health and illness.
- The most prevalent pattern for the native American is the alternate use of traditional medicine and Western medicine either independently of each other or simultaneously. In most instances the two systems are complementary and should be encouraged.
- Some tribes are not receptive to invasive bodily procedures and only reluctantly will agree to surgery.
- Offering food is a tangible expression of the link in a relationship and serves as something always to be remembered about that individual.
- Because of a history of inconsistent care and disrespectful treatment, native Americans often are not comfortable with Western health care providers.
- The pain threshold of native Americans is often considered high because stoicism is valued in their culture.
- When treatment is sought, medication generally is expected. If none is given, the native American may be disappointed because expectations for treatment were not met.

## Healing practices

- The traditional healer is the medicine person who is wise in the ways of the land and nature.
- There are different types of medicine men and women with specific roles.
  - The first type are those who assume a purely positive role. They cannot use their powers in a negative way. Their main role is to maintain cultural integration at a time of great cultural stress.

- The second type of healers are capable of both good and evil. They are expected to perform negative acts toward the tribe's enemies and have knowledge of witchcraft, poisoning, and other ways of doing evil to others.
  - The diviner-diagnosticians are the third type. They diagnose the cause of the disharmony and may indicate a cure but do not have the power or skill necessary to implement treatment.
  - Fourth are the medicine men and women who specialize in the use of herbs for curative and nonsacred medical procedures.
  - Fifth are those medicine men and women whose primary concern is to care for souls.
  - Last are the singers who are usually male. The singer is the medicine man who treats illnesses and disharmony.
- Native Americans believe an individual gets back in equal proportion what he gives in words and actions to another.
- Healing ceremonies differ from tribe to tribe with varying degrees of complexity.
- Purification is often practiced to maintain harmony with nature and to cleanse the body and spirit.
- Western physicians are regarded as a type of herbalist who can cure symptoms but cannot restore the individual's harmonious relationship with nature because they do not know the importance of rituals.

## Social organization

- Traditional native American families are generally very involved in making decisions about the member's health care and may often make the decision for the patient.
- As members of a matrilineal society, native American patients may not give consent for anything until permission is obtained from the mother, grandmother, or aunt.
- Native Americans rely on their family, tribe, and land to cope with stress.

## Communication

- Some tribes believe that a discussion with one individual about another is a sign of disrespect and could break a cultural taboo, leaving oneself or family vulnerable to harm.
- Limited ability to speak English may limit the understanding of the patient. It is common for native Americans to be silent rather than to admit to not understanding.
- Making direct eye contact may be viewed as looking into one's soul and could result in its loss.
- Who one speaks to, when the speaking occurs, how one speaks, and the sequence of speaking are very important.
- Native American communication generally emphasizes language that promotes the values of generosity, bravery, compassion, respect for elders, and concern for the tribal entity.
- The importance of observing periods of silence is a cultural trait. Silence helps formulate one's thoughts so that the spoken words will have significance.
- Native American individuals are very sensitive to body language.
- Native Americans are private people who do not readily volunteer information.
- It is common for native Americans to speak in a very soft voice.
- Note taking is considered taboo for some native Americans because traditionally their history is passed on through verbal story telling.
- Some native Americans consider a firm handshake a sign of agression.
- Using body language that is open without closing or crossing the arms is suggested. Loud speech may be viewed as rude or angry and speaking slowly may be perceived as condescending.
- Initiating a visit with casual conversation about family, social functions, and about the tribe they are from may be helpful since native Americans are very private.

## Space and time

- Personal space is very important to some native Americans who may have difficulty adapting to situations that place them in spaces that are not familiar such as clinics or hospitals.
- Modesty is very significant.
- Time is casual, present oriented, and relative to present needs that must be accomplished in a given time frame.

## Death and dying issues

- Existence is circular and continuous for most traditional native Americans.
- Navajos will not touch a person who is dying because they must let the person go; touching could delay the soul's journey to the next world.
- Attitudes and approaches to death and dying vary considerably among the tribes.

## Biological variations

- There is a high incidence of obesity and alcohol abuse in native Americans.

# NURSING ISSUES

## Cancer, Poverty, and Ethnicity

- The impact of poverty on cancer is felt in ethnic minorities since a disproportionate number of ethnic minorities comprises the poor of America.
- The "culture of poverty" includes economic factors, social factors, and psychological factors that increase cancer incidence and mortality by increasing risk factors.
- Secondary prevention may be absent because of a present orientation where survival needs take precedence over screening and early detection.
- Delayed tertiary prevention is due to a lack of insurance, inability to pay for service, or limited care access.
- There are many common elements between the culture of poverty and the cultures of the four ethnic groups discussed. Poverty is overrepresented in these groups.
- The many recommendations made in the American Cancer Society report on *Cancer in the Economically Disadvantaged* to reduce cancer incidence and mortality in the poor would be effective in many ethnic groups.

## Strategies to Enhance Access to Health Care

- Many programs focus on providing effective cancer screening for ethnic minority populations using culturally sensitive strategies. These strategies include the involvement of trusted and respected members of the community in the planning and delivery of health care services, provision of social support by women in the social network, and development of culturally sensitive patient education materials.
- Culturally appropriate strategies used in the development of effective cancer control programs are listed on text page 1726.

## Culturally Appropriate Public/Patient Education

### Strategies

- Strategies to provide culturally sensitive patient education interventions include: (1) culturally relevant and community-specific materials, (2) keeping educational messages simple, (3) determining the preferred language as well as learning process, and (4) identification of the preferred communication style of the individual.

### Use of interpreters

- The use of professional interpreters, if available, is the optimal choice. Family and/or friends may be used but the correct or complete message may not be relayed.
- Recommendations for using interpreters and what to do if there is no interpreter are listed in Table 62-10 on text page 1728.

### Translating written materials

- Translating material that is written in English into another language is not enough. The newly-translated material must be back-translated into English by independent translators.
- Analyses of the reading level of available cancer education materials have shown an average reading level that is much higher than the actual reading level of the general population.

### Preferred styles of learning

- The different styles include one-to-one versus group, oral tradition, story telling, peer educators, and receiving information from "powerful others."

## Clinical Trials and Cancer Research

- Historically, there has been underrepresentation of minorities in clinical trials.
- Two major barriers that have been identified are ethnic minorities' distrust of outsiders doing research in their communities and the lack of culturally sensitive and specific education materials.
- Additional barriers to accrual of ethnic minorities in clinical trials are listed on text page 1720.
- The Minority-Based (MB) Community Clinical Oncology Program (CCOP) has progressed as a result of the health care providers' respect for, and increased understanding of the unique cultures that they serve.
- Whether the issue is accrual of ethnic minorities to cancer treatment or cancer prevention trials, continued efforts directed toward overcoming the identified barriers are needed.
- Factors that facilitate participation in clinical trials among ethnic minorities who are socioeconomically disadvantaged are listed on text page 1799.

### Research studies

- Because of the heterogeneity of the major groups, study samples need to be selected carefully.
  - Knowing which subgroups were studied would make a difference in interpreting the research findings and distinguishing for whom the data are generalizable.
  - Knowing which particular ethnic group will be studied can make a difference in the development of appropriate instruments and the chosen research methodology.
- When research instruments are developed in English and translated into another language, subtle cultural nuances and conceptual equivalency may be compromised, leading to difficulties in retaining the validity of the instrument.

## Resources

- Three of the major resources available at the national level are the Office of Minority Health Resource Center (OMH-RC), the National Cancer Institute's Cancer Information Service (CIS), and the American Cancer Society (ACS).
- Several professional organizations also exist to promote cultural awareness in nurses and to provide support for ethnic minority nurses.

- ONS originally had two specific groups devoted to multicultural issues with an oncology focus: the Multicultural Advisory Council and the Transcultural Nursing Issues Special Interest Group (TNI SIG). The Council no longer exists.
- Specific local resources may vary in their availability from region to region as a reflection of the ethnic minority populations that are served.

## PRACTICE QUESTIONS

1. The SEER data is helpful in:
   a. reflecting cancer rates for the total U.S. population.
   b. carefully distinguishing cancer patterns in special subgroups among native American and Hispanic populations.
   c. identifying general ethnic patterns of cancer.
   d. a and c.

2. The highest overall cancer incidence rates occur among:
   a. young adult Asian/Pacific Islanders (APIs).
   b. native Americans on reservations in the northwest.
   c. African-American men.
   d. none of the above.

3. For breast cancer, the average annual rate per 100,000 individuals has been highest among _____ females.
   a. Japanese
   b. white
   c. Hawaiian
   d. black

4. The basic unit of society is the:
   a. family.
   b. social structure.
   c. religious structure.
   d. relationship of ethnicity and culture to role assignment.

5. Which of the following does not ascribe to the holistic health view?
   a. The native Americans' medicine wheel
   b. The Hispanic belief in the evil eye or *mal ojo*
   c. The concept of yin and yang from the Chinese
   d. The hot/cold theory of illness in Hispanic cultures

6. Among African-Americans, the most common and frequently cited method of treating illness is:
   a. some early screening but a fatalistic attitude toward pain and acquired disease.
   b. prayer.
   c. aggressive medical treatment whenever possible.
   d. holistic medicine.

7. Asian/Pacific Islanders (APIs) are:
   a. the slowest growing ethnic group in the United States.
   b. approximately 95% Pacific Islanders.
   c. approximately 95% Asian Americans.
   d. a and b.

8. Many Chinese believe that:
   a. a balance between hot and cold elements is essential for good health.
   b. a balance between *yin* and *yang* characteristics is essential for good health.
   c. cancer is a *yin* illness and should be treated with foods, herbs, and healing ceremonies that possess "hot" properties.
   d. all of the above.

9.  Categories of disease that exist in Hispanic culture include:
    a.  disorders caused by hot and cold imbalances.
    b.  disorders caused by magical interventions.
    c.  two types of emotional diseases: mental and moral illness.
    d.  all of the above.

10. The first line of treatment in Hispanic cultures is the use of:
    a.  home remedies.
    b.  prayer.
    c.  conventional Western medicine.
    d.  holistic medicine.

11. Among the high-risk behaviors in the Hispanic population are:
    a.  obesity.
    b.  heavy over-the-counter and street drug use.
    c.  voodoo practices.
    d.  all of the above.

12. Native Americans are at greatest risk for death due to:
    a.  environmental cancer.
    b.  liver cancer.
    c.  an accident.
    d.  cardiopulmonary disease.

13. In native American cultures, the singers are those healers who:
    a.  can transform themselves into other forms of life to maintain cultural integration at a time of great cultural stress.
    b.  diagnose the cause of disharmony and may indicate a cure; their primary interest is care for souls.
    c.  treat illnesses and disharmony by laying on of hands, massage, sweatbaths, and the use of herbs and roots.
    d.  all of the above.

14. In a culture of poverty, secondary prevention may be absent because of:
    a.  a lack of insurance, inability to pay for service.
    b.  a present orientation where survival needs take precedence over screening and early detection.
    c.  limited care access.
    d.  all of the above.

15. Helen is preparing to discuss options with a patient who speaks only Spanish; Helen speaks only English. If given a choice, Helen will probably want to choose the use of:
    a.  a professional interpreter.
    b.  a family member as interpreter because the family is an integral part of treatment delivery and involvement in most Hispanic cultures.
    c.  a friend as interpreter because of the emotional support friends lend in a Hispanic, extended-family social structure and because a friend is more likely than family to relay the complete message.
    d.  any of the above, as long as the interpreter is fluent in both languages.

# ANSWER EXPLANATIONS

1.  **The answer is c.** There are limitations in the SEER data because (1) SEER data does not reflect the total U.S. population; (2) cancer rates in smaller populations are less precise than rates in larger populations; (3) the native American population is represented by two separate groups: Alaska native and American Indian; and (4) individuals who classify themselves as being of Hispanic ethnicity may be of any race, resulting in some overlap. However, the SEER data are helpful in identifying general ethnic patterns of cancer. (p. 1694)

2.  **The answer is c.** The highest overall cancer incidence rates occur among African-American men. (p. 1694)

3.  **The answer is b.** For breast cancer, the average annual rate per 100,000 individuals has been highest among white females. (Table 62-2, p. 1695)

4.  **The answer is a.** The basic unit of society is the family. Cultural values can determine communication with the family, the norm for the family size, and the roles of specific family members. (p. 1703)

5.  **The answer is b.** The holistic health view is that the forces of nature must be in balance or harmony. Human life is one aspect of nature and must be in harmony with the rest of nature. Examples are the native Americans' medicine wheel, which balances the four aspects of the individual's nature; the concept of yin and yang from the Chinese; and the hot/cold theory of illness in Hispanic cultures. (p. 1704)

6.  **The answer is b.** Many African-Americans find it impossible to separate religious beliefs from health beliefs. The most common and frequently cited method of treating illness remains prayer. (p. 1711)

7.  **The answer is c.** Asian/Pacific Islanders (APIs) are the fastest growing ethnic group in the United States. Approximately 95% are Asian Americans, compared to 5% who are Pacific Islander Americans. (p. 1713)

8.  **The answer is d.** APIs believe that a balance between hot and cold elements is essential for good health. The Chinese believe that the human body, illnesses, and foods possess *yin* and *yang* characteristics and treatment is aimed at reestablishing the balance. Cancer is a yin or cold illness and would be treated with foods, herbs, and healing ceremonies that possess "hot" properties. (p. 1714)

9.  **The answer is d.** Several categories of disease exist in Hispanic culture; some are interpreted through the concept of maintaining an equilibrium between hot and cold elements in the body. Some diseases are thought to be caused by hot and cold imbalances; others by magical interventions; as well as some scientific diseases that must be treated by the Western health care system. Finally, the Hispanic culture often acknowledges two types of emotional diseases: mental and moral illness. (p. 1718)

10. **The answer is a.** Home remedies are the first line of treatment in Hispanic cultures. To cure a hot or cold imbalance, the opposite quality of the causative agent is applied. (p. 1718)

11. **The answer is a.** Among the high-risk behaviors in the Hispanic population are obesity, alcohol consumption, and sexual practices. (p. 1720)

12. **The answer is c.** Cancer is ranked as the third leading cause of death among native Americans, preceded by accidents and heart disease. Native Americans also have the lowest cancer incidence and rank mid to low in mortality rates of all U.S. minority populations. (p. 1720)

13. **The answer is c.** In native American cultures, the singers are those healers who treat illnesses and disharmony by laying on of hands, massage, sweatbaths, use of herbs and roots, and chanting. (p. 1723)

14. **The answer is b.** In a culture of poverty, secondary prevention may be absent because of a present orientation where survival needs take precedence over screening and early detection. Delayed tertiary prevention is due to a lack of insurance, inability to pay for service, or limited care access. (p. 1725)

15. **The answer is a.** The use of professional interpreters, if available, is the optimal choice. Family and/or friends may be used but the correct or complete message may not be relayed. (p. 1727)

# Chapter 62  Role of the Oncology Advanced Practice Nurse

This chapter corresponds to Chapter 64 in *Cancer Nursing: Principles and Practice*, **Fourth Edition.**

## HISTORY OF ADVANCED PRACTICE NURSING

### The Nurse Practitioner Movement

- A nurse practitioner (NP) is a registered nurse who has advanced education and clinical training in a specialty area such as adult health or women's health.
  - Nurse practitioners obtain medical histories, perform physical examinations, make medical and nursing diagnoses, and treat common health problems and chronic diseases.
  - The amount of autonomy the NP has in performing these functions varies from state to state.
- The NP role originated in 1965 with a demonstration project at the University of Colorado.
- In 1974, the American Nurses' Association (ANA) Congress on Nursing Practice published the first definitions of the roles of the NP.
- In 1979 the National League for Nursing, the agency that accredits schools of nursing, declared in their position statement on NP education that the NP should hold a master's degree in nursing.

### The Development of the Clinical Nurse Specialist Role

- While the NP role evolved with a strong focus on the medical model, the clinical nurse specialist (CNS) role was based on nursing models.
- A CNS is a master's-prepared registered nurse who has expert knowledge and skill in caring for a population of patients within a given specialty.
- Four functional components of the CNS role include clinical practice, education, consultation, and research. Administration and change agent have also been cited as functional components.
- The first master's degree program with a clinical specialty was developed by Hildegard Peplau at Rutgers University in 1954.
- Specialization in health care was the trend in the 1970s fostered by dramatic increases in knowledge and technology.
- The ANA Social Policy Statement (1980) further defined the title CNS as an expert in a defined area of knowledge and practice with advanced preparation at the graduate level.

### The Trend Toward Merged Roles

- NP practice traditionally has focused on primary care in an ambulatory setting while specialty-focused acute care has been within the domain of the CNS.
- The boundaries that have traditionally existed between the NP and CNS are becoming less distinct.

### Advanced Practice Nursing Defined

- According to the American Nurses' Association, "Advanced practice registered nurses have acquired the knowledge base and practice experiences to prepare them for specialization, expansion, and advancement in practice."
- The National Council of State Boards of Nursing's definition of advanced practice nursing includes nurse practitioners, nurse anesthetists, nurse-midwives, and clinical nurse specialists with a graduate

degree and a major in nursing or a graduate degree with a concentration in an advanced nursing practice category.
- The National League for Nursing (NLN) has recommended the merging of the CNS and NP roles under the title "advanced practice nurse" (APN).
- According to ONS's position statement, the inclusion of other nonclinically focused, master's-prepared nurses is not consistent with the generally accepted use of the term APN.
- In contrast, the ANA states, "The term advanced practice is used to refer exclusively to advanced clinical practice."
- The ANA Council of Clinical Nurse Specialists and Council of Primary Health Care Nurse Practitioners were merged in 1990 to form the Council of Nurses in Advanced Practice.

### The Evolution of the Oncology Advanced Practice Nurse

- *The Master's Degree with a Specialty in Advanced Practice Oncology Nursing* has a significantly different focus than previous editions. The current curriculum guide has been broadened to support a blended role of an advanced practice oncology nurse that combines both CNS and NP skills.
- Historically, the vast majority of master's degree programs focused on the preparation of the oncology CNS. Currently, the specialty title of several of these programs—"advanced practice oncology nursing"—reflects preparation in a blended or merged CNS/NP role.

## REGULATION OF ADVANCED PRACTICE NURSING

- There is inconsistency regarding the definition of an advanced practice registered nurse.
- An advanced practice nurse must obtain information regarding the regulatory requirements in the jurisdiction where the APN intends to practice.

### Levels of Regulation

- There are four levels of regulation—designation/recognition, registration, certification, and licensure.
  - Designation/recognition is the least restrictive method of regulation and consists of recognition of credentials by a state's board of nursing. It does not involve an inquiry.
  - Registration is the placement of names of APNs on an official board roster. It also does not involve an inquiry.
  - Certification involves title regulation. The APN must meet specified, predetermined requirements. Certification attempts to measure competence.
  - Licensure specifies scope of practice; applications for licensure are evaluated to ensure that predetermined requirements are met. Licensure also allows the grantor to take disciplinary action for violation of laws or rules.

### Certification Versus Second Licensure

- A topic of increasing concern and one for which there is no consensus is whether certification or second licensure is the appropriate regulatory mechanism for advanced practice.
- There are no standard criteria used by professional organizations that offer certification examinations to ensure that the examination has a clinical focus. Yet in many states, national certification is used to regulate advanced nursing practice.
- Many professional nursing organizations, including the ANA, have supported the regulation of advanced practice through the mechanism of voluntary certification.
- A *standardized* certification process for advanced practice nursing would eliminate much of the criticism of the current certification process and potentially abolish the need for a second license to regulate nursing practice.

- The ANA supports the following features to be included within a regulatory system for advanced practice: a definition of an APN, an educational standard of a graduate degree, recognition of professional certification, and a description of scope of practice.

## PRESCRIPTIVE AUTHORITY

- The authority for the APN to prescribe is regulated on the state level. Forty-seven states currently provide for some level of prescriptive authority.
- The level of authority varies from independent prescriptive authority, including controlled substances, to dependent authority, excluding controlled substances. (See Table 64-2 on text page 1760.)

### Controlled Substances

- In states where APNs are allowed to prescribe controlled substances, Drug Enforcement Administration (DEA) registration numbers are required.
- DEA registration allows a wide variety of acts including purchasing, storing, administering, dispensing, and prescribing controlled substances; however, the advanced practice nurse may engage in only those activities authorized by the state in which they practice.
- Figure 64-1 on text page 1761 provides information on obtaining a DEA registration number.

### Research Related to Prescriptive Authority

- As regulatory changes are made that grant APNs prescriptive authority, implementation of these changes and their effects on access to care, clinical practice, and patient outcomes need to be evaluated.

## REIMBURSEMENT OF ADVANCED PRACTICE NURSING SERVICES

- The effective utilization of an APN is, in part, tied to reimbursement of services provided.

### Medicare Payment

- Medicare is a federal health insurance program for individuals who are disabled or over the age of 65.
- Part A of the program pays for costs incurred during hospitalization; part B pays for physician services and for APN services under the following circumstances:
  - Service is usually furnished by an MD/DO.
  - Service is performed by a person who meets the Medicare definition of NP or CNS.
  - An NP or CNS is legally authorized to perform the service in the state in which it is performed.
  - Service is performed in collaboration with an MD/DO.
- Reimbursement for APNs varies considerably by the type of APN, the health care setting, and the payment rate.

### Medicaid Payment

- Medicaid is a joint state and federally funded health care program for lower income Americans. Direct reimbursement to pediatric and family nurse practitioners for services provided to children is federally mandated.

### Payment by Other Providers

- Health maintenance organizations may have contracts with Medicare. APNs who work in collaboration with a physician are eligible for reimbursement.
- The APN contracts directly with the HMO to provide services and is paid by the HMO.

- The Civilian and Medical Program of the Uniformed Services (CHAMPUS) is a federal program that provides services to members of the uniformed services and their families.
- The Federal Employee Health Benefit Plan (FEHBP) offers health insurance plans to federal employees and retirees. Coverage of APN services is mandated, and direct reimbursement is provided; however, prepaid health insurance plans are not required to include APNs in their provider network.

## COLLABORATION AND CONSULTATION—HALLMARKS OF ONCOLOGY ADVANCED PRACTICE

- The OAPN is expert in the process of patient and family education, skilled in the utilization of nursing research, and savvy in negotiating complex organizational structures. In addition to this clinical expertise, the OAPN also must be an expert consultant and skilled in the process of collaboration. The OAPN is on the cutting edge of practice.
- Oncology and oncology advanced practice nursing lends itself to a collaborative model of practice.
- Characteristics of a collaborative practice include mutual trust and understanding, as well as shared problem solving, decision making, and authority.
- In this practice, NPs function independently in caring for a caseload of patients, whether in the ambulatory or acute care setting.

## ONCOLOGY ADVANCED PRACTICE NURSING ROLES

- Although the OAPN specializes in the care of individuals and families with cancer, the OAPN also often develops a practice focus.
- Successful advanced practice is the expansion of nursing's traditional boundaries while preserving the essence of nursing.
- Appendix A on text page 1769 provides a sample of a position description for an oncology nurse practitioner.

### The OAPN in Primary Care

#### Prevention and early detection

- The OAPN is involved in many aspects of cancer screening from the identification of "at risk" individuals to performing physical examinations focusing on cancer screening. The OAPN also develops and implements educational programs in schools, community, and employment settings on cancer risk factors, prevention, and early detection practices.

#### Cancer genetic counseling

- OAPNs with knowledge and expertise in medical genetics and counseling are in an excellent position to provide screening, counseling, and education of individuals undergoing cancer genetic testing.

### The OAPN in Secondary Care

#### Active treatment

- OAPNs are involved in the care of patients receiving treatment for cancer as either direct care provider or consultant. As direct care provider, the OAPN obtains the initial history and performs the physical examination.
- The treatment plan and expected outcomes are discussed with the patient and family.
- During the phase active treatment, the OAPN meets both the patient's medical and nursing needs.
- As a consultant, the OAPN in secondary care is involved in planning and implementing initiatives aimed at patient and family education and support.

- The OAPN's expertise is also utilized in symptom management, and they are often an important member of a multidisciplinary pain and symptom management team. They also may act as consultants to the institution in establishing standards for oncology practice and developing critical pathways.

### Follow-up care

- The OAPN is responsible for performing physical examinations, ordering and interpreting laboratory and radiological studies, and referring patients for diagnostic studies as needed. Additionally, the OAPN maintains communication with the patient's primary care provider and referring physician. The OAPN also helps the individual become a cancer survivor.

## The OAPN in Tertiary Care

### Acute care

- The two major trends that have led to the development of the acute care NP role are changes in medical residency training programs and the shift from fee-for-service to capitated payment plans for health care.
- While both the CNS and NP are advanced practice nursing roles with a similar goal—ensuring the provision of outstanding patient care—their means differ.
  - The CNS affects care indirectly by working through the organization and the nursing staff to facilitate changes that improve patient care.
  - The NP affects care directly by managing the medical and nursing needs for a specific caseload of patients.
- The OAPN with a direct care emphasis is responsible for the management of a caseload of patients from admission through discharge. The OAPN has medical staff privileges and obtains the patient's health history, performs a physical examination, interprets laboratory and radiological studies, prescribes medications including chemotherapy, and coordinates discharge and follow-up care. In essence, this OAPN is responsible for the minute-to-minute care of the patient in collaboration with the attending physician.
- The OAPN with an organizational focus performs functions such as acting as a mentor to nursing staff, consulting with nursing staff on the care of patients with complex needs, developing staff and patient educational programs, facilitating support groups, and implementing research-based changes in practice.

### Blended role

- The OAPN role in this setting may incorporate components of both the traditional CNS and NP roles into one "blended" role.
- Descriptions of these blended roles vary in the literature, but have one common theme—the delivery of coordinated, comprehensive, and cost-effective care. The OAPN serves as the link between the attending physician, the patient and family, the inpatient medical and nursing staff, and, increasingly in today's fiscal climate, the insurer.
- The difference between this OAPN role and that of the direct care OAPN or organizational OAPN in tertiary care is the accountability for care across practice settings and the links with community providers including the insurer.

### Case manager

- The economic and clinical demands of case management in tertiary care require a master's degree.
- Again, the emphasis is on "the three Cs"—coordinated, comprehensive, and cost-effective care.

- The case manager usually does not provide direct care but rather coordinates the care provided by others.
- The focus is on ensuring the effective use of resources and meeting outcomes within an appropriate length of stay.

## The OAPN in Hospice and Bereavement Care

- Since OAPNs are not eligible for direct reimbursement of home visits, they usually are employed by the agency and utilized as a consultant for complex patients and families with difficult management issues.

## The OAPN in Industry and Research

### Industry

- OAPNs fill a multiplicity of roles in the health care industry. They bring to these positions an "insider's" knowledge of health care. This, coupled with clinical expertise, makes them a valuable asset to an organization.

### Research

- The OAPN is involved in research through utilizing research results, implementing an independent research agenda, and collaborating on medical research.

## ADVANCED PRACTICE NURSING—INTO THE TWENTY-FIRST CENTURY

- There are three forces that will continue to influence changes in nursing practice in the coming years—the health care insurance industry, medical education, and scientific advances.
- The traditional fee-for-service system of payment is being replaced by managed care systems in which providers agree to render services to a given group of patients for a predetermined fee.
- To compensate, physicians are seeing more patients in less time. The result is a physician/patient interaction that is limited to what is medically essential.
- Changes in medical education with its renewed emphasis on the preparation of primary care providers ultimately will result in fewer subspecialists, including oncologists.
- It is predicted that OAPNs soon will be eligible for direct reimbursement for home visits under Medicare. This will dramatically change the face of home and hospice care.

## PRACTICE QUESTIONS

1. Which of the following does *not* describe the clinical nurse specialist (CNS) role?
   a. It has evolved with a strong focus on the medical model.
   b. Its components include administration and change agent.
   c. Its components include clinical practice, education, consultation, and research.
   d. Boundaries between CNS and NP are becoming less distinct.

2. Attempts to regulate APNs through registration involves:
   a. recognition of credentials by a state's board of nursing with no inquiry into qualifications.
   b. title regulation after measuring the applicant's competence.
   c. the placement of names of APNs on an official board roster with no inquiry into qualifications.
   d. a and c.

3. Licensure involves:
   a. evaluation of the scope of practice and applications to determine that requirements are met.
   b. the placement of names of APNs on an official board roster.
   c. title regulation.
   d. all of the above.

4. DEA registration allows a wide variety of acts. Depending on the state in which one practices, these may include:
   a. the purchase and dispensing of controlled substances.
   b. administering controlled substances.
   c. prescribing controlled substances.
   d. all of the above.

5. Alex, a CNS, recently delivered services to a patient who has health insurance through Medicare. Alex will be paid under part B under each of the following circumstances *except when*:
   a. the service Alex performed is usually furnished by an AM/DO.
   b. Alex is legally authorized to perform the service within the state where he practices.
   c. the costs for Alex's services are incurred during hospitalization.
   d. Alex's service is performed in collaboration with an MD/DO.

6. Nurse practitioners or APNs are eligible for direct reimbursement under all of the following programs *except*:
   a. services to children covered under Medicaid.
   b. services to eligible members under the Federal Employee Health Benefit Plan (FEHBP).
   c. prepaid health insurance plans that are part of the FEHBP network.
   d. services provided under CHAMPUS.

7. Karen is an NP working in a collaborative practice. In general, in a collaborative practice, which of the following is *not* true?
   a. NPs function independently in caring for a caseload of patients in the ambulatory setting.
   b. NPs function independently in caring for a caseload of patients in the acute care setting.
   c. The skills of the provider are matched with the needs of the patient.
   d. All of the above are true.

8. Terrence has training as an oncology advanced practice nurse (OAPN). He chooses to work as a consultant rather than a direct care provider. As a consultant, the OAPN in secondary care may be involved in any of the following *except*:
   a. discussing the treatment plan and expected outcomes with the patients and family.
   b. planning and implementing initiatives aimed at patient and family education and support.
   c. pain and symptom management.
   d. establishing standards for oncology practice and developing critical pathways.

## ANSWER EXPLANATIONS

1. **The answer is a.** While the nurse practitioner (NP) role evolved with a strong focus on the medical model, the clinical nurse specialist (CNS) role was based on nursing models. Four components of the CNS role are clinical practice, education, consultation, and research. Administration and change agents have also been cited as functional components. Boundaries between the NP and CNS are becoming less distinct. (p. 1756)

2. **The answer is c.** Registration is the placement of names of APNs on an official board roster. It does not involve an inquiry. Designation/recognition is least restrictive and consists of recognition of credentials by a state's board of nursing. It does not involve an inquiry. Certification involves title regulation. The APN must meet specified, predetermined requirements; certification attempts to measure competence. Licensure specifies scope of practice, and applications are evaluated to determine that requirements are met. (p. 1759)

3. **The answer is a.** Licensure specifies scope of practice, and applications are evaluated to determine that requirements are met. Registration is the placement of names of APNs on an official board roster. It does not involve an inquiry. Designation/recognition is least restrictive and consists of recognition of credentials by a state's board of nursing. It does not involve an inquiry. Certification involves title regulation. The APN must meet specified, predetermined requirements; certification attempts to measure competence. (p. 1759)

4. **The answer is d.** DEA registration allows a wide variety of acts. Depending on the state in which one practices, these may include purchasing, storing, administering, dispensing, and prescribing controlled substances. (pp. 1760–1761)

5. **The answer is c.** Part A of the Medicare federal health insurance program pays for costs incurred during hospitalizations; part B pays for physician services and for APN services under the following circumstances: the service is usually furnished by an AM/DO; service is performed by someone who meets the Medicare definition of NP or CNS; the NP or CNS is legally authorized to perform the service within the specified state; service is performed in collaboration with an MD/DO. (p. 1761)

6. **The answer is c.** Nurse practitioners or APNs who are eligible for direct reimbursement include those nurse practitioners who provide services to children under Medicaid; NPs who provide services under CHAMPUS; and APNs providing services to eligible members under the Federal Employee Health Benefit Plan (FEHBP). Prepaid health insurance plans that are part of the FEHBP network are not required to include APNs in their provider network. (p. 1762)

7. **The answer is d.** In a collaborative practice, NPs function independently in caring for a caseload of patients, whether in the ambulatory or acute care setting. Care is provided based on competence: the skills of the provider are matched with the needs of the patient. (p. 1762)

8. **The answer is a.** As a consultant, the OAPN in secondary care is involved in planning and implementing initiatives aimed at patient and family education and support. The OAPN's expertise is also

utilized in symptom management, and they are often important members of a multidisciplinary pain and symptom management team. They also may act as a consultant to the institution in establishing standards for oncology practice and developing critical pathways. (p. 1764)